• *To all who use this textbook, that they may benefit from its use as much as we did in its preparation*

国家卫生和计划生育委员会"十三五"英文版规划教材

全国高等学校教材

供临床医学专业及来华留学生（MBBS）双语教学用

Medical Microbiology

医学微生物学 改编教学版
Annotated Edition

Patrick R. Murray   Ken S. Rosenthal
Michael A. Pfaller.

主 编　郭晓奎
Chief Editor　Xiaokui Guo

副主编　彭宜红
Vice Chief Editor　Yihong Peng

樊晓晖
Xiaohui Fan

钟照华
Zhaohua Zhong

人民卫生出版社
People's Medical Publishing House

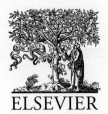

ELSEVIER

Elsevier (Singapore) Pte Ltd.

3 Killiney Road

#08-01 Winsland House I

Singapore 239519

Tel: (65) 6349-0200

Fax: (65) 6733-1817

1995 年,我国首次招收全英文授课医学留学生,到 2015 年,接收临床医学专业 MBBS (Bachelor of Medicine & Bachelor of Surgery)留学生的院校达到了 40 余家,MBBS 院校数量、规模不断扩张;同时,医学院校在临床医学专业五年制、长学制教学中陆续开展不同规模和范围的双语或全英文授课,使得对一套符合我国教学实际、成体系、高质量英文教材的需求日益增长。

为了满足教学需求,进一步落实教育部《关于加强高等学校本科教学工作提高教学质量的若干意见(教高 [2001]4 号)》和《来华留学生医学本科教育(英文授课)质量控制标准暂行规定(教外来 [2007]39 号)》等相关文件的要求,规范和提高我国高等医学院校临床医学专业五年制、长学制和来华留学生(MBBS)双语教学及全英文教学的质量,推进医学双语教学和留学生教育的健康有序发展,完善和规范临床医学专业英文版教材的体系,人民卫生出版社在充分调研的基础上,于 2015 年召开了全国高等学校临床医学专业英文版规划教材的编写论证会,经过会上及会后的反复论证,最终确定组织编写一套全国规划的、适合我国高等医学院校教学实际的临床医学专业英文版教材,并计划作为 2017 年春季和秋季教材在全国出版发行。

本套英文版教材的编写结合国家卫生和计划生育委员会、教育部的总体要求,坚持"三基、五性、三特定"的原则,组织全国各大医学院校、教学医院的专家编写,主要特点如下:

1. 教材编写应教学之需启动,在全国范围进行了广泛、深入调研和论证,借鉴国内外医学人才培养模式和教材建设经验,对主要读者对象、编写模式、编写科目、编者遴选条件等进行了科学设计。

2. 坚持"三基、五性、三特定"和"多级论证"的教材编写原则,组织全国各大医学院校及教学医院有丰富英语教学经验的专家一起编写,以保证高质量出版。

3. 为保证英语表达的准确性和规范性,大部分教材以国外英文原版教科书为蓝本,根据我国教学大纲和人民卫生出版社临床医学专业第八轮规划教材主要内容进行改编,充分体现科学性、权威性、适用性和实用性。

4. 教材内部各环节合理设置,根据读者对象的特点,在英文原版教材的基础上结合需要,增加本章小结、关键术语(英中对照)、思考题、推荐阅读等模块,促进学生自主学习。

本套临床医学专业英文版规划教材共 38 种,均为国家卫生和计划生育委员会"十三五"规划教材,计划于 2017 年全部出版发行。

In 1995, China recruited overseas medical students of full English teaching for the first time. Up to 2015, more than 40 institutions enrolled overseas MBBS (Bachelor of Medicine & Bachelor of Surgery) students. The number of MBBS institutions and overseas students are continuously increasing. At the meantime, medical colleges' application for bilingual or full English teaching in different size and range in five-year and long-term professional clinical medicine teaching results to increasingly demand for a set of practical, systematic and high-qualified English teaching material.

In order to meet the teaching needs and to implement the regulations of relevant documents issued by Ministry of Education including "Some Suggestions to Strengthen the Undergraduate Teaching and to Improve the Teaching Quality" and "Interim Provisions on Quality Control Standards of International Medical Undergraduate Education (English teaching)", as well as to standardize and improve the quality of the bilingual teaching and English teaching of the five-year, long-term and international students (MBBS) of clinical medicine in China's higher medical colleges so as to promote the healthy and orderly development of medical bilingual teaching and international students education and to improve and standardize the system of English clinical medicine textbooks, after full investigation, People's Medical Publishing House (PMPH) held the writing discussion meeting of English textbook for clinical medicine department of national colleges and universities in 2015. After the repeated demonstration in and after the meeting, PMPH ultimately determined to organize the compilation of a set of national planning English textbooks which are suitable for China's actual clinical medicine teaching of medical colleges and universities. This set will be published as spring and autumn textbooks of 2017.

This set of English textbooks meets the overall requirements of the Ministry of Education and National Health and Family Planning Commission, the editorial committee includes the experts from major medical colleges and universities as well as teaching hospitals, the main features are as follows:

1. Textbooks compilation is started to meet the teaching needs, extensive and deep research and demonstration are conducted across the country, the main target readers, the model and subject of compilation and selection conditions of authors are scientifically designed in accordance with the reference of domestic and foreign medical personnel training model and experience in teaching materials.

2. Adhere to the teaching materials compiling principles of "three foundations, five characteristics, and three specialties" and "multi-level demonstration", the organization of English teaching experts with rich experience from major medical schools and teaching hospitals ensures the high quality of publication.

3. In order to ensure the accuracy and standardization of English expression, most of the textbooks are modeled on original English textbooks, and adapted based on national syllabus and main content of the eighth round of clinical medicine textbooks which were published by PMPH, fully reflecting the scientificity, authority, applicability and practicality.

4. All aspects of teaching materials are arranged reasonably, based on original textbooks,the chapter summary, key terms (English and Chinese), review questions, and recommended readings are added to promote students' independent learning in accordance with teaching needs and the characteristics of the target readers.

This set of English textbooks for clinical medicine includes 38 species which are among "13th Five-Year" planning textbooks of National Health and Family Planning Commission, and will be all published in 2017.

全国高等学校临床医学专业第一轮英文版规划教材 · 教材目录

教材名称		主　审	主编
1 人体解剖学	Human Anatomy		刘学政
2 生理学	Physiology		闫剑群
3 医学免疫学	Medical Immunology		储以微
4 生物化学	Biochemistry		张晓伟
5 组织学与胚胎学	Histology and Embryology		李　和
6 医学微生物学	Medical Microbiology		郭晓奎
7 病理学	Pathology		陈　杰
8 医学分子生物学	Medical Molecular Biology		吕社民
9 医学遗传学	Medical Genetics		傅松滨
10 医学细胞生物学	Medical Cell Biology		刘　佳
11 病理生理学	Pathophysiology		王建枝
12 药理学	Pharmacology		杨宝峰
13 临床药理学	Clinical Pharmacology		李　俊
14 人体寄生虫学	Human Parasitology		李学荣
15 流行病学	Epidemiology		沈洪兵
16 医学统计学	Medical Statistics		郝元涛
17 核医学	Nuclear Medicine		黄　钢　李　方
18 医学影像学	Medical Imaging		申宝忠　龚启勇
19 临床诊断学	Clinical Diagnostics		万学红
20 实验诊断学	Laboratory Diagnostics		胡翊群　王　琳
21 内科学	Internal Medicine		文富强　汪道文
22 外科学	Surgery		陈孝平　田　伟
23 妇产科学	Obstetrics and Gynaecology	郎景和	狄　文　曹云霞
24 儿科学	Pediatrics		黄国英　罗小平
25 神经病学	Neurology		张黎明
26 精神病学	Psychiatry		赵靖平
27 传染病学	Infectious Diseases		高志良　任　红

全国高等学校临床医学专业第一轮英文版规划教材 · 教材目录

教材名称		主审	主编
28 皮肤性病学	Dermatovenereology	陈洪铎	高兴华
29 肿瘤学	Oncology		石远凯
30 眼科学	Ophthalmology		杨培增 刘奕志
31 康复医学	Rehabilitation Medicine		虞乐华
32 医学心理学	Medical Psychology		赵旭东
33 耳鼻咽喉头颈外科学	Otorhinolaryngology-Head and Neck Surgery		孔维佳
34 急诊医学	Emergency Medicine		陈玉国
35 法医学	Forensic Medicine		赵 虎
36 全球健康学	Global Health		吴群红
37 中医学	Chinese Medicine		王新华
38 医学汉语	Medical Chinese		李 骢

Preface

Our knowledge about microbiology and immunology is constantly growing, and by building a good foundation of understanding in the beginning, it will be much easier to understand the advances of the future.

Medical microbiology can be a bewildering field for the novice. We are faced with many questions when learning microbiology: How do I learn all the names? Which infectious agents cause which diseases? Why? When? Who is at risk? Is there a treatment? However, all these concerns can be reduced to one essential question: **What information do I need to know that will help me understand how to diagnose and treat an infected patient?**

Certainly, there are a number of theories about what a student needs to know and how to teach it, which supposedly validates the plethora of microbiology textbooks that have flooded the bookstores in recent years. Although we do not claim to have the one right approach to teaching medical microbiology (there is truly no one perfect approach to medical education), we have founded the revisions of this textbook on our experience gained through years of teaching medical students, residents, and infectious disease fellows, as well as on the work devoted to the seven previous editions. We have tried to present the basic concepts of medical microbiology clearly and succinctly in a manner that addresses different types of learners. The text is written in a straightforward manner with, it is hoped, uncomplicated explanations of difficult concepts. In this edition, we challenged ourselves to improve the learning experience even more. We are using the new technology on StudentConsult.com (e-version) to enhance access to the material. New to this edition, **chapter summaries** and learning aids are placed at the beginning of each of the microbe chapters, and on the e-version these are keyed to the appropriate sections in the chapter. In addition, many of the **figures** are enhanced to assist learning. **Details** are summarized in tabular format rather than in lengthy text, and there are colorful illustrations for the visual learner. **Clinical Cases** provide the relevance that puts reality into the basic science. **Important points** are emphasized in **boxes** to aid students, especially in their review, and the **study questions**, including Clinical Cases, address relevant aspects of each chapter. Each section (bacteria, viruses, fungi, parasites) begins with a chapter that summarizes microbial diseases, and this also provides **review material**.

Our understanding of microbiology and immunology is rapidly expanding, with new and exciting discoveries in all areas. We used our experience as authors and teachers to choose the most important information and explanations for inclusion in this textbook. Each chapter has been carefully updated and expanded to include new, medically relevant discoveries. In each of these chapters, we have attempted to present the material that we believe will help the student gain an interest in as well as a clear understanding of the significance of the individual microbes and their diseases.

With each edition of *Medical Microbiology* we refine and update our presentation. There are many changes to the eighth edition, both in the print and e-versions of the book. The book starts with a general introduction to microbiology and new chapters on the human microbiome and epidemiology of infectious diseases. The human microbiome (that is, the normal population of organisms that populate our bodies) can now be considered as another organ system with 10 times as many cells as human cells. This microbiota educates the immune response, helps digest our food, and protects us against more harmful microbes. Additional chapters in the introductory section introduce the techniques used by microbiologists and immunologists and are followed by chapters on the functional immune system. The immune cells and tissues are introduced, followed by an enhanced chapter on innate immunity and updated chapters on antigen-specific immunity, antimicrobial immunity, and vaccines. The sections on bacteria, viruses, fungi, and parasites have also been reorganized. Each section is introduced by the relevant basic science chapters and then the specific microbial disease summary chapter before proceeding into descriptions of the individual microbes, "the bug parade." Each chapter on the specific microbes begins with a summary (including trigger words), which is keyed to the appropriate part of the chapter in the e-version. As in previous editions, there are many summary boxes, tables, clinical photographs, and original clinical cases. **Clinical Cases** are included because we believe students will find them particularly interesting and instructive, and they are a very efficient way to present this complex subject. Each chapter in the "bug parade" is introduced by relevant questions to excite students and orient them as they explore the chapter. Finally, students are provided with access to the new Student Consult website, which provides links to additional reference materials, clinical photographs, animations (including new animations), and answers to the introductory and summary questions of each chapter. Many of the figures are presented in step-by-step manner to facilitate learning. A very important feature on the website is access to more than 200 **practice exam questions** that will help students assess their mastery of the subject matter and prepare for their course and licensure exams. In essence, this edition provides an understandable text, details, questions, examples, and a review book all in one.

● To Our Future Colleagues: The Students

On first impression, success in medical microbiology would appear to depend on memorization. Microbi-

ology may seem to consist of only innumerable facts, but there is also a logic to microbiology and immunology. Like a medical detective, the first step is to know your villain. Microbes establish a niche in our bodies; some are beneficial and help us to digest our food and educate our immune system, while others may cause disease. Their ability to cause disease, and the disease that may result, depend on how the microbe interacts with the host and the innate and immune protective responses that ensue.

There are many ways to approach learning microbiology and immunology, but ultimately the more you interact with the material using multiple senses, the better you will build memory and learn. A **fun** and **effective** approach to learning is to **think like a physician and treat each microbe and its diseases as if it were an infection in your patient. Create a patient for each microbial infection, and compare and contrast the different patients.** Perform role-playing and ask the seven basic questions as you approach this material: Who? Where? When? Why? Which? What? and How? For example: Who is at risk for disease? Where does this organism cause infections (both body site and geographic area)? When is isolation of this organism important? Why is this organism able to cause disease? Which species and genera are medically important? What diagnostic tests should be performed? How is this infection managed? Each organism that is encountered can be systematically examined. Use the following acronym to create a clinical case and learn the essential information for each microbe: **DIVIRDEPT**. How does the microbial *d*isease present in the patient and the differential diagnosis? How would you confirm the diagnosis and *i*dentify the microbial cause of disease? What are the *v*irulence properties of the organism that cause the disease? What are the helpful and harmful aspects of the *i*nnate and *i*mmune response to the infection? What are the specific conditions or mechanisms for *r*eplicating the microbe? What are all the *d*isease characteristics and consequences? What is the *e*pidemiology of infection? How can you *p*revent its disease? What is its *t*reatment? Answering the DIVIRDEPT questions will require that you jump around in the chapter to find the information, but this will help you learn the material. For each of the microbes, learn three to five words or phrases that are associated with the microbe—words that will stimulate your memory (**trigger words**, provided in the new chapter summary) and organize the diverse facts into a logical picture. Develop **alternative associations**. For example, this textbook presents organisms in the systematic taxonomic structure (frequently called a "bug parade," but which the authors think is the easiest way to introduce the organisms). Take a given virulence property (e.g., toxin production) or type of disease (e.g., meningitis) and list the organisms that share this property. Pretend that an imaginary patient is infected with a specific agent and create the case history. Explain the diagnosis to your imaginary patient and also to your future professional colleagues. In other words, do not simply attempt to memorize page after page of facts; rather, use techniques that stimulate your mind and challenge your understanding of the facts presented throughout the text and **it will be more fun**. Use the summary chapter at the beginning of each organism section to **review** and help refine your "differential diagnosis" and classify organisms into logical "boxes." Get familiar with the textbook and its bonus materials and you will not only learn the material but also have a review book to work from in the future.

No textbook of this magnitude would be successful without the contributions of numerous individuals. We are grateful for the valuable professional help and support provided by the staff at Elsevier, particularly Jim Merritt, Katie DeFrancesco, and Rhoda Howell. We also want to thank the many students and professional colleagues who have offered their advice and constructive criticism throughout the development of this eighth edition of *Medical Microbiology*.

Patrick R. Murray, PhD
Ken S. Rosenthal, PhD
and
Michael A. Pfaller, MD

Adaptation Preface

We are in an era of near instant communication. The past decade has seen a booming trend of global communication in medical science efficiently propelling medical advances. The need to incorporate international elements into medical education to expand students' learning of medicine on the global scale becomes paramount. Medical Microbiology is at the center of infectious disease control and management. We therefore embarked on the task of a textbook on medical microbiology in English targeting Chinese medical students as well as international students with a focus on the patterns and features of infectious diseases commonly seen in China.

Murray's Medical Microbiology is highly recognized among the renowned prescribed textbooks of medical microbiology worldwide which demonstrates microbial pathogens explicitly with tables and graphical illustrations, as well as combining basic microbial characteristics of physiology, structure, pathogenesis, etc. and clinical information including disease presentation, diagnosis, treatment and prevention, etc. Therefore, we adopted this book as our main reference and every modification was made in an effort to enhance its contents among students in China. We've retained key features of Murray's original version but modified the text to make it more user-friendly to suit students who are used to the educational system in China.

Specifically, new features of the revised textbook focus on the following three aspects:

1. The infectious diseases spectrum and epidemiological data vary between Eastern and Western countries, even among different regions in our country. For instance, some infectious diseases and their causative agents are of great significance specifically in our country, including hepatitis B caused by hepatitis B virus and tuberculosis caused by *M. tuberculosis*, etc., while the prevalence is much less in the Western world. We've therefore added these "ethnic-specific characteristics" or made certain updates and additions based on Murray's textbook so that our future medical doctors might respond more appropriately when confronted with patients from different cultural backgrounds.

2. In our textbook, chapters covering Immunology and Parasitology have been excluded to make the textbook focus on bacteriology, virology and mycology which are more pertinent to our students.

3. Rote learning in Medical microbiology is common but it's far more than simple enumeration of pathogens. Rather, infectious diseases display tremendous complexity in which multiple tissues and organs can be affected at the same time and multiple pathogens can be found in single focus of lesion. Various textbooks have endeavored on the appropriate coverage of all pathogens in appropriate order including classification by biological properties of the pathogens, clinical manifestations and body systems, etc., but unfortunately few managed to fully depict the relationship between pathogens and clinical diseases. In this book, we adopted the original biological classification system in the organization of pathogens, and supplemented these with medical classification systems. In addition, we've added a comprehensive map of all body systems and organs with their associated infectious diseases and microbial pathogens that cause such diseases, in the hope that students will be able to efficiently link infectious diseases with host anatomy and most importantly, pinpoint the pathogens that cause them.

Contents

SECTION 2

Virology

SECTION 3

Mycology

Chapter 1

Introduction to Medical Microbiology

In 1674, the Dutch biologist Anton van Leeuwenhoek most excitedly peered through his carefully ground microscopic lenses at a drop of water and discovered millions of tiny "animalcules". Almost 100 years later, the Danish biologist Otto Müller organized bacteria into genera and species. This was the beginning of the taxonomic classification of microbes. In 1840, the German pathologist Friedrich Henle proposed criteria for proving the liability of microorganisms in human diseases (the "germ theory" of disease). Robert Koch and Louis Pasteur confirmed this theory in the 1870s and 1880s proving that microorganisms were responsible for anthrax, rabies, plague, cholera, and tuberculosis. The era of chemotherapy began in 1910, when the German chemist Paul Ehrlich discovered the first antibacterial agent, a compound effective against syphilis. This was followed by Alexander Fleming's discovery of penicillin in 1928, Gerhard Domagk's discovery of sulfanilamide in 1935, and Selman Waksman's discovery of streptomycin in 1943. In 1946, the American microbiologist John Enders first cultivated viruses in cell cultures, leading the way to the large-scale production of virus cultures for vaccine development. Afterwards, thousands of scientists have expanded our understanding of microbes and their role in diseases.

Van Leeuwenhoek discovered a complex world consisting of protozoa and bacteria. However, the complexity of medical microbiology today rivals the limits of imagination. We now know that there are thousands of different types of microbes that live in, on, and around us—and hundreds that cause serious human diseases. To understand this, it is important to know some basic aspects of medical microbiology. To start, the microbes can be subdivided into there general groups: viruses, bacteria, fungi.

VIRUSES

Viruses are the smallest infectious particles, ranging in diameter from 18 to 600 nanometers (most viruses are less than 200 nm and cannot be seen with a light microscope). Viruses typically contain either deoxyribonucleic acid (DNA) or ribonucleic acid (RNA) but not both; however, some viral-like particles do not contain any detectable nucleic acids (e.g., prions), while the recently discovered Mimivirus contains both RNA and DNA. Viruses are true parasites, requiring host cells for replication. More than 2000 species of viruses have been described, with approximately 650 infecting humans and animals. Infection can lead to either rapid replication and cell destruction or to a long-term chronic relationship with possible integration of the viral genetic information into the host genome. The factors that determine which of these takes place are only partially understood. For example, infection with the human immunodeficiency virus, the etiologic agent of the acquired immunodeficiency syndrome (AIDS), can result in the latent infection of CD4 lymphocytes or the active replication and destruction of these immunologically important cells.

BACTERIA

Bacteria are **prokaryotic** organisms—simple unicellular organisms with no nuclear membrane, mitochondria, Golgi bodies, or endoplasmic reticulum—that reproduce by asexual division. The bacterial cell wall is classified into gram-positive with a thick peptidoglycan layer, or gram-negative with a thin peptidoglycan layer and an overlying outer membrane. Some bacteria lack this cell wall structure and compensate by surviving only inside host cells or in a hypertonic environment. The size (1 to 20 μm or larger), shape (spheres, rods, spirals), and spacial arrangement (single cells, chains, clusters) of the cells are used for the preliminary classification of bacteria, and the phenotypic and genotypic properties of the bacteria form the basis for the definitive classification. The human body is inhabited by thousands of different bacterial species—some living transiently, others in a permanent parasitic relationship. Likewise, the environment that surrounds us, including the air we breathe, water we drink, and food we eat, is populated with bacteria, many of which are relatively avirulent and some of which are capable of producing life-threatening disease.

FUNGI

Compared with bacteria, the cellular structure of fungi is more complex. These are **eukaryotic** organisms that contain a well-defined nucleus and organelles. Most fungi exist as either yeasts (a unicellular form that can replicate asexually) or molds (a filamentous form that can replicate asexually and sexually). However, some fungi can assume both morphology, known as **dimorphic** fungi and include *Histoplasma*, *Blastomyces*, and *Coccidioides*.

MICROBIAL DISEASE

It's important to understand the diseases microbes cause and ways to control them. Unfortunately, the relationship between many organisms and their diseases is not simple. Specifically, most organisms do not cause a single, well-defined disease, although there are certainly ones that do (e.g., *Clostridium tetani*, tetanus; Ebola virus, Ebola; *Plasmodium* species, malaria). Instead, it is more common for a particular

organism to produce many manifestations of disease (e.g., *Staphylococcus aureus*—endocarditis, pneumonia, wound infections, food poisoning) or for many organisms to produce the same disease (e.g., meningitis caused by viruses, bacteria, fungi, and parasites). In addition, relatively few organisms can be classified as always pathogenic, although some do belong in this category (e.g., rabies virus, *Bacillus anthracis*, *Sporothrix schenckii*, *Plasmodium* species). Instead, most organisms are able to establish disease only under well-defined circumstances (e.g., the introduction of an organism with a potential for causing disease into a normally sterile site, such as the brain, lungs, and peritoneal cavity). Some diseases arise when a person is exposed to organisms from external sources, known as **exogenous infections**. Most human diseases, however, are produced by organisms in the person's own microbial flora that spread to inappropriate body sites where disease can ensue (**endo-genous infections**).

The interaction between an organism and the human host is complex. The interaction can result in transient colonization, a long-term symbiotic relationship, or disease, determined by the virulence of the organism, the site of exposure, and the host's ability to respond to the organism. Thus the manifestations of disease can range from mild symptoms to organ failure and death. The role of microbial virulence and the host's immunologic response is discussed in depth in subsequent chapters.

The human body is remarkably adapted to controlling exposure to pathogenic microbes. Physical barriers prevent microbial invasion; innate responses recognize molecular patterns on the microbial components and activate local defenses and specific adapted immune responses that target the microbe for elimination. Unfortunately, the immune response is often too late or too slow. To improve the human body's ability to prevent infection, the immune system can be augmented either through the passive transfer of antibodies present in immune globulin preparations or through active immunization with components of the microbes (vaccines). Infections can also be controlled with a variety of chemotherapeutic agents. Unfortunately, microbes can mutate and share genetic information and those that cannot be recognized by the immune response due to **antigenic variation** or are resistant to antibiotics will be selected and will endure. Thus the battle for control between microbe and host continues, with neither side yet able to claim victory (although the microbes have demonstrated remarkable ingenuity). There clearly is no "magic bullet" that has eradicated infectious diseases.

DIAGNOSTIC MICROBIOLOGY

The clinical microbiology laboratory plays an important role in the diagnosis and control of infectious diseases. However, its functions are limited by the quality of the specimen collected from the patient, the means by which it is transported from the patient to the laboratory, and the techniques used to demonstrate the microbe in the sample.

The laboratory is also able to determine the antimicrobial activity of selected chemotherapeutic agents, although the value of these tests is limited. The laboratory must test only organisms capable of producing disease and only medically relevant antimicrobials. Testing all isolated organisms or an indiscriminate selection of drugs can yield misleading results with potentially dangerous consequences. Not only can a patient be treated inappropriately with unnecessary antibiotics, but also the true pathogenic organism may not be recognized among the plethora of organisms isolated and tested. Finally, the in vitro determination of an organism's susceptibility to a variety of antibiotics is only one aspect of a complex picture. The virulence of the organism, site of infection, and patient's ability to respond to the infection influence the host-microbes interaction and must also be considered when planning treatment.

SUMMARY

It is important to realize that our knowledge of the microbial world is evolving continually. Just as the early microbiologists built their discoveries on the foundations established by their predecessors, we and future generations will continue to discover new microbes, new diseases, and new therapies. The following chapters are intended as a foundation of knowledge that can be used to build your understanding of microbes and their diseases.

KEYWORDS

English	Chinese
Microbiology	微生物学
Medical Microbiology	医学微生物学
Bacteria	细菌
Fungi	真菌
Viruses	病毒

SECTION 1

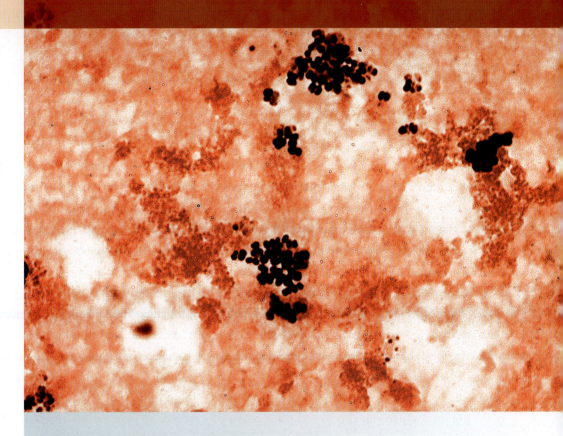

Bacteriology

Bacterial Classification, Structure, and Replication

Chapter 2

Cells from animals, plants, and fungi are **eukary-otes** (Greek for "true nucleus"), whereas bacteria, **archae**, and blue-green algae belong to the **prokaryotes** (Greek for "primitive nucleus"). Bacteria, the smallest cells, are visible only with the aid of a microscope. The smallest bacteria (*Chlamydia* and *Rickettsia*) are just 0.1 to 0.2 μm in diameter, whereas larger bacteria may be many microns in length. A newly described species is hundreds of times larger than the average bacterial cell and is visible to the naked eye. Most species, however, are approximately 1 μm in diameter and are therefore visible with the use of the light microscope, which has a resolution of 0.2 μm. In comparison, animal and plant cells are much larger, ranging from 7 μm (the diameter of a red blood cell) to several feet (the length of certain nerve cells).

BACTERIAL CLASSIFICATION

Bacteria can be classified by their macroscopic and microscopic appearance, by characteristic growth and metabolic properties, by their antigenicity, and finally by their genotype.

Macroscopic and Microscopic Distinction

The initial distinction between bacteria can be made by growth characteristics on different nutrient and selective media. The bacteria grow in colonies; each colony is like a city of as many as a million or more organisms. The sum of their characteristics provides the colony with distinguishing characteristics, such as color, size, shape, and smell. The ability to resist certain antibiotics, ferment specific sugars (e.g., lac-tose, to distinguish *E. coli* from *Salmonella*), to lyse erythrocytes (hemolytic properties), or to hydrolyze lipids (e.g., clostridial lipase) can also be determined using the appropriate growth media.

The microscopic appearance, including the size, shape, and configuration of the organisms (cocci, rods, curved, or spiral) and their ability to retain the Gram stain (gram-positive or gram-negative) are the primary means for distinguishing the bacteria. A spherical bacterium, such as *Staphylococcus*, is a coccus; a rod-shaped bacterium, such as *E. coli*, is a bacillus; and the snakelike treponeme is a spirillum. In addition, *Nocardia* and *Actinomyces* species have branched filamentous appearances similar to those of fungi. Some bacteria form aggregates, such as the grapelike clusters of *Staphylococcus aureus* or the dip-lococcus (two cells together) observed in *Streptococcus* or *Neisseria* species.

Gram stain is a rapid, powerful, easy test that allows clinicians to distinguish between the two major classes of bacteria, develop an initial diagnosis, and initiate therapy based on inherent differences in the bacteria (Figure 2-1,). Bacteria are heat fixed or otherwise dried onto a slide, stained with crystal violet (Figure 2-2), a stain that is precipitated with iodine, and then the unbound and excess stain is removed by washing with the acetone-based decolorizer and water. A red counterstain, safranin, is added to stain any decolor-ized cells. This process takes less than 10 minutes.

For gram-positive bacteria, which turn purple, the stain gets trapped in a thick, cross-linked, mesh-like structure, the peptidoglycan layer, which surrounds the cell. Gram-negative bacteria have a thin peptidoglycan layer that does not retain the crystal

6

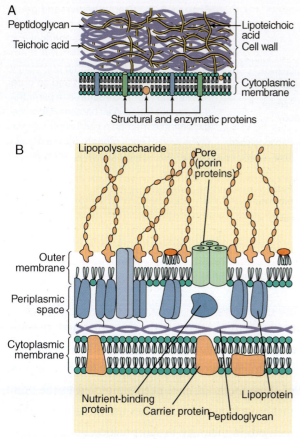

Figure 2-1   Comparison of the gram-positive and gram-negative bacterial cell walls. **A,** A gram-positive bacterium has a thick peptidoglycan layer that contains teichoic and lipoteichoic acids. **B,** A gram-negative bacterium has a thin peptidoglycan layer and an outer membrane that contains lipopolysaccharide, phospholipids, and proteins. The periplasmic space between the cytoplasmic and outer membranes contains transport, degradative, and cell wall synthetic proteins. The outer membrane is joined to the cytoplasmic membrane at adhesion points and is attached to the peptidoglycan by lipoprotein links.

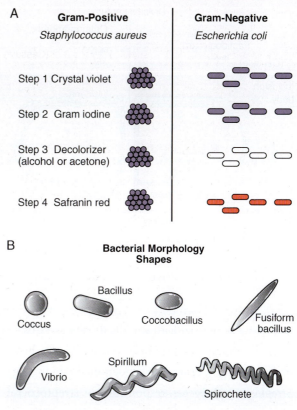

Figure 2-2   Gram-stain morphology of bacteria. **A,** The crystal violet of Gram stain is precipitated by Gram iodine and is trapped in the thick peptidoglycan layer in gram-positive bacteria. The decolorizer disperses the gram-negative outer membrane and washes the crystal violet from the thin layer of peptidoglycan. Gram-negative bacteria are visualized by the red counterstain. **B,** Bacterial morphologies.

violet stain; so the cells must be counterstained with safranin and turned red (Figure 2-3).

Due to degradation of the peptidoglycan, Gram staining is not a dependable test for bacteria that are starved (e.g., old or stationary-phase cultures) or treated with antibiotics. Bacteria that cannot be classified by Gram staining include mycobacteria, which have a waxy outer shell and are distinguished with the acid-fast stain, and mycoplasmas, which have no peptidoglycan.

Metabolic, Antigenic, and Genetic Distinction

The next level of classification is based on the metabolic signature of the bacteria, including requirement for anaerobic or aerobic environments, requirement for specific nutrients (e.g., ability to ferment specific carbohydrates or use different compounds as a source of carbon for growth), and production of characteristic metabolic products (acid, alcohols) and specific enzymes (e.g., staphylococcal catalase). Automated procedures for distinguishing enteric and other bacteria have been developed; they analyze the growth in different media and their microbial products and provide a numerical biotype for each of the bacteria.

A particular strain of bacteria can be distinguished using antibodies to detect characteristic antigens on the bacteria (serotyping). These serologic tests can also be used to identify organisms that are difficult (*Treponema pallidum*, the organism responsible for syphilis) or too dangerous (e.g., *Francisella*, the organism that causes tularemia) to grow in the labo-

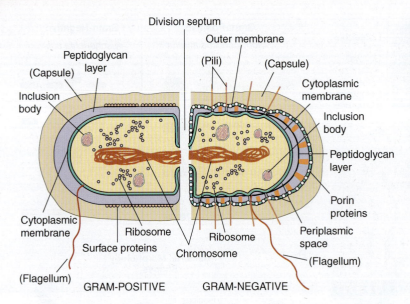

Figure 2-3 Gram-positive and gram-negative bacteria. A gram-positive bacterium has a thick layer of peptidoglycan (filling the purple space) *(left)*. A gram-negative bacterium has a thin peptidoglycan layer *(single black line)* and an outer membrane *(right)*. Structures in parentheses are not found in all bacteria. Upon cell division, the membrane and peptidoglycan grow toward each other to form a division septum to separate the daughter cells.

ratory, are associated with specific disease syndromes (e.g., *E. coli* serotype O157:H7, responsible for hemorrhagic colitis), or need to be identified rapidly (e.g., *Streptococcus pyogenes*, responsible for streptococcal pharyngitis). Serotyping is also used to subdivide bacteria below the species level for epidemiologic purposes.

The most precise method for classifying bacteria is by analysis of their genetic material. New methods distinguish bacteria by detection of specific characteristic DNA sequences. These techniques include DNA hybridization, polymerase chain reaction (PCR) amplification. These genetic techniques do not require living or growing bacteria and can be used for rapid detection and identification of slow-growing organisms, such as mycobacteria and fungi, or analysis of pathology samples of even very virulent bacteria. The technology is now available for rapid analysis of the nucleic acid sequence of specific segments or the entire bacterial chromosome. The most common application of this technique is analysis of sequences of ribosomal DNA to detect the highly conserved sequences that identify a family or genus and the highly variable sequences that distinguish a species or subspecies. It has also been used to define the evolutionary relationship among organisms and to identify organisms that are difficult or impossible to grow. Various other methods that have been used, primarily to classify organisms at the subspecies level

for epidemiologic investigations, include: plasmid analysis, ribotyping, and analysis of chromosomal DNA fragments. In recent years the technical aspects of these methods have been simplified to the point that most clinical laboratories use variations of these methods in their day-to-day practice.

BACTERIAL STRUCTURE

Cytoplasmic Structures

The cytoplasm of the bacterial cell contains the DNA chromosome, messenger RNA (mRNA), ribosomes, proteins, and metabolites (see Figure 2-3). Unlike eukaryotes, the bacterial chromosome is a single, double-stranded circle that is contained not in a nucleus, but in a discrete area known as the nucleoid. Histones are not present to maintain the conformation of the DNA, and the DNA does not form nucleosomes. Plasmids, which are smaller, circular, extrachromosomal DNAs, may also be present. Plasmids, although not usually essential for cellular survival, often provide a selective advantage: many confer resistance to one or more antibiotics.

The lack of a nuclear membrane simplifies the requirements and control mechanisms for the synthesis of proteins. Without a nuclear membrane, transcription and translation are coupled; in other words, ribosomes can bind to the mRNA, and protein can be made as the mRNA is being synthesized and still attached to the DNA.

The bacterial ribosome consists of 30S + 50S subunits, forming a 70S ribosome. This is unlike the eukaryotic 80S (40S + 60S) ribosome. The proteins and RNA of the bacterial ribosome are significantly different from those of eukaryotic ribosomes and are major targets for antibacterial drugs.

The cytoplasmic membrane has a lipid bilayer structure similar to the structure of the eukaryotic membranes, but it contains no steroids (e.g., cholesterol); mycoplasmas are the exception to this rule. The cytoplasmic membrane is responsible for many of the functions attributable to organelles in eukaryotes. These tasks include electron transport and energy production, which are normally achieved in the mitochondria. In addition, the membrane contains transport proteins that allow the uptake of metabolites and the release of other substances, ion pumps to maintain a membrane potential, and enzymes. The inside of the membrane is lined with actin-like protein filaments, which help determine the shape of the bacteria and the site of septum formation for cell division. These filaments determine the spiral shape of the treponemes.

Cell Wall

The structure (Table 2-1), components, and functions (Table 2-2) of the cell wall distinguish gram-positive

Table 2-1   Bacterial Membrane Structures

Structure	Chemical Constituents	Functions
Plasma membrane	Phospholipids, proteins, and enzymes	Containment, generation of energy, membrane potential, and transport
Cell Wall		
Gram-Positive Bacteria		
Peptidoglycan	Glycan chains of GlcNAc and MurNAc cross-linked by peptide bridge	Cell shape and structure; protection from environment and complement killing
Teichoic acid	Polyribitol phosphate or glycerol phosphate cross-linked to peptidoglycan	Strengthens cell wall; calcium ion sequestration; activator of innate host protections
Lipoteichoic acid	Lipid-linked teichoic acid	
Gram-Negative Bacteria		
Peptidoglycan	Thinner version of that found in gram-positive bacteria	Cell shape and structure
Periplasmic space		Enzymes involved in transport, degradation, and synthesis
Outer membrane		Cell structure; protection from host environment
Proteins	Porin channel	Permeation of small, hydrophilic molecules; restricts some antibiotics
	Secretory devices (types I, II, III, IV)	Penetrates and delivers proteins across membranes, including virulence factors
	Lipoprotein	Outer membrane link to peptidoglycan
LPS	Lipid A, core polysaccharide, O antigen	Outer membrane structure; potent activator of innate host responses
Phospholipids	With saturated fatty acids	
Other Structures		
Capsule	Polysaccharides (disaccharides and trisaccharides) and polypeptides	Antiphagocytic
Biofilm	Polysaccharides	Protection of colony from environment, antimicrobials and host response
Pili	Pilin, adhesins	Adherance, sex pili
Flagellum	Motor proteins, flagellin	Movement, chemotaxis
Proteins	M protein of streptococci (for example)	Various

GlcNAc, N-Acetylglucosamine; *LPS*, lipopolysaccharide; *MurNAc*, N-acetylmuramic acid.

from gram-negative bacteria. Cell wall components are also unique to bacteria, and their repetitive structures bind to Toll-like receptors on human cells to elicit innate protective responses. The important differences in membrane characteristics are outlined in Table 2-3. Rigid peptidoglycan (murein) layers surround the cytoplasmic membranes of most prokaryotes. The exceptions are *Archaea* organisms (which contain pseudoglycans or pseudomureins related to peptidoglycan) and mycoplasmas and chlamydia (which have no peptidoglycan). Because the peptidoglycan provides rigidity, it also helps to determine the shape of the particular bacterial cell. Gram-negative bacteria are also surrounded by outer membranes.

Mycobacteria have a peptidoglycan layer (slightly different structure), which is intertwined with and covalently attached to an arabinogalactan polymer and surrounded by a waxlike lipid coat of mycolic

Table 2-2 Functions of the Bacterial Envelope

Function	Component
Structure	
Rigidity	All
Packaging of internal contents	All
Bacterial Functions	
Permeability barrier	Outer membrane or plasma membrane
Metabolic uptake	Membranes and periplasmic transport proteins, porins, permeases
Energy production	Plasma membrane
Motility	Flagella
Mating	Pili
Host Interaction	
Adhesion to host cells	Pili, proteins, teichoic acid
Immune recognition by host	All outer structures and peptidoglycan
Escape from host immune protections	
Antibody	M protein
Phagocytosis	Capsule
Complement	Gram-positive peptidoglycan
Medical Relevance	
Antibiotic targets	Peptidoglycan synthesis, outer membrane
Antibiotic resistance	Outer membrane barrier

Table 2-3 Membrane Characteristics of Gram-Positive and Gram-Negative Bacteria

Characteristic	Gram-Positive	Gram-Negative
Outer membrane	−	+
Cell wall	Thicker	Thinner
Lipopolysaccharide	−	+
Endotoxin	−	+
Teichoic acid	Often present	−
Sporulation	Some strains	−
Capsule	Sometimes present	Sometimes present
Lysozyme	Sensitive	Resistant
Antibacterial activity of penicillin	More susceptible	More resistant
Exotoxin production	Some strains	Some strains

acid (large α-branched β-hydroxy fatty acids), cord factor (glycolipid of trehalose and two mycolic acids), wax D (glycolipid of 15 to 20 mycolic acids and sugar), and sulfolipids (Figure 2-4). These bacteria are described as staining acid-fast. The coat is responsible for virulence and is antiphagocytic. *Corynebacterium* and *Nocardia* organisms also produce mycolic acid lipids. Chlamydia and mycoplasmas have no peptidoglycan cell wall and mycoplasmas incorporate steroids from the host into their membranes.

Gram-Positive Bacteria

A gram-positive bacterium has a *thick, multilayered cell wall consisting mainly of peptidoglycan* (150 to 500 Å) surrounding the cytoplasmic membrane (Figure 2-5). The peptidoglycan is a meshlike exoskeleton similar in function to the exoskeleton of an insect. Unlike the exoskeleton of the insect, however, the peptidoglycan of the cell is sufficiently porous to allow diffusion of metabolites to the plasma membrane. A new model for peptidoglycan suggests that the glycan extends out from the plasma membrane like bristles that are cross-linked with short peptide chains. The peptidoglycan is essential for the structure, for replication, and for survival in the normally hostile conditions in which bacteria grow.

The peptidoglycan can be degraded by treatment with lysozyme. Lysozyme is an enzyme in human tears and mucus, but is also produced by bacteria

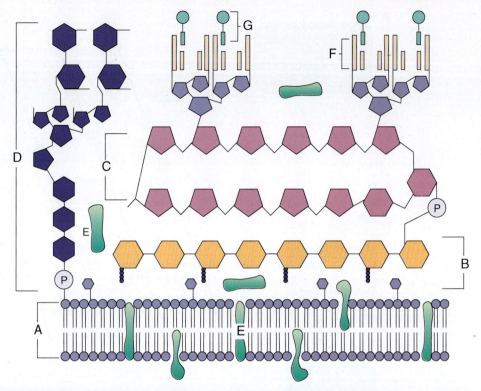

Figure 2-4 Mycobacterial cell wall structure. The components include the *(A)* plasma membrane, *(B)* peptidoglycans, *(C)* arabinogalactan, *(D)* mannose-capped lipoarabinomannan, *(E)* plasma-associated and cell wall-associated proteins, *(F)* mycolic acids, and *(G)* glycolipid surface molecules associated with the mycolic acids. (Modified from Karakousis, et al: *Mycobacterium tuberculosis* cell wall lipids and the host immune response, *Cell Microbiol* 6: 105-116, 2004.).

and other organisms. Lysozyme cleaves the glycan backbone of the peptidoglycan. Without the peptidoglycan, the bacteria succumb to the large osmotic pressure differences across the cytoplasmic membrane and lyse. Removal of the cell wall produces a protoplast that lyses, unless it is osmotically stabilized.

The gram-positive cell wall may also include other components such as proteins, teichoic and lipoteichoic acids, and complex polysaccharides (usually called C polysaccharides). The M protein of streptococci and R protein of staphylococci associate with the peptidoglycan. Teichoic acids are water-soluble, anionic polymers of polyol phosphates, which are covalently linked to the peptidoglycan and essential to cell viability. Lipoteichoic acids have a fatty acid and are anchored in the cytoplasmic membrane. These molecules are common surface antigens that distinguish bacterial serotypes and promote attachment to other bacteria and to specific receptors on mammalian cell surfaces (adherence). Teichoic acids are important factors in virulence. Lipoteichoic acids are

shed into the media and the host and although weaker, they can initiate innate protective host responses similar to endotoxin.

Gram-Negative Bacteria

Gram-negative cell walls are more complex than grampositive cell walls, both structurally and chemically (see Figure 2-1). Structurally, a gram-negative cell wall contains two layers external to the cytoplasmic membrane. Immediately external to the cytoplasmic membrane is a *thin peptidoglycan layer*, which accounts for only 5% to 10% of the gram-negative cell wall by weight. There are *no teichoic or lipoteichoic acids* in the gram-negative cell wall. External to the peptidoglycan layer is the outer membrane, which is unique to gram-negative bacteria. The area between the external surface of the cytoplasmic membrane and the internal surface of the outer membrane is referred to as the periplasmic space. This space is actually a compartment containing components of transport systems for iron, proteins, sugars and other

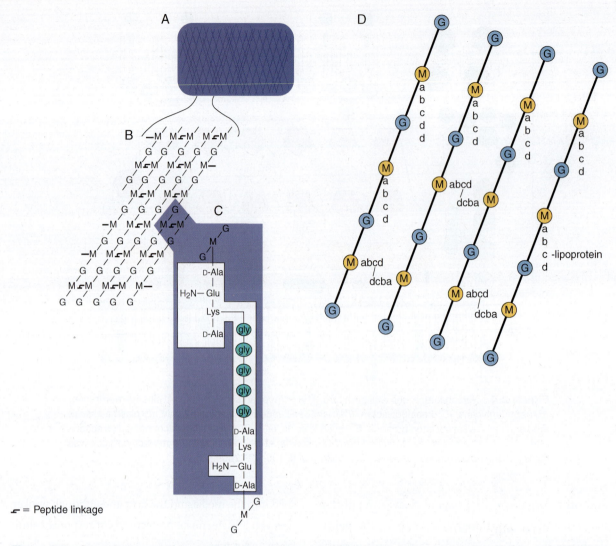

= Peptide linkage

Figure 2-5 General structure of the peptidoglycan component of the cell wall. **A,** The peptidoglycan forms a meshlike layer around the cell. **B,** The peptidoglycan mesh consists of a polysaccharide polymer that is cross-linked by peptide bonds. **C,** Peptides are cross-linked through a peptide bond between the terminal D-alanine (D-Ala) from one chain and a lysine (Lys) (or another diamino amino acid) from the other chain. A pentaglycine bridge (gly₅) expands the cross-link in *Staphylococcus aureus* (as shown). **D,** Representation of the *Escherichia coli* peptidoglycan structure. Diaminopimelic acid, the diamino amino acid in the third position of the peptide, is *directly linked* to the terminal alanine of another chain to cross-link the peptidoglycan. Lipoprotein anchors the outer membrane to the peptidoglycan. *G,* N-Acetylglucosamine; *Glu,* D-glutamic acid; *gly,* glycine; *M,* N-acetylmuramic acid. (**A** to **C,** Modified from Talaro K, Talaro A: *Foundations in microbiology,* ed 2, Dubuque, Iowa, 1996, William C Brown. **D,** Modified from Joklik KJ, et al: *Zinsser microbiology,* Norwalk, Conn, 1988, Appleton & Lange.).

metabolites, and a variety of hydrolytic enzymes that are important to the cell for the breakdown of large macromolecules for metabolism. These enzymes typically include proteases, phosphatases, lipases, nucleases, and carbohydrate-degrading enzymes. In the case of pathogenic gram-negative species, many of the lytic virulence factors, such as collagenases, hyaluronidases, proteases, and β-lactamase, are in the periplasmic space.

The gram-negative cell wall is also traversed by different transport systems, including the type I, II, III, IV, and V secretion devices. Transport systems provide mechanisms for the uptake and release of different metabolites and other compounds. Production of the secretion devices may be induced during infection and contribute to the virulence of the microbe by transporting molecules that facilitate bacterial adhesion or intracellular growth. The type III secretion device is a major virulence factor for some bacteria, with a complex structure that traverses both the inner and outer membranes and can act as a syringe to inject proteins into other cells.

As mentioned previously, outer membranes (see Figure 2-1) are unique to gram-negative bacteria. The outer membrane is like a stiff canvas sack around the bacteria. *The outer membrane maintains the bacterial structure and is a permeability barrier to large molecules* (e.g., proteins such as lysozyme) *and hydrophobic molecules* (e.g., some antimicrobials). It also provides protection from adverse environmental conditions, such as the digestive system of the host (important for *Enterobacteriaceae* organisms). The outer membrane has an asymmetric bilayer structure that differs from any other biologic membrane in the structure of the outer leaflet of the membrane. The inner leaflet contains phospholipids normally found in bacterial membranes. However, the outer leaflet is composed primarily of lipopoly-saccharide (LPS). Except for those LPS molecules in the process of synthesis, the outer leaflet of the outer membrane is the only location where LPS molecules are found.

LPS (endotoxin) consists of three structural sections: Lipid A, core polysaccharide (rough core), and O antigen (Figure 2-6). Lipid A is a basic component of LPS and is essential for bacterial viability. Lipid A is responsible for the endotoxin activity of LPS. It has a phosphorylated glucosamine disaccharide backbone with fatty acids attached to anchor the structure in the outer membrane.

LPS structure is used to classify bacteria. The basic structure of lipid A is identical for related bacteria and is similar for all gram-negative Enterobacteriaceae. The core region is the same for a species of bacteria. The O antigen distinguishes serotypes (strains) of a bacterial species. For example, the O157:H7 (O antigen:flagellin) serotype identifies the *E. coli* agent of hemolytic-uremic syndrome.

LPS is a powerful stimulator of innate and immune responses. LPS is shed from the bacteria into the media and host. LPS activates B cells and induces macrophage, dendritic, and other cells to release interleukin-1, interleukin-6, tumor necrosis factor, and other factors. LPS induces fever and can cause shock. The Shwartzman reaction (disseminated intravascular coagulation) follows the release of large amounts of endotoxin into the bloodstream. *Neisse-*

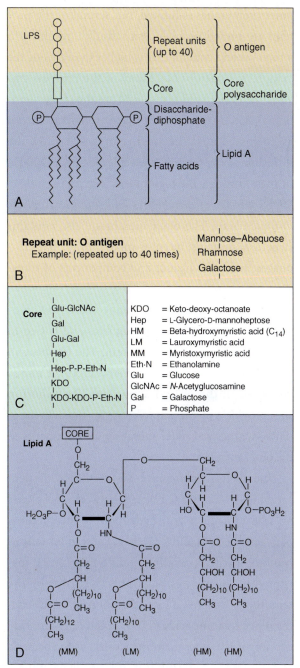

Figure 2-6 The lipopolysaccharide (*LPS*) of the gram-negative cell envelope. **A,** Segment of the molecule showing the arrangements of the major constituents. Each LPS molecule has one lipid A and one polysaccharide core unit but many repeats of O antigen. **B,** Typical O-antigen repeat unit (*Salmonella typhimurium*). **C,** Polysaccharide core. **D,** Structure of lipid A of *S. typhimurium*. (Modified from Brooks GF, Butel JS, Ornston LN: *Jawetz, Melnick, and Aldenberg's medical microbiology*, ed 19, Norwalk, Conn, 1991, Appleton & Lange.)

ria bacteria shed large amounts of a related molecule, lipooligosaccharide (LOS), resulting in fever and severe symptoms.

The variety of proteins found in gram-negative

outer membranes is limited, but several of the proteins are present in high concentration, resulting in a total protein content that is higher than that of the cytoplasmic membrane. Many of the proteins traverse the entire lipid bilayer and are thus transmembrane proteins. A group of these proteins is known as porins because they form pores that allow the diffusion of hydrophilic molecules less than 700 Da in mass through the membrane. *The porin channel allows passage of metabolites and small hydrophilic antimicrobials.* The outer membrane also contains structural proteins, receptor molecules for bacteriophages, and other ligands and components of transport and secretory systems.

The outer membrane is connected to the cytoplasmic membrane at adhesion sites and is tied to the peptidoglycan by lipoprotein. The lipoprotein is covalently attached to the peptidoglycan and is anchored in the outer membrane. The adhesion sites provide a membranous route for the delivery of newly synthesized outer membrane components to the outer membrane.

The outer membrane is held together by divalent cation (Mg^{+2} and Ca^{+2}) linkages between phosphates on LPS molecules and hydrophobic interactions between the LPS and proteins. These interactions produce a stiff, strong membrane that can be disrupted by antibiotics (e.g., polymyxin) or by the removal of Mg and Ca ions (chelation with ethylenediaminetetraacetic acid [EDTA] or tetracycline). Disruption of the outer membrane weakens the bacteria and allows the permeability of large, hydrophobic molecules. The addition of lysozyme to cells with a disrupted outer membrane produces spheroplasts, which, like protoplasts, are osmotically sensitive.

External Structures

Some bacteria (gram-positive or gram-negative) are closely surrounded by loose polysaccharide or protein layers called capsules. In cases in which it is loosely adherent and nonuniform in density or thickness, the material is referred to as a slime layer. The capsules and slime layers are also called the glycocalyx. *Bacillus anthracis*, the exception to this rule, produces a polypeptide capsule. The capsule is hard to see in a microscope, but its space can be visualized by the exclusion of India ink particles.

Capsules and slimes are unnecessary for the growth of bacteria, but are very important for survival in the host. *The capsule is poorly antigenic and antiphagocytic and is a major virulence factor* (e.g., *Streptococcus pneumoniae*). The capsule can also act as a barrier to toxic hydrophobic molecules, such as detergents, and can promote adherence to other bacteria or to host tissue surfaces. For *Streptococcus mutans*, the dextran and levan capsules are the means by which the bacteria attach and stick to the tooth enamel. Bacterial strains lacking a capsule may arise during growth under laboratory conditions, away from the selective pressures of the host, and are therefore less virulent. Some bacteria (e.g., *Pseudomonas aeruginosa*, *S. aureus*) will produce a polysaccharide biofilm when sufficient numbers of bacteria (quorum) are present and under conditions which support growth, which establishes a bacterial community and protects them from antibiotics and host defenses. Another example of a biofilm is tooth plaque produced by *S. mutans*.

Flagella are ropelike propellers composed of helically coiled protein subunits (flagellin) that are anchored in the bacterial membranes through hook and basal body structures and are driven by membrane potential. Bacterial species may have one or several flagella on their surfaces, and they may be anchored at different parts of the cell. Flagella are composed of an adenosine triphosphate (ATP)-driven protein motor connected to a whiplike propeller made of multiple subunits of flagellin. Flagella provide motility for bacteria, allowing the cell to swim (chemotaxis) toward food and away from poisons. Bacteria approach food by swimming straight and then tumbling in a new direction. The swimming period becomes longer as the concentration of chemoattractant increases. The direction of flagellar spinning determines whether the bacteria swim or tumble. Flagella express antigenic and strain determinants and are a ligand for Toll-like receptor 5 to activate innate host protections.

Fimbriae (pili) (Latin for "fringe") are hairlike structures on the outside of bacteria; they are composed of protein subunits (pilin). Fimbriae can be morphologically distinguished from flagella because they are smaller in diameter (3 to 8 nm versus 15 to 20 nm) and usually are not coiled in structure. In general, several hundred fimbriae are arranged peritrichously (uniformly) over the entire surface of the bacterial cell. They may be as long as 15 to 20 μm or many times the length of the cell.

Fimbriae promote adherence to other bacteria or to the host (alternative names are *adhesins*, *lectins*, *evasins*, and *aggressins*). As an adherence factor (adhesin), fimbriae are an important virulence factor for colonization and infection of the urinary tract by *E. coli*, *Neisseria gonorrhoeae*, and other bacteria. The tips of the fimbriae may contain proteins (lectins) that bind to specific sugars (e.g., mannose). F pili (sex pili) bind to other bacteria and are a tube for transfer of large segments of bacterial chromosomes between bacteria. These pili are encoded by a plasmid (F).

Some gram-positive, but never gram-negative, bacteria, such as members of the genera *Bacillus* (e.g., *Bacillus anthracis*) and *Clostridium* (e.g., *Clostridium tetani* or *botulinum*) (soil bacteria), are spore formers. Under harsh environmental conditions, such as the loss of a nutritional requirement, these bacteria can convert from a vegetative state to a dormant state, or spore. The location of the spore within a cell is a characteristic of the bacteria and can assist in identification of the bacterium.

The spore is a dehydrated, multishelled structure that protects and allows the bacteria to exist in "suspended animation". It contains a complete copy of the chromosome, the bare minimum concentrations of essential proteins and ribosomes, and a high concentration of calcium bound to dipicolinic acid. The spore has an inner membrane, two peptidoglycan layers, and an outer keratin-like protein coat. The spore looks refractile (bright) in the microscope. The structure of the spore protects the genomic DNA from intense heat, radiation, and attack by most enzymes and chemical agents. In fact, bacterial spores are so resistant to environmental factors that

they can exist for centuries as viable spores. Spores are also difficult to decontaminate with standard disinfectants.

CELL DIVISION

The cell division of bacteria follow the binary fission mode. The replication of the bacterial chromosome also triggers the initiation of cell division (Figure 2-7). The production of two daughter bacteria requires the growth and extension of the cell wall components, followed by the production of a septum (cross wall) to divide the daughter bacteria into two cells. The septum consists of two membranes separated by two layers of peptidoglycan. Septum formation is initiated at midcell, at a site defined by protein complexes affixed to a protein filament ring that lines the inside of the cytoplasmic membrane. The septum grows from opposite sides toward the center of the cell,

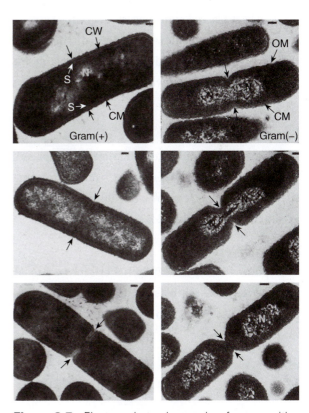

Figure 2-7   Electron photomicrographs of gram-positive cell division *(Bacillus subtilis) (left)* and gram-negative cell division *(Escherichia coli) (right)*. Progression in cell division from top to bottom. *CM*, Cytoplasmic membrane; *CW*, cell wall; *N*, nucleoid; *OM*, outer membrane; *S*, septum. Bar = 0.2 μm. (From Slots J, Taubman MA: *Contemporary oral biology and immunology*, St Louis, 1992, Mosby.)

causing cleavage of the daughter cells. This process requires special transpeptidases (PBPs) and other enzymes. For streptococci, the growth zone is located at 180 degrees from each other, producing linear chains of bacteria. In contrast, the growth zone of staphylococci is at 90 degrees. Incomplete cleavage of the septum can cause the bacteria to remain linked, forming chains (e.g., streptococci) or clusters (e.g., staphylococci).

SUMMARY

Bacterial Classification

Bacterial classification serves both academic and practical purposes. They help the differentiation and identification of unknown species in applied and medical bacterium.

Macroscopic and microscopic distinction is an important standard in bacterial classification, which presents the bacterium into two main groups: gram-positive bacteria and gram-negative bacteria.

Metabolic, antigenic, and genetic distinction is the classification standard maybe more suitable for clinical identification, owing to the little time cost and high veracity.

Bacterial Structure

Structures include **outer cell membrane, cytoplasm, chromosome and ribosome**. For bacterium, some special structures (capsule, flagellum, pili, spore) exist to play specific functions.

Bacterial Replication

The splitting of a parent bacterial cell into a pair of daughter cells is known as **replication process**. The duration of each replication process is called generation.

KEYWORDS

English	Chinese
Classification	分类
Gram stain	革兰染色
Gram-positive bacteria	革兰阳性菌
Gram-negative bacteria	革兰阴性菌
Polymerase chain reaction	聚合酶链式反应
Capsule	荚膜
Spore	芽胞
Biofilm	生物膜
Fimbriae	菌毛
Flagellum	鞭毛
Binary fission	二分裂

BIBLIOGRAPHY

1. Bower S, Rosenthal KS: Bacterial cell walls: the armor, artillery and Achilles heel, Infect Dis Clin Pract 14: 309-317, 2006.

2. Daniel RA, Errington J: Control of cell morphogenesis in bacteria: two distinct ways to make a rod-shaped cell, Cell 113: 767-776, 2003.

3. Lutkenhaus J: The regulation of bacterial cell division: a time and place for it, Curr Opin Microbiol 1: 210-215, 1998.

4. Meroueh SO, et al: Three-dimensional structure of the bacterial cell wall peptidoglycan, Proc Natl Acad Sci U S A 103: 4404-4409, 2006.

5. Nanninga N: Morphogenesis of *Escherichia coli*, Microbiol Mol Biol Rev 62: 110-129, 1998.

6. Talaro K: Foundations in microbiology, ed 6, New York, 2008, McGraw-Hill.

7. Willey J, Sherwood L, Woolverton C: Prescott/Harley/Klein's microbiology, ed 7, New York, 2007, McGraw-Hill.

Chapter 3

Bacterial Metabolism and Genetics

BACTERIAL METABOLISM

Metabolic Requirements

Bacterial growth requires a source of energy and the raw materials to build the proteins, structures, and membranes that make up and power the cell. Bacteria must obtain or synthesize the amino acids, carbohydrates, and lipids used as building blocks of the cell.

The minimum requirements for growth are a source of carbon and nitrogen, an energy source, water, and various ions. The essential elements include the components of proteins, lipids and nucleic acids (C, O, H, N, S, P), important ions (K, Na, Mg, Ca, Cl), and components of enzymes (Fe, Zn, Mn, Mo, Se, Co, Cu, Ni). Iron is so important that many bacteria secrete special proteins (siderophores) to concentrate iron from dilute solutions, and our bodies will sequester iron to reduce its availability as a means of protection.

Oxygen (O_2 gas), although essential for the human host, is actually a poison for many bacteria. Some organisms, such as *Clostridium perfringens*, which causes gas gangrene, cannot grow in the presence of oxygen. Such bacteria are referred to as obligate anaerobes. Other organisms, such as *Mycobacterium tuberculosis*, which causes tuberculosis, require the presence of molecular oxygen for metabolism and growth and are therefore referred to as obligate aerobes. Most bacteria, however, grow in either the presence or the absence of oxygen. These bacteria are referred to as facultative anaerobes. Aerobic bacteria produce superoxide dismutase and catalase enzymes, which can detoxify hydrogen peroxide and superoxide radicals that are the toxic byproducts of aerobic metabolism.

Growth requirements and metabolic byproducts may be used as a convenient means of classifying different bacteria. Some bacteria, such as certain strains of *Escherichia coli* (a member of the intestinal flora), can synthesize all the amino acids, nucleotides, lipids, and carbohydrates necessary for growth and division, whereas the growth requirements of the causative agent of syphilis, *Treponema pallidum*, are so complex that a defined laboratory medium capable of supporting its growth has yet to be developed. Bacteria that can rely entirely on inorganic chemicals for their energy and source of carbon (carbon dioxide [CO_2]) are referred to as autotrophs (lithotrophs), whereas many bacteria and animal cells that require organic carbon sources are known as heterotrophs (organotrophs). Clinical microbiology laboratories distinguish bacteria by their ability to grow on specific carbon sources (e.g., lactose) and the end products of metabolism (e.g., ethanol, lactic acid, succinic acid).

Metabolism, Energy, and Biosynthesis

All cells require a constant supply of energy to survive. This energy, typically in the form of adenosine triphosphate (ATP), is derived from the controlled breakdown of various organic substrates (carbohydrates, lipids, and proteins). This process of substrate breakdown and conversion into usable energy is known as catabolism. The energy produced may then be used in the synthesis of cellular constituents (cell walls, proteins, fatty acids, and nucleic acids), a process known as anabolism. Together these two processes, which are interrelated and tightly integrated, are referred to as intermediary metabolism.

The metabolic process generally begins with hydrolysis of large macromolecules in the external cellular environment by specific enzymes (Figure 3-1). The smaller molecules that are produced (e.g., monosaccharides, short peptides, and fatty acids) are transported across the cell membranes into the cytoplasm by active or passive transport mechanisms specific for the metabolite. These mechanisms may use specific carrier or membrane transport proteins to help concentrate metabolites from the medium. The metabolites are converted via one or more pathways to one common, universal intermediate, pyruvic acid. From pyruvic acid, the carbons may be channeled toward energy production or the synthesis of new carbohydrates, amino acids, lipids, and nucleic acids.

CATABOLISM

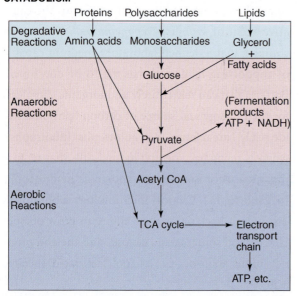

Figure 3-1 Catabolism of proteins, polysaccharides, and lipids produces glucose, pyruvate, or intermediates of the tricarboxylic acid *(TCA)* cycle and, ultimately, energy in the form of adenosine triphosphate *(ATP)* or the reduced form of nicotinamide adenine dinucleotide *(NADH)*. *CoA,* Coenzyme A.

Metabolism of Glucose

For the sake of simplicity, this section presents an overview of the pathways by which glucose is metabolized to produce energy or other usable substrates. Instead of releasing all of glucose's energy as heat (as for burning), the bacteria break down glucose in discrete steps to allow the energy to be captured in usable forms. *Bacteria can produce energy from glu-*

cose by—in order of increasing efficiency—fermentation, anaerobic respiration (both of which occur in the absence of oxygen), or aerobic respiration. Aerobic respiration can completely convert the six carbons of glucose to CO_2 and water (H_2O) plus energy, whereas two- and three-carbon compounds are the end products of fermentation. For a more complete discussion of metabolism, please refer to a textbook on biochemistry.

Embden-Meyerhof-Parnas Pathway

Bacteria use three major metabolic pathways in the catabolism of glucose. Most common among these is the glycolytic, or Embden-Meyerhof-Parnas (EMP), pathway (Figure 3-2,) for the conversion of glucose to pyruvate. These reactions, which occur under both aerobic and anaerobic conditions, begin with activation of glucose to form glucose-6-phosphate. This reaction, as well as the third reaction in the series, in which fructose-6-phosphate is converted to fructose-1,6-diphosphate, requires 1 mole of ATP per mole of glucose and represents an initial investment of cellular energy stores.

Energy is produced during glycolysis in two different forms, chemical and electrochemical. In the first, the high-energy phosphate group of one of the intermediates in the pathway is used under the direction of the appropriate enzyme (a kinase) to generate ATP from adenosine diphosphate (ADP). This type of reaction, termed substrate-level phosphorylation, occurs at two different points in the glycolytic pathway (i.e., conversion of 3-phosphoglycerol phosphate to 3-phosphoglycerate and 2-phosphoenolpyruvic acid to pyruvate).

This pathway yields four ATP molecules per molecule of glucose, but two ATP molecules were used in the initial glycolytic conversion of glucose to two molecules of pyruvic acid, resulting in a net production of two molecules of ATP, two molecules of reduced nicotinamide adenine dinucleotide (NADH) and two pyruvate molecules. NADH may then be converted to ATP by a series of oxidation reactions.

In the absence of oxygen, substrate-level phosphorylation represents the primary means of energy

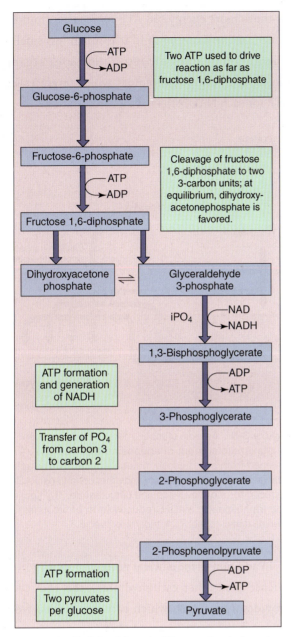

Figure 3-2   Embden-Meyerhof-Parnas glycolytic pathway results in conversion of glucose to pyruvate. *ADP*, Adenosine diphosphate; *ATP*, adenosine triphosphate; *iPO₄*, inorganic phosphate; *NAD*, nicotinamide adenine dinucleotide; *NADH*, reduced form of NAD.

conversion of pyruvate to ethanol plus CO_2. Alcoholic fermentation is uncommon in bacteria, which most commonly use the one-step conversion of pyruvic acid to lactic acid. This process is responsible for making milk into yogurt and cabbage into sauerkraut. Other bacteria use more complex fermentative pathways, producing various acids, alcohols, and often gases (many of which have vile odors). These products lend flavors to various cheeses and wines and odors to wound and other infections.

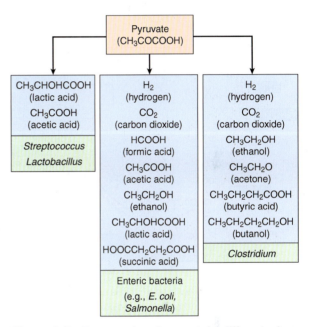

Figure 3-3   Fermentation of pyruvate by different microorganisms results in different end products. The clinical laboratory uses these pathways and end products as a means of distinguishing different bacteria.

production. The pyruvic acid produced from glycolysis is then converted to various end products, depending on the bacterial species, in a process known as fermentation. Many bacteria are identified on the basis of their fermentative end products (Figure 3-3). These organic molecules, rather than oxygen, are used as electron acceptors to recycle the NADH, which was produced during glycolysis, to NAD. In yeast, fermentative metabolism results in the

Tricarboxylic Acid Cycle

In the presence of oxygen, the pyruvic acid produced from glycolysis and from the metabolism of other substrates may be completely oxidized (controlled burning) to H_2O and CO_2 using the tricarboxylic acid (TCA) cycle (Figure 3-4), which results in production of additional energy. The process begins with the oxidative decarboxylation (release of CO_2) of pyruvate to the high-energy intermediate, acetyl coenzyme A (acetyl CoA); this reaction also produces two NADH molecules. The two remaining carbons derived from pyruvate then enter the TCA cycle in the form of acetyl CoA by condensation with oxaloacetate, with the formation of the six-carbon citrate molecule. In a stepwise series of oxidative reactions, the citrate is converted back to oxaloacetate. The theoretical yield from each pyruvate is 2 moles of CO_2, 3 moles of NADH, 1 mole of flavin adenine dinucleotide ($FADH_2$), and 1 mole of guanosine triphosphate (GTP).

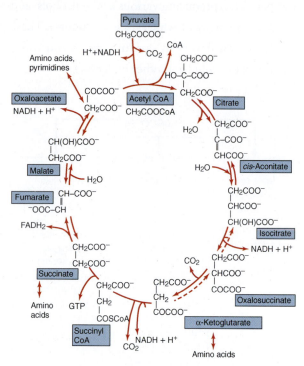

Figure 3-4 Tricarboxylic acid cycle is an amphibolic cycle. Precursors for the synthesis of amino acids and nucleotides are also shown. *CoA,* Coenzyme A; *FADH₂,* reduced form of flavin adenine dinucleotide; *GTP,* guanosine triphosphate; *NADH,* reduced form of nicotinamide adenine dinucleotide.

The TCA cycle allows the organism to generate substantially more energy per mole of glucose than is possible from glycolysis alone. In addition to the GTP (an ATP equivalent) produced by substrate-level phosphorylation, the NADH and $FADH_2$ yield ATP from the electron transport chain. In this chain the electrons carried by NADH (or $FADH_2$) are passed in a stepwise fashion through a series of donor-acceptor pairs and ultimately to oxygen (aerobic respiration) or other terminal electron acceptor (nitrate, sulfate, CO_2, ferric iron) (anaerobic respiration).

Anaerobic organisms are less efficient at energy production than aerobic organisms. Fermentation produces only two ATP molecules per glucose, whereas aerobic metabolism with electron transport and a complete TCA cycle can generate as much as

19 times more energy (38 ATP molecules) from the same starting material (and it is much less smelly) (Figure 3-5). Anaerobic respiration uses organic molecules as electron acceptors, which produces less ATP for each NADH than aerobic respiration.

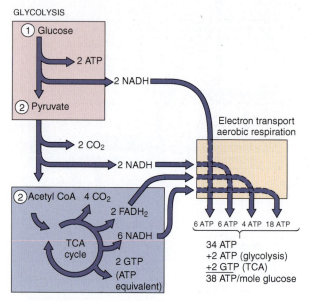

Figure 3-5 Aerobic glucose metabolism. The theoretical maximum amount of adenosine triphosphate *(ATP)* obtained from one glucose molecule is 38, but the actual yield depends on the organism and other conditions. *FADH₂,* Reduced form of flavin adenine dinucleotide; *GTP,* guanosine triphosphate; *NADH,* reduced form of nicotinamide adenine dinucleotide; *TCA,* tricarboxylic acid.

In addition to the efficient generation of ATP from glucose (and other carbohydrates), the TCA cycle provides a means by which carbons derived from lipids (in the form of acetyl CoA) may be shunted toward either energy production or the generation of biosynthetic precursors. Similarly, the cycle includes several points at which deaminated amino acids may enter (see Figure 3-4). For example, deamination of glutamic acid yields α-ketoglutarate, whereas deamination of aspartic acid yields oxaloacetate, both of which are TCA cycle intermediates. The TCA cycle therefore serves the following functions:

It is the most efficient mechanism for the generation of ATP.

It serves as the final common pathway for the complete oxidation of amino acids, fatty acids, and carbohydrates.

It supplies key intermediates (i.e., α-ketoglutarate,

pyruvate, oxaloacetate) for the ultimate synthesis of amino acids, lipids, purines, and pyrimidines.

The last two functions make the TCA cycle a so-called amphibolic cycle (i.e., it may function to break down and synthesize molecules).

Pentose Phosphate Pathway

The final pathway of glucose metabolism considered here is known as the pentose phosphate pathway, or the hexose monophosphate shunt. The function of this pathway is to provide nucleic acid precursors and reducing power in the form of nicotinamide adenine dinucleotide phosphate (reduced form) (NADPH) for use in biosynthesis. In the first half of the pathway, glucose is converted to ribulose-5-phosphate, with consumption of 1 mole of ATP and generation of 2 moles of NADPH per mole of glucose. The ribulose-5-phosphate may then be converted to ribose-5-phosphate (a precursor in nucleotide biosynthesis) or alternatively to xylulose-5-phosphate. The remaining reactions in the pathway use enzymes known as transketolases and transaldolases to generate various sugars, which may function as biosynthetic precursors or may be shunted back to the glycolytic pathway for use in energy generation.

BACTERIAL GENES AND EXPRESSION

The bacterial genome is the total collection of genes carried by a bacterium, both on its chromosome and on its extrachromosomal genetic elements, if any. Genes are sequences of nucleotides that have a biologic function; examples are protein-structural genes (cistrons, which are coding genes), ribosomal ribonucleic acid (RNA) genes, and recognition and binding sites for other molecules (promoters and operators). Each genome contains many operons, which are made up of genes. Genes may also be grouped in islands, such as the pathogenicity islands, which share function or to coordinate their control.

Bacteria usually have only one copy of their chromosomes (they are therefore haploid), whereas eukaryotes usually have two distinct copies of each chromosome (they are therefore diploid). With only one chromosome, alteration of a bacterial gene (mutation) will have a more obvious effect on the cell. In addition, the structure of the bacterial chromosome is maintained by polyamines, such as spermine and spermidine, rather than by histones.

Bacteria may also contain extrachromosomal genetic elements such as plasmids or bacteriophages (bacterial viruses). These elements are independent of the bacterial chromosome and, in most cases, can be transmitted from one cell to another.

Transcription

The information carried in the genetic memory of the deoxyribonucleic acid (DNA) is transcribed into a useful messenger RNA (mRNA) for subsequent translation into protein. RNA synthesis is performed by a DNA-dependent RNA polymerase. The process begins when the sigma factor recognizes a particular sequence of nucleotides in the DNA (the promoter) and binds tightly to this site. Promoter sequences occur just before the start of the DNA that actually encodes a protein. Sigma factors bind to these promoters to provide a docking site for the RNA polymerase. Some bacteria encode several sigma factors to allow transcription of a group of genes under special conditions, such as heat shock, starvation, special nitrogen metabolism, or sporulation.

Once the polymerase has bound to the appropriate site on the DNA, RNA synthesis proceeds with the sequential addition of ribonucleotides complementary to the sequence in the DNA. Once an entire gene or group of genes (operon) has been transcribed, the RNA polymerase dissociates from the DNA, a process mediated by signals within the DNA. The bacterial DNA-dependent RNA polymerase is inhibited by rifampin, an antibiotic often used in the treatment of tuberculosis. The transfer RNA (tRNA), which is used in protein synthesis, and ribosomal RNA (rRNA), a component of the ribosomes, are also transcribed from the DNA. Promoters and operators control the expression of a gene by influencing which sequences will be transcribed into mRNA. Operons are groups of one or more structural genes expressed from a particular promoter and ending at a transcriptional terminator. Thus all the genes coding for the enzymes of a particular pathway can be coordinately regulated. Operons with many structural genes are polycistronic. The *E. coli lac* operon includes all the genes necessary for lactose metabolism, as well as the control mechanisms for turning off (in the presence of glucose) or turning on (in the presence of galactose or an inducer) these genes only when they are needed. The *lac* operon includes a repressor sequence, a promoter sequence, and structural genes for the β-galactosidase enzyme, a permease, and an acetylase (Figure 3-6). The *lac* operon is discussed later in this chapter.

Translation

Translation is the process by which the language of the genetic code, in the form of mRNA, is converted (translated) into a sequence of amino acids, the protein product. Each amino acid word and the punctuation of the genetic code is written as sets of three nucleotides, known as codons. There are 64 different codon combinations encoding the 20 amino acids, plus start and termination codons. Some of the amino acids are encoded by more than one triplet codon. This feature is known as the *degeneracy of the genetic code* and may function in protecting the cell

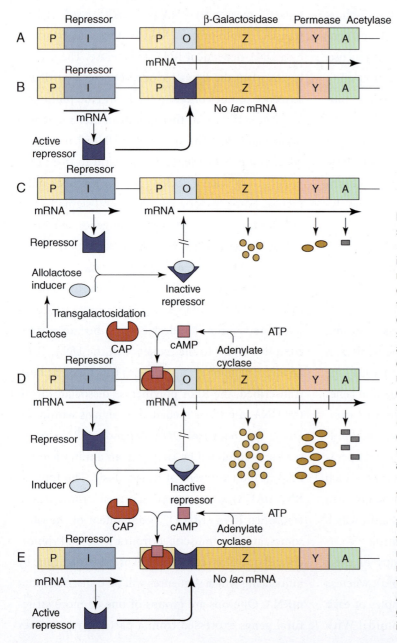

Figure 3-6   A, The lactose operon is transcribed as a polycistronic messenger RNA *(mRNA)* from the promoter *(P)* and translated into three proteins: β-galactosidase *(Z),* permease *(Y),* and acetylase *(A).* The *(I)* gene encodes the repressor protein. **B,** The lactose operon is not transcribed in the absence of an allolactose inducer because the repressor competes with the RNA polymerase at the operator site *(O).* **C,** The repressor, complexed with the inducer, does not recognize the operator because of a conformation change in the repressor. The *lac* operon is thus transcribed at a low level. **D,** *Escherichia coli* is grown in a poor medium in the presence of lactose as the carbon source. Both the inducer and the CAP-cAMP complex are bound to the promoter, which is fully "turned on," and a high level of *lac* mRNA is transcribed and translated. **E,** Growth of *E. coli* in a poor medium without lactose results in the binding of the CAP-cAMP complex to the promoter region and binding of the active repressor to the operator sequence because no inducer is available. The result will be that the *lac* operon will not be transcribed. *ATP,* Adenosine triphosphate; *CAP,* catabolite gene-activator protein; *cAMP,* cyclic adenosine monophosphate.

from the effects of minor mutations in the DNA or mRNA. Each tRNA molecule contains a three-nucleotide sequence complementary to one of the codon sequences. This tRNA sequence is known as the anticodon; it allows base pairing and binds to the codon sequence on the mRNA. Attached to the opposite end of the tRNA is the amino acid that corresponds to the particular codon-anticodon pair.

The process of protein synthesis (Figure 3-7) begins with the binding of the 30S ribosomal subunit and a special initiator tRNA for formyl methionine (fMet) at the methionine codon (AUG) start codon to form the initiation complex. The 50S ribosomal subunit binds to the complex to initiate mRNA synthesis. The ribosome contains two tRNA binding sites, the A (aminoacyl) site and the P (peptidyl) site, each of which allows base pairing between the bound tRNA and the codon sequence in the mRNA. The tRNA corresponding to the second codon occupies the A site. The amino group of the amino acid attached to the A site forms a peptide bond with the carboxyl group of the amino acid in the P site in a reaction known as transpeptidation, and the empty

tRNA in the P site (uncharged tRNA) is released from the ribosome. The ribosome then moves down the mRNA exactly three nucleotides, thereby transferring the tRNA with attached nascent peptide to the P site and bringing the next codon into the A site. The appropriate charged tRNA is brought into the A site, and the process is then repeated. Translation continues until the new codon in the A site is one of the three termination codons, for which there is no corresponding tRNA. At that point the new protein is released to the cytoplasm and the translation complex may be disassembled, or the ribosome shuffles to the next start codon and initiates a new protein. The ability to shuffle along the mRNA to start a new protein is a characteristic of the 70S bacterial but not of the 80S eukaryotic ribosome. The eukaryotic constraint has implications for the synthesis of proteins for some viruses.

The process of protein synthesis by the 70S ribosome represents an important target of antimicrobial action. The aminoglycosides (e.g., streptomycin and gentamicin) and the tetracyclines act by binding to the small ribosomal subunit and inhibiting normal ribosomal function. Similarly, the macrolide (e.g., erythromycin) and lincosamide (e.g., clindamycin) groups of antibiotics act by binding to the large ribosomal subunit. Also, formyl methionine peptides (e.g., fmet-leu-phe) attract neutrophils to the site of an infection.

Control of Gene Expression

Bacteria have developed mechanisms to adapt quickly and efficiently to changes and triggers from the environment. This allows them to coordinate and regulate the expression of genes for multicomponent structures or the enzymes of one or more metabolic pathways. For example, temperature change could signify entry into the human host and indicate the need for a global change in metabolism and up-regulation of genes important for parasitism or virulence. Many bacterial genes are controlled at multiple levels and by multiple methods.

A coordinated change in the expression of many genes, as would be required for sporulation, occurs

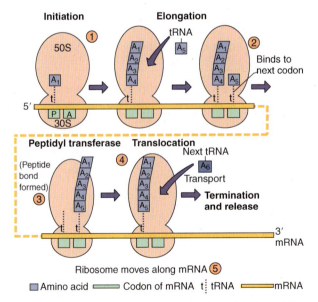

Figure 3-7 Bacterial protein synthesis. *1,* Binding of the 30S subunit to the messenger RNA *(mRNA)* with the formyl methionine transfer RNA (fMet-tRNA) at the AUG start codon allows assembly of the 70S ribosome. The fMet-tRNA binds to the peptidyl site *(P). 2,* The next *tRNA* binds to its codon at the *A* site and "accepts" the growing peptide chain. *3* and *4,* Before translocation to the peptidyl site. *5,* The process is repeated until a stop codon and the protein are released.

through use of a different sigma factor for the RNA polymerase. This would change the specificity of the RNA polymerase and allow mRNA synthesis for the necessary genes while ignoring unnecessary genes. Bacteria might produce more than six different sigma factors to provide global regulation in response to stress, shock, starvation, or to coordinate production of complicated structures such as flagella.

Coordination of a large number of processes on a global level can also be mediated by small molecular activators, such as cyclic adenosine monophosphate (cAMP). Increased cAMP levels indicate low glucose levels and the need to utilize alternative metabolic pathways. Similarly, in a process called quorum sensing, when a sufficient number of bacteria are present and producing a specific small molecule, virulence and other genes are turned on. The trigger for biofilm production by *Pseudomonas* spp. is triggered by a critical concentration of *N*-acyl homoserine lactone (AHL) produced when sufficient numbers of bacteria (a quorum) are present. Activation of toxin production and more virulent behavior by *Staphylococcus aureus* accompanies the increase in concentration of a cyclic peptide.

To coordinate the expression of a more limited group of genes, such as for a specific metabolic process, the genes for the necessary enzymes would be organized into an operon. The operon would be under the control of a promoter or repressor DNA sequence that can activate or turn off the expression of a gene or a group of genes to coordinate production of the necessary enzymes and allow the bacteria to react to changes in concentrations of nutrients. The genes for some virulence mechanisms are organized into a pathogenicity island under the control of a single promoter to allow their expression under appropriate (to the bacteria) conditions. The many components of the type III secretion devices of *E. coli*, *Salmonella*, or *Yersinia* are grouped together within a pathogenicity island.

Transcription can also be regulated by the translation process. Unlike eukaryotes, the absence of a nuclear membrane in prokaryotes allows the ribosome to bind to the mRNA as it is being transcribed from the DNA. The position and speed of ribosomal movement along the mRNA can affect the presence of loops in the mRNA and the ability of the polymerase to transcribe new mRNA. This allows control of gene expression at both the transcriptional and translational levels.

Initiation of transcription may be under positive or negative control. Genes under negative control are expressed unless they are switched off by a repressor protein. This repressor protein prevents gene expression by binding to a specific DNA sequence called the operator, blocking the RNA polymerase from initiating transcription at the promoter sequence. Inversely, genes whose expression is under positive control are not transcribed unless an active regulator protein, called an apoinducer, is present. The apoinducer binds to a specific DNA sequence and assists the RNA polymerase in the initiation steps by an unknown mechanism.

Operons can be inducible or repressible. Introduction of a substrate (inducer) into the growth medium may induce an operon to increase the expression of the enzymes necessary for its metabolism. An abundance of the end products (co-repressors) of a pathway may signal that a pathway should be shut down or repressed by reducing the synthesis of its enzymes.

The lactose *(lac)* operon responsible for the degradation of the sugar lactose is an inducible operon under positive and negative regulation. Normally the bacteria use glucose and not lactose. In the absence of lactose the operon is repressed by the binding of the repressor protein to the operator sequence, thus impeding the RNA polymerase function. In the absence of glucose, however, the addition of lactose reverses this repression. Full expression of the *lac* operon also requires a protein-mediated, positive-control mechanism. In *E. coli*, when glucose decreases in the cell, cAMP increases to promote usage of other sugars for metabolism. Binding of cAMP to a protein called the catabolite gene-activator protein (CAP) allows it to bind to a specific DNA sequence present in the promoter. The CAP-cAMP complex enhances binding of the RNA polymerase to the promoter, thus allowing an increase in the frequency of transcription initiation.

The tryptophan operon (*trp* operon) contains the structural genes necessary for tryptophan biosynthesis and is under dual transcriptional control mechanisms (Figure 3-8). Although tryptophan is essential for protein synthesis, too much tryptophan in the cell can be toxic; therefore its synthesis must be regulated. At the DNA level the repressor protein is activated by an increased intracellular concentration of tryptophan to prevent transcription. At the protein synthesis level, rapid translation of a "test peptide" at the beginning of the mRNA in the presence of tryptophan allows the formation of a double-stranded loop in the RNA, which terminates transcription. The same loop is formed if no protein synthesis is occurring, a situation in which tryptophan synthesis would similarly not be required. This regulates tryptophan synthesis at the mRNA level in a process termed attenuation, in which mRNA synthesis is prematurely terminated.

The expression of the components of virulence mechanisms are also coordinately regulated from an operon. Simple triggers, such as temperature, osmolarity, pH, nutrient availability, or the concentration of specific small molecules, such as oxygen or iron, can turn on or turn off the transcription of a single gene or a group of genes. *Salmonella* invasion genes within a pathogenicity island are turned on by high osmolarity and low oxygen, conditions present in the gastrointestinal tract or an endosomal vesicle within a macrophage. *E. coli* senses its exit from the gut of a host by a drop in temperature and inactivates its adherence genes. Low iron levels can activate expression of hemolysin in *E. coli* or diphtheria toxin from *Corynebacterium diphtheriae*, potentially to kill cells

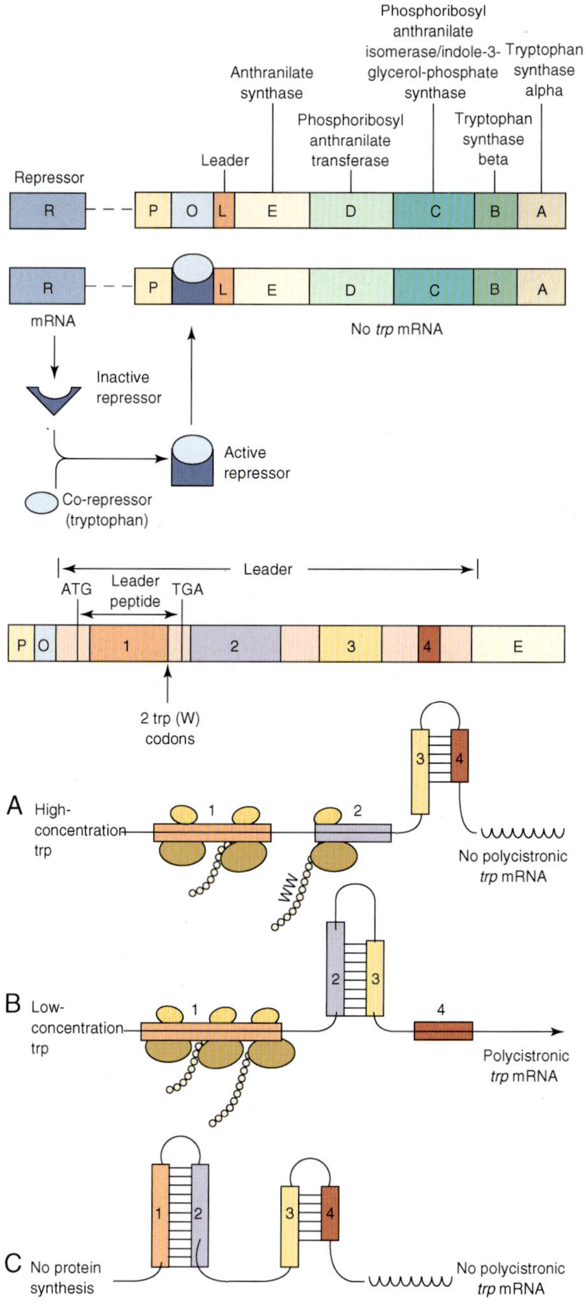

Figure 3-8 Regulation of the tryptophan (*trp*) operon. **A,** The *trp* operon encodes the five enzymes necessary for tryptophan biosynthesis. This *trp* operon is under dual control. **B,** The conformation of the inactive repressor protein is changed after its binding by the co-repressor tryptophan. The resulting active repressor (*R*) binds to the operator (*O*), blocking any transcription of the *trp* mRNA by the RNA polymerase. **C,** The *trp* operon is also under the control of an attenuation-antitermination mechanism. Upstream of the structural genes are the promoter (*P*), the operator, and a leader (*L*), which can be transcribed into a short peptide containing two tryptophans (*W*), near its distal end. The leader mRNA possesses four repeats (1, 2, 3, and 4), which can pair differently according to the tryptophan availability, leading to an early termination of transcription of the *trp* operon or its full transcription. In the presence of a high concentration of tryptophan, regions 3 and 4 of the leader mRNA can pair, forming a terminator hairpin, and no transcription of the *trp* operon occurs. However, in the presence of little or no tryptophan the ribosomes stall in region 1 when translating the leader peptide because of the tandem of tryptophan codons. Then regions 2 and 3 can pair, forming the antiterminator hairpin and leading to transcription of the *trp* genes. Finally, the regions 1:2 and 3:4 of the free leader mRNA can pair, also leading to cessation of transcription before the first structural gene *trpE*. *A*, Adenine; *G*, guanine; *T*, thymidine.

and provide iron. Quorum sensing for virulence factors of *S. aureus* and biofilm production by *Pseudomonas* spp. were discussed above. An example of coordinated control of virulence genes for *S. aureus* based on the growth rate, availability of metabolites, and the presence of a quorum is presented in Figure 3-9.

Replication of DNA

Replication of the bacterial genome is triggered by a cascade of events linked to the growth rate of the cell. Replication of bacterial DNA is initiated at a specific sequence in the chromosome called *oriC*. The replication process requires many enzymes, including an enzyme (helicase) to unwind the DNA at the origin to expose the DNA, an enzyme (primase) to synthesize primers to start the process, and the enzyme or enzymes (DNA-dependent DNA polymerases) that synthesize a copy of the DNA, but only if there is a primer sequence to add onto and only in the 5′ to 3′ direction.

New DNA is synthesized semiconservatively, using both strands of the parental DNA as templates. New DNA synthesis occurs at growing forks and proceeds bidirectionally. One strand (the leading strand) is copied continuously in the 5′ to 3′ direction, whereas the other strand (the lagging strand) must be synthesized as many pieces of DNA using RNA primers (Okazaki fragments). The lagging-strand DNA must be extended in the 5′ to 3′ direction as its template becomes available. Then the pieces are ligated together by the enzyme DNA ligase. To maintain the high degree of accuracy required for replication, the DNA polymerases possess "proofreading" functions, which allow the enzyme to confirm that the appropriate nucleotide was inserted and to correct any errors that were made. During log-phase growth in rich medium, many initiations of chromosomal replication may occur before cell division. This process produces a series of nested bubbles of new daughter chromosomes, each with its pair of growth forks of new DNA synthesis. The polymerase moves down the DNA strand, incorporating the appropriate (complementary) nucleotide at each position. Replication is complete when the two replication forks meet 180 degrees from the origin. The process of DNA replication puts great torsional strain on the chromosomal circle of DNA; this strain is relieved by topoisomerases (e.g., gyrase), which supercoil the DNA. Topoisomerases are essential to the bacteria and are targets for the quinolone antibiotics.

Population Dynamics

When bacteria are added to a new medium, they require time to adapt to the new environment before they begin dividing (Figure 3-10). This hiatus is known as the lag phase of growth. During the logarithmic (log) or exponential phase, the bacteria will grow and divide with a doubling time characteristic of the strain and determined by the conditions. The number of bacteria will increase to 2^n, in which n is the number of generations (doublings). The culture eventually runs out of metabolites, or a toxic substance builds up in the medium; the cell growth slows to a stop (stationary phase) and eventually enters decline phase (death).

BACTERIAL GENETICS

Mutation, Repair, and Recombination

Accurate replication of DNA is important to the survival of the bacteria, but mistakes and accidental damage to the DNA occurs. The bacteria have efficient DNA repair systems, but mutations and alterations to the DNA still occur. Most of these mutations have little effect on the bacteria or are detrimental, but some mutations may provide a selective advantage for survival of the bacteria when challenged by the environment, the host, or therapy.

Mutations and Their Consequences

A mutation is any change in the base sequence of the DNA. A single base change can result in a transition in which one purine is replaced by another purine, or in which a pyrimidine is replaced by another pyrimidine. A transversion, in which, for example, a purine is replaced by a pyrimidine and vice versa, may also result. A silent mutation is a change at the DNA level that does not result in any change

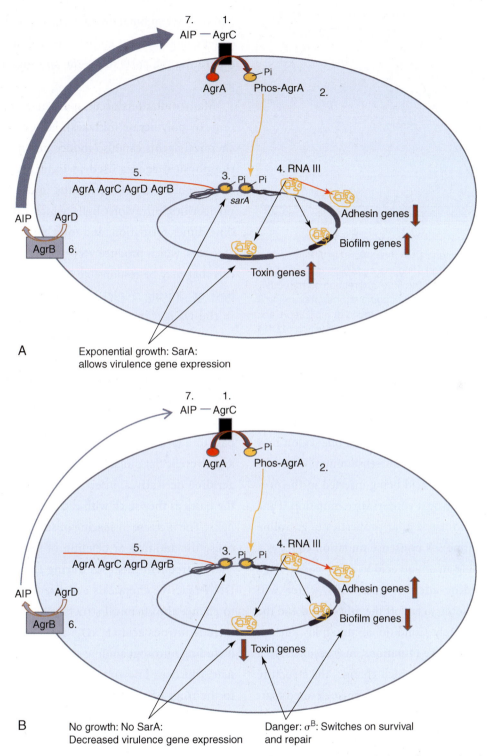

Figure 3-9   Control of virulence genes in *Staphylococcus aureus*. *S. aureus* switches on virulence factors when in exponential growth and when their numbers increase to a quorum. Toxin and protease are produced to kill host cells and supply the colony with food, and the colony produces a biofilm for protection. Cell wall thickness and adhesion factors are less important within the colony and are repressed. Quorum sensing is mediated and autoinduced by the **Agr (A-D)** proteins. **A,** *1.* The autoinducing peptide **(AIP)** binds to AgrC. *2,* **AgrC** is a receptor that phosphorylates **AgrA**. *3,* **Phosphorylated AgrA** activates the promoter for the *agr* operon and the promoter for a regulatory RNA called **RNA III**. *4,* RNA III contains the 26-amino acid δ-hemolysin RNA sequence. In addition, RNA III activates toxin and other virulence genes while decreasing expression of adhesion and cell wall synthesis genes. *5,* **AgrD** interacts with **AgrB,** in the membrane, to be converted into the AIP. As long as the bacteria are in exponential phase growth, they produce **SarA,** which also binds and activates the promoters for the *agr* and *RNA III* genes. **B,** Upon metabolic problems and danger, SarA production is decreased and a new sigma factor, σ^B is produced to decrease production of these virulence factors and σ^B turns on DNA and cellular repair mechanisms. *Large red arrows* indicate increases or decreases in expression.

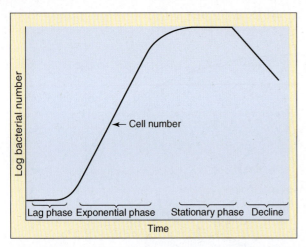

Figure 3-10 Bacterial DNA replication. New DNA synthesis occurs at growing forks and proceeds bidirectionally. DNA synthesis progresses in the 5′ to 3′ direction continuously (leading strand) or in pieces (lagging strand). Assuming it takes 40 minutes to complete one round of replication, and assuming new initiation every 20 minutes, initiation of DNA synthesis precedes cell division. Multiple growing forks may be initiated in a cell before complete septum formation and cell division. The daughter cells are "born pregnant".

of amino acid in the encoded protein. This type of mutation occurs because more than one codon may encode an amino acid. A missense mutation results in a different amino acid being inserted in the protein, but this may be a conservative mutation if the new amino acid has similar properties (e.g., valine replacing alanine). A nonsense mutation changes a codon encoding an amino acid to a stop codon (e.g., TAG [thymidine-adenine-guanine]), which will cause the ribosome to fall off the mRNA and end the protein prematurely. Conditional mutations, such as temperature-sensitive mutations, may result from a conservative mutation which changes the structure or function of an important protein at elevated temperatures.

More drastic changes can occur when numerous bases are involved. A small deletion or insertion that *is not in multiples of three* produces a frameshift mutation. This results in a change in the reading frame, usually leading to a useless peptide and premature truncation of the protein. Null mutations, which completely destroy gene function, arise when there is an extensive insertion, deletion, or gross rearrangement of the chromosome structure. Insertion of long sequences of DNA (many thousands of base

pairs) by recombination, by transposition, or during genetic engineering can produce null mutations by separating the parts of a gene and inactivating the gene.

Many mutations occur spontaneously in nature (e.g., by polymerase mistakes); however, physical or chemical agents can also induce mutations. Among the physical agents used to induce mutations in bacteria are heat, which results in deamination of nucleotides; ultraviolet light, which causes pyrimidine dimer formation; and ionizing radiation, such as x-rays, which produce very reactive hydroxyl radicals that may be responsible for opening a ring of a base or causing single- or double-stranded breaks in the DNA. Chemical mutagens can be grouped into three classes. Nucleotide-base analogues lead to mispairing and frequent DNA replication mistakes. For example, incorporation of 5-bromouracil into DNA instead of thymidine allows base pairing with guanine instead of adenine, changing a T-A base pair to a G-C base pair. Frameshift mutagens, such as polycyclic flat molecules like ethidium bromide or acridine derivatives, insert (or intercalate) between the bases as they stack with each other in the double helix. The increase in spacing of successive base pairs cause the addition or deletion of a single base and lead to frequent mistakes during DNA replication. DNA-reactive chemicals act directly on the DNA to change the chemical structure of the base. These include nitrous acid (HNO_2) and alkylating agents, including nitrosoguanidine and ethyl methane sulfonate, which are known to add methyl or ethyl groups to the rings of the DNA bases. The modified bases may pair abnormally or not at all. The damage may also cause the removal of the base from the DNA backbone.

Repair Mechanisms of DNA

A number of repair mechanisms have evolved in bacterial cells to minimize damage to DNA. These repair mechanisms can be divided into the following five groups:

Direct DNA repair is the enzymatic removal of damage, such as pyrimidine dimers and alkylated bases.

Excision repair is the removal of a DNA segment containing the damage, followed by synthesis of a new DNA strand. Two types of excision-repair mechanisms, generalized and specialized, exist.

Recombinational or postreplication repair is the retrieval of missing information by genetic recombination when both DNA strands are damaged.

The SOS response is the induction of many genes (approximately 15) after DNA damage or interruption of DNA replication.

Error-prone repair is the last resort of a bacterial cell before it dies. It is used to fill in gaps with a random sequence when a DNA template is not available for directing an accurate repair.

Gene Exchange in Prokaryotic Cells

Many bacteria, especially many pathogenic bacterial species, are promiscuous with their DNA. The exchange of DNA between cells allows the exchange of genes and characteristics between cells, thus producing new strains of bacteria. This exchange may be advantageous for the recipient, especially if the exchanged DNA encodes antibiotic resistance. The transferred DNA can be integrated into the recipient chromosome or stably maintained as an extrachromosomal element (plasmid) or a bacterial virus (bacteriophage) and passed on to daughter bacteria as an autonomously replicating unit.

Plasmids are small genetic elements that replicate independently of the bacterial chromosome. Most plasmids are circular, double-stranded DNA molecules varying from 1500 to 400,000 base pairs. However, *Borrelia burgdorferi*, the causative agent of Lyme disease, and the related *Borrelia hermsii* are unique among all eubacteria because they possess linear plasmids. Like the bacterial chromosomal DNA, plasmids can autonomously replicate and, as such, are referred to as replicons. Some plasmids, such as the *E. coli* F plasmid, are episomes, which means that they can integrate into the host chromosome.

Plasmids carry genetic information, which may not be essential but can provide a selective advantage to the bacteria. For example, plasmids may encode the production of antibiotic resistance mechanisms, bacteriocins, toxins, virulence determinants, and other genes that may provide the bacteria with a unique growth advantage over other microbes or within the host. The number of copies of plasmid produced by a cell is determined by the particular plasmid. The copy number is the ratio of copies of the plasmid to the number of copies of the chromosome. This may be as few as one in the case of large plasmids or as many as 50 in smaller plasmids.

Large plasmids (20 to 120 kb), such as the fertility factor F found in *E. coli* or the resistance transfer factor (80 kb), can often mediate their own transfer from one cell to another by a process called conjugation (see the section on conjugation later in this chapter). These conjugative plasmids encode all the necessary factors for their transfer. Other plasmids can be transferred into a bacterial cell by means other than conjugation, such as transformation or transduction. These terms are also discussed later in the chapter.

Bacteriophages are bacterial viruses with a DNA or RNA genome usually protected by a protein shell. These extrachromosomal genetic elements can survive outside of a host cell and be transmitted from one cell to another. Bacteriophages infect bacterial cells and either replicate to large numbers and cause the cell to lyse (lytic infection) or, in some cases, integrate into the host genome without killing the host (the lysogenic state), such as the *E. coli* bacteriophage lambda. Some lysogenic bacteriophages carry toxin genes (e.g., corynephage beta carries the gene for the diphtheria toxin). Bacteriophage lambda remains lysogenic as long as a repressor protein is synthesized and prevents the phage genome from becoming unintegrated in order to replicate and exit the cell. Damage to the host cell DNA by radiation or by another means or inability to produce the repressor protein is a signal that the host cell is unhealthy and is no longer a good place for "freeloading."

Transposons (jumping genes) are mobile genetic elements (Figure 3-11) that can transfer DNA within a cell, from one position to another in the genome, or between different molecules of DNA (e.g., plasmid to plasmid or plasmid to chromosome). Transposons are present in prokaryotes and eukaryotes. The sim-

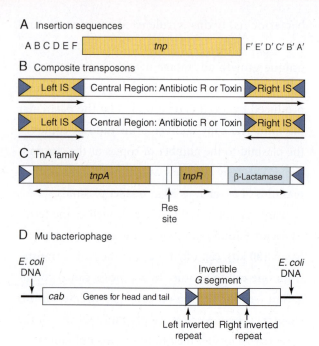

A Insertion sequences

A B C D E F   *tnp*   F' E' D' C' B' A'

B Composite transposons

Left IS◁ Central Region: Antibiotic R or Toxin ▷Right IS◁

Left IS◁ Central Region: Antibiotic R or Toxin ▷Right IS◁

C TnA family

tnpA   *tnpR*   β-Lactamase

Res
site

D Mu bacteriophage

E. coli
DNA

cab   Genes for head and tail

Invertible
G segment

E. coli
DNA

Left inverted   Right inverted
repeat   repeat

Figure 3-11 Bacterial cell division. Replication requires extension of the cell wall and replication of the chromosome and septum formation. Membrane attachment of the DNA pulls each daughter strand into a new cell.

plest transposons are called *insertion sequences* and range in length from 150 to 1500 base pairs, with inverted repeats of 15 to 40 base pairs at their ends and the minimal genetic information necessary for their own transfer (i.e., the gene coding for the transposase). Complex transposons carry other genes, such as genes that provide resistance against antibiotics. Transposons sometimes insert into genes and inactivate those genes. If insertion and inactivation occur in a gene that encodes an essential protein, the cell dies.

Some pathogenic bacteria use a transposon-like mechanism to coordinate the expression of a system of virulence factors. The genes for the activity may be grouped together in a pathogenicity or virulence island, which is surrounded by transposon-like mobile elements, allowing them to move within the chromosome and to other bacteria. The entire genetic unit can be triggered by an environmental stimulus (e.g., pH, heat, contact with the host cell surface) as a way to coordinate the expression of a complex process. For example, the SPI-1 island of *Salmonella* encodes 25 genes for a type III secretion device that allow the bacteria to enter nonphagocytic cells.

Mechanisms of Genetic Transfer between Cells

The exchange of genetic material between bacterial cells may occur by one of three mechanisms (Figure 3-12): (1) conjugation, which is the mating or quasisexual exchange of genetic information from one bacterium (the donor) to another bacterium (the recipient); (2) transformation, which is an active uptake and incorporation of exogenous or foreign DNA; or (3) transduction, which is the transfer of genetic information from one bacterium to another by a bacteriophage. Once inside a cell, a transposon can jump between different DNA molecules (e.g., plasmid to plasmid or plasmid to chromosome).

Transformation

Transformation is the process by which bacteria take up fragments of naked DNA and incorporate them into their genomes. Transformation was the first mechanism of genetic transfer to be discovered in bacteria. In 1928, Griffith observed that pneumococcus virulence was related to the presence of a polysaccharide capsule and that extracts of encapsulated bacteria producing smooth colonies could transmit this trait to nonencapsulated bacteria, normally appearing with rough edges. Griffith's studies led to Avery, MacLeod, and McCarty's identification of DNA as the transforming principle some 15 years later.

Gram-positive and gram-negative bacteria can take up and stably maintain exogenous DNA. Certain species are naturally capable of taking up exogenous DNA (such species are then said to be competent), including *Haemophilus influenzae*, *Streptococcus pneumoniae*, *Bacillus* species, and *Neisseria* species. Competence develops toward the end of logarithmic growth. *E. coli* and most other bacteria lack the natural ability for DNA uptake, and competence must be induced or chemical methods or electroporation (the use of high-voltage pulses), used to facilitate uptake of plasmid and other DNA.

Conjugation

Conjugation results in one-way transfer of DNA from a donor (or male) cell to a recipient (or female)

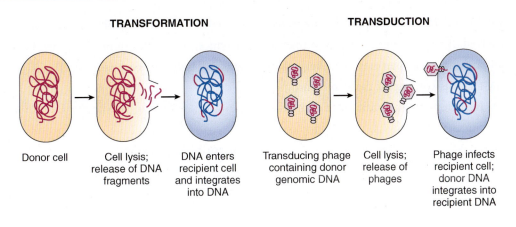

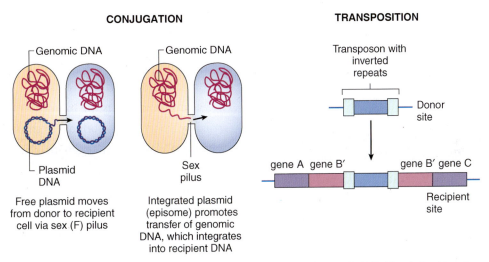

Figure 3-12   Mechanisms of bacterial gene transfer. (From Rosenthal KS, Tan J: *Rapid reviews microbiology and immunology*, St Louis, 2002, Mosby.)

cell through the sex pilus. Conjugation occurs with most, if not all, eubacteria, usually between members of the same or related species, but it has also been demonstrated to occur between prokaryotes and cells from plants, animals, and fungi. Many of the large conjugative plasmids specify colicins or antibiotic resistance.

The mating type (sex) of the cell depends on the presence (male) or absence (female) of a conjugative plasmid, such as the F plasmid of *E. coli*. The F plasmid is defined as conjugative because it carries all the genes necessary for its own transfer, including the ability to make sex pili and to initiate DNA synthesis at the transfer origin *(oriT)* of the plasmid. The sex pili is a specialized type IV secretion device. Upon transfer of the F plasmid, the recipients become F⁺ male cells. If a fragment of chromosomal DNA has been incorporated into the plasmid, it is designated an

F prime (F′) plasmid. When it transfers into the recipient cell, it carries that fragment with it and converts it into an F′ male. If the F plasmid sequence is integrated into the bacterial chromosome, the cell is designated an Hfr (high-frequency recombination) cell.

The DNA that is transferred by conjugation is not a double helix but a single-stranded molecule. Mobilization begins when a plasmid-encoded protein makes a single-stranded, site-specific cleavage at the oriT. The nick initiates rolling circle replication, and the displaced linear strand is directed to the recipient cell. The transferred single-stranded DNA is recircularized and its complementary strand synthesized. Conjugation results in transfer of a part of the plasmid sequence and some portion of the bacterial chromosomal DNA. Because of the fragile connection between the mating pairs, the transfer is usually aborted before being completed such that only the chromosomal sequences adjacent to the integrated F are transferred. Artificial interruption of a mating between an Hfr and an F⁻ pair has been helpful in constructing a consistent map of the *E. coli* chromosomal DNA. In such maps, the position of each gene is given in minutes (based on 100 minutes for complete transfer at 37°C), according to its time of entry into a recipient cell in relation to a fixed origin.

Transduction

Genetic transfer by transduction is mediated by bacterial viruses (bacteriophages), which pick up fragments of DNA and package them into bacteriophage particles. The DNA is delivered to infected cells and becomes incorporated into the bacterial genomes. Transduction can be classified as specialized if the phages in question transfer particular genes (usually those adjacent to their integration sites in the genome) or generalized if incorporation of DNA sequences is random because of accidental packaging of host DNA into the phage capsid. For example, a nuclease from the P1 phage degrades the host *E. coli* chromosomal DNA, and some of the DNA fragments are packaged into phage particles. The encapsulated DNA, instead of phage DNA, is injected into a new host cell, where it can recombine with the homologous host DNA. Generalized transducing particles are valuable in the genetic mapping of bacterial chromosomes. The closer two genes are within the bacterial chromosome, the more likely it is that they will be co-transduced in the same fragment of DNA.

Recombination

Incorporation of extrachromosomal (foreign) DNA into the chromosome occurs by recombination. There are two types of recombination: homologous and nonhomologous. Homologous (legitimate) recombination occurs between closely related DNA sequences and generally substitutes one sequence for another. The process requires a set of enzymes produced (in *E. coli*) by the *rec* genes. Nonhomologous (illegitimate) recombination occurs between dissimilar DNA sequences and generally produces insertions or deletions or both. This process usually requires specialized (sometimes site-specific) recombination enzymes, such as those produced by many transposons and lysogenic bacteriophages.

SUMMARY

Bacterial Metabolism

The minimum requirements for growth are a source of carbon and nitrogen, an energy source, water, and various ions. Bacteria can produce energy from glucose by fermentation, anaerobic respiration, or aerobic respiration. The phases of bacterial growth include lag phase, logarithmic phase, stationary phase and decline phase.

Bacterial Genes and Expression

The bacterial genome is the total collection of genes carried by a bacterium, both on its chromosome and on its extra chromosomal genetic elements including plasmids, transposons and bacteriophages. The information carried in the DNA is transcribed into mRNA for subsequent translation into protein. Bacteria have developed mechanisms to coordinate and regulate the expression of genes for multicomponent structures or the enzymes of one or more metabolic pathways.

Bacterial Genetics

The bacteria have efficient DNA repair systems, but mutations and alterations to the DNA still occur. The exchange of genetic material between bacterial cells may occur by conjugation, transformation or transduction.

In transformation, a competent recipient prokaryote takes up DNA from its environment. Competency is found naturally or can be created artificially in some cells.

In transduction, a virus such as a bacteriophage, or phage, carries DNA from a donor cell to a recipient cell. Donor DNA is accidentally incorporated in such transducing phages.

In conjugation, the two bacterial cells mating with each other, which lead to DNA transfer from the donor to the recipient. The mating process is controlled by an F (fertility) plasmid.

KEYWORDS

English	Chinese
Metabolism	新陈代谢
Obligate anaerobes	专性厌氧菌
Obligate aerobes	专性需氧菌
Facultative anaerobes	兼性厌氧菌
Catabolism	分解代谢
Anabolism	合成代谢
Tricarboxylic Acid Cycle	三羧酸循环
Pentose Phosphate Pathway	戊糖磷酸途径
Operons	操纵子
Cistrons	顺反子
Anticodon	反密码子
Sigma factor	转录起始因子
Plasmid	质粒
Bacteriophage	噬菌体
Mutation	突变
Transposon	转座子
Transformation	转化
Transduction	转导
Conjugation	接合

BIBLIOGRAPHY

1. Alberts B: Molecular biology of the cell, ed 4, New York, 2002, Garland Science.

2. Berg JM, Tymoczko JL, Stryer L: Biochemistry, ed 6, New York, 2006, WH Freeman.

3. Cotter PA, Miller JF: In vivo and ex vivo regulation of bacterial virulence gene expression, Curr Opin Microbiol 1: 17-26, 1998.

4. Lewin B: Genes IX, Sudbury, Mass, 2007, Jones and Bartlett.

5. Lodish H, et al: Molecular cell biology, ed 6, New York, 2007, WH Freeman.

6. Nelson DL, Cox M: Lehninger principles of biochemistry, ed 4, New York, 2004, Worth.

7. Novick RP, Geisinger E: Quorum sensing in staphylococci, Ann Rev Genet 42: 541-546, 2008.

8. Patel SS, Rosenthal KS: Microbial adaptation: putting the best team on the field, Infect Dis Clin Pract 15: 330-334, 2007.

9. Watson JD, et al: Molecular biology of the gene, ed 4, Menlo Park, Calif, 1987, Benjamin-Cummings.

10. Weigel LM, et al: Genetic analysis of a high-level vanco-mycin-resistant isolate of *Staphylococcus aureus*, Science 302: 1569-1571, 2003.

Commensal and Pathogenic Microbial Flora in Humans

Although the primary interest of medical microbiology is in diseases caused by microbes, it must also be appreciated that microorganisms play a critical role in human survival. The normal commensal population of microbes participates in the metabolism of food products, provides essential growth factors, protects against infections with highly virulent microorganisms, and stimulates the immune response. In the absence of these organisms, life as we know it would be impossible.

The microbial flora in and on the human body is in a continual state of flux determined by a variety of factors, such as age, diet, hormonal state, health, and personal hygiene. Whereas the human fetus lives in a protected, sterile environment, the newborn human is exposed to microbes from the mother and the environment. The infant's skin is colonized first, followed by the oropharynx, gastrointestinal tract, and other mucosal surfaces. Throughout the life of a human being, this microbial population continues to change. Changes in health can drastically disrupt the delicate balance that is maintained among the heterogeneous organisms coexisting within us. For example, hospitalization can lead to the replacement of normally avirulent organisms in the oropharynx with gram-negative rods (e.g., *Klebsiella*, *Pseudomonas*) that can invade the lungs and cause pneumonia. Likewise, the indigenous bacteria present in the intestines restrict the growth of *Clostridium difficile* in the gastrointestinal tract. In the presence of antibiotics, however, this indigenous flora is eliminated, and *C. difficile* is able to proliferate and produce diarrheal disease and colitis.

Exposure of an individual to an organism can lead to one of three outcomes. The organism can (1) transiently colonize the person, (2) permanently colonize the person, or (3) produce disease. It is important to understand the distinction between **colonization** and **disease**. (Note: Many people use the term *infection* inappropriately as a synonym for both terms.) Organisms that colonize humans (whether for a short period, such as hours or days [transient], or permanently) do not interfere with normal body functions. In contrast, disease occurs when the interaction between microbe and human leads to a pathologic process characterized by damage to the human host. This process can result from microbial factors (e.g., damage to organs caused by the proliferation of the microbe or the production of toxins or cytotoxic enzymes) or the host's immune response to the organism (e.g., the pathology of severe acute respiratory syndrome [SARS] coronavirus infections is primarily caused by the patient's immune response to the virus).

An understanding of medical microbiology requires knowledge not only of the different classes of microbes but also of their propensity for causing disease. A few infections are caused by **strict pathogens** (i.e., organisms always associated with human disease). A few examples of strict pathogens and the diseases they cause include *Mycobacterium tuberculosis* (tuberculosis), *Neisseria gonorrhoeae* (gonorrhea), *Clostridium tetani* (tetani), *Bacillus anthracis* (anthrax), and rabies virus (rabies). Most human infections are caused by **opportunistic pathogens**, organisms that are typically members of the patient's normal microbial flora (e.g., *Staphylococcus aureus*, *Escherichia coli*, *Candida albicans*). These organisms do not produce disease in their normal setting but establish disease when they are introduced into unprotected sites (e.g., blood, tissues). The specific factors responsible for the virulence of strict and opportunistic pathogens are discussed in later chapters. If a patient's immune system is defective, that patient is more susceptible to disease caused by opportunistic pathogens.

The microbial population that colonizes the human body is numerous and diverse (Table 4-1). Our knowledge of the composition of this population is currently based on comprehensive culture methods; however, it is estimated that only a small proportion of the microbes can be cultivated. To better understand the microbial population, a large scale project called the **Human Microbiome Project (HMP)** has been initiated to characterize comprehensively the human microbiota and analyze its role in human health and disease. The skin and all mucosal surfaces of the human body are currently being analyzed systematically by genomic techniques. The initial phase of this study was completed in 2012, and it is apparent that the human microbiome is complex, composed of many organisms not previously recognized, and undergoes dynamic changes in disease. For the most current information about this study, please refer to the HMP website: http://nihroadmap.nih.gov/hmp/. For this edition of *Medical Microbiology*, the information discussed in this chapter will be based on data collected from systematic cultures, with the understanding that much of what we currently know may be very different from what we will learn in the next 5 years.

UPPER RESPIRATORY TRACT

The upper respiratory tract is colonized with numerous organisms, with 10 to 100 anaerobes for every aerobic bacterium. The most common anaerobic bacteria are *Peptostreptococcus* and related anaerobic cocci, *Veillonella*, *Actinomyces*, and *Fusobacterium* spp. The most common aerobic bacteria are *Streptococcus*, *Haemophilus*, and *Neisseria* spp. The relative proportion of these organisms varies at different anatomic sites; for example, the microbial flora on the surface of a tooth is quite different from the flora in saliva or in the subgingival spaces. Most of the common organisms in the upper respiratory tract are relatively avirulent and are rarely associated with disease unless they are introduced into normally sterile sites (e.g., sinuses, middle ear, brain). Potentially pathogenic organisms, including *Streptococcus pyogenes*, *Streptococcus pneumoniae*, *S. aureus*, *Neisseria meningitidis*, *Haemophilus influenzae*, *Moraxella catarrhalis*, and Enterobacteriaceae, can also be found in the upper airways. Isolation of these organisms from an upper respiratory tract specimen does not

Table 4-1   Most Common Microbes That Colonize the Human Body

Location	Main bacterial flora	Fungi
Upper Respiratory Tract	*Acinetobacter, Actinobacillus, Actinomyces, Cardiobacterium, Corynebacterium, Eikenella,* Enterobacteriaceae, *Eubacterium, Fusobacterium, Haemophilus, Kingella, Moraxella, Mycoplasma, Neisseria, Peptostreptococcus, Porphyromonas, Prevotella, Propionibacterium, Staphylococcus, Streptococcus, Stomatococcus, Treponema, Veillonella*	*Candida*
Gastrointestinal Tract and Rectum	*Acinetobacter, Actinomyces, Bacteroides, Bifidobacterium, Campylobacter, Clostridium, Corynebacterium,* Enterobacteriaceae, *Enterococcus, Eubacterium, Fusobacterium, Haemophilus, Helicobacter, Lactobacillus, Mobiluncus, Peptostreptococcus, Porphyromonas, Prevotella, Propionibacterium, Pseudomonas, Staphylococcus, Streptococcus, Veillonella*	*Candida*
Genitourinary Tract	*Actinomyces, Bacteroides, Bifidobacterium, Clostridium, Corynebacterium,* Enterobacteriaceae, *Enterococcus, Eubacterium, Fusobacterium, Gardnerella, Haemophilus, Lactobacillus, Mobiluncus, Mycoplasma, Peptostreptococcus, Porphyromonas, Prevotella, Propionibacterium, Staphylococcus, Streptococcus, Treponema, Ureaplasma*	*Candida*
Skin	*Acinetobacter, Aerococcus, Bacillus, Clostridium, Corynebacterium, Micrococcus, Peptostreptococcus, Propionibacterium, Staphylococcus, Streptococcus*	*Candida, Malassezia*

define their pathogenicity (remember the concept of colonization versus disease). Their involvement with a disease process must be demonstrated by the exclusion of other pathogens. For example, with the exception of *S. pyogenes*, these organisms are rarely responsible for pharyngitis, even though they can be isolated from patients with this disease. *S. pneumoniae*, *S. aureus*, *H. influenzae*, and *M. catarrhalis* are organisms commonly associated with infections of the sinuses.

Ear

The most common organism colonizing the outer ear is coagulase-negative *Staphylococcus*. Other organisms colonizing the skin have been isolated from this site, as well as potential pathogens such as *S. pneumoniae*, *Pseudomonas aeruginosa*, and members of the Enterobacteriaceae family.

Eye

The surface of the eye is colonized with coagulase-negative staphylococci, as well as rare numbers of organisms found in the nasopharynx (e.g., *Haemophilus* spp., *Neisseria* spp., viridans streptococci). Disease is typically associated with *S. pneumoniae*, *S. aureus*, *H. influenzae*, *N. gonorrhoeae*, *Chlamydia trachomatis*, *P. aeruginosa*, and *Bacillus cereus*.

Lower Respiratory Tract

The larynx, trachea, bronchioles, and lower airways are generally sterile, although transient colonization with secretions of the upper respiratory tract may occur. More virulent bacteria present in the mouth (e.g., *S. pneumoniae*, *S. aureus*, members of the family Enterobacteriaceae such as *Klebsiella*) cause acute disease of the lower airway. Chronic aspiration may lead to a polymicrobial disease in which anaerobes are the predominant pathogens, particularly *Peptostreptococcus*, related anaerobic cocci, and anaerobic gram-negative rods. Fungi such as *C. albicans* are a rare cause of disease in the lower airway, and invasion of these organisms into tissue must be demonstrated to exclude simple colonization. In contrast, the presence of the dimorphic fungi (e.g.,

Histoplasma, *Coccidioides*, and *Blastomyces* spp.) is diagnostic, because asymptomatic colonization with these organisms never occurs.

GASTROINTESTINAL TRACT

The gastrointestinal tract is colonized with microbes at birth and remains the home for a diverse population of organisms throughout the life of the host. Although the opportunity for colonization with new organisms occurs daily with the ingestion of food and water, the population remains relatively constant, unless exogenous factors such as antibiotic treatment disrupt the balanced flora.

Esophagus

Oropharyngeal bacteria and yeast, as well as the bacteria that colonize the stomach, can be isolated from the esophagus; however, most organisms are believed to be transient colonizers that do not establish permanent residence. Bacteria rarely cause disease of the esophagus (esophagitis); *Candida* spp. and viruses, such as herpes simplex virus and cytomegalovirus, cause most infections.

Stomach

Because the stomach contains hydrochloric acid and pepsinogen (secreted by the parietal and chief cells lining the gastric mucosa), the only organisms present are small numbers of acid-tolerant bacteria, such as the lactic acid-producing bacteria (*Lactobacillus* and *Streptococcus* spp.) and *Helicobacter pylori*. *H. pylori* is a cause of gastritis and ulcerative disease. The microbial population can dramatically change in numbers and diversity in patients receiving drugs that neutralize or reduce the production of gastric acids.

Small Intestine

In contrast with the anterior portion of the digestive tract, the small intestine is colonized with many different bacteria, fungi, and parasites. Most of these organisms are anaerobes, such as *Peptostreptococcus*, *Porphyromonas*, and *Prevotella*. Common causes of gastroenteritis (e.g., *Salmonella* and *Campylobacter* spp.) can be present in small numbers as asymptomatic residents; however, their detection in the clinical laboratory generally indicates disease. If the small intestine is obstructed, such as after abdominal surgery, then a condition called blind loop syndrome can occur. In this case, stasis of the intestinal contents leads to the colonization and proliferation of the organisms typically present in the large intestine, with a subsequent malabsorption syndrome.

Large Intestine

More microbes are present in the large intestine than anywhere else in the human body. It is estimated that more than 10^{11} bacteria per gram of feces can be found, with anaerobic bacteria in excess by more than 1000-fold. Various yeasts and nonpathogenic parasites can also establish residence in the large intestine. The most common bacteria include *Bifidobacterium*, *Eubacterium*, *Bacteroides*, *Enterococcus*, and the Enterobacteriaceae family. *E. coli* is present in virtually all humans from birth until death. Although this organism represents less than 1% of the intestinal population, it is the most common aerobic organism responsible for intraabdominal disease. Likewise, *Bacteroides fragilis* is a minor member of the intestinal flora, but it is the most common anaerobe responsible for intraabdominal disease. In contrast, *Eubacterium* and *Bifidobacterium* are the most common bacteria in the large intestine but are rarely responsible for disease. These organisms simply lack the diverse virulence factors found in *B. fragilis*.

Antibiotic treatment can rapidly alter the population, causing the proliferation of antibiotic-resistant organisms, such as *Enterococcus*, *Pseudomonas*, and fungi. *C. difficile* can also grow rapidly in this situation, leading to diseases ranging from diarrhea to pseudomembranous colitis. Exposure to other enteric pathogens, such as *Shigella*, enterohemorrhagic *E. coli*, and *Entamoeba histolytica*, can also disrupt the colonic flora and produce significant intestinal disease.

Anterior Urethra

The commensal population of the urethra consists of a variety of organisms, with lactobacilli, streptococci, and coagulase-negative staphylococci the most numerous. These organisms are relatively avirulent and are rarely associated with human disease. In contrast, the urethra can be colonized transiently with fecal organisms, such as *Enterococcus*, Enterobacteriaceae, and *Candida*—all of which can invade the urinary tract, multiply in urine, and lead to significant disease. Pathogens such as *N. gonorrhoeae* and *C. trachomatis* are common causes of urethritis and can persist as asymptomatic colonizers of the urethra. The isolation of these two organisms in clinical specimens should always be considered significant, regardless of the presence or absence of clinical symptoms.

Vagina

The microbial population of the vagina is more diverse and is dramatically influenced by hormonal factors. Newborn girls are colonized with lactobacilli at birth, and these bacteria predominate for approximately 6 weeks. After that time, the levels of maternal estrogen have declined, and the vaginal flora changes to include staphylococci, streptococci, and Enterobacteriaceae. When estrogen production is initiated at puberty, the microbial flora again changes. Lactobacilli reemerge as the predominant organisms, and many other organisms are also isolated, including staphylococci (*S. aureus* less commonly than the coagulase-negative species), streptococci (including group B *Streptococcus*), *Enterococcus*, *Gardnerella*, *Mycoplasma*, *Ureaplasma*, Enterobacteriaceae, and a variety of anaerobic bacteria. *N. gonorrhoeae* is a common cause of vaginitis. In the absence of this organism, significant numbers of cases develop when the balance of vaginal bacteria is disrupted, resulting in decreases in the number of lactobacilli and increases in the number of *Mobiluncus* and *Gardnerella*. *Trichomonas vaginalis*, *C. albicans*, and *Candida glabrata* are also important causes of vaginitis. Although herpes simplex virus and papillomavirus would not be considered normal flora of the genitourinary tract, these viruses can establish persistent infections.

SKIN

Although many organisms come into contact with the skin surface, this relatively hostile environment does not support the survival of most organisms. Gram-positive bacteria (e.g., coagulase-negative *Staphylococcus* and, less commonly, *S. aureus*, corynebacteria, and propionibacteria) are the most common organisms found on the skin surface. *Clostridium perfringens* is isolated on the skin of approximately 20% of healthy individuals, and the fungi *Candida* and *Malassezia* are also found on skin surfaces, particularly in moist sites. Streptococci can colonize the skin transiently, but the volatile fatty acids produced by the anaerobe propionibacteria are toxic for these organisms. Gram-negative rods with the exception of *Acinetobacter* and a few other less common genera are not commonly cultured from the human skin. It was felt that the environment was too hostile to allow survival of these organisms; however, the HMP has revealed that uncultureable gram-negative rods may be the most common organisms on the skin surface.

SUMMARY

Microbes live with their hosts in symbiotic relationships, including mutualism, in which both members benefit; parasitism, in which a parasite benefits while the host is harmed; and more rarely commensalism, in which one member benefits while the other is relatively unaffected. Any parasite that cause disease is called a pathogen.

Organisms called microbial flora live in and on the body. Some of these microbes are resident, whereas others are transient.

Opportunistic pathogens cause disease when the immune system is suppressed, when normal microbial antagonism is affected by certain changes in the body, and when a member of the microbial flora is introduced into an area of the body unusual for that microbe.

KEYWORDS

English	Chinese
Microbial flora	微生物群
Colonization	定植
Pathogens	病原菌
Opportunistic pathogens	机会致病病原
Commensal	共生

BIBLIOGRAPHY

1. Patrick R, Murray. Medical microbiology, ed 7, 2012, Saunders. US

2. Jawetz. Medical microbiology, ed 26, 2013, McGraw-Hill Medical. US

3. Murray P, Shea Y. Pocket guide to clinical microbiology, ed 3, Washington, DC, 2004, American Society for Microbiology Press.

Chapter 5

Mechanisms of Bacterial Pathogenesis

Pathogenicity is the ability of a microorganism to cause infection and disease in host. When bacteria enter into human body, not all bacteria or bacterial infections cause disease; however, some always cause disease. Bacteria can be classified into three major groups: **virulent bacteria**, **opportunistic bacteria** and **normal flora**. **Virulent bacteria** have mechanisms that promote their growth in the host at the expense of the host's tissue or organ function. **Opportunistic bacteria** take advantage of preexisting conditions, such as immunosuppression, to grow and cause serious disease. **Normal flora** bacteria cause disease if they enter normally sterile sites of the body. The ability of bacteria to cause disease is described in terms of the number of infecting bacteria, the route of entry into the body, the effects of host defense mechanisms, and intrinsic characteristics of the bacteria called virulence factors. Many virulence factors are so-called effector proteins that are injected into the host cells by special secretion machines such as the type 3 secretion system. The virulence factors of bacteria are typically proteins or other molecules that are synthesized by enzymes. These proteins are coded for by genes in chromosomal DNA, bacteriophage DNA or plasmids. The pathogenesis of bacterial infection includes initiation of the infectious process and the mechanisms that lead to the development of signs and symptoms of disease. Although many bacteria cause disease by directly destroying tissue, some release toxins, which are then disseminated by the blood to cause system-wide pathogenesis (Box 5-1). The surface structures of bacteria are powerful stimulators of host responses (acute phase: interleukin-1 [IL-1], IL-6, tumor necrosis factor-α [TNF-α]), which

can be protective but are often major contributors to the disease symptoms (e.g., sepsis). Production of disease results from the combination of damage caused by the bacteria and the consequences of the innate and immune responses to the infection (Box 5-2). The biochemical, structural, and genetic factors that play important roles in bacterial pathogenesis are introduced in this chapter and may be revisited in the organism-specific sections.

Box 5-1

Bacterial Virulence Mechanisms

Adherence
Invasion
Byproducts of growth (gas, acid)
Toxins
Degradative enzymes
Cytotoxic proteins
Endotoxin
Superantigen
Induction of excess inflammation
Evasion of phagocytic and immune clearance
Capsule
Resistance to antibiotics
Intracellular growth

Box 5-2

Bacterial Disease Production

Disease is caused by damage produced by the bacteria plus the consequences of innate and immune responses to the infection.

The signs and symptoms of a disease are determined by the function and importance of the affected tissue.

The length of the incubation period is the time required for the bacteria and/or the host response to cause sufficient damage to initiate discomfort or interfere with essential functions.

ENTRY INTO THE HUMAN BODY

For infection to become established, bacteria must first gain entry into the body (Table 5-1; Figure 5-1). Natural defense mechanisms and barriers, such as skin, mucus, ciliated epithelium, and secretions containing antibacterial substances (e.g., lysozyme, defensins) make it difficult for bacteria to gain entry into the body. However, these barriers are sometimes broken (e.g., a tear in the skin, a tumor or ulcer in the bowel), providing a portal of entry for the bacteria, or the bacteria may have the means to compromise the barrier and invade the body. On invasion, the bacteria can travel in the bloodstream to other sites in the body.

COLONIZATION, ADHESION, AND INVASION

Different bacteria colonize different parts of the body. This may be closest to the point of entry or due to the presence of optimal growth conditions at the site. Colonization of sites that are normally sterile implies the existence of a defect in a natural defense mechanism or a new portal of entry. Patients with cystic fibrosis have such defects because of the reduction in their ciliary mucoepithelial function and altered mucosal secretions; as a result, their lungs are colonized by *S. aureus* and *P. aeruginosa*. In some cases, colonization requires special structures and functions to remain at the site, survive, and obtain food.

Bacteria may use specific mechanisms to adhere to and colonize different body surfaces (Table 5-2).

If the bacteria can adhere to epithelial or endothelial cell linings of the bladder, intestine, and blood vessels, they cannot be washed away, and this adherence allows them to colonize the tissue. Although bacteria do not have mechanisms that enable them to cross intact skin, several bacteria can cross mucosal membranes and other tissue barriers to enter normally sterile sites and more susceptible tissue. These invasive bacteria either destroy the barrier or penetrate into the cells of the barrier. The effector proteins can facilitate uptake and invasion, promote the intracellular survival and replication of the bacteria, or the apoptotic death of the host cell.

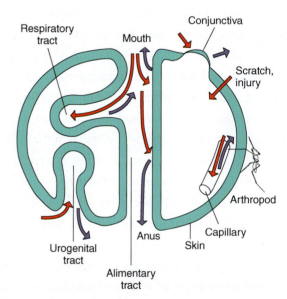

Figure 5-1 Body surfaces as sites of microbial infection and shedding. Red arrows indicate infection; purple arrows indicate shedding. (Modified from Mims C, et al: *Medical microbiology*, London, 1993, Mosby-Wolfe.)

Table 5-1 Bacterial Port of Entry

Route	Examples
Ingestion	*Salmonella* spp., *Shigella* spp., *Yersinia enterocolitica*, enterotoxigenic *Escherichia coli*, *Vibrio* spp., *Campylobacter* spp., *Clostridium botulinum*, *Bacillus cereus*, *Listeria* spp., *Brucella* spp.
Inhalation	*Mycobacterium* spp., *Nocardia* spp., *Mycoplasma pneumoniae*, *Legionella* spp., *Bordetella*, *Chlamydophila psittaci*, *Chlamydophila pneumoniae*, *Streptococcus* spp.
Trauma	*Clostridium tetani*
Needlestick	*Staphylococcus aureus*, *Pseudomonas* spp.
Arthropod bite	*Rickettsia*, *Ehrlichia*, *Coxiella*, *Francisella*, *Borrelia* spp., *Yersinia pestis*
Sexual transmission	*Neisseria gonorrhoeae*, *Chlamydia trachomatis*, *Treponema pallidum*

Table 5-2 Examples of Bacterial Adherence Mechanisms

Microbe	Adhesin	Receptor
Staphylococcus aureus	LTA	Unknown
Staphylococcus spp.	Slime	Unknown
Streptococcus, group A	LTA-M protein complex	Fibronectin
Streptococcus pneumoniae	Protein	*N*-Acetylhexosamine-galactose
Escherichia coli	Type 1 fimbriae	D-Mannose
	Colonization factor antigen fimbriae	GM ganglioside 1
	P fimbriae	P blood group glycolipid
Neisseria gonorrhoeae	Fimbriae	GD_1 ganglioside
Treponema pallidum	P_1, P_2, P_3	Fibronectin
Chlamydia trachomatis	Cell surface lectin	*N*-Acetylglucosamine
Mycoplasma pneumoniae	Protein P1	Sialic acid
Vibrio cholerae	Type 4 pili	Fucose and mannose

LTA, Lipoteichoic acid.

PATHOGENIC ACTIONS OF BACTERIA

Tissue Destruction

Byproducts of bacterial growth, especially fermentation, include acids, gas, and other substances that are toxic to tissue. In addition, *many bacteria release degradative enzymes* to break down tissue, thereby providing food for the growth of the organisms and promoting the spread of the bacteria. For example, *Clostridium perfringens* organisms are part of the normal flora of the GI tract but are also opportunistic pathogens that can establish infection in oxygen-depleted tissues and cause gas gangrene. These anaerobic bacteria produce enzymes (e.g., phospholipase C, collagenase, protease, and hyaluronidase), several toxins, and acid and gas from bacterial metabolism, which destroy the tissue. *Staphylococci* produce many different enzymes that modify the tissue environment. These enzymes include hyaluronidase, fibrinolysin, and lipases. *Streptococci* also produce enzymes, including streptolysins S and O, hyaluronidase, DNAases, and streptokinases.

Toxins

Toxins are bacterial products that directly harm tissue or trigger destructive biologic activities. Toxins and toxin-like activities are degradative enzymes that cause lysis of cells or specific receptor-binding proteins that initiate toxic reactions in a specific target tissue. In addition, endotoxin (lipid A portion of lipopolysaccharide) and superantigen proteins promote excessive or inappropriate stimulation of innate or immune responses. In many cases, the toxin is completely responsible for causing the characteristic symptoms of the disease.

Exotoxins

Exotoxins are proteins that can be produced by gram-positive or gram-negative bacteria and include cytolytic enzymes and receptor-binding proteins that alter a function or kill the cell. In many cases, the toxin gene is encoded on a plasmid (tetanus toxin of *C. tetani*, heat-labile [LT] and heat-stabile [ST] toxins of enterotoxigenic *E. coli*), or a lysogenic phage (*Corynebacterium diphtheriae* and *C. botulinum*).

Cytolytic toxins include membrane-disrupting enzymes, such as the α-toxin (phospholipase C) produced by *C. perfringens*, which breaks down sphingomyelin and other membrane phospholipids. Hemolysins insert into and disrupt erythrocyte and other cell membranes. Pore-forming toxins, including streptolysin O, can promote leakage of ions and water from the cell and disrupt cellular functions or cell lysis.

Many toxins are dimeric with A and B subunits (**A-B toxins**). The **B** portion of the A-B toxins binds to a specific cell surface receptor, and then the A subunit is transferred into the interior of the cell, where it acts to promote cell injury (B for binding, A for action). The tissues targeted by these toxins are very defined and limited (Figure 5-2; Table 5-3). **Superantigens** are a special group of toxins (Figure 5-3). These molecules activate T cells by binding simultaneously to a T-cell receptor and a major histocom-

Table 5-3 Properties of A-B-Type Bacterial Toxins

Toxin	Organism	Gene Location	Subunit Structure	Target Cell Receptor	Biologic Effects
Anthrax toxins	*Bacillus anthracis*	Plasmid	Three separate proteins (EF, LF, PA)	Tumor endothelial marker-8 (TEM-8); capillary morphogenesis protein 2 (CMG2)	EF + PA: increase in target cell cAMP level, localized edema; LF + PA: death of target cells and experimental animals
Bordetella	*Bordetella* spp.	Chromosomal	A-B	Unknown, probably glycolipid	Adenylate cyclase toxin. Increase in target cell cAMP level, modified cell function, or cell death
Botulinum toxin	*Clostridium botulinum*	Phage	A-B	Polysialogangliosides plus synaptotagmin (co-receptors)	Decrease in peripheral presynaptic acetylcholine release, flaccid paralysis
Cholera toxin	*Vibrio cholerae*	Chromosomal	A-B$_5$	Ganglioside (GM$_1$)	Activation of adenylate cyclase, increase in cAMP level, secretory diarrhea
Diphtheria toxin	*Corynebacterium diphtheriae*	Phage	A-B	Growth factor receptor precursor	Inhibition of protein synthesis, cell death
Heat-labile enterotoxins	*Escherichia coli*	Plasmid	Similar or identical to cholera toxin		
Pertussis toxin	*Bordetella pertussis*	Chromosomal	A-B$_5$	Surface glycoproteins with terminal sialic acid residues	Block of signal transduction mediated by target G proteins
Pseudomonas exotoxin A	*Pseudomonas aeruginosa*	Chromosomal	A-B	α_2-Macroglobulin receptor (α_2-MR)	Similar or identical to diphtheria toxin
Shiga toxin	*Shigella dysenteriae*	Chromosomal	A-B$_5$	Globotriaosylceramide (Gb3)	Inhibition of protein synthesis, cell death
Shiga-like toxins	*Shigella* spp., *E. coli*	Phage	Similar or identical to Shiga toxin		
Tetanus toxin	*Clostridium tetani*	Plasmid	A-B	Polysialogangliosides plus 15-kDa glycoprotein (co-receptors)	Decrease in neurotransmitter release from inhibitory neurons, spastic paralysis

cAMP, Cyclic adenosine monophosphate, *EF*, edema factor; *LF*, lethal factor; *PA*, protective antigen.
Modified from Mandell G, Douglas G, Bennett J: *Principles and practice of infectious disease*, ed 3, New York, 1990, Churchill Livingstone.

A **Inhibition of protein synthesis**

B **Hyperactivation**

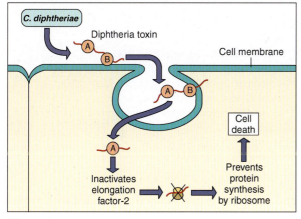

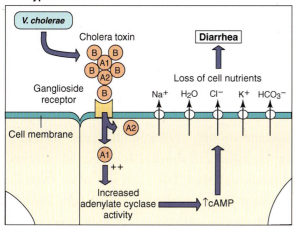

C **Effects on nerve–muscle transmission**

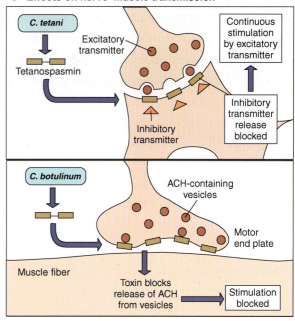

Figure 5-2   A-C, The mode of action of dimeric A-B exotoxins. The bacterial A-B toxins often consist of a two-chain molecule. The B chain binds and promotes entry of the A chain into cells, and the A chain has inhibitory activity against some vital function. *ACH,* Acetylcholine; *cAMP,* cyclic adenosine monophosphate. (Modified from Mims C, et al: *Medical microbiology,* London, 1993, Mosby-Wolfe.)

Figure 5-3   Superantigen binding to the external regions of the T-cell receptor and the major histocompatibility complex *(MHC)* class II molecules.

patibility complex class II (MHC II) molecule on an antigen-presenting cell without requiring antigen. This superantigen stimulation of T cells can also lead to death of the activated T cells, resulting in the loss of specific T-cell clones and the loss of their immune responses. Superantigens include the toxic shock syndrome toxin of *S. aureus,* staphylococcal enterotoxins, and the erythrogenic toxin A or C of *S. pyogenes.*

Endotoxin and Other Cell Wall Components

The presence of bacterial cell wall components acts as a signal of infection that provides a powerful multialarm warning to the body to activate the host's protective systems. The molecular patterns in these structures (**pathogen-associated molecular patterns [PAMPs]**) bind to Toll-like receptors (TLRs) and other molecules and stimulate the production of cytokines (see Chapters 8 and 10). In some cases, the host response is excessive and may even be life threatening. The **lipid A portion of lipopolysaccharide (LPS)** produced by gram-negative bacteria is a powerful activator of acute-phase and inflammatory reactions and is termed **endotoxin**. It is important to appreciate that endotoxin is not the same as exotoxin and that *only gram-negative bacteria make endotoxin.* Weaker, endotoxin-like responses may occur to gram-positive bacterial structures, including **teichoic** and **lipoteichoic acids**.

Gram-negative bacteria release endotoxin during infection. Endotoxin binds to specific receptors (CD14 and TLR4) on macrophages, B cells, and other cells and stimulates the production and release of **acute-phase cytokines**, such as IL-1, TNF-α, IL-6, and prostaglandins (Figure 5-4). Endotoxin also stimulates the growth (mitogenic) of B cells.

At low concentrations, endotoxin stimulates the development of protective responses, such as fever, vasodilation, and the activation of immune and inflammatory responses (Box 5-3). However, the

Box 5-3

Endotoxin-Mediated Toxicity

Fever
Leukopenia followed by leukocytosis
Activation of complement
Thrombocytopenia
Disseminated intravascular coagulation
Decreased peripheral circulation and perfusion to major organs
Shock
Death

endotoxin levels in the blood of patients with **gram-negative bacterial sepsis** (bacteria in the blood) can be very high, and the systemic response to these can be overpowering, resulting in shock and possibly death. High concentrations of endotoxin can also activate the alternative pathway of complement and production of anaphylotoxins (C3a, C5a), contributing to vasodilation and capillary leakage. In combination with TNF-α and IL-1, this can lead to **hypotension** and **shock. Disseminated intravascular coagulation (DIC)** can also result from the activation of blood coagulation pathways. The high fever, petechiae (skin lesions resulting from capillary leakage), and potential symptoms of shock (resulting from increased vascular permeability) associated with *Neisseria meningitidis* infection can be related to the large amounts of endotoxin released during infection.

IMMUNOPATHOGENESIS

In many cases, the symptoms of a bacterial infection are produced by excessive innate, immune, and inflammatory responses triggered by the infection. When limited and controlled, the acute-phase response to cell wall components is a protective antibacterial response. However, these responses also cause fever and malaise, and when systemic and out of control, the acute-phase response and inflammation can cause life-threatening symptoms associated with sepsis and meningitis (see Figure 5-4). Autoimmune responses can be triggered by bacterial proteins, such as the M protein of *S. pyogenes*, which antigenically mimics heart tissue. The anti-M protein

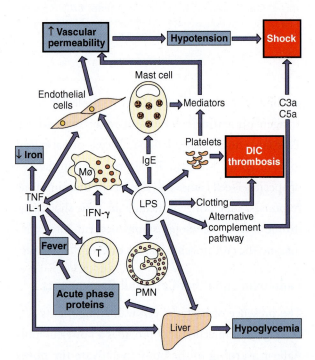

Figure 5-4   The many activities of lipopolysaccharide *(LPS)*. This bacterial endotoxin activates almost every immune mechanism, as well as the clotting pathway, which together make LPS one of the most powerful immune stimuli known. *DIC,* Disseminated intravascular coagulation; *IFN-γ,* interferon-γ; *IgE,* immunoglobulin E; *IL-1,* interleukin-1; *PMN,* polymorphonuclear (neutrophil) leukocytes; *TNF,* tumor necrosis factor. (Modified from Mims C, et al: *Medical microbiology,* London, 1993, Mosby-Wolfe.)

antibodies cross-react with and can initiate damage to the heart to cause rheumatic fever. Immune complexes deposited in the glomeruli of the kidney cause poststreptococcal glomerulonephritis. For *Chlamydia*, *Treponema* (syphilis), *Borrelia* (Lyme disease), and other bacteria, the host immune response is the principal cause of disease symptoms in patients.

MECHANISMS FOR ESCAPING HOST DEFENSES

Bacteria are parasites, and evasion of host protective responses is a selective advantage. Logically, the longer a bacterial infection remains in a host, the more time the bacteria have to grow and also cause damage. Therefore bacteria that can evade or incapacitate the host defenses have a greater potential for causing disease. Bacteria evade recognition and killing by phagocytic cells, inactivate or evade the complement system and antibody, and even grow inside cells to hide from host responses (Box 5-4).

The capsule is one of the most important virulence factors (Box 5-5). These slime layers function by shielding the bacteria from immune and phagocytic responses. The capsule also acts like a slimy football jersey, in that it is hard to grasp and tears away when grabbed by a phagocyte. The capsule also protects a bacterium from destruction within the phagolysosome of a macrophage or leukocyte. All of these properties can extend the time bacteria spend in blood (bacteremia) before being eliminated by host responses. Mutants of normally encapsulated bacteria that lose the ability to make a capsule also

---

Box 5-4

Microbial Defenses against Host Immunologic Clearance

Encapsulation
Antigenic mimicry
Antigenic masking
Antigenic shift
Production of anti-immunoglobulin proteases
Destruction of phagocyte
Inhibition of chemotaxis
Inhibition of phagocytosis
Inhibition of phagolysosome fusion
Resistance to lysosomal enzymes
Intracellular replication

Box 5-5

Examples of Encapsulated Microorganisms

Staphylococcus aureus
Streptococcus pneumoniae
Streptococcus pyogenes (group A)
Streptococcus agalactiae (group B)
Bacillus anthracis
Bacillus subtilis
Neisseria gonorrhoeae
Neisseria meningitidis
Haemophilus influenzae
Escherichia coli
Klebsiella pneumoniae
Salmonella spp.
Yersinia pestis
Campylobacter fetus
Pseudomonas aeruginosa
Bacteroides fragilis
Cryptococcus neoformans (yeast)

Box 5-6

Examples of Intracellular Pathogens

Mycobacterium spp.
Brucella spp.
Francisella spp.
Rickettsia spp.
Chlamydia spp.
Listeria monocytogenes
Salmonella typhi
Shigella dysenteriae
Yersinia pestis
Legionella pneumophila

---

lose their virulence; examples of such bacteria are *Streptococcus pneumoniae* and *N. meningitidis*. A **biofilm**, which is made from capsular material, can prevent antibody and complement from getting to the bacteria.

Bacteria can evade antibody responses by **antigenic variation**, by **inactivation of antibody** or **by intracellular growth**. *N. gonorrhoeae* can vary the structure of surface antigens to evade antibody responses and also produces a protease that degrades immunoglobulin A (IgA). *S. aureus* makes an IgG-binding protein, protein A, which prevents antibody from activating complement or being an opsonin and masks the bacteria from detection. Bacteria that grow intracellularly include mycobacteria, francisellae, brucellae, chlamydiae, and rickettsiae (Box 5-6. Bacteria evade complement action by preventing access of the components to the membrane, masking themselves, and by inhibiting activation of the cascade. The thick peptidoglycan of gram-positive bacteria and the long O antigen of LPS of most gram-negative bacteria (not *Neisseria* species) prevent the complement from gaining access and protects the bacterial membrane from being damaged. By degrading the C5a component of complement, *S. pyogenes* can limit the chemotaxis of leukocytes to the site of infection. To compensate for the lack of O antigen, *N. gonorrhoeae* attaches sialic acid to its lipooligosaccharide (LOS) to inhibit complement activation.

Phagocytes (neutrophil, macrophage) are the most important antibacterial defense, but many bacteria can circumvent phagocytic killing in various ways. They can produce enzymes capable of lysing phagocytic cells (e.g., the streptolysin produced by *S. pyogenes* or the α-toxin produced by *C. perfringens*). They can inhibit phagocytosis (e.g., the effects of the **capsule** and the **M protein** produced by *S. pyogenes)* or block intracellular killing. Bacterial mechanisms for protection from intracellular killing include blocking phagolysosome fusion to prevent contact with its bactericidal contents (*Mycobacterium* species), capsule-mediated or enzymatic resistance to the bactericidal lysosomal enzymes or substances, and the ability to exit the phagosome into the host cytoplasm before being exposed to lysosomal enzymes (Table 5-4 and Figure 5-5). Production of catalase by staphylococci can break down the hydrogen peroxide produced by the myeloperoxidase system. Many of the bacteria that are internalized but survive phagocytosis can use the cell as a place to grow and hide from immune responses and as a means of being disseminated throughout the body.

Table 5-4 Methods That Circumvent Phagocytic Killing

Method	Example
Inhibition of phagolysosome fusion	*Legionella* spp., *Mycobacterium tuberculosis*, *Chlamydia* spp.
Resistance to lysosomal enzymes	*Salmonella typhimurium*, *Coxiella* spp., *Ehrlichia* spp., *Mycobacterium leprae*, *Leishmania* spp.
Adaptation to cytoplasmic replication	*Listeria*, *Francisella*, and *Rickettsia* spp.

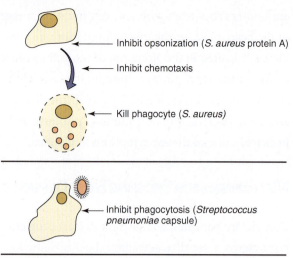

- Inhibit opsonization (*S. aureus* protein A)
- Inhibit chemotaxis
- Kill phagocyte (*S. aureus*)

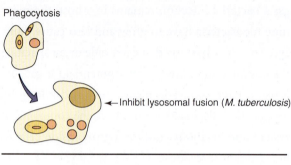

- Inhibit phagocytosis (*Streptococcus pneumoniae* capsule)

Phagocytosis

- Inhibit lysosomal fusion (*M. tuberculosis*)

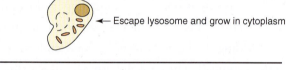

- Escape lysosome and grow in cytoplasm

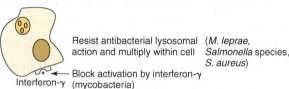

Resist antibacterial lysosomal action and multiply within cell (*M. leprae, Salmonella* species, *S. aureus*)

Interferon-γ — Block activation by interferon-γ (mycobacteria)

Figure 5-5 Bacterial mechanisms for escaping phagocytic clearance. Selected examples of bacteria that use the indicated antiphagocytic mechanisms are given.

SUMMARY

The primary virulence factors of bacteria are the capsule, adhesins, invasins, degradative enzymes, toxins, and mechanisms for escaping elimination by host defenses.

The capsule functions by shielding the bacteria from immune and phagocytic responses.

The adhesins of bacteria will bind to specific receptors on the tissue surface and keep the organisms from being wash away.

The bacteria have invasins that can cross the

mucosal membranes and other tissue barrier to enter human body.

The bacteria release degradative enzymes to break down tissue, thereby promoting the spread of the bacteria.

Toxins are bacterial products that directly harm tissue or trigger destructive biologic activities, in which exotoxin and endotoxin are included. Exotoxins are proteins that can be produced by gram-positive or gram-negative bacteria and include cytolytic enzymes and receptor-binding proteins that alter a function or kill the cell. Lipid A portion of lipopolysaccharide (LPS) produced by gram-negative bacteria is termed endotoxin, which is a powerful activator of acute-phase and inflammatory reactions.

Bacteria evade recognition and killing by phagocytic cells, inactivate or evade the complement system and antibody, and even grow inside cells to hide from host responses. Bacteria can evade antibody responses by antigenic variation, by inactivation of antibody or by intracellular growth. Many bacteria can circumvent phagocytic killing in various ways.

KEYWORDS

English	Chinese
Opportunistic bacteria	机会致病菌
Disseminated intravascular coagulation (DIC)	弥散性血管内凝血
adhesin	黏附素
Invasin	侵袭素
Exotoxin	外毒素
Endotoxin	内毒素
Biofilm	生物膜

BIBLIOGRAPHY

1. Bisno AL, Brito MO, Collins CM: Molecular basis of group A streptococcal virulence, Lancet Infect Dis 3: 191-200, 2003.

2. Bower S, Rosenthal KS: Bacterial cell walls: the armor, artillery and Achilles heel, Infect Dis Clin Pract 14: 309-317, 2006.

3. Brodell LA, Rosenthal KS: Skin structure and function: the body's primary defense against infection, Infect Dis Clin Pract 16: 113-117, 2008.

4. Cohen J, Powderly WC: Infectious diseases, ed 2, London, 2004, Mosby.

5. Desvaux M, et al: Type III secretion: what's in a name? Trends Microbiol 14: 157-160, 2006.

6. Finlay BB, Falkow S: Common themes in microbial pathogenicity revisited, Microbiol Mol Biol Rev 61: 136-169, 1997.

7. Groisman EA, Ochman H: How *Salmonella* became a pathogen, Trends Microbiol 5: 343-349, 1997.

8. Lee CA: Pathogenicity islands and the evolution of bacterial pathogens, Infect Agents Dis 5: 1-7, 1996.

9. Mandell GL, Bennet JE, Dolin R, editors: Principles and practice of infectious diseases, ed 6, Philadelphia, 2005, Churchill Livingstone.

10. McClane BA, et al: Microbial pathogenesis: a principles-oriented approach, Madison, Conn, 1999, Fence Creek.

11. Papageorgiou AC, Acharya KR: Microbial superantigens: from structure to function, Trends Microbiol 8: 369-375, 2000.

12. Reading N, Sperandio V: Quorum sensing: the many languages of bacteria, FEMS Microbiol Lett 254: 1-11, 2006.

13. Rosenthal KS: Are microbial symptoms "self-inflicted"? The consequences of immunopathology, Infect Dis Clin Pract 13: 306-310, 2005.

14. Excellent videos, prepared by the Howard Hughes Medical Institute, of the action of *E. coli* and *Salmonella* type III secretion devices promoting adhesion and intracellular growth can be seen at: www.hhmi.org/biointeractive/disease/ecoli.html/www.hhmi.org/biointeractive/disease/salmonella.html A video of *Salmonella* virulence mechanisms: www.youtube.com/watch?v=j5GvvQJVD_Y.

Immune Responses to Bacteria

6

Most infections are controlled by innate responses before immune responses can be initiated, but immune responses are necessary to resolve the more troublesome infections. The importance of each of the components of the host response differs for different infectious agents (Table 6-1).

Antibacterial responses are initiated by activation of innate and inflammatory responses on a local basis and progresses to acute-phase and antigen-specific responses on a systemic scale. The response progresses from soluble antibacterial factors (peptides and complement) to cellular responses and then soluble antibody responses. The most important antibacterial host response is phagocytic killing by neutrophils and macrophages. Complement and antibody facilitate the uptake of microbes by phagocytes and TH17, and TH1 CD4 T-cell responses enhance and regulate their function. Figure 6-1 illustrates the progression of protective responses to a bacterial challenge.

THE BASIC LINES OF PROTECTION AGAINST INFECTION

Human beings have three basic lines of protection against infection by microbes to block entry, spread in the body, and inappropriate colonization.

Natural barriers, such as skin, mucus, ciliated epithelium, gastric acid, and bile, restrict entry of the agent. The **skin** and **mucous membranes** serve as barriers to most infectious agents (Figure 6-2). Free fatty acids produced in sebaceous glands and by organisms on the skin surface, lactic acid in perspiration, and the low pH and relatively dry environment of the skin all form unfavorable conditions for the survival of most organisms.

The mucosal epithelium covering the orifices of the body is protected by mucus secretions and cilia. Antimicrobial substances (cationic peptides [**defensins**], lysozyme, lactoferrin, and secretory [IgA]) found in secretions at mucosal surfaces (e.g., tears, mucus, and saliva) also provide protection (Table 6-2).

Table 6-1 Importance of Antimicrobial Defenses for Infectious Agents

	Bacteria	Intracellular Bacteria	Viruses	Fungi	Parasites
Complement	+++	−	−	−	−
Interferon-α/β	−	−	++++	−	−
Neutrophils	++++	−	+	+++	++
Macrophages	+++	+++[*]	++	++	+
Natural killer cells	−	−	+++	−	−
CD4 TH1	+	++	+++	++	+
TH17	++	++	++	++++	+
CD8 cytotoxic T lymphocytes	−	++	++++	−	−
Antibody	+++	+	++	++	++ (IgE)[†]

[*]By activation of macrophages.
[†]Immunoglobulin E and mast cells are especially important for worm infections.

48

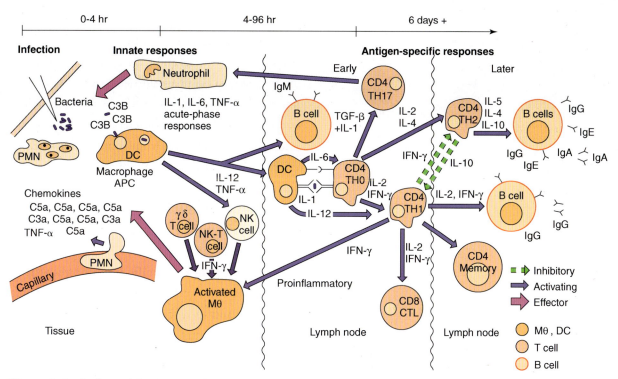

Figure 6-1 Antibacterial responses. First, innate antigen-nonspecific responses attract and promote polymorphonuclear neutrophil *(PMN)* and macrophage *(Mθ)* responses. Dendritic cells *(DCs)* and antigen reach the lymph node to activate early immune responses (TH17, TH1, and IgM). Later, TH2 systemic antibody responses and memory cells are developed. **The time course of events is indicated at the top of the figure.** *APC,* Antigen-presenting cell; *CTL,* cytotoxic T lymphocyte; *IFN-γ,* interferon-γ; *IL,* interleukin; *TGF-β,* transforming growth factor-β; *TH,* T helper (cell); *TNF-α,* tumor necrosis factor-α.

Table 6-2 Soluble Innate Defense Mediators

Factor	Function	Source
Lysozyme	Catalyzes hydrolysis of bacterial peptidoglycan	Tears, saliva, nasal secretions, body fluids, lysosomal granules
Lactoferrin, transferrin	Bind iron and compete with microorganisms for it	Specific granules of PMNs
Lactoperoxidase	May be inhibitory to many microorganisms	Milk and saliva
β-Lysin	Is effective mainly against gram-positive bacteria	Thrombocytes, normal serum
Chemotactic factors	Induce directed migration of PMNs, monocytes, and other cells	Complement and chemokines
Properdin	Activates complement in the absence of antibody-antigen complex	Normal plasma
Lectins	Bind to microbial carbohydrates to promote phagocytosis	Normal plasma
Cationic peptides	Disrupt membranes, block cell transport activities	Polymorphonuclear granules, epithelial cells, etc. (defensins, etc.)

PMNs, Polymorphonuclear neutrophils (leukocytes).

The acidic environment of the stomach, bladder, and kidneys and the bile of the intestines inactivate many bacteria and viruses. Urinary flow also limits the establishment of infection.

Innate, antigen-nonspecific immune defenses such as fever, interferon, complement, neutrophils,

macrophages, dendritic cells (DCs), and natural killer (NK) cells provide rapid local responses to act at the infection site in order to restrict the growth and spread of the agent.

Soluble components of innate responses include antimicrobial peptides and complement. Defensins

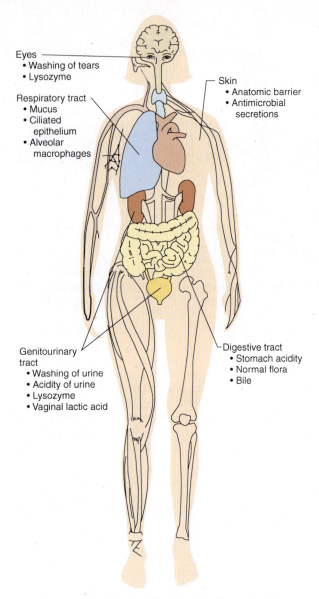

Eyes
• Washing of tears
• Lysozyme

Respiratory tract
• Mucus
• Ciliated
  epithelium
• Alveolar
  macrophages

Skin
• Anatomic barrier
• Antimicrobial
  secretions

Genitourinary
tract
• Washing of urine
• Acidity of urine
• Lysozyme
• Vaginal lactic acid

Digestive tract
• Stomach acidity
• Normal flora
• Bile

Figure 6-2 Barrier defenses of the human body.

and cathelicidins are peptides produced by neutrophils, epithelial cells, and other cells that are toxic to many microbes. Defensins are small (approximately 30 amino acids), cationic peptides that can disrupt membranes, kill bacteria and fungi and inactivate viruses. The complement system is an alarm and a weapon against bacterial infection. The complement system is activated directly by bacteria and bacterial products (alternate or properdin pathway), by lectin binding to sugars on the bacterial cell surface (mannose-binding protein), or by complexes of antibody and antigen (classical pathway).

Cellular components of innate responses include phagocytes, macrophages, NKT cells and γ/δ T cells.

Neutrophils play a major role in antibacterial protections. Macrophages can be activated by IFN-γ produced by NK cells and CD4 and CD8 T cells and are then able to kill phagocytosed bacteria. NKT cells and γ/δ T cells sense nonpeptide antigens, including bacterial glycolipids (mycobacteria) and phosphorylated amine metabolites from some bacteria (*Escherichia coli*, *mycobacteria*) but not others (*streptococci*, *staphylococci*). These T cells and NK cells produce IFN-γ, which activate macrophages and DCs to enforce a protective TH1 cycle of cytokines and local cellular inflammatory reactions.

Adaptive, antigen-specific immune responses, such as antibody and T cells, reinforce the innate protections and specifically target, attack, and eliminate the invaders that succeed in passing the first two defenses.

Antigen-specific immune responses provided by T cells and antibody expand the host protections provided by innate responses. The antigen-specific immune system is a randomly generated, coordinately regulated, inducible, and activatible system that ignores self-proteins but specifically responds to and protects against infection. Once specifically activated by exposure to a new antigen, the immune response rapidly expands in strength, cell number, and specificity. For proteins, immune memory develops to allow more rapid recall upon rechallenge.

Usually, barrier functions and innate responses are sufficient to control most infections before symptoms or disease occurs. Initiation of a new antigen-specific immune response takes time, and infections can grow and spread during this time period. Prior immunity and immune memory elicited by infection or vaccination can activate quickly enough to control most infections.

INITIATION OF THE ANTIBACTERIAL RESPONSE

Once past the barriers, bacterial cell surfaces activate the alternative or lectin pathways of complement that are present in interstitial fluids and serum. The **complement system** is a very early and important antibacterial defense. The **alternative complement** pathway (**properdin**) can be activated by teichoic acid, peptidoglycan, and lipopolysaccharide (LPS) in the absence of antibody and, with **mannose-binding protein,** can activate the lectin complement pathway. Later, when immunoglobulin (Ig) M or IgG is present, the classical complement pathway is activated. C3b promotes its phagocytosis as an opsonin. The membrane attack complex (MAC) can directly kill gram-negative bacteria and, to a much lesser extent, gram-positive bacteria (the thick peptidoglycan of gram-positive bacteria shields them from the components). *Neisseria* are especially sensitive to complement lysis due to the truncated structure of lipooligosaccharide in the outer membrane. Complement facilitates elimination of all bacteria by producing

1. chemotactic factors (C5a) to attract neutrophils and macrophages to the site of infection;

2. anaphylotoxins (C3a, C4a, and C5a) to stimulate

mast cell release of histamine and thereby increase vascular permeability, allowing access to the infection site;

3. opsonins (C3b), which bind to bacteria and promote their phagocytosis;

4. a B-cell activator (C3d) to enhance antibody production.

Bacterial cell wall molecules (teichoic acid and peptidoglycan fragments of gram-positive bacteria and lipid A of LPS of gram-negative bacteria) also activate **pathogen-associated molecular pattern (PAMP) receptors,** including the cell surface **Toll-like receptors (TLRs)** (Table 6-3 and Figure 6-3) and the cytoplasmic peptidoglycan receptors—nucleotide-binding oligomerization domain protein (NOD)1, NOD2, and cryopyrin (Box 6-1). **Lipid A (endotoxin)** binds to TLR4 and other PAMP receptors and is a very strong activator of DCs, macrophages, B cells,

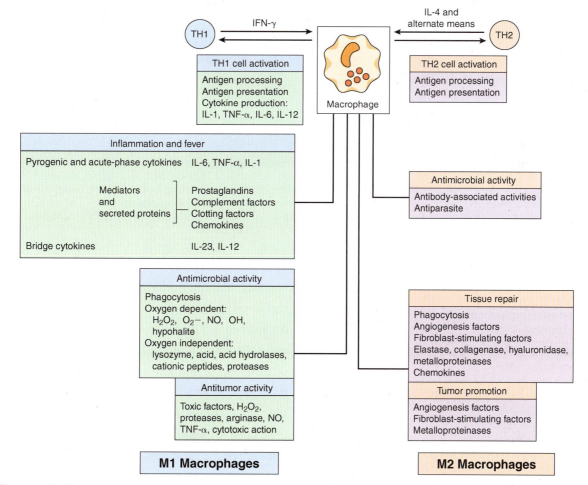

Figure 6-3　The many functions of macrophages and members of the macrophage family. *H₂O₂*, Hydrogen peroxide; *IFN-γ*, interferon-γ; *IL*, interleukin; *NO*, nitric oxide; ·*O⁻*, oxygen radical; *OH*, hydroxyl radical; *TH*, T helper (cell); *TNF-α*, tumor necrosis factor-α. (From Roitt I, et al: *Immunology*, ed 4, St Louis, 1996, Mosby.)

Table 6-3   Pathogen Pattern Receptors

Receptor[*]	Microbial Activators	Ligand
Cell Surface		
TLR1	Bacteria, mycobacteria *Neisseria meningitidis*	Lipopeptides Soluble factors
TLR2	Bacteria Fungi Cells	LTA, LPS, PG, etc. Zymosan Necrotic cells
TLR4	Bacteria, parasites, host proteins Viruses, parasites, host proteins	**LPS**, fungal mannans, viral glycoproteins, parasitic phospholipids, host heat shock proteins, LDL
TLR5	Bacteria	Flagellin
TLR6	Bacteria Fungi	LTA, lipopeptides, zymosan
Lectins	Bacteria, fungi, viruses	Specific carbohydrates (e.g., mannose)
N-Formyl methionine receptor	Bacteria	Bacterial proteins
Endosome		
TLR3	Viruses	Double-stranded RNA
TLR7	Viruses	Single-stranded RNA Imidazoquinolines
TLR8	Viruses	Single-stranded RNA Imidazoquinolines
TLR9	Bacteria Viruses	Unmethylated DNA (CpG)
Cytoplasm		
NOD1, NOD2, NALP3	Bacteria	Peptidoglycan
Cryopyrin	Bacteria	Peptidoglycan
RIG-1	Viruses	RNA
MDA5	Viruses	RNA
DAI	Viruses, cytoplasmic DNA	DNA

Activators: *DAI*, DNA-dependent activator of interferon regulatory factors; *DNA*, deoxyribonucleic acid; *dsRNA*, double-stranded RNA; *LDL*, minimally modified low-density lipoprotein; *LPS*, lipopolysaccharide; *LTA*, lipoteichoic acid; *MDA5*, melanoma differentiation-associated gene 5; *NALP3*, Nacht, leucine-rich repeat and pyrin domain-containing protein 3; *NOD*, nucleotide-binding oligomerization domain; *PG*, peptidoglycan; *RIG-1*, retinoic acid-inducible gene-1; *TLR*, Toll-like receptor.
[*]Information about Toll-like receptors from Takeda A, Kaisho T, Akira S: Toll-like receptors, *Annu Rev Immunol* 21: 335-376, 2003; and Akira S, Takeda K: Toll-like receptor signalling, *Nat Rev Immunol* 4: 499-511, 2003.

Box 6-1

Bacterial Components That Activate Protective Responses

Direct Activation through Pathogen-Associated Pattern Receptors
Lipopolysaccharide (endotoxin)
Lipoteichoic acid
Lipoarabinomannan
Glycolipids and glycopeptides
Polyanions
N-Formyl peptides (formyl-methionyl-leucyl-phenylalanine)
Peptidoglycan fragments

Chemotaxis via C3a, C5a, and Other Mechanisms
Peptidoglycan fragments
Cell surface activation of alternative pathways of complement

---

and selected other cells (e.g., epithelial and endothelial cells). Binding of these PAMPs to receptors on epithelial cells, macrophages, Langerhans cells, and DCs activate kinase cascades that activate the inflammasome and also promote cytokine production (including the **acute-phase cytokines, interleukin (IL)-1, IL-6, and tumor necrosis factor [TNF]**), protective responses, and maturation of DCs. The inflammasome promotes the cleavage of IL-1β and IL-18 to reinforce local inflammation. NK cells, NKT cells, and γ/δ T cells residing in tissue also respond, produce cytokines, and reinforce cellular responses.

IL-1 and TNF-α enhance the inflammatory response by locally stimulating changes in the tissue, promoting diapedesis of neutrophils and macrophages to the site, and activating these cells and activating systemic responses. IL-1 and TNF-α are endogenous pyrogens, inducing fever, and also induce the **acute-phase response.** The acute-phase response can also be triggered by inflammation, tissue injury, prostaglandin E$_2$, and interferons associated with infection. The acute-phase response promotes changes that support host defenses and include fever, anorexia, sleepiness, metabolic changes, and production of proteins. Acute-phase proteins that are produced and released into the serum include C-reactive protein, complement components, coagulation proteins, LPS-binding proteins, transport proteins, protease inhibitors, and adherence proteins. **C-reactive protein** complexes with the polysaccharides of numerous bacteria and fungi and activates the complement pathway, facilitating removal of these organisms from the body through greater phagocytosis. The acute-phase proteins reinforce the innate defenses against infection.

Antimicrobial peptides, including defensins, are released by activated epithelial cells, neutrophils, and other cells to protect skin and mucoepithelial surfaces. Their release is reinforced by TH17 responses. Antimicrobial peptides are very important for regulating the species of bacteria in the gastrointestinal tract. In addition, chelating peptides are released as part of the inflammatory response to sequester essential metal ions, such as iron and zinc, to limit microbial growth.

Immature DCs (iDCs), macrophages, and other cells of the macrophage lineage will produce IL-23 and IL-12 in addition to the acute-phase cytokines. IL-12 activates NK cells at the site of infection, which can produce interferon-γ (IFN-γ) to further activate macrophages and DCs. IL-12 and IL-23 activate TH1 and TH17 immune responses, respectively, to reinforce macrophages and neutrophil function. Epithelial cells also respond to PAMPs and release cytokines to promote natural protections.

These actions initiate **local, acute inflammation**. Expansion of capillaries and increased blood flow brings more antimicrobial agents to the site. Increase in permeability and alteration of surface molecules of the microvasculature structure attract and facilitate leukocyte entry and provides access for fluid and plasma proteins into the site of infection. Kinins and clotting factors induced by tissue damage (e.g., factor XII [Hageman factor], bradykinin, fibrinopeptides) are also involved in inflammation. These factors increase vascular permeability and are chemotactic for leukocytes. Products of arachidonic acid metabolism also affect inflammation. Cyclooxygenase-2 (COX-2) and 5-lipooxygenase convert arachidonic acid to **prostaglandins and leukotrienes,** respectively, which can mediate essentially every aspect of acute inflammation. The course of inflammation can be followed by rapid increases in serum levels of acute-phase proteins, especially C-reactive protein (which can increase a thousand fold within 24 to 48 hours) and serum amyloid A. Although these processes are beneficial, they also cause **pain, redness, heat, and swelling and promote tissue damage**. Inflammatory damage is caused to some extent by complement and macrophages but mostly by neutrophils.

Phagocytic Responses

C3a, C5a, bacterial products (e.g., formyl-methionyl-leucyl-phenylalanine [f-met-leu-phe]), and chemokines produced by epithelial cells, Langerhans cells, and other cells in skin and mucous epithelium are powerful chemoattractants for neutrophils, macrophages, and later in the response, lymphocytes. The chemokines and **tumor necrosis factor-α (TNF-α)** cause the endothelial cells lining the capillaries (near the inflammation) and the leukocytes passing by to express complementary adhesion molecules (molecular "Velcro") to promote diapedesis (Figure 6-4). Polymorphonuclear neutrophils (PMNs) provide a major antibacterial response and contribution to inflammation. **Neutrophils** are the first cells to arrive at the site in response to infection; they are followed later by monocytes and macrophages. An increased number of neutrophils in the blood, body fluids (e.g., cerebrospinal fluid), or tissue indicates a bacterial infection. Recruitment of immature band forms of neutrophils from the bone marrow during infection

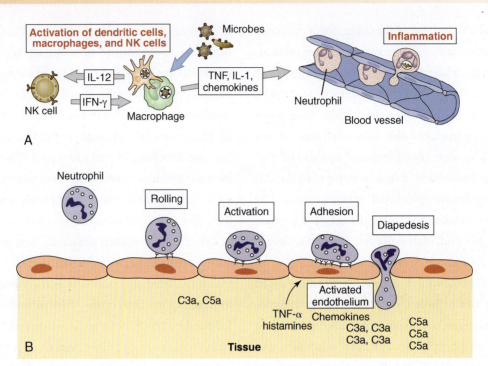

Figure 6-4 **A** and **B,** Neutrophil diapedesis in response to inflammatory signals. Tumor necrosis factor-α *(TNF-α)* and chemokines activate the expression of selectins and intercellular adhesion molecules on the endothelium near the inflammation and their ligands on the neutrophil: integrins, L-selectin, and leukocyte function-associated antigen-1. The neutrophil binds progressively tighter to the endothelium until it finds its way through the endothelium. Epithelial cells, Langerhans cells, and macrophages activated by microbes and interferon-γ *(IFN-γ)* make TNF-α and other cytokines and chemokines to enhance diapedesis. *IL,* Interleukin; *NK,* natural killer. (**A,** From Abbas AK, Lichtman AH: *Basic immunology: functions and disorders of the immune system,* ed 3, Philadelphia, 2008, WB Saunders.)

is indicated by a "left shift" in the complete blood count (*left* refers to the beginning of a chart of neutrophil development). Neutrophils are recruited and activated by the TH17 response and macrophages, and DCs are activated by IFN-γ produced by NK cells and the TH1 T response. **Phagocytosis** of bacteria by macrophages and neutrophils involves three steps: attachment, internalization, and digestion. Bacteria are bound to the neutrophils and macrophages with receptors for bacterial carbohydrates (**lectins** [specific sugar-binding proteins]), fibronectin receptors (especially for *Staphylococcus aureus*), and **receptors for opsonins,** including complement (C3b), C-reactive protein, mannose-binding protein, and the Fc portion of antibody.

After attachment, a section of plasma membrane surrounds the particle, which forms a **phagocytic vacuole** around the microbe. This vacuole fuses with the **primary lysosomes** (macrophages) or **granules** (PMNs) to allow inactivation and digestion of the vacuole contents.

Phagocytic killing may be oxygen dependent or oxygen independent, depending on the antimicrobial chemicals produced by the granules (Figure 6-5). Neutrophils do not need special activation to kill internalized microbes, but their response is reinforced by IL-17-mediated activities. Activation of macrophages is promoted by IFN-γ (best) and GM-CSF, which are produced early in the infection by NK and NKT cells or later by CD4 T cells, and sustained by TNF-α and lymphotoxin (TNF-*β*). Activation of macrophages is required for macrophages to kill internalized microbes.

Oxygen-dependent killing is activated by a powerful oxidative burst that culminates in the formation of hydrogen peroxide and other antimicrobial substances (ROS) (Box 6-2). In the neutrophil, but not the macrophage, hydrogen peroxide with myeloperoxidase (released by primary granules during fusion to the phagolysosome) transforms chloride ions into hypochlorous ions that kill the microorganisms. Nitric oxide produced by neutrophils and activated macrophages has antimicrobial activity and is

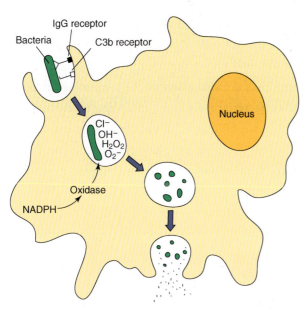

Figure 6-5 Phagocytosis and killing of bacteria. Bacteria are bound directly or are opsonized by mannose-binding protein, immunoglobulin G *(IgG)*, and/or C3b receptors, promoting their adherence and uptake by phagocytes. Within the phagosome, oxygen-dependent and oxygen-independent mechanisms kill and degrade the bacteria. *NADPH*, Nicotinamide adenine dinucleotide phosphate reduced.

Box 6-2

Antibacterial Compounds of the Phagolysosome

Oxygen-Dependent Compounds
Hydrogen peroxide: NADPH oxidase and NADH oxidase
Superoxide
Hydroxyl radicals (OH⁻)
Activated halides (Cl⁻, I⁻, Br⁻): myeloperoxidase (neutrophil)
Nitrous oxide

Oxygen-Independent Compounds
Acids
Lysosome (degrades bacterial peptidoglycan)
Lactoferrin (chelates iron)
Defensins and other cationic proteins (damage membranes)
Proteases: Elastase, Cathepsin G

NADH, Nicotinamide adenine dinucleotide reduced; *NADPH,* nicotinamide adenine dinucleotide phosphate reduced.

---

also a major second messenger molecule (like cyclic adenosine monophosphate [cAMP]) which enhances the inflammatory and other responses.

The **neutrophil** can also mediate **oxygen-independent killing** upon fusion of the phagosome with azurophilic granules containing cationic proteins (e.g., cathepsin G) and specific granules containing lysozyme and lactoferrin. These proteins kill gram-negative bacteria by disrupting their cell membrane integrity, but they are far less effective against gram-

positive bacteria, which are killed principally through the oxygen-dependent mechanism.

The neutrophils contribute to the inflammation in several ways. Prostaglandins and leukotrienes are released and increase vascular permeability, cause swelling (edema) and stimulate pain receptors. In addition, during phagocytosis, the granules may leak their contents to cause tissue damage. The neutrophils have short lives, and upon death, neutrophils release a sticky DNA net (neutrophil extracellular trap) and become **pus**.

In contrast to neutrophils, macrophages have long lives. Resting macrophages are phagocytic and will internalize microbes but do not have the preformed granules of antimicrobial molecules to kill them. Activation of the macrophage by IFN-γ, making the macrophages "angry," promotes production of inducible nitric oxide synthase (iNOS) and nitric oxide, other ROS, and antimicrobial enzymes to kill internalized microbes. Activated macrophages also make acute-phase cytokines (IL-1, IL-6, and TNF-α) and possibly IL-23 or IL-12. Intracellular infection can occur upon infection of a resting macrophage or if the microbe can counteract the antimicrobial activities of an activated macrophage. In addition to the tissue macrophages, splenic macrophages are important for clearing bacteria, especially encapsulated bacteria, from blood. Asplenic (congenitally or surgically) individuals are highly susceptible to pneumonia, meningitis, and other manifestations of *Streptococcus pneumoniae*, *Neisseria meningitidis*, and other encapsulated bacteria.

Antigen-Specific Response to Bacterial Challenge

On ingestion of bacteria and after stimulation of TLRs by bacterial components, Langerhans cells and iDCs become mature, cease to phagocytize, and move to the lymph nodes to process and deliver their internalized antigen for presentation to T cells. Antigenic peptides (having more than 11 amino acids) produced from phagocytosed proteins (exogenous route) are bound to class II major histocompatibility complex (MHC) molecules and presented by these antigen-presenting cells (APCs) to naïve **CD4 TH0**

T cells. The CD4 T cells are activated by a combination of (1) antigenic peptide in the cleft of the MHC II molecule with the T-cell antigen receptor (TCR) and with CD4, (2) co-stimulatory signals provided by the interaction of B7 molecules on the DC with CD28 molecules on the T cells, and (3) IL-6, and other cytokines produced by the DC. The TH0 cells produce IL-2, IFN-γ, and IL-4. Simultaneously, bacterial molecules with repetitive structures (e.g., capsular polysaccharide) interact with B cells expressing surface IgM and IgD specific for the antigen and activate the cell to grow and produce IgM. Microbial cell wall polysaccharides, especially LPS and also the C3d component of complement, activate B cells and promote the specific IgM antibody responses. Swollen lymph nodes are an indication of lymphocyte activation in response to antigenic challenge.

Early responses are also provided by γ/δ T cells, NKT cells and innate lymphoid cells (including NK cells). **γ/δ T cells** in tissue and in the blood sense phosphorylated amine metabolites from some bacteria (*Escherichia coli*, mycobacteria) but not others (streptococci, staphylococci). DCs can present bacterial glycolipids to activate **NKT** cells. These T cells and **innate lymphoid cells** produce IFN-γ, which activate macrophages and DCs to enforce local cellular inflammatory reactions.

The conversion of TH0 cells to TH17 and TH1 cells initiates the expansion of the host response. Acute-phase cytokines IL-1 and TNF-α together with TGF-β promote the development of **CD4 TH17 T cells**. TH17 cells produce IL-17 and TNF-α to activate epithelial cells and neutrophils and also promote production of antimicrobial peptides. TH17 responses are important for early antibacterial responses and antimycobacterial responses. A balance of TH17 and Treg responses are also important to regulate the populations of intestinal flora.

DCs producing IL-12 promote TH1 responses. **CD4 TH1 T cells** (1) promote and reinforce inflammatory responses (e.g., IFN-γ activation of macrophage) and growth of T and B cells (IL-2) to expand the immune response, and (2) promote B cells to produce complement-binding antibodies (IgM, IgG

upon class switching) and mature into plasma cells and memory cells. These responses are important for the early phases of an antibacterial defense. TH1 responses are also essential for combating intracellular bacterial infections, including mycobacteria, which are hidden from antibody. IFN-γ activates macrophage to kill the phagocytized microbe. Upon chronic stimulation by macrophages expressing microbial (e.g., mycobacterial or histoplasma) antigen, CD4 TH1 T cells will produce IFN-γ and TNF-α and cause the transformation of other macrophages into epithelioid cells and giant cells, which can surround the infection and produce a granuloma. Granulomas wall off intracellular infections arising either because the microbe can evade antimicrobial responses (e.g., Mycobacterium tuberculosis), the macrophages are not activated and cannot kill them (normal alveolar macrophages), or a genetic defect prevents generation of antimicrobial reactive oxygen substances, as in chronic granulomatous disease. CD8 T cells facilitate clearance of intracellular infections by producing cytokines but are not essential for antibacterial immunity. **CD4 TH2 T-cell** responses occur in the absence of IL-12 at more distant lymph nodes. These responses are also initiated by DCs and are sustained by the B-cell presentation of antigen. TH2 responses can occur at the same time as TH1 responses when antigen is delivered in lymph fluid to lymph nodes other than the draining lymph node. The DCs act a sewage inspectors who promote a response to clear out excess and damaged protein. This is the same type of response that occurs to injection of a bolus of antigen for an inactivated vaccine. Binding of antigen to the cell surface antibody on B cells activates the B cells and also promotes uptake, processing of the antigen, and presentation of antigenic peptides on class II MHC molecules to the CD4 TH2 cell. The TH2 cell produces IL-4, IL-5, IL-6, IL-10, and IL-13, which enhance IgG production and, depending on other factors, the production of IgE or IgA. CD4TFH cells are a conduit for the TH1 or TH2 responses to promote memory cell production and terminal differentiation of B cells to plasma-cell antibody factories. **CD4$^+$CD25$^+$ regula-**

tory T cells (Treg) prevent spurious activation of naive T cells, curtail both TH1 and TH2 responses, and promote the development of some of the antigen-specific cells into memory T cells. Only DCs can override the Treg block to naive T cell activation. **Antibodies** are the primary protection against extracellular bacteria and reinfection and promotes the clearance and prevents the spread of bacteria in the blood (bacteremia). Antibody promotes complement activation, opsonizes bacteria for phagocytosis, blocks bacterial adhesion, and neutralizes (inactivates) exotoxins (e.g., tetanospasmin, botulinum toxin) and other cytotoxic proteins produced by bacteria (e.g., degradative enzymes). Vaccine immunization with inactivated exotoxins (toxoids) is the primary means of protection against the potentially lethal effects of exotoxins.

IgM antibodies are produced early in the antibacterial response. IgM bound to bacteria activates the classical complement cascade, promoting both the direct killing of gram-negative bacteria and the inflammatory responses. IgM is usually the only antibody produced against capsular carbohydrates and promotes opsonization of the bacteria with complement. Splenic macrophages depend upon IgM bound to capsular polysaccharides to activate complement and opsonize the encapsulated bacteria so they can be recognized, phagocytized, and eliminated. The large size and limited transport mechanisms for IgM limits its ability to spread into the tissue. IgM produced in response to polysaccharide vaccines (as for Streptococcus pneumonia) can prevent bacteremia but not infection of the interstitium of the lung. Approximately a week later, T-cell help promotes differentiation of the B cell and immunoglobulin class switching to produce IgG. **IgG** antibodies are the predominant antibody, especially on rechallenge. IgG antibodies fix complement and promote phagocytic uptake of the bacteria through Fc receptors on macrophages. The production of **IgA** requires TH2 cytokines and other factors. IgA is the primary secretory antibody and is important for protecting mucosal membranes. Large amounts of secretory IgA are released to regulate the normal flora population, prevent adhesion of bacteria, and neutralize toxins at epithelial cell surfaces.

A primary antigen-specific response to bacterial infection takes at least 5 to 7 days. Movement of the DC to the lymph node may take 1 to 3 days, followed by activation, expansion, and maturation of the response. On rechallenge to infection, long-lived plasma cells may still be producing antibody. Memory T cells can respond quickly to antigen presentation by DC, macrophage, or B cells, not just DC; memory B cells are present to respond quickly to antigen; and the secondary antibody response occurs within 2 to 3 days.

Skin, Intestinal and Mucosal Immunity

The skin, intestine, and mucous membranes are populated with bacteria upon traversing the birth canal and soon thereafter. The immune response matures, and a balance develops between regulatory and inflammatory cells in response to this normal flora.

The intestinal flora is constantly interacting with and being regulated by the innate and immune systems of the gut-associated lymphoid tissue (Figure 6-6). Similarly, the immune response is shaped by its interaction with intestinal flora as regulatory cells limit the development of autoimmune responses and inflammation. DCs, innate lymphoid cells, Treg, TH17, TH1, and other T cells and B cells in the lamina propria, Peyer patches, and intestinal lymphoid follicles monitor and control the bacteria within the gut. These cells and epithelial and other cells lining the gut produce antimicrobial peptides, and plasma cells secrete IgA into the gut to maintain a healthy mixture of bacteria. At the same time, regulatory cells prevent the development of detrimental or excessive immune responses to the contents of the gut. Alterations in the microbial flora and its interaction with the innate and immune cells can disrupt the system and result in inflammatory bowel diseases. For example, absence or a mutation in the IL-23 receptor or NOD2 receptor for peptidoglycan enhances chances for certain types of Crohn disease.

In the skin, Langerhans cells are sentinel DCs responsive to trauma and infection. Memory CD4

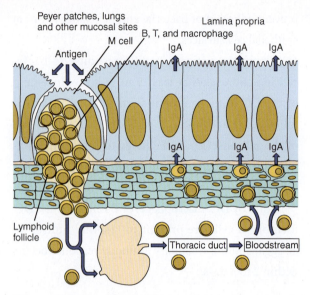

Peyer patches, lungs
and other mucosal sites
Lamina propria
M cell
B, T, and macrophage
Antigen
IgA   IgA   IgA
IgA   IgA   IgA
Lymphoid
follicle
Thoracic duct → Bloodstream

Figure 6-6 Lymphoid cells stimulated with antigen in Peyer patches (or the lungs or another mucosal site) migrate via the regional lymph nodes and thoracic duct into the bloodstream, then to the lamina propria of the gut and probably other mucosal surfaces. Thus lymphocytes stimulated at one mucosal surface may become distributed throughout the MALT (mucosa-associated lymphoid tissue) system. *IgA*, Immunoglobulin A. (From Roitt I, et al: Immunology, ed 4, St Louis, 1996, Mosby.)

and CD8 T cells constantly cycle into the skin from the blood. In the respiratory tract, antimicrobial peptides and secreted IgA control bacteria, mucus traps, and cilia move the mucus and bacteria out of the lungs. Inflammatory responses are controlled by alveolar macrophages (M2 macrophages) to prevent tissue damage to normal flora. Like in the gastrointestinal tract, DCs monitor the epithelium for normal and abnormal microbes.

Bacterial Immunopathogenesis

Activation of the inflammatory and acute-phase responses can initiate significant tissue and systemic damage. Activation of macrophages and DCs in the liver, spleen, and blood by endotoxin can promote release of TNF-α into the blood, causing many of the symptoms of **sepsis**, including hemodynamic failure, shock, and death. Although IL-1, IL-6, and TNF-α promote protective responses to a local infection, these same responses can be life threatening when activated by systemic infection. Increased blood flow and fluid leakage can lead to shock when it occurs throughout the body. Antibodies produced

against bacterial antigens that share determinants with human proteins can initiate autoimmune tissue destruction (e.g., antibodies produced in poststreptococcal glomerulonephritis and rheumatic fever). Nonspecific activation of CD4 T cells by **superantigens** (e.g., toxic shock syndrome toxin of *S. aureus*) promotes the production of large amounts of cytokines and, eventually, the death of large numbers of T cells. The sudden, massive release of cytokines ("cytokine storm") can cause shock and severe tissue damage (e.g., toxic shock syndrome) (see Cytokine Storm section).

Bacterial Evasion of Protective Responses

The mechanisms used by bacteria to evade host-protective responses are discussed in Chapter 14 as virulence factors. These mechanisms include (1) the inhibition of phagocytosis and intracellular killing in the phagocyte, (2) inactivation of complement function, (3) binding of the Fc portion of IgG and cleavage of IgA, (4) intracellular growth (avoidance of antibody), and (5) change in bacterial antigenic appearance. Some microorganisms, including but not limited to mycobacteria (also *Listeria* and *Brucella* species), survive and multiply within macrophages and use the macrophages as a protective reservoir or transport system to help spread the organisms throughout the body. However, cytokine-activated macrophages can kill the intracellular pathogens.

Sepsis and Cytokine Storm

Cytokine storms are generated by an overwhelming release of cytokines in response to bacterial cell wall components (especially LPS), toxic shock toxins, and certain viral infections. Strong innate responses are triggered by the presence of microbes in the blood during bacteremia and viremia. During bacteremia, large amounts of complement C5a and cytokines are produced and distributed throughout the body (Figure 6-7). C5a and TNF-α promote vascular leakage, neutrophil activation, and activation of the coagulation pathway. Plasmacytoid DCs in the blood produce large amounts of inflammatory cytokines and IL-12 in response to bacterial PAMPs. Endotoxin

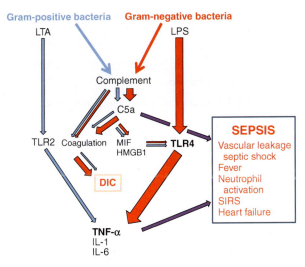

Figure 6-7 Gram-positive and gram-negative bacteria inducesepsis by shared and separate pathways. Bacterial surface lipopolysaccharides (LPS) activate complement, producing C5a, which promotes inflammation and activates coagulation. LPS, lipoteichoic acid (LTA), and other pathogen-associated molecular patterns interact with Toll-like receptors (TLRs) and other pathogen pattern receptors to activate inflammation and proinflammatory cytokine production. These add up to sepsis. The thickness of the arrow indicates the strength of the response. Red is for gram-negative and blue is for gram-positive bacteria. *DIC*, Disseminated intravascular coagulation; *IL*, interleukin; *SIRS*, systemic inflammatory responsesyndrome; *TNF-α*, tumor necrosis factor-α. (Modified from Rittirsch D, Flierl MA, Ward PA: Harmful molecular mechanisms in sepsis, *Nat Rev Immunol* 8: 776-787, 2008.)

is an especially potent activator of cells and inducer of cytokine production and sepsis (see Figure 5-4). Cytokine storms can also occur upon the abnormal stimulation of T cells and antigen-presenting cells (DCs, macrophages, and B cells) by superantigens produced by *S. aureus* or *Streptococcus pyogenes*.

Although beneficial on a limited and local basis, excess cytokines in the blood induce life-threatening inflammatory trauma throughout the entire body. Most significantly, increases in vascular permeability can result in leakage of fluids from the bloodstream into tissue and cause shock. Septic shock is a consequence of cytokine storm and can be attributed to the systemic action of large quantities of C5a and TNF-α.

SUMMARY

For complement, the alternative and lectin pathways are activated by bacterial surfaces. The classical path-

way activated later by antibody-antigen complexes. The production of chemotactic and anaphylotoxic proteins (C3a, C5a) attracts phagocytic and inflammatory cells to the site, and activates the response. C3b could help the opsonization of bacteria and promote killing gram-negative bacteria. The complement (C3d) could activate B cells.

The neutrophils cells are important antibacterial phagocytic cell which kill the bacteria by oxygen-dependent and oxygen-independent mechanisms.

The dendritic cells could produce acute phase cytokines (TNF-α, IL-6, IL-1), IL-23, IL-12, IFN-α, present antigen to CD4 and CD8 T cells, and initiate immune responses in naive T cells.

The macrophage is a kind of important antibacterial phagocytic cell which kills the bacteria by oxygen-dependent and oxygen-independent mechanisms. The macrophage could produce TNF-α, IL-1, IL-6, IL-23, IL-12, activate acute-phase and inflammatory responses, and present antigen to CD4 T cell.

The γ/δ T-cell responses to bacterial metabolites. Natural killer-1 T-cell response to CD1 presentation of mycobacterial glycolipids. The TH1 CD4 response is important for bacterial, especially intracellular, infections. The TH2 CD4 response important for antibody protections. The TH17 CD4 response activates neutrophils.

The antibodies could bind to surface structures of bacteria (fimbriae, lipoteichoic acid, capsule), block bacteria attachment, opsonize bacteria phagocytosis, promote complement action, bacteria clearance, neutralize toxins and toxic enzymes.

KEYWORDS

English	Chinese
Natural barriers	天然屏障
Antigen-nonspecific immune defenses	抗原非特异性免疫防御
Antimicrobial peptides	抗菌肽
Antigen-specific immune responses	抗原特异性免疫应答
Pathogen-associated molecular pattern (PAMP)	病原相关分子模式
Toll-like receptors (TLRs)	Toll 样受体

C-reactive protein	C 反应蛋白
Phagocytic responses	吞噬反应
Oxygen-independent killing	氧非依赖性杀伤作用
Oxygen-dependent killing	氧依赖性杀伤作用
Phagocytic vacuole	吞噬泡
Innate lymphoid cells	固有淋巴样细胞
Cytokine storms	细胞因子风暴
Bacterial evasion	细菌逃逸

BIBLIOGRAPHY

1. Abbas AK, et al: Cellular and molecular immunology, ed 7, Philadelphia, 2011, WB Saunders.

2. Akira S, Takeda K: Toll-like receptor signaling, Nat Rev Immunol 4: 499-511, 2004.

3. DeFranco AL, Locksley RM, Robertson M: Immunity: the immune response in infectious and inflammatory disease, Sunderland, Mass, 2007, Sinauer Associates.

4. Janeway CA, et al: Immunobiology: the immune system in health and disease, ed 6, New York, 2004, Garland Science.

5. Kindt TJ, Goldsby RA, Osborne BA: Kuby immunology, ed 7, New York, 2011, WH Freeman.

6. Kumar V, Abbas AK, Fausto N: Robbins and Cotran pathologic basis of disease, ed 7, Philadelphia, 2005, Elsevier.

7. Lamkanfi M: Emerging inflammasome effector mechanisms, Nat Rev Immunol 11: 213-220, 2011.

8. Male D: Immunology, ed 4, London, 2004, Elsevier.

9. Mims C, et al: Medical microbiology, ed 3, London, 2004, Elsevier.

10. Novak R: Crash course immunology, Philadelphia, 2006, Mosby.

11. Rittirsch, D, Flierl MA, Ward PA: Harmful molecular mechanisms in sepsis, Nat Rev Immunol 8: 776-787, 2008.

12. Rosenthal KS: Are microbial symptoms "self-inflicted"? The consequences of immunopathology, Infect Dis Clin Pract 13: 306-310, 2005.

13. Sompayrac L: How the immune system works, ed 2, Malden, Mass, 2003, Blackwell Scientific.

14. Trends Immunol: Issues contain understandable reviews on current topics in immunology.

15. Spits H, DiSanto JP: The expanding family of innate lymphoid cells: regulators and effectors of immunity and tissue remodeling, Nat Immunol 12: 21-27, 2011.

Chapter 7

Laboratory Diagnosis of Bacterial Diseases

The laboratory diagnosis of bacterial diseases requires that the appropriate specimen is collected, delivered expeditiously to the laboratory in the appropriate transport system, and processed in a manner that will maximize detection of the most likely pathogens. Collection of the proper specimen and its rapid delivery to the clinical laboratory are primarily the responsibility of the patient's physician, whereas the clinical microbiologist selects the appropriate transport systems and detection method (i.e., microscopy, culture, antigen or antibody detection, nucleic acid-based tests). These responsibilities are not mutually exclusive. The microbiologist should be prepared to instruct the physician about what specimens should be collected if a particular diagnosis is suspected, and the physician must provide the microbiologist with information about the clinical diagnosis so that the right tests are selected. This chapter is designed to provide an overview of specimen collection and transport, as well as the methods used in the microbiology laboratory for the detection and identification of bacteria. Because it is beyond the scope of this chapter to cover this subject exhaustedly, the student is referred to the citations in the Bibliography and the individual chapters that follow for more detailed information.

SPECIMEN COLLECTION, TRANSPORT, AND PROCESSING

Guidelines for the proper collection and transport of specimens are summarized in Table 7-1.

BACTERIAL DETECTION AND IDENTIFICATION

Detection of bacteria in clinical specimens is accomplished by five general procedures: (1) microscopy, (2) detection of bacterial antigens, (3) detection of specific bacterial nucleic acids, (4) culture, and (5) detection of an antibody response to the bacteria (serology). The specific techniques used for these procedures were presented in the preceding chapters and will not be repeated in this chapter. However, Table 7-2 summarizes the relative value of each procedure for the detection of organisms.

MICROSCOPY

In general, microscopy is used in microbiology for two basic purposes: the initial detection of microbes and the preliminary or definitive identification of microbes. The microscopic examination of clinical specimens is used to detect bacterial cells. Characteristic morphologic properties can be used for the preliminary identification of most bacteria. The microscopic detection of organisms stained with antibodies labeled with fluorescent dyes or other markers has proved to be very useful for the specific identification of many organisms. Five general microscopic methods are used (Box 7-1).

Box 7-1

Microscopic Methods
Brightfield (light) microscopy
Darkfield microscopy
Phase-contrast microscopy
Fluorescent microscopy
Electron microscopy

Table 7-1 Bacteriology Specimen Collection for Bacterial Pathogens.

Specimen	Transport System	Specimen Volume	Other Considerations
Blood: routine bacterial culture	Blood culture bottle with nutrient media	Adults: 20 ml/culture Children: 5-10 ml/culture Neonates: 1-2 ml/culture	Skin should be disinfected with 70% alcohol followed by 2% iodine; 2-3 cultures collected every 24 hr unless patient is in septic shock or antibiotics will be started immediately; blood collections should be separated by 30-60 min; blood is divided equally into two bottles of nutrient media.
Blood: intracellular bacteria (e.g., *Brucella*, *Francisella*, *Neisseria* spp.)	Same as that for routine blood cultures; lysis-centrifugation system	Same as that for routine blood cultures	Considerations are same as those for routine blood cultures; release of intracellular bacteria may improve the organism's recovery; *Neisseria* sp. are inhibited by some anticoagulants (sodium polyanethoesulfonate).
Blood: *Leptospira* sp.	Sterile heparinized tube	1-5 ml	The specimen is useful only during the first week of illness; afterward, urine should be cultured.
Cerebrospinal fluid	Sterile screw-capped tube	Bacteria culture: 1-5 ml Mycobacterial culture: as large a volume as possible	The specimen must be collected aseptically and delivered immediately to the laboratory; it should not be exposed to heat or refrigeration.
Other normally sterile fluids (e.g., abdominal, chest, synovial, pericardial)	Small volume: sterile screw-capped tube Large volume: blood culture bottle with nutrient medium	As large a volume as possible	Specimens are collected with a needle and syringe; a swab is not used because the quantity of collected specimen is inadequate; air should not be injected into culture bottle because it will inhibit growth of anaerobes.
Catheter	Sterile screw-capped tube or specimen cup	N/A	The entry site should be disinfected with alcohol; the catheter should be aseptically removed on receipt of the specimen in the laboratory; the catheter is rolled across a blood agar plate and then discarded.
Respiratory: throat	Swab immersed in transport medium	N/A	The area of inflammation is swabbed; exudate is collected if present; contact with saliva should be avoided because it can inhibit recovery of group A streptococci.
Respiratory: epiglottis	Collection of blood for culture	Same as for blood culture	Swabbing the epiglottis can precipitate complete airway closure; blood cultures should be collected for specific diagnosis.
Respiratory: sinuses	Sterile anaerobic tube or vial	1-5 ml	Specimens must be collected with a needle and syringe; culture of nasopharynx or oropharynx has no value; the specimen should be cultured for aerobic and anaerobic bacteria.
Respiratory: lower airways	Sterile screw-capped bottle; anaerobic tube or vial only for specimens collected by avoiding upper tract flora	1-2 ml	Expectorated sputum: If possible, the patient rinses mouth with water before collection of the specimen; the patient should cough deeply and expectorate lower airway secretions directly into a sterile cup; the collector should avoid contamination with saliva. Bronchoscopy specimen: Anesthetics can inhibit growth of bacteria; so, specimens should be processed immediately; if a "protected" bronchoscope is used, anaerobic cultures can be performed; direct lung aspirate: specimens can be processed for aerobic and anaerobic bacteria.

Table 7-1   Bacteriology Specimen Collection for Bacterial Pathogens. (Continued)

Specimen	Transport System	Specimen Volume	Other Considerations
Ear	Capped, needleless syringe; sterile screw-capped tube	Whatever volume is collected	The specimen should be aspirated with a needle and syringe; culture of the external ear has no predictive value for otitis media.
Eye	Inoculate plates at bedside (seal and transport to laboratory immediately)	Whatever volume is collected	For infections on surface of eye, specimens are collected with a swab or by corneal scrapings; for deep-seated infections, aspiration of aqueous or vitreous fluid is performed; all specimens should be inoculated onto appropriate media at collection; delays will result in significant loss of organisms.
Exudates (transudates, drainage, ulcers)	Swab immersed in transport medium; aspirate in sterile screw-capped tube	Bacteria: 1-5 ml Mycobacteria: 3-5 ml	Contamination with surface material should be avoided; specimens are generally unsuitable for anaerobic culture.
Wounds (abscess, pus)	Aspirate in sterile screw-capped tube or sterile anaerobic tube or vial	1-5 ml of pus	Specimens should be collected with a sterile needle and syringe; a curette is used to collect specimen at base of wound; swabbed specimens should be avoided.
Tissues	Sterile screw-capped tube; sterile anaerobic tube or vial	Representative sample from center and border of lesion	The specimen should be aseptically placed into appropriate sterile container; an adequate quantity of specimen must be collected to recover small numbers of organisms.
Urine: midstream	Sterile urine container	Bacteria: 1 ml Mycobacteria: ≥10 ml	Contamination of the specimen with bacteria from the urethra or vagina should be avoided; the first portion of the voided specimen is discarded; organisms can grow rapidly in urine; so, specimens must be transported immediately to the laboratory, held in bacteriostatic preservative, or refrigerated.
Urine: catheterized	Sterile urine container	Bacteria: 1 ml Mycobacteria: ≥10 ml	Catheterization is not recommended for routine cultures (risk of inducing infection); the first portion of collected specimen is contaminated with urethral bacteria, so it should be discarded (similar to midstream voided specimen); the specimen must be transported rapidly to the laboratory.
Urine: suprapubic aspirate	Sterile anaerobic tube or vial	Bacteria: 1 ml Mycobacteria: ≥10 ml	This is an invasive specimen, so urethral bacteria are avoided; it is the only valid method available for collecting specimens for anaerobic culture; it is also useful for collection of specimens from children or adults unable to void uncontaminated specimens.
Genitals	Specially designed swabs for *Neisseria gonorrhoeae* and *Chlamydia* probes	N/A	The area of inflammation or exudate should be sampled; the endocervix (not vagina) and urethra should be cultured for optimal detection.
Feces (stool)	Sterile screw-capped container	N/A	Rapid transport to the laboratory is necessary to prevent production of acid (bactericidal for some enteric pathogens) by normal fecal bacteria; it is unsuitable for anaerobic culture; because a large number of different media will be inoculated, a swab should not be used for specimen collection.

N/A, Not applicable.

Table 7-2　Detection Methods for Bacteria.

Organism	Detection Methods				
	Microscopy	Antigen Detection	Nucleic Acid-Based Tests	Culture	Antibody Detection
Gram-Positive Cocci					
Staphylococcus aureus	A	B	C	A	D
Streptococcus pyogenes	B	A	A	A	B
Streptococcus agalactiae	B	B	B	A	D
Streptococcus pneumoniae	A	B	C	A	C
Enterococcus spp.	A	D	B	A	D
Gram-Positive Rods					
Bacillus anthracis	B	C	B	A	D
Bacillus cereus	B	D	D	B	D
Listeria monocytogenes	A	D	D	A	D
Erysipelothrix rhusiopathiae	A	D	D	A	D
Corynebacterium diphtheriae	B	D	C	A	D
Corynebacterium, other spp.	A	D	D	A	D
Tropheryma whipplei	B	D	A	D	D
Acid-Fast and Partially Acid-Fast Rods					
Nocardia spp.	A	D	D	A	D
Rhodococcus equi	A	D	D	A	D
Mycobacterium tuberculosis	A	B	B	A	C
Mycobacterium leprae	B	D	D	D	B
Mycobacterium, other spp.	A	D	B	A	D
Gram-Negative Cocci					
Neisseria gonorrheae	A	D	A	A	D
Neisseria meningitidis	A	B	D	A	D
Moraxella catarrhalis	A	D	D	A	D
Gram-Negative Rods					
Escherichia coli	A	B	C	A	D
Salmonella spp.	B	D	D	A	B
Shigella spp.	B	D	D	A	D
Yersinia pestis	B	C	B	A	C
Yersinia enterocolitica	B	D	D	A	B
Enterobacteriaceae, various genera	A	D	D	A	D
Vibrio cholerae	B	D	D	A	D
Vibrio, other spp.	B	D	D	A	D
Aeromonas spp.	B	D	D	A	D
Campylobacter spp.	B	A	D	A	D
Helicobacter pylori	B	A	C	B	A
Pseudomonas aeruginosa	A	D	D	A	D
Burkholderia spp.	A	D	D	A	D
Acinetobacter spp.	A	D	D	A	D
Haemophilus influenzae	A	B	C	A	D
Haemophilus ducreyi	B	D	C	A	D
Bordetella pertussis	B	C	A	B	A
Brucella spp.	B	C	D	A	B

Table 7-2 Detection Methods for Bacteria. (Continued)

Organism	Microscopy	Antigen Detection	Nucleic Acid-Based Tests	Culture	Antibody Detection
Francisella tularensis	B	C	D	A	B
Legionella spp.	B	A	B	A	B
Bartonella spp.	C	D	B	A	A
Anaerobes					
Clostridium perfringens	A	D	D	A	D
Clostridium tetani	B	D	D	A	D
Clostridium botulinum	B	A	D	B	D
Clostridium difficile	B	A	B	B	D
Anaerobic gram-positive cocci	A	D	D	A	D
Anaerobic gram-positive rods	A	D	D	A	D
Anaerobic gram-negative rods	A	D	D	A	D
Spiral-Shaped Bacteria					
Treponema pallidum	B	D	D	D	A
Borrelia burgdorferi	C	D	A	B	A
Borrelia, other spp.	A	D	D	B	D
Leptospira spp.	B	D	D	B	A
Mycoplasma and Obligate Intracellular Bacteria					
Mycoplasma pneumoniae	D	C	A	B	A
Rickettsia spp.	B	D	C	D	A
Orientia spp.	B	C	C	C	A
Ehrlichia spp.	B	C	C	C	A
Anaplasma spp.	B	C	C	C	A
Coxiella burnetii	C	C	C	C	A
Chlamydia trachomatis	B	B	A	B	D
Chlamydophila pneumoniae	D	D	B	C	B
Chlamydophila psittaci	D	D	B	D	A

A, Test generally useful for diagnosis; *B*, test useful under certain circumstances or for the diagnosis of specific forms of disease; *C*, test generally not used in diagnostic laboratories or used only in specialty reference laboratories; *D*, test generally not useful.

Clinical specimens or suspensions of microorganisms can be placed on a glass slide and examined under the microscope. The specimen or organism can be stained by a variety of methods (Table 7-3).

DETECTION OF SPECIFIC BACTERIAL NUCLEIC ACIDS

Like the evidence left at the scene of a crime, the DNA (deoxyribonucleic acid), RNA (ribonucleic acid) of an infectious agent in a clinical sample can be used to help identify the agent. In many cases, the agent can be detected and identified in this way. New techniques and adaptations of older techniques are being developed for the analysis of infectious agents.

The advantages of molecular techniques are their sensitivity, specificity, and safety. From the standpoint of safety, these techniques do not require isolation of the infectious agent and can be performed on chemically fixed (inactivated) samples or extracts. Because of their sensitivity, very dilute samples of microbial DNA can be detected in a tissue, even if the agent is not replicating or producing other evidence of infection. These techniques can distinguish related strains on the basis of differences in their genotype (i.e., mutants).

Table 7-3   Microscopic Preparations and Stains Used in the Clinical Microbiology Laboratory

Staining Method	Principle and Applications
Direct Examination	
Wet mount	Unstained preparation is examined by brightfield, darkfield, or phase-contrast microscopy.
10% KOH	KOH is used to dissolve proteinaceous material and facilitate detection of fungal elements that are not affected by strong alkali solution. Dyes such as lactophenol cotton blue can be added to increase contrast between fungal elements and background.
India ink	Modification of KOH procedure in which ink is added as contrast material. Dye primarily used to detect *Cryptococcus* spp. in cerebrospinal fluid and other body fluids. Polysaccharide capsule of *Cryptococcus* spp. excludes ink, creating halo around yeast cell.
Lugol's iodine	Iodine is added to wet preparations of parasitology specimens to enhance contrast of internal structures. This facilitates differentiation of ameba and host white blood cells.
Differential Stains	
Gram stain	Most commonly used stain in microbiology laboratory, forming basis for separating major groups of bacteria (e.g., gram-positive, gram-negative). After fixation of specimen to glass slide (by heating or alcohol treatment), specimen is exposed to crystal violet, and then iodine is added to form complex with primary dye. During decolorization with alcohol or acetone, complex is retained in gram-positive bacteria but lost in gram-negative organisms; counterstain safranin is retained by gram-negative organisms (hence their red color). The degree to which organism retains stain is function of organism, culture conditions, and staining skills of the microscopist.
Iron hematoxylin stain	Used for detection and identification of fecal protozoa. Helminth eggs and larvae retain too much stain and are more easily identified with wet-mount preparation.
Methenamine silver	In general, performed in histology laboratories rather than in microbiology laboratories. Used primarily for stain detection of fungal elements in tissue, although other organisms, such as bacteria, can be detected. Silver staining requires skill, because nonspecific staining can render slides unable to be interpreted.
Toluidine blue O stain	Used primarily for detection of *Pneumocystis* organisms in respiratory specimens. Cysts stain reddish-blue to dark purple on light-blue background. Background staining is removed by sulfation reagent. Yeast cells stain and are difficult to distinguish from *Pneumocystis* cells. Trophozoites do not stain. Many laboratories have replaced this stain with specific fluorescent stains.
Trichrome stain	Alternative to iron hematoxylin for staining protozoa. Protozoa have bluish-green to purple cytoplasms with red or purplish-red nuclei and inclusion bodies; specimen background is green.
Wright-Giemsa stain	Used to detect blood parasites; viral and chlamydial inclusion bodies; and *Borrelia, Toxoplasma, Pneumocystis,* and *Rickettsia* spp. This is a polychromatic stain that contains a mixture of methylene blue, azure B, and eosin Y. Giemsa stain combines methylene blue and eosin. Eosin ions are negatively charged and stain basic components of cells orange to pink, whereas other dyes stain acidic cell structures various shades of blue to purple. Protozoan trophozoites have a red nucleus and grayish-blue cytoplasm; intracellular yeasts and inclusion bodies typically stain blue; rickettsiae, chlamydiae, and *Pneumocystis* spp. stain purple.
Acid-Fast Stains	
Ziehl-Neelsen stain	Used to stain mycobacteria and other acid-fast organisms. Organisms are stained with basic carbolfuchsin and resist decolorization with acid-alkali solutions. Background is counterstained with methylene blue. Organisms appear red against light-blue background. Uptake of carbolfuchsin requires heating specimen (hot acid-fast stain).
Kinyoun stain	Cold acid-fast stain (does not require heating). Same principle as Ziehl-Neelsen stain.
Auramine-rhodamine	Same principle as other acid-fast stains, except that fluorescent dyes (auramine and rhodamine) are used stain for primary stain and potassium permanganate (strong oxidizing agent) is the counterstain and inactivates unbound fluorochrome dyes. Organisms fluoresce yellowish-green against a black background.
Modified acid-fast stain	Weak decolorizing agent is used with any of three acid-fast stains listed. Whereas mycobacteria are strongly acid-fast, other organisms stain weaker (e.g., *Nocardia, Rhodococcus, Tsukamurella, Gordonia, Cryptosporidium, Isospora, Sarcocystis,* and *Cyclospora*). These organisms can be stained more efficiently by using a weak decolorizing agent. Organisms that retain this stain are referred to as partially acid-fast.

Table 7-3 Microscopic Preparations and Stains Used in the Clinical Microbiology Laboratory (Continued)

Staining Method	Principle and Applications
Fluorescent Stains	
Acridine orange stain	Used for detection of bacteria and fungi in clinical specimens. Dye intercalates into nucleic acid (native and denatured). At neutral pH, bacteria, fungi, and cellular material stain reddish-orange. At acid pH (4.0), bacteria and fungi remain reddish-orange, but background material stains greenish-yellow.
Auramine-rhodamine stain	Same as acid-fast stains.
Calcofluor white stain	Used to detect fungal elements and *Pneumocystis* spp. Stain binds to cellulose and chitin in cell walls; microscopist can mix dye with KOH. (Many laboratories have replaced traditional KOH stain with this stain.)
Direct fluorescent antibody stain	Antibodies (monoclonal or polyclonal) are complexed with fluorescent molecules. Specific binding to an organism is detected by presence of microbial fluorescence. Technique has proved useful for detecting or identifying many organisms (e.g., *Streptococcus pyogenes*, *Bordetella*, *Francisella*, *Legionella*, *Chlamydia*, *Pneumocystis*, *Cryptosporidium*, *Giardia*, influenza virus, herpes simplex virus). Sensitivity and specificity of the test are determined by the number of organisms present in the test sample and quality of antibodies used in reagents.

KOH, Potassium hydroxide.

Electrophoretic Analysis of DNA and Restriction Fragment Length Polymorphism

The genome structure and genetic sequence are major distinguishing characteristics of the family, type, and strain of microorganism. Specific strains of microorganisms can be distinguished on the basis of their DNA or RNA or by the DNA fragments produced when the DNA is cleaved by specific restriction endonucleases (**restriction enzymes**). The differences in the length of the DNA fragments among the different strains of a specific organism produced on cleavage with one or more restriction endonucleases is termed **restriction fragment length polymorphism (RFLP)**.

DNA or RNA fragments of different sizes or structures can be distinguished by their electrophoretic mobility in an agarose or polyacrylamide gel. Smaller fragments (fewer than 20,000 base pairs), such as those from bacterial plasmids or from viruses, can be separated and distinguished by normal electrophoretic methods. Larger fragments, such as those from whole bacteria, can be separated only by using a special electrophoretic technique called *pulsed-field gel electrophoresis*.

RFLP has been used to show the spread of necrotizing fasciitis produced by a strain of *Streptococcus* from one patient to other patients, an emergency medical technician, and the emergency department and attending physicians (Figure 7-1). Often, comparison of the 16S ribosomal RNA is used to identify different bacteria.

Nucleic Acid Detection, Amplification, and Sequencing

DNA probes can be used like antibodies as sensitive and specific tools to detect, locate, and quantitate specific nucleic acid sequences in clinical specimens. Because of the specificity and sensitivity of DNA probe techniques, individual species or strains of an infectious agent can be detected, even if they are not growing or replicating.

The DNA probes are labeled with radioactive or chemically modified nucleotides (e.g., biotinylated uridine) so that they can be detected and quantitated. The DNA probes can detect specific genetic sequences in fixed, permeabilized tissue biopsy specimens by **in situ hybridization**. When fluorescent detection is used, it is called **FISH: fluorescent in situ hybridization**. There are now many commercially available microbial probes and kits for detecting bacteria.

The **polymerase chain reaction (PCR)** amplifies single copies of bacterial DNA millions of times over and is one of the newest techniques of genetic analy-

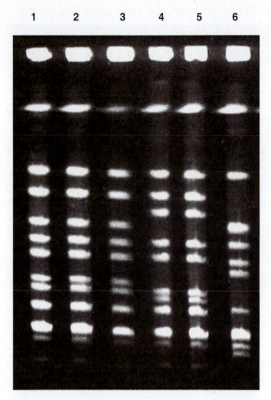

Figure 7-1 Restriction fragment length polymorphism distinction of DNA from bacterial strains separated by pulsed-field gel electrophoresis. Lanes 1 to 3 show Sma 1 restriction endonuclease-digested DNA from bacteria from two family members with necrotizing fasciitis and from their physician (pharyngitis). Lanes 4 to 6 are from unrelated *Streptococcus pyogenes* strains. (Courtesy Dr. Joe DiPersio, Akron, Ohio.)

DNA **sequencing** has become sufficiently fast and inexpensive to allow laboratory determination of microbial sequences for identification of microbes. Sequencing of the 16S ribosomal subunit can be used to identify specific bacteria.

The molecular techniques used to identify infectious agents are summarized in Table 7-4.

DETECTION OF BACTERIAL ANTIGENS

Immunologic techniques are used to detect, identify, and quantitate antigen in clinical samples. Antibodies can be used as sensitive and specific tools to detect, identify, and quantitate the antigens from a bacterium. The specificity of the antibody-antigen interaction and the sensitivity of many of the immunologic techniques make them powerful laboratory tools (Table 7-5). *In most cases, the same technique can be adapted to evaluate antigen and antibody.*

Antibody-antigen complexes can be detected directly, by precipitation techniques, or by labeling the antibody with a radioactive, fluorescent, or enzyme probe, or they can be detected indirectly through measurement of an antibody-directed reaction, such as complement fixation.

Specific antigen-antibody complexes and cross-reactivity can be distinguished by immunoprecipitation techniques. **Single radial immunodiffusion** can be used to detect and quantify an antigen. The **Ouchterlony immuno-double-diffusion** technique is used to determine the relatedness of different anti-

sis. The **real-time PCR** can be used to quantitate the amount of DNA or RNA in a sample after it is converted to DNA by reverse transcriptase. PCR assays are especially useful for detecting bacterial sequences, such as in *N gonorrhoeae*, *M tuberculosis*, and other bacteria.

Table 7-4 Molecular Techniques Used to Identify Bacteria

Technique	Purpose	Clinical Examples
RFLP	Comparison of DNA	Molecular epidemiology, comparison of DNA from bacterial strains
FISH: fluorescent in situ hybridization	Comparison of DNA	Detection of bacteria and other microbes
Pulsed-field gel electrophoresis	Comparison of DNA (large pieces of DNA)	Streptococcal strain comparisons
PCR	Amplification of very dilute DNA samples	Detection of *N gonorrhoeae*, *M tuberculosis*
Real-time PCR	Quantification of very dilute DNA and RNA samples	Quantitation of bacterial DNA
DNA sequencing	Comparison of DNA	Sequencing of the 16S ribosomal subunit can be used to identify specific bacteria

DNA, Deoxyribonucleic acid; *PCR*, polymerase chain reaction; *RFLP*, restriction fragment length polymorphism; *RNA*, ribonucleic acid.

Table 7-5 Selected Immunologic Techniques

Technique	Purpose	Clinical Examples
Ouchterlony immuno-double-diffusion	Detect and compare antigen and antibody	Fungal antigen and antibody
Immunofluorescence	Detection and localization of antigen	Viral antigen in biopsy (e.g., rabies, herpes simplex virus)
Enzyme immunoassay (EIA)	Same as immunofluorescence	Same as immunofluorescence
Immunofluorescence flow cytometry	Population analysis of antigen-positive cells	Immunophenotyping
ELISA	Quantitation of antigen or antibody	Viral antigen (rotavirus); viral antibody (anti-HIV)
Western blot	Detection of antigen-specific antibody	Confirmation of anti-HIV seropositivity
Radioimmunoassay (RIA)	Same as ELISA	Same as for ELISA
Complement fixation	Quantitate specific antibody titer	Fungal, viral antibody
Hemagglutination inhibition	Antiviral antibody titer; serotype of virus strain	Seroconversion to current influenza strain; identification of influenza
Latex agglutination	Quantitation and detection of antigen and antibody	Rheumatoid factor; fungal antigens; streptococcal antigens

ELISA, Enzyme-linked immunosorbent assay; *HIV*, human immunodeficiency virus.

gens. **Agglutination tests** can be used to detect bacterial antigens present in clinical specimens. **Latex agglutination** is a rapid, technically simple assay for detecting antibody or soluble antigen.

The enzyme immunoassay (EIA), including **enzyme-linked immunosorbent assay (ELISA)** can be used to quantitate the soluble bacterial antigen and antibody in a patient's sample. The many variations of ELISAs differ in the way in which they capture or detect antibody or antigen. **Western blot analysis** is a variation of an ELISA. This technique shows the proteins recognized by the patient serum. For example, Western blot analysis is used to distinguish antibody of Lyme disease.

Complement fixation is a standard but technically difficult serologic test. Antibodies measured by this system generally develop slightly later in an illness than those measured by other techniques.

VITRO CULTURE

The success of culture methods is defined by the biology of the organism, the site of the infection, the patient's immune response to the infection, and the quality of the culture media. The bacterium *Legionella* is an important respiratory pathogen; however, it was never grown in culture until it was recognized that recovery of the organism required using media supplemented with iron and L-cysteine. *Campylobacter*, an important enteric pathogen, was not recovered in stool specimens until highly selective media were incubated at 42°C in a microaerophilic atmosphere. *Staphylococcus aureus*, the cause of staphylococcal toxic shock syndrome, produces disease by release of a toxin into the circulatory system. Culture of blood will almost always be negative, but culture of the site where the organism is growing will detect the organism. In many infections (e.g., gastroenteritis, pharyngitis, urethritis), the organism responsible for the infection will be present among many other organisms that are part of the normal microbial population at the site of infection. Many media have been developed that suppress the normally present microbes and allow easier detection of clinically important organisms. The patient's innate and adaptive immunity may suppress the pathogen; so highly sensitive culture techniques are frequently required. Likewise, some infections are characterized by the presence of relatively few organisms. Finally, the quality of the media must be carefully monitored to demonstrate it will perform as designed.

Types of Culture Media

Culture media can be subdivided into four general categories: (1) enriched nonselective media, (2) selective media, (3) differential media, and (4) specialized media. Some examples of these media are summarized below (Table 7-6).

Antimicrobial Susceptibility Tests

The results of in vitro antimicrobial susceptibility testing are valuable for selecting chemotherapeutic agents active against the infecting organism. The selection of an antibiotic and the patient's outcome are influenced by a variety of interrelated factors, including the pharmacokinetic properties of the antibiotic, drug toxicity, the clinical disease, and the patient's general medical status. Thus some organisms that are "susceptible" to an antibiotic will persist in an infection, and some organisms that are "resistant" to an antibiotic will be eliminated.

Two general forms of antimicrobial susceptibil-ity tests are performed in clinical laboratory: **broth dilution tests** and **agar diffusion tests**. For the broth dilution tests, serial dilutions of an antibiotic are prepared in a nutrient medium and then inoculated with a standardized concentration of the test bacterium. After overnight incubation, the lowest concentration of antibiotic that is able to inhibit the growth of the bacteria is referred to as the **minimum inhibitory concentration (MIC)**. For the agar diffusion tests, a standardized concentration of bacteria is spread over the surface of an agar medium and then paper disks or strips impregnated with antibiotics are placed on the agar surface. After overnight incubation, an area of inhibited growth is observed surrounding the paper disks or strips. The size of the area of inhibition corresponds to the activity of the antibiotic—the more susceptible the organism is to the antibiotic, the larger the area of inhibited growth. By standardizing the test conditions for the agar diffusion tests, the area of inhibition corresponds to the MIC value.

Table 7-6 Types of Culture Media

Type	Media (examples)	Purpose
Nonselective	Blood agar	Recovery of bacteria and fungi
	Chocolate agar	Recovery of bacteria including *Haemophilus* and *Neisseria gonorrheae*
	Mueller-Hinton agar	Bacterial susceptibility test medium
	Thioglycolate broth	Enrichment broth for anaerobic bacteria
	Sabouraud dextrose agar	Recovery of fungi
Selective, differential	MacConkey agar	Selective for gram-negative bacteria; differential for lactose-fermenting species
	Mannitol salt agar	Selective for staphylococci; differential for *Staphylococcus aureus*
	Xylose lysine deoxycholate agar	Selective, differential agar for *Salmonella* and *Shigella* in enteric cultures
	Lowenstein-Jensen medium	Selective for mycobacteria
	Middlebrook agar	Selective for mycobacteria
	CHROMagar	Selective, differential for yeast
	Inhibitory mold agar	Selective for molds
Specialized	Buffered charcoal yeast extract (BCYE) agar	Recovery of *Legionella* and *Nocardia*
	Cystine-tellurite agar	Recovery of *Corynebacterium diphtheriae*
	Lim broth	Recovery of *Streptococcus agalactiae*
	MacConkey sorbitol agar	Recovery of *Escherichia coli* O157
	Regan Lowe agar	Recovery of *Bordetella pertussis*
	Thiosulfate citrate bile salts sucrose (TCBS) agar	Recovery of *Vibrio* species

Broth dilution tests were originally performed in test tubes and were very labor intensive. Commercially prepared systems are now available where the antibiotic dilutions are prepared in microtiter trays, and the inoculation of the trays and interpretation of the MICs are automated. The disadvantages of these systems are the range of different antibiotics is determined by the manufacturer, and the number of dilutions of an individual antibiotic is limited. Thus results may not be available for newly introduced antibiotics. Diffusion tests are labor intensive and the interpretation of the size of the area of inhibition can be subjective; however, the advantage of these tests is that virtually any antibiotic can be tested. The ability of both susceptibility testing methods to predict clinical response to an antibiotic is equivalent; so, the selection of the tests is determined by practical considerations.

SEROLOGIC DIAGNOSIS

The humoral immune response provides a history of a patient's infections. Serology can be used to identify the infecting agent, evaluate the course of an infection, or determine the nature of the infection— whether it is a primary infection or a reinfection, and whether it is acute or chronic. The antibody type and titer and the identity of the antigenic targets provide serologic data about an infection. Serologic testing is used to identify bacteria and other agents that are difficult to isolate and grow in the laboratory or that cause diseases that progress slowly.

The relative antibody concentration is reported as a titer. A **titer** is the inverse of the greatest dilution, or lowest concentration (e.g., dilution of 1:64 = titer of 64), of a patient's serum that retains activity in one of the immunoassays just described. Serology is used to determine the time course of an infection. **Seroconversion** occurs when antibody is produced in response to a primary infection. *Specific IgM antibody, found during the first 2 to 3 weeks of a primary infection, is a good indicator of a recent primary infection.* Reinfection or recurrence later in life causes an **anamnestic** (secondary or booster) response. Anti-

body titers may remain high, however, in patients whose disease recurs frequently. Seroconversion or reinfection is indicated by the finding *of at least a fourfold increase in the antibody titer between serum obtained during the acute phase of disease and that obtained at least 2 to 3 weeks later during the convalescent phase.* A twofold serial dilution will not distinguish between samples with 512 and 1023 units of antibody, both of which would give a reaction on a 512-fold dilution but not on a 1024-fold dilution, and both results would be reported as titers of 512. On the other hand, samples with 1020 and 1030 units are not significantly different but would be reported as titers of 512 and 1024, respectively.

Although many organisms can be specifically identified by a variety of techniques, the most common procedure used in diagnostic laboratories is to identify an organism isolated in culture by biochemical tests. In large teaching hospital laboratories and reference laboratories, many of the biochemical test procedures have been replaced recently with sequencing bacterial specific genes (e.g., 16S rRNA gene) or using proteomic tools, such as mass spectrometry, to identify organisms. However, we believe most students using this textbook are not interested in the details of microbial identification. Those who are interested should refer to textbooks such as *Bailey and Scott's Diagnostic Microbiology*, the *ASM Manual of Clinical Microbiology*, and reviews that specifically cover this topic.

It is important for all students to appreciate that empiric antimicrobial therapy can be refined based on the preliminary identification of an organism using microscopic and macroscopic morphology and selected, rapid biochemical tests. Refer to Table 7-7 for specific examples.

SUMMARY

For laboratory diagnosis of bacteria diseases, collection of the proper specimen is very important. After sampling, rapidly deliver the specimen to the clinical laboratory. The general procedure of detection methods include microscopy, detection of bacterial

Table 7-7   Preliminary Identification of Bacteria Isolated in Culture

Organism	Properties
Staphylococcus aureus	Gram-positive cocci in clusters; large, β-hemolytic colonies; catalase-positive, coagulase-positive
Streptococcus pyogenes	Gram-positive cocci in long chains; small colonies with large zone of β-hemolysis; catalase-negative, PYR-positive (*L*-pyrrolidonyl arylamidase)
Streptococcus pneumoniae	Gram-positive cocci in pairs and short chains; small, α-hemolytic colonies; catalase-negative, soluble in bile
Enterococcus spp.	Gram-positive cocci in pairs and short chains; large, α- or nonhemolytic colonies; catalase-negative, PYR-positive
Listeria monocytogenes	Small, gram-positive rods; small, weakly β-hemolytic colonies; characteristic (tumbling) motility
Nocardia spp.	Weakly staining (Gram and modified acid-fast), thin, filamentous, branching rods; slow growth; fuzzy colonies (aerial hyphae)
Rhodococcus equi	Weakly staining (Gram and modified acid-fast); initially nonbranching rods, cocci in older cultures; slow growth; pink-red colonies
Mycobacterium tuberculosis	Strongly acid-fast rods; slow growth; nonpigmented colonies; identified using specific molecular probes
Enterobacteriaceae	Gram-negative rods with "bipolar" staining (more intense at ends); typically single cells; large colonies; growth on MacConkey agar (may/may not ferment lactose); oxidase-negative
Pseudomonas aeruginosa	Gram-negative rods with uniform staining; typically in pairs; large spreading, fluorescent green colonies, usually β-hemolytic, fruity smell (grapelike); growth on MacConkey agar (nonfermenter); oxidase-positive
Stenotrophomonas maltophila	Gram-negative rods with uniform staining; typically in pairs; lavender-green color on blood agar; growth on MacConkey agar (nonfermenter); oxidase-negative
Acinetobacter spp.	Large, gram-negative coccobacilli arranged as single cells or pairs; will retain crystal violet and may resemble fat, gram-positive cocci in pairs; growth on blood agar and MacConkey agar (may oxidize lactose and resemble weakly purple); oxidase-negative
Campylobacter spp.	Thin, curved, gram-negative rods, arranged in pairs (S-shaped pairs); growth on highly selective media for *Campylobacter*; no growth on routine media (blood, chocolate, or MacConkey agars)
Haemophilus spp.	Small, gram-negative coccobacilli, arranged as single cells; growth on chocolate agar but not blood or MacConkey agars; oxidase-positive
Brucella spp.	Very small, gram-negative coccobacilli, arranged as single cells; slow-growing; no growth on MacConkey agar; biohazard
Francisella spp.	Very small, gram-negative coccobacilli, arranged as single cells; slow-growing, no growth on blood or MacConkey agars; biohazard
Legionella spp.	Weakly staining, thin, gram-negative rods; slow-growing; growth on specialized agar; no growth on blood, chocolate, or MacConkey agars
Clostridium perfringens	Large, rectangular rods with spores not observed; rapid growth of spreading colonies with "double zone" of hemolysis (large zone of α-hemolysis with inner zone of β-hemolysis); strict anaerobe
Bacteroides fragilis group	Weakly staining, pleomorphic (variable lengths), gram-negative rods; rapid growth stimulated by bile in media; strict anaerobe

antigens, nucleic acid-based tests and culture. The detection of antibody response to the bacteria is also useful. The *new experimental techniques* include sequencing bacterial specific genes (e.g., 16S rRNA gene), mass spectrometry (MS), etc.

KEYWORDS

English	Chinese
Culture media	培养基
Enriched nonselective media	非选择性增菌培养基
Antimicrobial susceptibility tests	抗菌药物敏感试验

Minimum inhibitory concentration 最小抑菌浓度
(MIC)
Serologic diagnosis 血清学诊断

BIBLIOGRAPHY

1. Chapin K: Principles of stains and media. In Murray P, et al, editors: Manual of clinical microbiology, ed 9, Washington, DC, 2007, American Society for Microbiology Press.

2. DiPersio JR, et al: Spread of serious disease-producing M3 clones of group A *Streptococcus* among family members and health care workers, Clin Infect Dis 22: 490-495, 1996.

3. Forbes BA, Sahm DF, Weissfeld AS: Bailey and Scott's diagnostic microbiology, ed 12, St Louis, 2007, Mosby.

4. Fredericks DN, Relman DA: Application of polymerase chain reaction to the diagnosis of infectious diseases, Clin Infect Dis 29: 475-486, 1999.

5. Mandell G, Bennett J, Dolin R: Principles and practice of infectious diseases, ed 7, New York, 2009, Churchill Livingstone.

6. Millar BC, Xu J, Moore JE: Molecular diagnostics of medically important bacterial infections, Curr Issues Mol Biol 9: 21-40, 2007.

7. Murray PR: ASM pocket guide to clinical microbiology, ed 3, Washington, DC, 2004, American Society for Microbiology Press.

8. Murray PR, et al: Manual of clinical microbiology, ed 9, Washington, DC, 2007, American Society for Microbiology Press.

9. Persing DS, et al: Molecular microbiology, diagnostic principles and practice, ed 2, Washington, DC, 2011, American Society for Microbiology Press.

10. Snyder J, Atlas R: Handbook of media for clinical microbiology, ed 2, Boca Raton, Fla, 2006, CRC Press.

11. Wiedbrauk D: Microscopy. In Murray P, et al, editors: Manual of clinical microbiology, ed 9, Washington, DC, 2007, American Society for Microbiology.

12. Zimbro M, Power D: Difco and BBL manual: manual of microbiological culture media, Sparks, Md, 2003, Becton Dickinson and Company.

13. Versalovic J, et al: Manual of clinical microbiology, ed 10, Washington, DC, 2011, American Society for Microbiology Press.

Antimicrobial Vaccines

Chapter

8

Immunity, whether generated in reaction to immunization or administered as therapy, can prevent or lessen the serious symptoms of disease by **blocking the spread** of a bacterium, bacterial toxin, or other microbe to its target organ or by acting rapidly at the site of infection. The memory immune responses activated upon challenge of an immunized individual are faster and stronger than for an unimmunized individual. The immunization of a population, like personal immunity, stops the spread of the infectious agent by reducing the number of susceptible hosts.

ACTIVE IMMUNIZATION

Active immunization occurs when an immune response is stimulated because of challenge with an immunogen, such as exposure to an infectious agent (**natural immunization**) or through exposure to microbes or their antigens in **vaccines**.

Classical vaccines can be subdivided into two groups on the basis of whether they elicit an immune response on infection (**live attenuated vaccines** such as vaccinia) or not (**inactivated-subunit-killed vaccines**) (Figure 8-1). **Deoxyribonucleic acid (DNA) vaccines** represent a new means of immunization. In this approach, plasmid DNA is injected into muscle or skin, then taken up by dendritic, muscle, or macrophage cells, which express the gene for the immunogen as if for a natural infection. DNA vaccination stimulates T-cell immune responses, which can be boosted with antigen to elicit mature antibody responses.

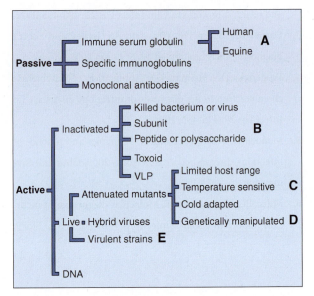

Figure 8-1 Types of immunizations. Antibodies (passive immunization) can be provided to block the action of an infectious agent, or an immune response can be elicited (active immunization) by natural infection or vaccination. The different forms of passive and active immunization are indicated. **A,** Equine antibodies can be used if human antibody is not available. **B,** Vaccine can consist of components purified from the infectious agent or can be developed through genetic engineering (virus-like particle [VLP]). **C,** Vaccine selected by passage at low or high temperature, in animals, embryonated eggs, or tissue culture cells. **D,** Deletion, insertion, reassortment, and other laboratory-derived mutants. **E,** Vaccine composed of a virus from a different species, which has a common antigen with the human virus.

Inactivated Vaccines

Inactivated vaccines (killed vaccines) can be produced by chemical (e.g., formalin) or heat inactivation of bacteria, bacterial toxins, or by purification or synthesis of the components or subunits of the infectious agents. There are three major types of inactivated bacterial vaccines: **toxoid** (inactivated toxins), **inactivated (killed)** bacteria, and **capsule or protein subunits** of the bacteria. Inactivated vaccines utilize a large amount of antigen to produce a protective antibody response but without the risk of infection by the agent. These vaccines usually generate antibody (TH2 responses) and limited cell-mediated immune responses.

Inactivated vaccines are generally safe, except in people who have allergic reactions to vaccine components. Inactivated vaccines of *Salmonella typhi*, *Vibrio cholerae*, *Neiseria meningitis*, and *Leptospira interrogans* are available.

Live attenuated vaccines

Live attenuated vaccines are prepared with organisms limited in their ability to cause disease (e.g., **avirulent** or **attenuated** organisms). Immunization with a live vaccine resembles the natural infection in that the immune response progresses through the natural innate, TH1, and then TH2 immune responses, and humoral, cellular, and memory immune responses are developed. Immunity is generally long lived and, depending on the route of administration, can mimic the normal immune response to the infecting agent. The advantages and disadvantages of live attenuated vaccines are compared to inactivated vaccines in Table 8-1.

Live attenuated vaccines consist of less virulent mutants (**attenuated**) of the wild-type organisms, or genetically engineered strains lacking virulence properties. BCG, plaque, or anthrax vaccines are representative for typical live attenuated vaccines.

Subunit vaccines

A **subunit vaccine** consists of the bacterial components that elicit a protective immune response. The immunogenic component can be isolated from the bacterium by biochemical means, or the vaccine can be prepared through genetic engineering approaches. For example, the subunit vaccine against *H. influenzae* B, *Neisseria meningitidis*, *Salmonella typhi*, and *S. pneumoniae* (23 strains) are prepared from capsular polysaccharides. Unfortunately, polysaccharides are generally poor immunogens (T-independent antigens). The meningococcal vaccine contains the polysaccharides of four major serotypes (A, C, Y, and

Table 8-1 Advantages and Disadvantages of Live versus Inactivated Vaccines

Property	Live	Inactivated
Route of administration	Natural[*] or injection	Injection
Dose of virus, cost	Low	High
Number of doses, amount	Single,[†] low	Multiple, high
Need for adjuvant	No	Yes[‡]
Duration of immunity	Long-term	Short-term
Antibody response	IgG, IgA[§]	IgG
Cell-mediated immune response	Good	Poor
Heat lability in tropics	Yes[‖]	No
Interference[¶]	Occasional	None
Side effects	Occasional mild symptoms[**]	Occasional sore arm
Reversion to virulence	Rarely	None

Ig, Immunoglobulin.
[*]Oral or respiratory, in certain cases.
[†]A single booster may be required (yellow fever, measles, rubella) after 6 to 10 years.
[‡]However, the commonly used alum is inefficient.
[§]IgA if delivered via the oral or respiratory route.
[‖]Magnesium chloride and other stabilizers and cold storage assist preservation.
[¶]Interference from other viruses or diseases may prevent sufficient infection and immunity.
[**]Especially rubella and measles.
From White DO, Fenner FJ: *Medical virology*, ed 3, New York, 1986, Academic.

W-135). The pneumococcal vaccine contains polysaccharides from 23 serotypes. The immunogenicity of polysaccharides can be enhanced by chemical linkage to a protein carrier (**conjugate vaccine**) (e.g., diphtheria toxoid, *N. meningitidis* outer membrane protein, or *Corynebacterium diphtheriae* protein) (Figure 8-2). The *H. influenzae* B (Hib) polysaccharide-diphtheria toxoid carrier complex is approved for administration to infants and children. An *S. pneumoniae* "pneumococcal" conjugate vaccine has been developed in which polysaccharide from the thirteen most prevalent strains in the United States is attached to a nontoxic form of the diphtheria toxin. This vaccine is available for use in infants and young children. The other polysaccharide vaccines are less immunogenic and should be administered to individuals older than 2 years.

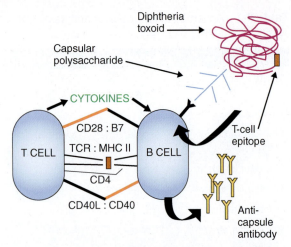

Figure 8-2 Capsular polysaccharide conjugate vaccines. Capsular polysaccharides are poor immunogens, do not elicit T-cell help, and only elicit IgM without memory. Capsule polysaccharide conjugated to a protein (e.g., diphtheria toxoid) binds to surface antipolysaccharide IgM on the B cell, the complex is internalized, processed and then a peptide is presented on major histocompatibility complex II (MHC II) to CD4 T cells. The T cells become activated, produce cytokines, and promote immunoglobulin class switching for the polysaccharide specific B cell. The B cell can become activated, make IgG, and memory cells will develop. TCR, T-cell receptor.

Genetically Engineered Subunit Vaccines

Genetically engineered subunit vaccines are being developed through cloning of genes that encode immunogenic proteins into bacterial and eukaryotic vectors. The greatest difficulties in the development of such vaccines are (1) identifying the appropriate subunit or peptide immunogen that can elicit protective antibody and, ideally, T-cell responses and (2) presenting the antigen in the correct conformation. Once identified, the gene can be isolated, cloned, and expressed in bacteria or yeast cells, and then large quantities of these proteins can be produced. The surface antigen of *Shigella sonnei* has been cloned into a plasmid vector and the proteins has been generated in *Salmonella typhi* Ty21a for use as subunit vaccines.

Recombinant Vector Vaccine

Molecular biology techniques are being used to develop new vaccines. New live attenuated vaccines can be created by genetic engineering mutations to inactivate or delete a virulence gene instead of through random attenuation of the virus by passage through tissue culture. Genes from infectious agents that cannot be properly attenuated can be inserted into safe viruses (e.g., vaccinia, canarypox, attenuated adenovirus) to form **hybrid virus vaccines**. This approach holds the promise of allowing the development of a polyvalent vaccine to many agents in a single, safe, inexpensive, and relatively stable vector. On infection, the hybrid virus vaccine need not complete a replication cycle but simply promote the expression of the inserted gene to initiate an immune response to the antigens.

Peptide Subunit Vaccines

Peptide subunit vaccines contain *specific epitopes* of microbial proteins that elicit neutralizing antibody or desired T-cell responses. To generate such a response, the peptide must contain sequences that bind to MHC I or MHC II (class I or class II major histocompatibility complex) proteins on DCs for presentation and recognition by T cells to initiate an immune response. The immunogenicity of the peptide can be enhanced by its covalent attachment to a carrier protein (e.g., tetanus toxoid or keyhole limpet hemocyanin [KLH]), a ligand for a Toll-like receptor (e.g., flagellin) or an immunologic peptide that can specifically present the epitope to the appropriate immune response. Better vaccines are being developed as the mechanisms of antigen presentation and T-cell receptor-specific antigens are better understood.

DNA Vaccines

DNA vaccines offer great potential for immunization against infectious agents that require T-cell responses but are not appropriate for use in live attenuated vaccines. For these vaccines, the gene for a protein that elicits protective responses is cloned into a plasmid that allows the protein to be expressed in eukaryotic cells. The naked DNA is injected into the muscle or skin of the vaccine recipient, where the DNA is taken up by cells, the gene is expressed, and the protein is produced, presented to, and activates T-cell responses. DNA vaccines usually require a boost with antigenic protein to produce antibody.

Future Directions for Vaccination

A new approach, termed *reverse vaccinology*, was used to develop a vaccine for *N. meningitidis B*. Based on protein properties predicted from the gene sequence, thousands of proteins were tested for their ability to confer protection against infection to identify protein candidates. With the advent of this and other new technology, it should be possible to develop vaccines against infectious agents, such as *Streptococcus mutans* (to prevent tooth decay). In fact, it should be possible to produce a vaccine to almost any infectious agent once the appropriate protective immunogen is identified and its gene isolated.

The bacterial vaccines currently available are listed in Table 8-2.

Passive Immunization

The injection of purified antibody or antibody-containing serum to provide rapid, temporary protection or treatment of a person is termed **passive immunization**. Newborns receive natural passive immunity from maternal immunoglobulin that crosses the placenta or is present in the mother's milk.

Passive immunization may be used to prevent disease after a known exposure (e.g., injury contaminated with *Clostridium tetanus*); or to ameliorate the symptoms of an ongoing disease; or to protect immunodeficient individuals; or to block the action of bacterial toxins and prevent the diseases they cause (i.e., as therapy).

Immune serum globulin preparations derived from seropositive humans or animals (e.g., horses) are available as prophylaxis for several bacterial diseases (e.g., tetanus, botulism, diphtheria). Human serum globulin is prepared from pooled plasma and contains the normal repertoire of antibodies for an adult. Special high-titer immune globulin preparation is available for tetanus. Human immunoglobulin is preferable to animal immunoglobulin because there is little risk of a hypersensitivity reaction (serum sickness).

Monoclonal antibody preparations are being

Table 8-2 Bacterial Vaccines*

Bacteria (Disease)	Vaccine Components	Who Should Receive Vaccinations
Corynebacterium diphtheriae (diphtheria)	Toxoid	Children and adults
Clostridium tetani (tetanus)	Toxoid	Children and adults
Bordetella pertussis (pertussis)	Acellular	Children and teens
Haemophilus influenzae B (Hib)	Capsule polysaccharide-protein conjugate	Children
Neisseria meningitidis A and C (meningococcal disease)	Capsule polysaccharide-protein conjugate, capsule polysaccharide	People at high risk (e.g., those with asplenia), travelers to epidemic areas (e.g., military personnel), children
Streptococcus pneumoniae (pneumococcal disease; meningitis)	Capsule polysaccharides; capsule polysaccharide-protein conjugate	Children, people at high risk (e.g., those with asplenia), the elderly
Vibrio cholerae (cholera)	Killed cell	Travelers at risk to exposure
Salmonella typhi (typhoid)	Killed cell; polysaccharide	Travelers at risk to exposure, household contacts, sewage workers
Bacillus anthracis (anthrax)	Killed cell	Handlers of imported fur, military personnel
Yersinia pestis (plague)	Killed cell	Veterinarians, animal handlers
Francisella tularensis (tularemia)	Live attenuated	Animal handlers in endemic areas
Coxiella burnetii (Q fever)	Inactivated	Sheep handlers, laboratory personnel working with *C. burnetii*
Mycobacterium tuberculosis (tuberculosis)	Live attenuated bacillus Calmette-Guérin *Mycobacterium bovis*	Not recommended in United States

*Listed in order of frequency of use.

developed for protection against various agents and diseases. In addition to infectious diseases, monoclonal antibodies are being used as therapy to block overzealous cytokine responses in inflammation and sepsis and for other therapies.

IMMUNIZATION PROGRAMS

An effective vaccine program can greatly save health care costs. Such a program not only protects each vaccinated person against infection and disease but also reduces the number of susceptible people in the population, thereby preventing the spread of the infectious agent within the population. Although immunization may be the best means of protecting people against infection, vaccines cannot be developed for all infectious agents. One reason is that it is very time consuming and costly to develop vaccines. Box 8-1 lists the considerations that are weighed in the choice of a candidate for a vaccine program.

Box 8-1

Properties of a Good Candidate for Vaccine Development

Organism causes significant illness
Organism exists as only one serotype
Antibody blocks infection or systemic spread
Organism does not have oncogenic potential
Vaccine is heat stable so that it can be transported to endemic areas

---

From the standpoint of the individual, the ideal vaccine should elicit dependable, lifelong immunity to infection without serious side effects. Factors that influence the success of an immunization program include not only the composition of the vaccine but also the timing, site, and conditions of its administration. Misinformation regarding safety issues with vaccines has deterred some individuals from being vaccinated putting them at risk to disease.

SUMMARY

Host defense to a certain bacterial agent can be achieved by either **active immunization** or **passive immunization**.

Active immunization occurs when an immune response is stimulated by exposure to an infectious agent (**natural immunization**) or their **vaccines**. **Passive immunization** can be acquired by injection of purified antibody or antibody-containing serum.

Inactivated vaccines (killed vaccine) can be produced by chemical or heat inactivation of bacteria, bacterial toxins, or by purification or synthesis of the components or subunits of the infectious agents.

Toxoid (inactivated toxins), **inactivated (killed)** bacteria, and **capsule or protein subunits** of the bacteria are three major types of inactivated bacterial vaccines.

Live attenuated vaccines are prepared with organisms limited in their ability to cause disease (e.g., **avirulent** or **attenuated** organisms). Immunization with a live vaccine resembles the natural infection. BCG, plaque, or anthrax vaccines are representative for typical live attenuated vaccines.

A **subunit vaccine** consists of the bacterial components that elicit a protective immune response.

Genetically engineered subunit vaccines are being developed through cloning of genes that encode immunogenic proteins into bacterial and eukaryotic vectors.

Recombinant vector vaccine is a new live vaccine containing genetic engineering mutations to inactivate or delete a virulence gene.

Peptide subunit vaccines contain *specific epitopes* of microbial proteins that elicit neutralizing antibody or desired T-cell responses. In **DNA vaccines**, the gene for a protein that elicits protective responses is cloned into a plasmid that allows the protein to be expressed in eukaryotic cells.

KEYWORDS

English	Chinese
Active immunization	主动免疫
DNA vaccines	DNA 疫苗
Genetically engineered subunit vaccines	基因工程疫苗
Inactivated vaccines	灭活疫苗
Live attenuated vaccines	减毒活疫苗
Passive immunization	被动免疫

Recombinant vector vaccine   重组载体疫苗

Subunit vaccines   亚单位疫苗

Toxoid   类毒素

BIBLIOGRAPHY

1. Chinese Center for Disease Control and Prevention: National Immunization Program http://www.chinanip.org.cn/

2. Centers for Disease Control and Prevention: Vaccines & immunizations (website) http://www.cdc.gov/vaccines/acip/index.html Accessed June 23, 2016.

3. Centers for Disease Control and Prevention: Vaccines & immunizations (website). http://www.cdc.gov/vaccines/default.htm. Accessed June 23, 2016.

4. Centers for Disease Control and Prevention, Atkinson W, Wolfe S, Hamborsky J, editors: Epidemiology and prevention of vaccine-preventable diseases (the pink book), ed 12, Washington, DC, 2011, Public Health Foundation.

5. World Health Organization: Immunization service delivery (website). www.who.int/vaccines-diseases/index.html. Accessed June 23, 2016.

Sterilization and Disinfection

An important aspect of the control of infections is an understanding of the following definitions.

Sterilization: Use of physical procedures or chemical agents to destroy all microbial forms, including bacterial spores.

Disinfection: Use of physical procedures or chemical agents to destroy most microbial forms; bacterial spores and other relatively resistant organisms (e.g., mycobacteria, viruses, fungi) may remain viable.

Antisepsis: Use of chemical agents on skin or other living tissue to inhibit or eliminate microbes; no sporicidal action is implied.

STERILIZATION

Sterilization is the total destruction of all microbes, including the more resilient forms such as bacterial spores, mycobacteria, nonenveloped (nonlipid) viruses, and fungi. This can be accomplished by using physical, gas vapor, or chemical sterilants (Table 9-1).

Moist and Dry Heat are the most common sterilizing methods used in hospitals and are indicated for most materials, except those that are heat sensitive or consist of toxic or volatile chemicals.

Attempts to sterilize items using boiling water are inefficient, because only a relatively low temperature (100°C) can be maintained. Indeed, spore formation by a bacterium is commonly demonstrated by boiling a solution of organisms and then subculturing the solution. Boiling vegetative organisms kills them, but the spores remain viable. In contrast, steam under pressure in an autoclave (autoclaving sterilization) is a very effective form of sterilization; the higher temperature causes denaturation of microbial proteins. The rate of killing organisms during the autoclave process is rapid but is influenced by the temperature and duration of autoclaving, size of the autoclave, flow rate of the steam, density and size of the load, and placement of the load in the chamber. In general, most autoclaves are operated at 121°C to 132°C for 15 minutes or longer.

Filtration is useful for removing bacteria and fungi from air or from solutions. However, these filters are unable to remove viruses and some small bacteria.

Sterilization by **ultraviolet** or **ionizing radiation** (e.g., microwave or gamma rays) is also commonly used. The limitation of ultraviolet radiation is that direct exposure is required.

Table 9-1 Methods of Sterilization

Method	Concentration or Level
Physical Sterilants	
Steam under pressure	121°C or 132°C for various time intervals
Filtration	0.22- to 0.45-μm pore size; HEPA filters
Ultraviolet radiation	Variable exposure to 254-nm wavelength
Ionizing radiation	Variable exposure to micro-wave or gamma radiation
Gas Vapor Sterilants	
Ethylene oxide	450-1200 mg/L at 29°C to 65°C for 2-5 hr
Formaldehyde vapor	2%-5% at 60°C to 80°C
Hydrogen peroxide vapor	30% at 55°C to 60°C
Plasma gas	Highly ionized hydrogen per-oxide gas
Chemical Sterilants	
Peracetic acid	0.2%
Glutaraldehyde	2%

HEPA, High-efficiency particulate air.

DISINFECTION

Chemical disinfectants which can destroy microbes are most common used in disinfection. Disinfectants are subdivided into high-, intermediate-, and low-level agents. High-level disinfectant kills all microbial pathogens except large numbers of bacterial spores. Intermediate-level disinfectant kills all microbial pathogens except bacterial endospores. Low-level disinfectant kills most vegetative bacteria and lipid-enveloped or medium-size viruses. High-level disinfection can generally approach sterilization in effectiveness, whereas spore forms can survive intermediate-level disinfection, and many microbes can remain viable when exposed to low-level disinfection.

The effectiveness of these procedures is influenced by the nature of the item to be disinfected, number and resilience of the contaminating organisms, amount of organic material present (which can inactivate the disinfectant), type and concentration of disinfectant, and duration and temperature of exposure.

High-level disinfectants

High-level disinfectants are used for items involved with invasive procedures that cannot withstand sterilization procedures (e.g., certain types of endoscopes and surgical instruments with plastic or other components that cannot be autoclaved).

Chlorine compounds are used extensively as disinfectants. Aqueous solutions of chlorine are rapidly bactericidal, although their mechanisms of action are not defined. Three forms of chlorine may be present in water: elemental chlorine (Cl_2), which is a very strong oxidizing agent; hypochlorous acid (HOCl); and hypochlorite ion (OCl_2). Chlorine also combines with ammonia and other nitrogenous compounds to form chloramines, or N-chloro compounds. Chlorine can exert its effect by the irreversible oxidation of sulfhydryl (SH) groups of essential enzymes. Hypochlorites are believed to interact with cytoplasmic components to form toxic N-chloro compounds, which interfere with cellular metabolism.

The efficacy of chlorine is inversely proportional to the pH, with greater activity observed at acid pH levels. This is consistent with greater activity associated with hypochlorous acid rather than with hypochlorite ion concentration. The activity of chlorine compounds also increases with concentration and temperature. Organic matter and alkaline detergents can reduce the effectiveness of chlorine compounds. These compounds demonstrate good germicidal activity, although spore-forming organisms are 10- to 1000-fold more resistant to chlorine than are vegetative bacteria.

Ethylene oxide is a commonly used **gas vapor sterilant**. Ethylene oxide is a colorless gas (soluble in water and common organic solvents) that is used to sterilize heat-sensitive items. The sterilization process is relatively slow and is influenced by the concentration of gas, relative humidity and moisture content of the item to be sterilized, exposure time, and temperature. Sterilization with ethylene oxide is optimal in a relative humidity of approximately 30%, with decreased activity at higher or lower humidity. This is particularly problematic if the contaminated organisms are dried onto a surface or lyophilized. Ethylene oxide exerts its sporicidal activity through the alkylation of terminal hydroxyl, carboxyl, amino, and sulfhydryl groups. This process blocks the reactive groups required for many essential metabolic processes.

Examples of other strong alkylating gases used as sterilants are formaldehyde and β-propiolactone. Because ethylene oxide can damage viable tissues, the gas must be dissipated before the item can be used. This aeration period is generally 16 hours or longer.

Although it is highly efficient, strict regulations limit its use, because ethylene oxide is flammable, explosive, and carcinogenic to laboratory animals. Sterilization with **formaldehyde gas** is also limited, because the chemical is carcinogenic. Its use is restricted primarily to sterilization of HEPA filters.

Hydrogen peroxide vapors are effective sterilants because of the oxidizing nature of the gas. This sterilant is used for the sterilization of instruments. Hydrogen peroxide effectively kills most bacteria at a concentration of 3% to 6% and kills all organisms, including spores, at higher concentrations (10% to 25%). The active oxidant form is not hydrogen peroxide but rather the free hydroxyl radical formed by the decomposition of hydrogen peroxide. Hydrogen peroxide is used to disinfect plastic implants, contact lenses, and surgical prostheses.

A variation is **plasma gas sterilization**, in which hydrogen peroxide is vaporized, and then reactive free radicals are produced with either microwave-frequency or radio-frequency energy. Because this is an efficient sterilizing method that does not produce toxic byproducts, plasma gas sterilization has replaced many of the applications for ethylene oxide. However, it cannot be used with materials that absorb hydrogen peroxide or react with it.

Peracetic acid, an oxidizing agent, has excellent activity, and the end products (i.e., acetic acid and oxygen) are nontoxic. In contrast, safety is a concern with **glutaraldehyde**, and care must be used when handling this chemical.

The two best-known **aldehydes** are **formaldehyde** and **glutaraldehyde**, both of which can be used as sterilants or high-level disinfectants. Formaldehyde gas can be dissolved in water (creating a solution called *formalin*) at a final concentration of 37%. Stabilizers, such as methanol, are added to formalin. Low concentrations of formalin are bacteriostatic (i.e., they inhibit but do not kill organisms), whereas higher concentrations (e.g., 20%) can kill all organisms. Combining formaldehyde with alcohol (e.g., 20% formalin in 70% alcohol) can enhance this microbicidal activity. Exposure of skin or mucous membranes to formaldehyde can be toxic. Glutaraldehyde is less toxic for viable tissues, but it can still cause burns on the skin or mucous membranes. Glutaraldehyde is more active at alkaline pH levels ("activated" by sodium hydroxide) but is less stable. Glutaraldehyde is also inactivated by organic material; so items to be treated must first be cleaned.

Intermediate-level Disinfectants

Intermediate-level disinfectants are used to clean surfaces or instruments where contamination with bacterial spores and other highly resilient organisms is unlikely. These have been referred to as semicritical instruments and devices and include flexible fiberoptic endoscopes, laryngoscopes, vaginal specula, anesthesia breathing circuits, and other items.

Iodophors are excellent skin antiseptic agents, having a range of activity similar to that of alcohols. They are slightly more toxic to the skin than is alcohol, have limited residual activity, and are inactivated by organic matter. Iodophors and iodine preparations are frequently used with alcohols for disinfecting the skin surface.

Iodine is a highly reactive element that precipitates proteins and oxidizes essential enzymes. It is microbicidal against virtually all organisms, including spore-forming bacteria and mycobacteria. Neither the concentration nor the pH of the iodine solution affects the microbicidal activity, although the efficiency of iodine solutions is increased in acid solutions because more free iodine is liberated. Iodine acts more rapidly than do other halogen compounds or quaternary ammonium compounds.

Alcohols have excellent activity against all groups of organisms, except spores, and are nontoxic, although they tend to dry the skin surface because they remove lipids. They also do not have residual activity and are inactivated by organic matter. Thus the surface of the skin should be cleaned before alcohol is applied.

The germicidal activity of alcohols increases with increasing chain length (maximum of five to eight carbons). The two most commonly used alcohols are **ethanol** and **isopropanol**. These alcohols are rapidly bactericidal against vegetative bacteria, mycobacteria, some fungi, and lipid-containing viruses. Unfortunately, alcohols have no activity against bacterial spores and have poor activity against some fungi and non-lipid-containing viruses. Activity is greater in the presence of water. Thus 70% alcohol is more active than 95% alcohol. Alcohol is a common disinfectant for skin surfaces and, when followed by treatment with an iodophor, is extremely effective for this purpose. Alcohols are also used to disinfect items such as thermometers.

Low-level Disinfectants

Low-level disinfectants (i.e., quaternary ammonium compounds) are used to treat noncritical instruments and devices, such as blood pressure cuffs, electrocardiogram electrodes, and stethoscopes. Although these items come into contact with patients, they do not penetrate through mucosal surfaces or into sterile tissues.

Quaternary ammonium compounds consist of four organic groups covalently linked to nitrogen. The germicidal activity of these cationic compounds is determined by the nature of the organic groups, with the greatest activity observed with compounds having 8- to 18-carbon long groups. Examples of quaternary ammonium compounds include **benzalkonium chloride** and **cetylpyridinium chloride**. These compounds act by denaturing cell membranes to release the intracellular components. Quaternary ammonium compounds are bacteriostatic at low concentrations and bactericidal at high concentrations; however, organisms such as *Pseudomonas*, *Mycobacterium*, and the fungus *Trichophyton* are resistant to these compounds. Indeed, some *Pseudomonas* strains can grow in quaternary ammonium solutions. Many viruses and all bacterial spores are also resistant. Ionic detergents, organic matter, and dilution neutralize quaternary ammonium compounds.

Chlorhexidine has broad antimicrobial activity, although it kills organisms at a much slower rate than alcohol. Its activity persists, although organic material and high pH levels decrease its effectiveness.

The activity of **parachlorometaxylenol (PCMX)** is limited primarily to gram-positive bacteria. Because it is nontoxic and has residual activity, it has been used in handwashing products. **Triclosan** is active against bacteria but not against many other organisms. It is a common antiseptic agent in deodorant soaps and some toothpaste products.

Antiseptic agents (Table 9-2) are used to reduce the number of microbes on skin surfaces. These compounds are selected for their safety and efficacy. A summary of their germicidal properties is presented in Table 9-3.

Table 9-2   Antiseptic Agents

Antiseptic Agent	Concentration
Alcohol (ethyl, isopropyl)	70%-90%
Iodophors	1-2 mg of free iodine/L; 1%-2% available iodine
Chlorhexidine	0.5%-4.0%
Parachlorometaxylenol	0.50%-3.75%
Triclosan	0.3%-2.0%

Table 9-3   Germicidal Properties of Disinfectants and Antiseptic Agents

Agents	Bacteria	Bacterial Spores	Fungi	Viruses
Disinfectants				
Alcohol	+	−	+	+/−
Hydrogen peroxide	+	+/−	+	+
Formaldehyde	+	+	+	+
Phenolics	+	−	+	+/−
Chlorine	+	+/−	+	+
Iodophors	+/−	−	+	+
Glutaraldehyde	+	+	+	+
Quaternary ammonium compounds	+/−		+/−	+/−
Antiseptic Agents				
Alcohol	+	−	+	+
Iodophors	+	−	+	+
Chlorhexidine	+	−	+	+
Parachlorometaxylenol	+/−	−	+	+/−
Triclosan	+/−	−	+/−	+

SUMMARY

Sterilization is the total destruction of all microbes, including bacterial spores, mycobacteria, viruses, and fungi. This can be accomplished by using physical procedures or chemical agents. Moist and dry heat are the most common sterilizing methods used in hospitals and are indicated for most materials, except those that are heat sensitive or consist of toxic or volatile chemicals.

Most autoclaves are operated at 121℃ to 132℃ for 15 minutes or longer.

Filtration is useful for removing bacteria and fungi from air or from solutions.

Ultraviolet or **ionizing radiation** (e.g., microwave or gamma rays) is also commonly used.

Disinfection is the procedure to destroy most microbial forms using physical procedures or chemical agents; bacterial spores and other relatively resistant organisms (e.g., mycobacteria, viruses, fungi) may remain viable.

Disinfectants are subdivided into high-, intermediate-, and low-level agents. High-level disinfectant kills all microbial pathogens except large numbers of bacterial spores. Intermediate-level disinfectant kills all microbial pathogens except bacterial endospores. Low-level disinfectant kills most vegetative bacteria and lipid-enveloped or medium-size viruses.

Chlorine compounds, ethylene oxide, hydrogen peroxide, peracetic acid and aldehydes are all common used high-level disinfectants.

Iodophors and alcohols are representatives for intermediate-level disinfectants.

Common low-level disinfectants includes quaternary ammonium compounds and chlorhexidine.

Antisepsis is to inhibit or eliminate microbes by using chemical agents on skin or other living tissue. Antiseptic agents are used to reduce the number of microbes on skin surfaces.

KEYWORDS

English	Chinese
Antisepsis	防腐
Disinfection	消毒
Disinfectant	消毒剂
Sterilization	灭菌
Autoclaving sterilization	高压蒸汽灭菌法

BIBLIOGRAPHY

1. Block SS: Disinfection, sterilization, and preservation, ed 2, Philadelphia, 1977, Lea & Febiger.

2. Brody TM, Larner J, Minneman KP: Human pharmacology: molecular to clinical, ed 3, St Louis, 1998, Mosby.

3. Widmer A, Frei R: Decontamination, disinfection, and sterilization. In Murray P, et al, editors: Manual of clinical microbiology, ed 9, Washington, DC, 2007, American Society for Microbiology.

Chapter 10

Antibacterial Agents

Antibacterial agents have been used for the treatment of infectious diseases and have greatly reduced the motility of many life-threatened infectious diseases. Antibacterial agents kill microorganisms or inhibit their growth. These drugs include antibiotics, which are natural substances produced by certain groups of microorganisms, and chemotherapeutic agents, which are chemically synthesized. However, the wide use of these drugs has accelerated the development of antimicrobial resistance, making the drugs less effective. This chapter provides an overview of the classification and mechanisms of action of the commonly used antibacterial antibiotics, and the mechanisms by which bacteria might exhibit resistance to these drugs.

CLASSES OF ANTIBACTERIAL AGENTS

Classification Based on the Molecular Structure and Chemical Properties of Antibacterial Agents (Table 10-1).

β-Lactam Antibiotics

β-lactam antibiotics contain a beta-lactam ring in their molecular structures. The β-lactam family of antibiotics includes many of the most widely used antibacterial agents in clinical medicine. These agents exhibit variable pharmacological properties and their antibacterial spectrum is largely related to the side chain in their molecular structure.

Penicillin: Penicillin antibiotics are highly effective antibiotics with an extremely low toxicity.

NATURAL: penicillin G, penicillin V.

PENICILLINASE-RESISTANT PENICILLLIN: methicillin; oxacillin.

EXTENDED SPECTRUM PENICILLIN: ampicillin, amoxicillin, carbenicillin.

Cephalosporin: Cephalosporins are grouped into generations based on their spectrum of gram-negative antimicrobial activity. Each newer generation of cephalosporins has significantly greater spectrum than the preceding generation, and in most cases decreased activity against gram-positive organisms. Fourth generation cephalosporins have true broad spectrum activity.

FIRST-GENERATION: cephalexin, cephalothin, cefazolin, cephradine, etc. First generation cephalosporins have relatively narrow spectrum of activity focused primarily on the penicillinase-producing *Staphylococcus*. They also have modest activity on some gram-negative bacteria.

SECOND-GENERATION: cefuroxime, cefamandole, cefaclor, etc. The second generation cephalosporins have enhanced activity against gram-negative bacilli.

Table 10-1 Antibiotics Grouping by Mechanism

Cell Wall Synthesis	Cell Membrane function	Protein synthesis	Nucleic Acid Synthesis
β-lactams	Polymyxins	chloramphenicol	sulfonamides
Vancomycin	amphotericin B	tetracyclines	trimethoprim
Bacitracin	Nystatin	erythromycin	rifampicin
Cycloserine	Ketoconazole	lincomycins aminoglycosides	quinolones

THIRD-GENERATION: ceftazimine, cefotaxime, ceftriaxone, cefoperazone, etc. The third generation cephalosporins have a marked activity against gram-negative bacteria due to enhanced beta-lactamase stability.

FOURTH- GENERATION: cefepime, cefpirome, etc. Fourth generation cephalosporins have the broadest spectrum of activity and a greater resistance to beta-lactamases than the third generation cephalosporins.

Fifth-generation cephalosporins including ceftaroline fosamil and ceftobiprole, have activity against a wide range of both gram-positive and gram-negative bacteria including methicillin resistant Staphylococcus aureus (MRSA). These agents are sometimes referred to as advanced generation rather than fifth generation cephalosporins.

Cephamycin: cefoxitin (Mefoxin).

Monobactam: aztreonam, carumonam. They are active against selected aerobic gram-negative rods but inactive against anaerobes or gram-positive cocci.

Carbapenem: imipenem, meropenem, ertapenem, doripenem. Carbapenem are broad-spectrum antibiotics active against most aerobic and anaerobic gram-positive and gram-negative bacteria except oxacillin-resistant staphylococci, most *Enterococcus faecium*, and selected gram-negative rods (e.g., some *Burkholderia*, *Stenotrophomonas*, some *Pseudomonas*).

β-lactamase inhibitors: clavulanic acid, sulbactam, tazobactam. Although having little antibacterial activity, beta-lactamase inhibitors block the activity of beta-lactamase enzymes and thus extend the range of bacteria the drugs are effective against.

Macrolide antibiotics

Examples: erythromycin, spiramycin, roxithromycin, josamycin, azithromycin.

Aminoglycosides

Examples: gentamicin, tobramycin, amikacin, kanamycin.

Tetracyclines

Examples: tetracycline, doxycycline, minocycline.

Chloramphenicol

Representatives includes chloramphenicol and thiamphenicol.

Chemically Synthesized Antibiotics

This class of antibiotics primarily includes sulfa antibiotics and quinolones.

Example for sulfa agents: sulfisoxazole.

Example for quinolones: norfloxacin, ciprofloxacin, ofloxacin, levofloxacin.

Miscellaneous

Examples include antituberculosis drugs such as rifampin, isoniazid, ethambutol, pyrazinamide; cyclic peptides (vancomycin, streptogramins, polymyxins); lincosamides (clindamycin); oxazolidinoes (linezolid).

Classification Based on the Microbiological Source of Antibacterial Agents

Most of the natural antibiotics are derived from eucaryotic molds, Actinomycetes, and bacteria.

Antibiotics Produced by Molds

Penicillium and Cephalosporium molds produce beta-lactam antibiotics such as penicillin and cephalosporin. They also produce the base molecule for development of semisynthetic beta-lactam antibiotics.

Antibiotics Produced by Actinomycetes

Actinomycetes are the mainstay of the antibiotics industry. Streptomyces species are the primary sources to produce tetracyclines, aminoglycosides, macrolides, chloramphenicol, rifamycins, and most other clinically-useful antibiotics except for beta-lactams.

Antibiotics Produced by Bacteria

Bacillus species, such as *B. polymyxa* and *B. subtilis*, produce polypeptide antibiotics (e.g. polymyxin and bacitracin).

Mechanisms of Action

The most important property of an antimicrobial agent is its selective toxicity, which means that when the drug is administered with a proper dose, it is highly effective against the bacteria but have minimal or no toxicity to the host. Selective toxicity may be a function of a specific receptor essential to drug attachment, or it may depend on the inhibition of biochemical events required for the pathogen but not to the host. Antibacterial agents act in one of several ways: by inhibition of cell wall synthesis, by inhibition of cell membrane function, by inhibition of synthesis of protein or nucleic acid (Figure 10-1). Antibiotics can also grouped by different mode of action (see Table 10-1).

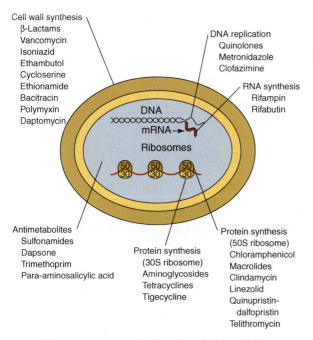

Cell wall synthesis
β-Lactams
Vancomycin
Isoniazid
Ethambutol
Cycloserine
Ethionamide
Bacitracin
Polymyxin
Daptomycin

DNA replication
Quinolones
Metronidazole
Clofazimine

RNA synthesis
Rifampin
Rifabutin

DNA
mRNA
Ribosomes

Antimetabolites
Sulfonamides
Dapsone
Trimethoprim
Para-aminosalicylic acid

Protein synthesis
(30S ribosome)
Aminoglycosides
Tetracyclines
Tigecycline

Protein synthesis
(50S ribosome)
Chloramphenicol
Macrolides
Clindamycin
Linezolid
Quinupristin-
  dalfopristin
Telithromycin

Figure 10-1 Basic sites of antibiotic activity.

Inhibition of Cell Wall

All bacteria (except for mycoplasma) have the rigid cell wall that protects them. The most common mechanism of antibiotic activity is interference with bacterial cell wall synthesis. Beta-lactams disrupt the synthesis of the peptidoglycan layer of bacterial cell walls, which causes the walls to break down and eventually the bacterial cellular death.

Peptidoglycan is a heteropolymeric component of the cell wall that maintains bacterial mechanical stability and rigidity. The final transpeptidation step in the synthesis of the peptidoglycan is facilitated by transpeptidases known as penicillin binding proteins (PBPs). PBPs bind to the D-Ala-D-Ala at the end of muropeptides (peptidoglycan precursors) to crosslink the peptidoglycan. Beta-lactams bind to the active site of PBPs, disrupting the cross-linking process and thus the cell wall loses its strength which

results in cell lysis.

Most of the cell wall-active antibiotics are classified as beta-lactam antibiotics. Other antibiotics that interfere with construction of the bacterial cell wall include vancomycin, daptomycin, bacitracin, and the following anti-mycobacterial agents: isoniazid, ethambutol, cycloserine, and ethionamide.

Inhibition of Cell Membrane Function

The **polymyxins** are a group of cyclic polypeptides that insert into bacterial membranes like detergents, by interacting with lipopolysaccharides and the phospholipids in the outer membrane, producing increased cell permeability and eventual cell death. These antibiotics are most active against gram-negative rods, because gram-positive bacteria do not have an outer membrane.

Amphotericin B and nystatin binds to ergosterol, a major component of the fungal cell membrane. When present in sufficient concentrations, it forms pores in the membrane that lead to K^+ leakage, acidification, and death of the fungus. Ketoconazole inhibits the synthesis of fungal ergosterol and blocks cell membrane synthesis.

Inhibition of Protein Synthesis

Many antibiotics can inhibit protein synthesis in bacteria. The precise mechanisms of action differ among different classes of drugs. Aminoglycosides and tetracyclines act the 30S subunit of the microbial ribosome. Chloramphenicol, erythromycin and lincomycins act the 50S subunit of the ribosome.

Inhibition of Nucleic Acids Synthesis

Rifampin inhibits bacterial RNA synthesis by binding to the DNA-dependent RNA polymerase of bacteria. Quinolones inhibit bacterial DNA synthesis by blocking DNA gyrases, topoisomerase which are required for DNA replication, recombination, and repair.

Sulfonamides are structural analogs of p-aminobenzoic acid (PABA) and compete for the active center of dihydropteroate synthetase. PABA is an essential bacterial metabolite involved in the synthesis of folic acid, an important precursor to the synthesis of nucleic acids. As a result, nonfunctional analogs of folic acid are formed, preventing further growth of the bacterial cell.

Trimethoprim (3,4,5-trimethoxybenzylpyrimidine) inhibits dihydrofolic acid reductase, leading to the inhibition of synthesis of purines and ultimately of DNA. Sulfonamides and trimethoprim each can be used alone to inhibit bacterial growth. If used together, they produce sequential blocking, resulting in a marked enhancement (synergism) of activity.

Mechanisms of Antimicrobial Resistance

Bacteria can become resistant to antibiotics. Bacterial drug resistance is the ability of bacteria to resist the effects of an antibiotic or a disinfectant to which they were once sensitive. Minimum inhibitory concentration (MIC) is the lowest concentration of an antibiotic required to inhibit the growth of a microorganism. "Susceptible" implies that isolates are inhibited by the usually achievable concentrations of antimicrobial agent with normal dosage schedules. "Resistant" implies that isolates are not inhibited by the usually achievable concentrations.

Antimicrobial resistance is an increasingly serious threat to global public health. It threatens the effective prevention and treatment of an ever-increasing range of infections. The cost of health care for patients with resistant infections is higher than care for patients with non-resistant infections due to longer duration of illness, additional tests and use of more expensive drugs.

One of the main reasons of bacterial drug resistance is antimicrobial agent overuse, abuse, and in some cases, misuse, due to incorrect diagnosis. Antibiotic use in animal husbandry also leads to rise of resistance. However, antimicrobial resistance can also arise from bacterial genetic ways. The molecular mechanisms of resistance to antibiotics have been studied extensively. With the significant progress of biochemistry, genetics, pharmacology and molecular biology, we have a chance to understand the bacterial resistance on the molecular level of cellular structure, physiological metabolism.

I. Genetic Mechanisms of Resistance

Intrinsic Resistance

Intrinsic resistance is also called natural resistance. It means that the bacteria are "naturally" resistant to some antimicrobial agents. Intrinsic resistance often arises from chromosomal resistant genes and could be transferred to offspring cells. This kind of resistance has genus and species-specificity. Examples include vancomycin and methicillin resistance in most Gram negative bacilli, cephalosporin resistance of *Entercoccus*. In other cases, the resistance can arise from outer membrane barrier or lack of a transport system or a target for the antibiotics.

Acquired Resistance

Acquired resistance refers to bacteria that are usually sensitive to antibiotics develop resistance by alteration of DNA. Resistant genes can derive from mutations in chromosomal genes, or the acquisition of exogenous genes from plasmids, transposons or integrons, which carry the antibiotic resistance genes, by ways of conjugation, transduction or transformation. Occurrence of acquired bacterial resistance is impacted by antibiotic dosages, spontaneous resistant mutation rate and resistant gene transfer.

Chromosomal Mutation

This develops as a result of spontaneous mutation in a locus that controls susceptibility to a given antimicrobial drug. The presence of the antimicrobial drug serves as a selecting mechanism to inhibit susceptible organisms and favor the growth of drug-resistant mutants.

Transferable Antibiotic Resistance

Resistant genes could be horizontally transferred mediated by mobile genetic elements, such as plasmids, transposons or integrons.

Transmission of Antibiotic Resistant Plasmid

Bacteria have special DNA elements called R plasmids that contain resistance genes and are easily passed to other bacteria. Plasmids are physically separated from a chromosomal DNA and can replicate independently. Resistance plasmids represent a medically important means of acquisition of antibiotic resistance by bacterial pathogens, due to their important roles in horizontal gene transfer between bacteria. Genes of many antibiotic modified enzymes are located in plasmid and could be transmitted between bacteria by means of conjugation or transduction. Resistance plasmids often carry multiple resistance-encoding genes. As a result, bacteria can simultaneously acquire resistance to multiple antibiotics due to acquisition of only a single resistance plasmid.

Transposon Mediated Resistance

Transposon, also named as "jumping genes", is a class of genetic elements that can change its position within a genome. Transposons in bacteria can carry an additional gene for functions other than transposition, often for antibiotic resistance. Transposons can jump from chromosomal DNA to plasmid DNA and back, allowing for the transfer and permanent addition of the resistant genes.

Integron

Integrons are exogenous gene acquisition elements that allow bacteria to express new genes. Integrons may be found as part of mobile genetic elements such as plasmids and transposons. Integrons can also be located in chromosomes. They can carry a variety of cassettes containing different resistance genes.

Multiple Drug Resistance

Multidrug resistance (MDR) is defined as insensitivity or resistance of a microorganism to the administered antimicrobial medicines (which are structurally unrelated and have different molecular targets) despite earlier sensitivity to it.

Cross resistance refers to microorganisms resistant to a certain drug may also be resistant to other drugs that share a mechanism of action. Such relationships exist mainly between agents that are closely related chemically (eg, different aminoglycosides) or that have a similar mode of binding or action (eg, macrolides and lincosamides).

Pan-drug resistance refers to a pathogen resistant to all antimicrobial agents available at the time of use.

Many different bacteria now exhibit multi-drug resistance, including staphylococci, enterococci, gonococci, streptococci, salmonella, as well as numerous other gram-negative bacteria and *Mycobacterium tuberculosis*. Antibiotic resistant bacteria are able to transfer copies of DNA that code for a mechanism of resistance to other bacteria even distantly related to them, which then are also able to pass on the resistance genes and so generations of antibiotics resistant bacteria are produced.

II. Biochemical Mechanisms of Resistance

Biochemical mechanisms of bacterial resistance include primarily production of modified enzyme, alteration of drug target, permeability barrier, active efflux, and bacterial metabolic alterations.

Production of Modified Enzyme

Microorganisms produce enzymes that destroy the active drug. *Staphylococci* resistant to penicillin G produce a β-lactamase that destroys the drug. Other β-lactamases are produced by gram-negative rods. Gram-negative bacteria resistant to aminoglycosides (by virtue of a plasmid) produce adenylating, phosphorylating, or acetylating enzymes that destroy the drug. Clinical important modified enzymes are listed as following.

(1) β-Lactamase

β-lactamase provides antibiotic resistance by breaking the four-atom ring, known as a β-ring, in β-lactam antibiotics' structure. β-lactamases found in most gram-negative rods (e.g., *Escherichia*, *Klebsiella*) are **extended-spectrum β-lactamases (ESBLs), metalloenzymes and AmpC β-lactamases. Most extended-spectrum β-lactamases (ESBLs)** are encoded on plasmids that can be transferred from organism to organism. Metalloenzymes have a broad spectrum of activity against all β-lactam antibiotics, including the cephamycins and carbapenems. **AmpC** β-lactamases are primarily cephalosporinases that are encoded on the bacterial chromosome and are active against the most potent expanded-spectrum cephalosporins. Plasmid coded AmpC β-lactamases have also been found.

(2) Aminoglycoside-modified Enzymes

Over 50 different aminoglycoside-modified enzymes have been identified. These enzymes can phosphorylate, adenylate or acetylate the aminoglycosides. The encoding genes are usually found on plasmids and transposons. Most enzyme-mediated resistance in gram-negative bacilli is due to multiple genes.

(3) Chloramphenicol Acetyl Transferase

This enzyme is encoded by plasmid and can acetylate chloramphenicol.

Alteration of Drug Target

Microorganisms develop an altered structural target for the drug. Resistance to some penicillins and cephalosporins may be a function of the loss or alteration of PBPs. Penicillin resistance in *Streptococcus pneumoniae* and enterococci is attributable to altered PBPs.

Reduced Permeability or Uptake

Microorganisms change their permeability to the drug. Examples: Tetracyclines accumulate in susceptible bacteria but not in resistant bacteria. Resistance to polymyxins is also associated with a change in permeability to the drugs. Streptococci have a natural permeability barrier to aminoglycosides. This can be partly overcome by the simultaneous presence of a cell wall-active drug such as a penicillin. Resistance to amikacin and to some other aminoglycosides may depend on a lack of permeability to the drugs caused by an outer membrane change that impairs active transport into the cell.

Increased Efflux Activity

Microorganisms can develop efflux pumps that transport the antibiotics out of the cell. Many gram positive and especially gram-negative organisms have developed this mechanism for tetracyclines (common), macrolides, fluoroquinolones, and even β-lactam agents.

Formation of Biofilm

Bacteria can adhere to implanted medical devices or damaged tissue and encase themselves in a hydrated matrix of polysaccharide and protein, and form a slimy layer known as a biofilm. Bacterial biofilms cause chronic infections because they show increased tolerance to antibiotics and disinfectant chemicals. Inside the biofilm, antimicrobial agents must overcome high cell density, an increased number of resistant mutants, substance delivery, molecular exchanges, such as high levels of beta-lactamases or inducers of efflux pump expression, and specific adaptive cells, so-called persisters.

Miscellaneous

Microorganisms can develop an altered metabolic pathway that bypasses the reaction inhibited by the drug. Example: Some sulfonamide-resistant bacteria do not require extracellular PABA but can use preformed folic acid. Other resistant mechanisms such as bacterial persisters, nutritional deficiency and metabolic antagonists, have also been found contributing to antimicrobial resistance.

Prevention and Control of Antimicrobial Resistance

Proper Use of Antimicrobial Agents

The improper use of antibiotics acts as a natural selection pressure that favors the survival and reproduction of resistant bacteria. To help combating resistance, health workers and pharmacists should use antibiotics properly: only prescribe and dispense antibiotics when they are truly needed; prescribe and dispense the right antibiotic(s) to treat the illness according to the susceptibility test, prophylactic policy, infection features. Antibiotic treatment duration should be based on the infection and other health problems a person may have. In most cases stopping the antibiotic treatment early may be reasonable.

Enhancing Infection Prevention and Control

Hospital infection control is an effective way to slow escalating antimicrobial resistance in all human pathogens. Powerful improvements include separation of patients infected with resistant bacteria to avoid cross infection, and regular inspection of carrier-state in healthcare staffs to prevent spread of nosocomial infection.

Antibiotic Administration Management

Policymakers can help tackle resistance by strengthening laboratory capacity of detection and resistance tracking. It is necessary to establish integrated, national and regional database of bacterial resistance data to support decision-making processes of antibiotics. Regulating and promoting appropriate use of antibiotic by implement restriction policy for antibiotics is also important.

To prevent the development and spread of antibiotic resistance, it is of great importance to regulation antibiotic use in farm animals by restrict and reduce the use of medically important antibiotic as growth enhancers or therapeutic agents. Because antibiotic resistant bacteria are at a selective disadvantage, their incidence decreases when antibiotics are not present. Therefore, regulation of antibiotics would slow and even reverse the increase in antibiotic resistant bacterial populations.

Development of New Antimicrobial Agents

It is a potential solution of antibiotic resistance to study and develop novel classes of antibacterial agents having activity against resistant bacteria, to screen and identify compounds that inhibit the antibiotic modifying enzymes.

Destruction of Resistance Determinants

Scientists found that antimicrobial sensitivity could be restored by damaging antibiotic resistance genes. Developing antimicrobial agents that can restrain transmission of resistant plasmid is also a promising solution due to the important role of R plasmid in production and dissemination of resistance.

SUMMARY

Based on the mechanisms of action, antibacterial agents are classified as (1) inhibition of cell wall synthesis (e.g., beta-lactams and glycopeptide agents), (2) inhibition of cell membrane function (e.g., poly-

myxins and daptomycin), (3) inhibition of protein synthesis (macrolides and tetracyclines) and (4) inhibition of nucleic acid synthesis (fluoroquinolones and rifampin). In addition, some antimicrobial agents acts as inhibition of a metabolic pathway (trimethoprim-sulfamethoxazole).

Genetic mechanisms of antimicrobial resistance can be divided into natural (intrinsic) resistance and acquired resistance. Acquired resistance can derive from mutations in chromosomal genes, or the acquisition of exogenous resistant genes from plasmids, transposons or integrons. Biochemical mechanisms of bacterial resistance include primarily production of modified enzyme, alteration of drug target, permeability barrier, active efflux, bacterial metabolic alterations.

Measures to prevent and control antimicrobial resistance include proper use of antimicrobial agents, enhancing infection control, antibiotic administration stewardship, developing new antimicrobial agents, and destruction of resistance determinant.

KEYWORDS

English	Chinese
Penicillin-binding proteins (PBPs)	青霉素结合蛋白
Cephalosporin	头孢菌素
Cephamycin	头霉素
Monobactam	单环酰胺
Carbapenem	碳青霉烯
β-Lactamase inhibitors	β内酰胺酶抑制剂
Macrolide	大环内酯
Aminoglycosides	氨基糖胺类
Tetracyclines	四环素类
Chloramphenicol	氯霉素
p-Aminobenzoic acid (PABA)	对氨基苯甲酸
Multidrug resistance (MDR)	多重耐药性
Cross resistance	交叉耐药性
Pan-drug resistance	泛耐药
β-Lactamase	β内酰胺酶
Extended-spectrum β-lactamases (ESBLs)	超广谱β内酰胺酶

BIBLIOGRAPHY

1. Bryskier A: Antimicrobial agents: antibacterials and antifungals, Washington, DC, 2005, American Society for

Microbiology Press.

2. Kucers A, Bennett NM: The use of antibiotics: a comprehensive review with clinical emphasis, ed 4, Philadelphia, 1989, Lippincott.

3. Mandell GL, Bennett JE, Dolin R: Principles and practice of infectious diseases, ed 7, Philadelphia, 2010, Churchill Livingstone.

4. Versalovic J, et al: Manual of clinical microbiology, ed 10, Washington, DC, 2011, American Society for Microbiology Press.

5. Dever LA, Dermody TS. Mechanisms of bacterial resistance to antibiotics. Arch Intern Med. 1991 May; 151(5): 886-895.

Chapter 11

Staphylococcus and Related Gram-Positive Cocci

The gram-positive cocci are a heterogeneous collection of bacteria. Features that they have in common are their spherical shape, their Gram-stain reaction, and an absence of endospores. The presence or absence of **catalase** activity is a simple test that is used to subdivide the various genera. Catalases are enzymes that convert **hydrogen peroxide** into water and oxygen gas. If a drop of a peroxide solution is placed on a catalase-producing bacterial colony, bubbles appear when the oxygen gas is formed. The aerobic catalase-positive genera (e.g., *Staphylococcus*, *Micrococcus*, and related organisms) are discussed in this chapter.

The genus name *Staphylococcus* refers to the fact that these gram-positive cocci grow in a pattern resembling a cluster of grapes (Table 11-1; Figure 11-1). These bacteria are present on the skin and mucous membranes of humans, many of which are found on humans. Some species are commonly found in very specific niches. Staphylococci are important pathogens in humans, causing a wide spectrum of life-threatening systemic diseases (Table 11-2). The species most commonly associated with human diseases are **S. aureus** (the most virulent and best-known member of the genus), **S. epidermidis**, **S. haemolyticus**, **S. lugdunensis**, and **S. saprophyticus.** Methicillin-resistant **S. aureus** (**MRSA**) is notorious for producing serious infections in hospitalized patients and outside the hospital. When a colony of S. aureus is suspended in plasma, coagulase_binds to a serum factor, and this complex converts fibrinogen to fibrin, resulting in the formation of a clot. Other staphylococcal species that do not produce coagulase are referred to collectively as **coagulase-negative staphylococci.** *Micrococcus* were subdivided into six genera, with **Micrococcus, Kocuria,** and **Kytococcus** most commonly colonizing the human skin surface. These cocci resemble staphylococci and can be confused with the coagulase-negative staphylococci.

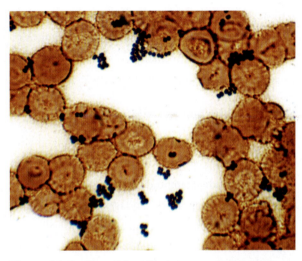

Figure 11-1   Gram stain of *Staphylococcus* in a blood culture.

Table 11-1   Important Staphylococci

Organism	Historical Derivation
Staphylococcus	*staphylé*, bunch of grapes; *coccus*, grain or berry (grapelike cocci)
S. aureus	*aureus*, golden (golden or yellow)
S. epidermidis	*epidermidis*, outer skin (of the epidermis or outer skin)
S. lugdunensis	*Lugdunum*, Latin name for Lyon, France, where the organism was first isolated
S. saprophyticus	*sapros*, putrid; *phyton*, plant (saprophytic or growing on dead tissues)

Table 11-2   Common *Staphylococcus* Species and Their Diseases

Organism	Diseases
S. aureus	Toxin mediated (food poisoning, scalded skin syndrome, toxic shock syndrome); cutaneous (carbuncles, folliculitis, furuncles, impetigo, wound infections); other (bacteremia, endocarditis, pneumonia, empyema, osteomyelitis, septic arthritis)
S. epidermidis	Bacteremia; endocarditis; surgical wounds; urinary tract infections; opportunistic infections of catheters, shunts, prosthetic devices, and peritoneal dialysates
S. saprophyticus	Urinary tract infections; opportunistic infections
S. lugdunensis	Endocarditis; arthritis; bacteremia; opportunistic infections; and urinary tract infections
S. haemolyticus	Bacteremia; endocarditis; bone and joint infections; urinary tract infections; wound infections; and opportunistic infections

PHYSIOLOGY AND STRUCTURE

Capsule and Slime Layer

The outermost layer of the cell wall of many staphylococci is covered with a **polysaccharide capsule**. The capsule protects the bacteria by inhibiting phagocytosis of the organisms by polymorphonuclear leukocytes (PMNs). A loose-bound, water-soluble film (**slime layer or biofilm**) consisting of monosaccharides, proteins, and small peptides is produced by most staphylococci in varying amounts.

Peptidoglycan and Associated Enzymes

The glycan chains in *S. aureus* are cross-linked with pentaglycine bridges that are attached to *L*-lysine in one oligopeptide chain and to *D*-alanine in an adjacent chain. The peptidoglycan layer consists of **many cross-linked layers**, which makes the cell wall more rigid. The enzymes that catalyze construction of the peptidoglycan layer are called penicillin-binding proteins because these are the targets of penicillins and other β-lactam antibiotics. Bacterial resistance to methicillin and related penicillins is mediated by acquisition of a gene (*mecA*) that codes for a novel penicillin-binding protein, PBP2a.

Teichoic Acids and Lipoteichoic Acids

Teichoic acids are **species-specific**, phosphate-containing polymers that are bound covalently to *N*-acetylmuramic acid residues of the peptidoglycan layer or to the lipids in the cytoplasmic membrane (**lipoteichoic acids**). Although the teichoic acids are poor immunogens, a specific antibody response is stimulated when they are bound to peptidoglycan.

Surface Adhesion Proteins

A large collection of surface proteins have been identified in *S. aureus* that are important for adherence to host matrix proteins bound to host tissues (e.g., fibronectin, fibrinogen, elastin, collagen). Most of these surface adhesion proteins are covalently bound to the cell wall peptidoglycan in staphylococci and have been designated **MSCRAMM (microbial surface components recognizing adhesive matrix molecules)** proteins. The best characterized MSCRAMM proteins are staphylococcal protein A, fibronectin-binding proteins A and B, and clumping factor proteins A and B. The clumping factor proteins (also called **coagulase**) bind fibrinogen and convert it to insoluble fibrin, causing the staphylococci to clump or aggregate. Detection of these proteins is the primary **identification test** for *S. aureus*. Two recently described MSCRAMM proteins, *S. aureus* surface proteins G and H, have been associated with invasive diseases.

Cytoplasmic Membrane

The **cytoplasmic membrane** is made up of a complex of proteins, lipids, and a small amount of carbohydrates. It serves as an osmotic barrier for the cell and provides an anchor for the cellular biosynthetic and respiratory enzymes.

PATHOGENESIS AND IMMUNITY

The pathology of staphylococcal infections depends on the ability of the bacteria to **evade** phagocytosis, produce surface proteins that mediate **adherence** of the bacteria to host tissues, and produce **tissue destruction** through the elaboration of specific toxins and hydrolytic enzymes (Table 11-3).

Defenses against Innate Immunity

Encapsulated staphylococci bind opsonins (IgG, complement factor C3) in serum, but the **capsule** covers these opsonins and protects the bacteria by inhibiting phagocytosis of the organisms by polymorphonuclear leukocytes. In the presence of specific antibodies directed against the staphylococci, increased C3 is bound to the bacteria, leading to phagocytosis. The extracellular **slime layer** also interferes with phagocytosis of bacteria. The ability of **protein A** to bind immunoglobulins effectively prevents antibody-mediated immune clearance of the *S. aureus*. Extracellular protein A can also bind antibodies, thereby forming immune complexes with the subsequent consumption of the complement.

Staphylococcal Toxins

S. aureus produces many toxins, including five cytolytic or membrane-damaging toxins (alpha, beta, delta, gamma, and Panton-Valentine [P-V] leukocidin), two exfoliative toxins (A and B), 18 enterotoxins (A to R), and toxic shock syndrome toxin-1 (TSST-1). The cytolytic toxins have been described as hemolysins, but this is a misnomer because the activities of the first four toxins are not restricted solely to red blood cells, and P-V leukocidin is unable to lyse erythrocytes.

Exfoliative toxin A, the enterotoxins, and TSST-1 belong to a class of polypeptides known as **superantigens**. These toxins bind to class II major histocompatibility complex (MHC II) molecules on macrophages. This results in a massive release of cytokines by both macrophages (IL-1β and tumor necrosis factor [TNF]-α) and T cells (IL-2, interferon-γ, and TNF-β).

Table 11-3 *Staphylococcus aureus* Virulence Factors

Virulence Factors	Biologic Effects
Structural Components	
Capsule	Inhibits chemotaxis and phagocytosis; inhibits proliferation of mononuclear cells
Slime layer	Facilitates adherence to foreign bodies; inhibits phagocytosis
Peptidoglycan	Provides osmotic stability; stimulates production of endogenous pyrogen (endotoxin-like activity); leukocyte chemoattractant (abscess formation); inhibits phagocytosis
Teichoic acid	Binds to fibronectin
Protein A	Inhibits antibody-mediated clearance by binding IgG$_1$, IgG$_2$, and IgG$_4$ Fc receptors; leukocyte chemoattractant; anticomplementary
Toxins	
Cytotoxins	Toxic for many cells, including erythrocytes, fibroblasts, leukocytes, macrophages, and platelets
Exfoliative toxins (ETA, ETB)	Serine proteases that split the intercellular bridges in the stratum granulosum epidermis
Enterotoxins (A-R)	Superantigens (stimulate proliferation of T cells and release of cytokines); stimulate release of inflammatory mediators in mast cells, increasing intestinal peristalsis and fluid loss, as well as nausea and vomiting
Toxic shock syndrome toxin-1	Superantigen (stimulates proliferation of T cells and release of cytokines); produces leakage or cellular destruction of endothelial cells
Enzymes	
Coagulase	Converts fibrinogen to fibrin
Hyaluronidase	Hydrolyzes hyaluronic acids in connective tissue, promoting the spread of staphylococci in tissue
Fibrinolysin	Dissolves fibrin clots
Lipases	Hydrolyzes lipids
Nucleases	Hydrolyzes DNA

Cytotoxins

Alpha toxin, which is a 33,000-Da polypeptide that is produced by most strains of *S. aureus* that cause human disease. The toxin disrupts the smooth muscle in blood vessels and is toxic to many types of cells, including erythrocytes, leukocytes, hepatocytes, and platelets. It becomes integrated in the hydrophobic regions of host cell membrane, leading to formation of 1- to 2-nm pores. Alpha toxin is believed to be an important mediator of tissue damage in staphylococcal disease.

Beta toxin, also called **sphingomyelinase C,** is a 35,000 Da heat-labile protein produced by most strains of *S. aureus* responsible for disease in humans and animals. This enzyme has a specificity for sphingomyelin and lysophosphatidylcholine and is toxic to a variety of cells, including erythrocytes, fibroblasts, leukocytes, and macrophages. It catalyzes the hydrolysis of membrane phospholipids in susceptible cells, with lysis proportional to the concentration of sphingomyelin exposed on the cell surface. This is believed to be responsible for the differences in species susceptibility to the toxin.

Delta toxin is a 3,000-Da polypeptide produced by almost all *S. aureus* strains and other staphylococci (e.g., *S. epidermidis, S. haemolyticus*). The toxin has a wide spectrum of cytolytic activity, affecting erythrocytes, many other mammalian cells, and intracellular membrane structures. This relatively nonspecific membrane toxicity is consistent with the belief that the toxin acts as a surfactant disrupting cellular membranes by means of a detergent-like action.

Gamma toxin (made by almost all *S. aureus* strains) and **P-V leukocidin** are bicomponent toxins, composed of two polypeptide chains: the S (slow-eluting proteins) component and F (fast-eluting proteins) component. Three S proteins (HlgA [hemolysin gamma A], HlgC, LukS-PV) and two F proteins (HlgB, LukF-PV) have been identified. Bacteria capable of producing both toxins can encode all these proteins, with the potential for producing six distinct toxins. All six toxins can lyse neutrophils and macrophages. The P-V leukocidin toxin (LukS-PV/LukF-PV) is leukotoxic but has no hemolytic activity. Cell lysis by the gamma and P-V leukocidin toxins is mediated by pore formation.

Exfoliative Toxins

Staphylococcal scalded skin syndrome (SSSS), a spectrum of diseases characterized by exfoliative dermatitis, is mediated by exfoliative toxins. The prevalence of toxin production in *S. aureus* strains varies geographically but is generally between less than 5%. Two distinct forms of exfoliative toxin (ETA and ETB) have been identified, and either can produce disease. ETA is heat stable, whereas ETB is heat labile. The toxins are **serine proteases** that are not associated with cytolysis or inflammation, so neither staphylococci nor leukocytes are typically present in the involved layer of the epidermis (this is an important **diagnostic clue**). SSSS is seen mostly in young children and only rarely in older children and adults.

Enterotoxins

Eighteen distinct **staphylococcal enterotoxins** (A to R) have been identified, with enterotoxin A most commonly associated with food poisoning. The enterotoxins are designed perfectly for causing foodborne disease—stable to heating at 100°C for 30 minutes and resistant to hydrolysis by gastric and jejunal enzymes. These toxins are produced by 30% to 50% of all *S. aureus* strains. Characteristic histologic changes in the stomach and jejunum include infiltration of neutrophils into the epithelium and underlying lamina propria, with loss of the brush border in the jejunum.

Toxic Shock Syndrome Toxin-1

TSST-1 is a 22,000-Da heat- and proteolysis-resistant, chromosomally mediated exotoxin. It is estimated that 90% of *S. aureus* strains responsible for menstruation-associated toxic shock syndrome (TSS), and half of the strains responsible for other forms of TSS, produce TSST-1. Enterotoxin B and, rarely, enterotoxin C are responsible for approximately half the cases of nonmenstruation-associated TSS. TSST-1 is a superantigen that stimulates release of cytokines, producing leakage of endothelial cells at low concentrations and a cytotoxic effect to the cells at high concentrations. The ability of TSST-1 to penetrate mucosal barriers, is responsible for the systemic effects of TSS. Death in patients with TSS is cause by hypovolemic shock, leading to multiorgan failure.

Staphylococcal Enzymes

S. aureus strains possess two forms of **coagulase: bound and free**. Coagulase bound to the staphylococcal cell wall can directly convert fibrinogen to insoluble fibrin and cause the staphylococci to clump. The cell-free coagulase accomplishes the same result by reacting with a globulin plasma factor (**coagulase-reacting factor**) to form staphylothrombin, a thrombin-like factor. This factor catalyzes the conversion of fibrinogen to insoluble fibrin. Coagulase may cause the formation of a fibrin layer around a staphylococcal abscess, thus localizing the infection and protecting the organisms from phagocytosis. Some other species of staphylococci produce coagulase, but these are primarily animal pathogens and uncommonly recovered in human infections.

Staphylococci produce a variety of other enzymes that hydrolyze host tissue components and aid in the spread of the bacteria. **Hyaluronidase** hydrolyzes hyaluronic acids, present in the acellular matrix of connective tissue. **Fibrinolysin,** also called *staphylokinase* can dissolve fibrin clots. All strains of *S. aureus* and more than 30% of the strains of coagulase-negative *Staphylococcus* produce several different **lipases** that hydrolyze lipids and ensure the survival of staphylococci in the sebaceous areas of the body. *S. aureus* also produce a thermostable **nuclease** that can hydrolyze viscous DNA.

CLINICAL DISEASES

Staphylococcus aureus

The clinical manifestations of some staphylococcal diseases are almost exclusively the result of toxin activity (e.g., SSSS, staphylococcal food poisoning, and TSS), whereas other diseases result from the proliferation of the organisms, leading to abscess formation and tissue destruction (e.g., cutaneous infections, endocarditis, pneumonia, empyema, osteomyelitis, septic arthritis) (Figure 11-2). In the presence of a foreign body (e.g., splinter, catheter, shunt, prosthetic valve or joint), significantly fewer staphylococci are necessary to establish disease. Likewise, patients with congenital diseases associated with an impaired chemotactic or phagocytic response (e.g., Job syndrome, Wiskott-Aldrich syndrome, chronic granulomatous disease) are more susceptible to staphylococcal diseases.

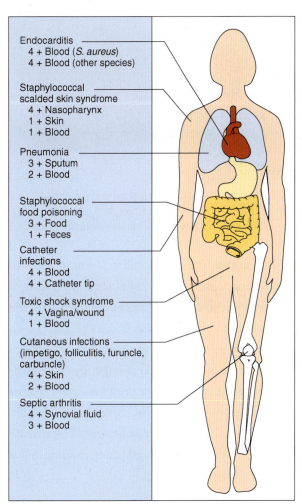

Figure 11-2 Staphylococcal diseases. Isolation of staphylococci from sites of infection. *1+,* Less than 10% positive cultures; *2+,* 10% to 50% positive cultures; *3+,* 50% to 90% positive cultures; *4+,* more than 90% positive cultures.

Staphylococcal Scalded Skin Syndrome

Ritter disease or SSSS, is characterized by the abrupt onset of a localized perioral erythema (redness and inflammation around the mouth) that spreads over the entire body within 2 days. Slight pressure displaces the skin (a positive Nikolsky sign), and large bullae or **cutaneous blisters** form soon thereafter, followed by desquamation of the epithelium (Figure 11-3). The blisters contain clear fluid but no organisms or leukocytes. This is a disease primarily of neonates and young children, with a mortality rate of less than 5%. Infections in adults usually occur in immunocompromised hosts or patients with renal disease, and mortality is as high as 60%.

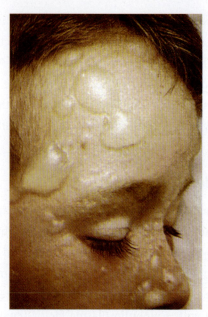

Figure 11-4 Bullous impetigo, a localized form of staphylococcal scalded skin syndrome. (From Emond RT, Rowland HAK: *A color atlas of infectious diseases*, London, 1987, Wolfe.)

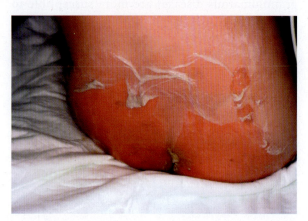

Figure 11-3 Staphylococcal scalded skin syndrome. (From Mandell GL, et al: *Principles and practice of infectious disease*, ed 6, Philadelphia, 2004, Churchill Livingstone.)

Bullous impetigo is a localized form of SSSS. In this syndrome, specific strains of toxin-producing *S. aureus* (e.g., phage type 71) are associated with the formation of superficial skin blisters (Figure 11-4). Unlike patients with the disseminated manifestations of SSSS, patients with bullous impetigo have localized blisters that are culture positive. The erythema does not extend beyond the borders of the blister, and the Nikolsky sign is not present. The disease occurs primarily in infants and young children and is highly communicable.

Staphylococcal Food Poisoning

Staphylococcal food poisoning is an **intoxication** rather than an infection. Disease is caused by bacterial toxin present in food, rather than from a direct effect of the organisms on the patient. The most commonly contaminated foods are **processed meats** such as ham and salted pork, **custard-filled pastries, potato salad**, and **ice cream**. Unlike many other forms of food poisoning in which an animal reservoir is important, staphylococcal food poisoning results from contamination of the food by a human carrier. The contaminated food will not appear or taste tainted. Subsequent heating of the food will kill the bacteria but not inactivate the **heat-stable toxin**.

After ingestion of contaminated food, the onset of disease is abrupt and rapid, with a mean incubation period of 4 hours, which again is consistent with a disease mediated by preformed toxin. The disease has a rapid course, with symptoms generally lasting less than 24 hours. Severe vomiting, diarrhea, and abdominal pain or nausea are characteristic of staphylococcal food poisoning. Sweating and headache may occur, but fever is not seen. The diarrhea is watery and nonbloody, and dehydration may result from the considerable fluid loss.

Certain strains of *S. aureus* can also cause **enterocolitis**, which is manifested clinically by watery diarrhea, abdominal cramps, and fever. The majority of strains producing this disease produce both enterotoxin A and the bicomponent leukotoxin LukE/LukD. Enterocolitis occurs primarily in patients who have received broad-spectrum antibiotics, which suppress the normal colonic flora and permit the growth of *S. aureus*.

Toxic Shock Syndrome

The disease is initiated with the localized growth of toxin-producing strains of *S. aureus* in the vagina or a wound, followed by release of the toxin into blood. Clinical manifestations start abruptly and include fever, hypotension, and a diffuse, macular erythematous rash. Multiple organ systems (e.g., central nervous, gastrointestinal, hematologic, hepatic, musculature, renal) are also involved, and the entire skin, including the palms and soles, desquamates (Figure 11-5). A particularly virulent form of TSS is **purpura fulminans**. This disease is characterized by large purpuric skin lesion, fever, hypotension, and disseminated intravascular coagulation. Previously, purpura fulminans was primarily associated with overwhelming *Neisseria meningitidis* infections.

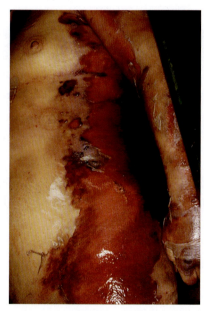

Figure 11-5 Toxic shock syndrome. A case of fatal infection with cutaneous and soft-tissue involvement is shown.

Cutaneous Infections

Localized, **pyogenic staphylococcal infections** include impetigo, folliculitis, furuncles, and carbuncles. **Impetigo**, a superficial infection that mostly affects young children, occurs primarily on the face and limbs. Initially, a small macule (flattened red spot) is seen, and then a pus-filled vesicle (pustule) on an erythematous base develops. Crusting occurs after the pustule ruptures. Multiple vesicles at different stages of development are common, owing to the secondary spread of the infection to adjacent skin sites (Figure 11-6). Impetigo is usually caused by *S. aureus*, although group A streptococci, either alone or with *S. aureus*, are responsible for 20% of cases.

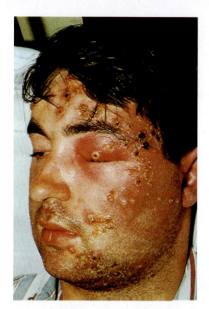

Figure 11-6 Pustular impetigo. Note the vesicles at different stages of development, including pus-filled vesicles on an erythematous base and dry, crusted lesions. (From Emond RT, Rowland HAK: *A color atlas of infectious diseases*, London, 1987, Wolfe.)

Folliculitis is a pyogenic infection in the hair follicles. The base of the follicle is raised and reddened, and there is a small collection of pus beneath the epidermal surface. If this occurs at the base of the eyelid, it is called a **stye. Furuncles** (boils), an extension of folliculitis, are large, painful, raised nodules that have an underlying collection of dead and necrotic tissue. These can drain spontaneously or after surgical incision.

Carbuncles occur when furuncles coalesce and extend to the deeper subcutaneous tissue (Figure 11-7). Multiple sinus tracts are usually present. Patients with carbuncles have chills and fevers, indicating the systemic spread of staphylococci via bacteremia to other tissues.

Staphylococcal **wound infections** can also occur in patients after a surgical procedure or after trauma, with organisms colonizing the skin introduced into the wound. The staphylococci are generally not able to establish an infection in an immunocompetent

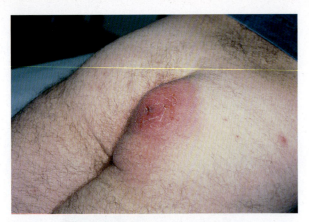

Figure 11-7 *Staphylococcus aureus* carbuncle. This carbuncle developed on the buttock over a 7- to 10-day period and required surgical drainage plus antibiotic therapy. (From Cohen J, Powderly WG: *Infectious diseases*, ed 2, St Louis, 2004, Mosby.)

person unless a foreign body (e.g., stitches, a splinter, dirt) is present in the wound. Infections are characterized by edema, erythema, pain, and an accumulation of purulent material. The infection can be easily managed if the wound is reopened, the foreign matter removed, and the purulence drained.

With the spread of **MRSA strains in the community**, these organisms are now the most common cause of skin and soft-tissue infections in patients presenting to hospital emergency departments in the United States. This problem is complicated by the fact that the majority of these patients are initially treated with a penicillin, cephalosporin, or other ineffective antibiotics.

Bacteremia and Endocarditis

S. aureus is a common cause of **bacteremia**. Most likely, the infection spreads to the blood from an innocuous-appearing skin infection. More than 50% of the cases of *S. aureus* bacteremia are acquired in the hospital after a surgical procedure or result from the continued use of a contaminated intravascular catheter. *S. aureus* bacteremias, particularly prolonged episodes, are associated with dissemination to other body sites, including the heart.

Acute **endocarditis** caused by *S. aureus* is a serious disease, with a mortality rate approaching 50%. Although patients with *S. aureus* endocarditis may initially have nonspecific influenza-like symptoms,

their condition can deteriorate rapidly and include disruption of cardiac output and peripheral evidence of septic embolization. The initial symptoms may be mild, but fever, chills, and pleuritic chest pain caused by pulmonary emboli are generally present. Clinical cure of the endocarditis is the rule, although it is common for complications to occur as the result of secondary spread of the infection to other organs.

Pneumonia and Empyema

S. aureus respiratory disease can develop after the aspiration of oral secretions or from the hematogenous spread of the organism from a distant site. **Aspiration pneumonia** is seen primarily in the very young, the elderly, and patients with cystic fibrosis, influenza, chronic obstructive pulmonary disease, and bronchiectasis. Radiographic examination reveals the presence of patchy infiltrates with consolidation or abscesses, the latter consistent with the organism's ability to secrete cytotoxic toxins and enzymes and to form localized abscesses. **Hematogenous pneumonia** is common for patients with bacteremia or endocarditis. Community-acquired MRSA is responsible for a severe form of **necrotizing pneumonia** with massive hemoptysis, septic shock, and a high mortality rate. Although this disease is reported most commonly in children and young adults, it is not restricted to these age groups.

Empyema occurs in 10% of patients with pneumonia, and *S. aureus* is responsible for one third of all cases.

Osteomyelitis and Septic Arthritis

S. aureus **osteomyelitis** can result from the hematogenous dissemination to bone, or it can be a secondary infection resulting from trauma or the extension of disease from an adjacent area. Hematogenous spread in children generally results from a cutaneous staphylococcal infection and usually involves the metaphyseal area of long bones, a highly vascularized area of bony growth. This infection is characterized by the sudden onset of localized pain over the involved bone and by high fever. Blood cultures are positive in approximately 50% of cases.

The hematogenous osteomyelitis that is seen in adults commonly occurs in the form of vertebral osteomyelitis and rarely in the form of an infection of the long bones. Intense back pain with fever is the initial symptom. Radiographic evidence of osteomyelitis in children and adults is not seen until 2 to 3 weeks after the initial symptoms appear. A **Brodie abscess** is a sequestered focus of staphylococcal osteomyelitis that arises in the metaphyseal area of a long bone and occurs only in adults. The staphylococcal osteomyelitis that occurs after trauma or a surgical procedure is generally accompanied by inflammation and purulent drainage from the wound or the sinus tract overlying the infected bone. Because the staphylococcal infection may be restricted to the wound, isolation of the organism from this site is not conclusive evidence of bony involvement. With appropriate antibiotic therapy and surgery, the cure rate for staphylococcal osteomyelitis is excellent.

S. aureus is the primary cause of **septic arthritis** in young children and in adults who are receiving intraarticular injections or who have mechanically abnormal joints. Secondary involvement of multiple joints is indicative of hematogenous spread from a localized focus. *S. aureus* is replaced by *Neisseria gonorrhoeae* as the most common cause of septic arthritis in sexually active persons. Staphylococcal arthritis is characterized by a painful, erythematous joint, with purulent material obtained on aspiration. Infection is usually demonstrated in the large joints (e.g., shoulder, knee, hip, elbow). The prognosis in children is excellent, but in adults it depends on the nature of the underlying disease and the occurrence of any secondary infectious complications.

Staphylococcus epidermidis and Other Coagulase-Negative Staphylococci

Endocarditis

S. epidermidis, *S. lugdunensis*, and related coagulase-negative staphylococci can infect prosthetic and, less commonly, native heart valves. Infections of native valves are believed to result from the inoculation of organisms onto a damaged heart valve (e.g., a congenital malformation, damage resulting from rheumatic heart disease). ***S. lugdunensis*** is the staphylococcal species most commonly associated with native valve endocarditis, although this disease is more commonly caused by streptococci. In contrast, staphylococci are a major cause of **endocarditis of artificial valves**. The infection characteristically has an indolent course, with clinical signs and symptoms not developing for as long as 1 year after the procedure. Although the heart valve can be infected, more commonly the infection occurs at the site where the valve is sewn to the heart tissue. Thus infection with abscess formation can lead to separation of the valve at the suture line and to mechanical heart failure.

Catheter and Shunt Infections

More than 50% of all infections of catheters and shunts are caused by coagulase-negative staphylococci. A persistent bacteremia is generally observed in patients with infections of shunts and catheters because the organisms have continual access to the blood. Immune complex-mediated glomerulonephritis occurs in patients with long-standing disease.

Prosthetic Joint Infections

Infections of artificial joints, particularly the hip, can be caused by coagulase-negative staphylococci. The patient usually experiences only localized pain and mechanical failure of the joint. Systemic signs, such as fever and leukocytosis, are not prominent, and blood cultures are usually negative. Treatment consists of joint replacement and antimicrobial therapy.

Urinary Tract Infections

S. saprophyticus has a predilection for causing urinary tract infections in young, sexually active women and is rarely responsible for infections in other patients. It is also infrequently found as an asymptomatic colonizer of the urinary tract. Infected women usually have dysuria (pain on urination), pyuria (pus in urine), and numerous organisms in the urine. Typically, patients respond rapidly to antibiotics and reinfection is uncommon.

EPIDEMIOLOGY

Staphylococci are **ubiquitous**. All persons have coagulase-negative staphylococci on their skin, and transient colonization of moist skin folds with *S. aureus* is common. Colonization of the umbilical stump, skin, and perineal area of neonates with *S. aureus* is common. *S. aureus* and coagulase-negative staphylococci are also found in the oropharynx, gastrointestinal tract, and urogenital tract. Approximately 15% of normal healthy adults are persistent nasopharyngeal carriers of *S. aureus*, with a higher incidence reported for hospitalized patients, medical personnel, persons with eczematous skin diseases, and those who regularly use needles, either illicitly (e.g., drug abusers) or for medical reasons (e.g., patients with insulin-dependent diabetes, patients receiving allergy injections, or those undergoing hemodialysis).

The bacteria is responsible for many hospital-acquired infections and susceptible to high temperatures and disinfectants and antiseptic solutions. However, the organisms can survive on dry surfaces for long periods. Therefore medical personnel must use proper hand-washing techniques to prevent the transfer of staphylococci from themselves to patients or among patients. Beginning in the 1980s, MRSA strains spread rapidly in susceptible hospitalized patients, dramatically changing the therapy available for preventing and treating staphylococcal infections.

LABORATORY DIAGNOSIS

Microscopy

Staphylococci are **gram-positive cocci** that form **clusters** when grown on agar media but commonly appear as single cells or small groups of organisms in clinical specimens. The successful detection of organisms in a clinical specimen depends on the type of the infection (e.g., abscess, bacteremia, impetigo) and the quality of the material submitted for analysis. If the clinician scrapes the base of the abscess with a swab or curette, then an abundance of organisms should be observed in the Gram-stained specimen. Aspirated pus or superficial specimens collected with

swabs consists primarily of necrotic material with relatively few organisms, so these specimens are not as useful. Relatively few organisms are generally present in the blood of bacteremic patients (an average of less than 1 organism per milliliter of blood), so blood specimens should be cultured, but blood examined by Gram stain is not useful. Staphylococci are seen in the nasopharynx of patients with SSSS and in the vagina of patients with TSS, but these staphylococci cannot be distinguished from the organisms that normally colonize these sites. Diagnosis of these diseases is made by the clinical presentation of the patient, with isolation of *S. aureus* in culture confirmatory. Staphylococci are implicated in food poisoning by the clinical presentation of the patient (e.g., rapid onset of vomiting and abdominal cramps) and a history of specific food ingestion (e.g., salted ham). Gram stains of the food or patient stool specimens are generally not useful.

Nucleic Acid-Based Tests

Commercial nucleic acid amplification tests are available for the direct detection and identification of *S. aureus* in clinical specimens. These tests are useful for the detection of MRSA in wound specimens and screening nasal specimens for carriage of these bacteria.

Culture

Clinical specimens should be inoculated onto nutritionally enriched agar media supplemented with sheep blood. Staphylococci grow rapidly on nonselective media incubated aerobically or anaerobically, with large, smooth colonies seen within 24 hours (Figure 11-8). As noted earlier, *S. aureus* colonies will gradually turn **yellow**, particularly when the cultures are incubated at room temperature. Almost all isolates of *S. aureus* and some strains of coagulase-negative staphylococci produce hemolysis on sheep blood agar. If there is a mixture of organisms in the specimen (e.g., wound or respiratory specimen), *S. aureus* can be isolated selectively on a variety of special media, including **mannitol-salt agar**, which is supplemented with mannitol (fermented by *S. aureus* but not by most other staphylococci) and 7.5% sodium chloride (inhibits the growth of most other organisms).

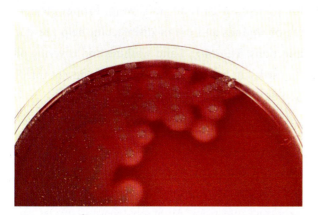

Figure 11-8 *Staphylococcus aureus* grown on a sheep blood agar plate. Note the colonies are large and β hemolytic.

Identification

Relatively simple biochemical tests (e.g., positive reactions for **coagulase**, protein A, heat-stable nuclease, and mannitol fermentation) can be used to identify *S. aureus*. Identification of the coagulase-negative staphylococci is more complex, requiring the use of commercial identification systems or detection of species-specific genes by nucleic acid sequencing techniques. Colonies resembling *S. aureus* are identified in most laboratories by mixing a suspension of organisms with a drop of plasma and observing clumping of the organisms (positive coagulase test). Alternatively, plasma placed in a test tube can be inoculated with the organism and examined at 4 and 24 hours for formation of a clot (positive tube coagulase test). These coagulase tests cannot be performed when staphylococci are initially detected in culture (e.g., in a blood culture broth) or a clinical specimen. This problem of differentiating the more virulent *S. aureus* from the coagulase-negative staphylococci was resolved with the commercial development of a novel method of **fluorescent in situ hybridization (FISH)**. Fluorescent-labeled artificial probes can bind specifically to *S. aureus* and be detected by fluorescent microscopy.

Antibody Detection

Antibodies to cell wall teichoic acids are present in many patients with long-standing *S. aureus* infec-

tions. However, this test has been discontinued in most hospitals because it is less sensitive than culture and nucleic acid-based tests.

TREATMENT, PREVENTION, AND CONTROL

Staphylococci quickly developed drug resistance after penicillin was introduced, and today less than 10% of the strains are susceptible to this antibiotic. This resistance is mediated by **penicillinase** (β-lactamase-specific for penicillins), that hydrolyzes the β-lactam ring of penicillin. Because of the problems with penicillin-resistant staphylococci, **semisynthetic penicillins** resistant to β-lactamase hydrolysis (e.g., methicillin, nafcillin, oxacillin, dicloxacillin) were developed. Unfortunately, the staphylococci developed resistance to these antibiotics as well. Currently, the majority of *S. aureus* responsible for hospital- and community-acquired infections are resistant to these semisynthetic penicillins, and these MRSA strains are resistant to all β-lactam antibiotics (i.e., penicillins, cephalosporins, carbapenems). Not all bacteria in a resistant population may express their resistance in traditional susceptibility tests (**heterogeneous resistance**); therefore, the definitive method for identifying a resistant isolate is detection of the *MecA* gene that codes for the penicillin-binding protein *(PBP2a)* that confers resistance.

Patients with localized skin and soft-tissue infections can generally be managed by incision and drainage of the abscesses. If the infection involves a larger area or systemic signs are present, then antibiotic therapy is indicated. Staphylococci have demonstrated the remarkable ability to develop resistance to most antibiotics. Until recently, the one antibiotic that remained uniformly active against staphylococci was vancomycin, the current antibiotic of choice for treating serious infections caused by staphylococci resistant to methicillin. Unfortunately, isolates of *S. aureus* have now been found with two forms of **resistance to vancomycin**. Presently, this resistance is uncommon.

Staphylococci are ubiquitous organisms present on the skin and mucous membranes, and their introduction through breaks in the skin occurs often. However, the number of organisms required to establish an infection (**infectious dose**) is generally large unless a foreign body (e.g., dirt, a splinter, stitches) is present in the wound. Proper cleansing of the wound and the application of an appropriate disinfectant (e.g., germicidal soap, iodine solution, hexachlorophene) will prevent most infections in healthy individuals.

The spread of staphylococci from person to person is more difficult to prevent. An example of this is surgical wound infections, which can be caused by relatively few organisms, because foreign bodies and devitalized tissue may be present. The risk of contamination during an operative procedure can be minimized through proper hand washing and the covering of exposed skin surfaces. The spread of methicillin-resistant organisms can also be difficult to control because asymptomatic nasopharyngeal carriage is the most common source of these organisms.

SUMMARY

Staphylococcus aureus

Staphylococcus aureus strains are catalase-positive, gram-positive cocci arranged in clusters.

The species are characterized by the presence of coagulase, protein A, and species-specific ribitol teichoic acid with *N*-acetylglucosamine residues ("polysaccharide A"). Virulence factors of *Staphylococcus aureus* include structural components that facilitate adherence to host tissues and avoid phagocytosis, and a variety of toxins and hydrolytic enzymes (refer to Table 11-3). *Staphylococcus aureus* can cause toxin-mediated diseases (food poisoning, TSS, scalded skin syndrome), pyogenic diseases (impetigo, folliculitis, furuncles, carbuncles, wound infections), and other systemic diseases. Hospital- and community-acquired infections with MRSA are a significant worldwide problem. MRSA now is the most common cause of community-acquired skin and soft-tissue infections.

Microscopy is useful for pyogenic infections but not blood infections or toxin-mediated infections.

Empiric therapy should include antibiotics active against MRSA strains. Treatment is symptomatic for patients with food poisoning. Proper cleansing of wounds and use of disinfectant help prevent infections. Thorough hand washing and covering of exposed skin helps medical personnel prevent infection or spread to other patients.

Coagulase-Negative Staphylococci

Coagulase-negative staphylococci are relatively avirulent, and can cause infections including subacute endocarditis, infections of foreign bodies, and urinary tract infections. All Staphylococcus species can cause wound infections, urinary tract infections, catheter and shunt infections and prosthetic device infections.

KEYWORDS

English	Chinese
Staphylococcus	葡萄球菌属
Staphylococcus aureus	金黄色葡萄球菌
Staphylococcus epidermidis	表皮葡萄球菌
Staphylococcus haemolyticus	溶血葡萄球菌
Staphylococcus saprophyticus	腐生葡萄球菌
Coagulase-negative staphylococci	凝固酶阴性葡萄球菌
Scalded skin syndrome	烫伤样皮肤综合征
Toxic shock syndrome toxin-1	毒素休克综合征毒素-1
Enterotoxins	肠毒素
Coagulase	凝固酶
Leukocidin	杀白细胞素
Staphylococcal protein A	葡萄球菌 A 蛋白

BIBLIOGRAPHY

1. Dinges MM, et al: Exotoxins of *Staphylococcus aureus*, Clin Microbiol Rev 13: 16-34, 2000.

2. Fournier B, Philpott D: Recognition of *Staphylococcus aureus* by the innate immune system. Clin Microbiol Rev 18: 521-540, 2005.

3. Frank K, del Pozo J, Patel R: From clinical microbiology to infection pathogenesis: how daring to be different works for *Staphylococcus lugdunensis*, Clin Microbiol Rev 21: 111-133, 2008.

4. Gravet A, et al: Predominant *Staphylococcus aureus* isolated from antibiotic-associated diarrhea is clinically rel-

evant and produces enterotoxin A and the biocomponent toxin LukE-5. LukD, J Clin Microbiol 37: 4012-4019, 1999.

5. Ippolito G, et al: Methicillin-resistant *Staphylococcus aureus*: the superbug, Int J Infect Dis 14(Suppl 4): S7-S11, 2010.

6. Kurlenda J, Grinholc M: Current diagnostic tools for methicillin-resistant *Staphylococcus aureus* infections, Mol Diagn Ther 14: 73-80, 2010.

7. Lowy FD: *Staphylococcus aureus* infections, N Engl J Med 339: 520-532, 1998.

8. Moran G, et al: Methicillin-resistant *S. aureus* infections among patients in the emergency department, N Engl J Med 355: 666-674, 2006.

9. Novick RP: Autoinduction and signal transduction in the regulation of staphylococcal virulence, Mol Microbiol 48: 1429-1449, 2003.

10. Nygaard T, Deleo F, Voyich J: Community-associated methicillin-resistant *Staphylococcus aureus* skin infections: advances toward identifying the key virulence factors, Curr Opin Infect Dis 21: 147-152, 2008.

11. Otto M: Basis of virulence in community-associated meth-icillin-resistant *Staphylococcus aureus*, Annu Rev Micro-biol 64: 143-162, 2010.

12. Pannaraj P, et al: Infective pyomyositis and myositis in children in the era of community-acquired, methicillin-resistant *Staphylococcus aureus* infection, Clin Infect Dis 43: 953-960, 2006.

13. Seybold U, et al: Emergence of community-associated methicillin-resistant *Staphylococcus aureus* USA300 geno-type as a major cause of health care associated blood stream infections, Clin Infect Dis 42: 647-656, 2006.

14. Silversides J, Lappin E, Ferguson A: Staphylococcal toxic shock syndrome: mechanisms and management, Curr Infect Dis Rep 12: 392-400, 2010.

15. Srinivasan A, Dick JD, Perl TM: Vancomycin resistance in staphylococci, Clin Microbiol Rev 15: 430-438, 2002.

16. Stanley J, Amagai M: Pemphigus, bullous impetigo, and the staphylococcal scalded-skin syndrome, N Engl J Med 355: 1800-1810, 2006.

17. Tang Y, Stratton C: *Staphylococcus aureus*: an old pathogen with new weapons, Clin Lab Med 30: 179-208, 2010.

Streptococcus

Chapter 12

The genus *Streptococcus* is a diverse collection of **gram-positive cocci** typically arranged in **pairs or chains** (in contrast to the clusters formed by *Staphylococcus*). Their nutritional requirements are complex, necessitating the use of blood- or serum-enriched media for isolation. Streptococci are **catalase-negative**.

Numerous streptococci are recognized as important human pathogens, the most common of which are discussed in this chapter (Table 12-1). Unfortunately, the classification of species within the genus is complicated because three different, overlapping schemes are used: (1) serologic properties: **Lancefield groupings** (originally A to W); (2) **hemolytic patterns:** complete (beta [β]) hemolysis, incomplete (alpha [α]) hemolysis, and no (gamma [γ]) hemolysis; and (3) **biochemical (physiologic) properties**.

Although this is an oversimplification, it is practical to think that the streptococci are divided into two groups: (1) the β-hemolytic streptococci, which are classified by Lancefield grouping and (2) the α-hemolytic and γ-hemolytic streptococci, which are classified by biochemical testing. The latter group is referred to collectively as **viridans streptococci**, a name derived from *viridis* (Latin for "green"), referring to the green pigment formed by the partial hemolysis of blood agar.

The Lancefield typing scheme is primarily used today for only a few species of streptococci (e.g., those classified in groups A, B, C, F, and G; Table 12-2). The viridans streptococci are subdivided into five clinically distinct groups (Table 12-3). Some species of the viridans streptococci can be β-hemolytic as well as α-hemolytic and nonhemolytic, which

Table 12-1 Important Streptococci

Organism	Historical Derivation
Streptococcus	*streptus*, pliant; *coccus*, grain or berry (a pliant berry or coccus; refers to the appearance of long, flexible chains of cocci)
S. agalactiae	*agalactia*, want of milk (original isolate [called *S. mastitidis*] was responsible for bovine mastitis)
S. anginosus	*anginosus*, pertaining to angina
S. constellatus	*constellatus*, studded with stars (original isolate embedded in agar with smaller colonies surrounding the large colony; satellite formation does not occur around colonies on the surface of an agar plate)
S. dysgalactiae	*dys*, ill, hard; galactia, pertaining to milk (loss of milk secretion; isolates associated with bovine mastitis)
S. gallolyticus	*gallatum*, gallate; *lyticus*, to loosen (able to digest or hydrolyze methyl gallate)
S. intermedius	*intermedius*, intermediate (initial confusion about whether this was an aerobic or an anaerobic bacterium)
S. mitis	*mitis*, mild (incorrectly thought to cause mild infections)
S. mutans	*mutans*, changing (cocci that may appear rodlike, particularly when initially isolated in culture)
S. pneumoniae	*pneumon*, the lungs (causes pneumonia)
S. pyogenes	*pyus*, pus; *gennaio*, beget or producing (pus producing; typically associated with formation of pus in wounds)
S. salivarius	*salivarius*, salivary (found in the mouth in saliva)

Table 12-2 Classification of Common β-Hemolytic Streptococci

Group	Representative Species	Diseases
A	S. pyogenes	Pharyngitis, skin and soft-tissue infections, bacteremia, rheumatic fever, acute glomerulonephritis
	S. anginosus group	Abscesses
B	S. agalactiae	Neonatal disease, endometritis, wound infections, urinary tract infections, bacteremia, pneumonia, skin and soft-tissue infections
C	S. dysgalactiae	Pharyngitis, acute glomerulonephritis
F, G	S. anginosus group	Abscesses
	S. dysgalactiae	Pharyngitis, acute glomerulonephritis

Table 12-3 Classification of Viridans Group of *Streptococcus*

Group	Representative Species	Diseases
Anginosus	S. anginosus, S. constellatus, S. intermedius	Abscesses in brain, oropharynx, or peritoneal cavity
Mitis	S. mitis, S. pneumoniae, S. oralis	Subacute endocarditis; sepsis in neutropenic patients; pneumonia; meningitis
Mutans	S. mutans, S. sobrinus	Dental caries; bacteremia
Salivarius	S. salivarius	Bacteremia; endocarditis
Bovis	S. gallolyticus subsp. gallolyticus, subsp. pasteurianus	Bacteremia associated with gastrointestinal cancer (subsp. gallolyticus); meningitis (subsp. pasteurianus)
Ungrouped	S. suis	Meningitis; bacteremia; streptococcal toxic shock syndrome

unfortunately has resulted in classifying these bacteria by both their Lancefield grouping and as viridans streptococci.

STREPTOCOCCUS PYOGENES

Physiology and Structure

Isolates of *S. pyogenes* are spherical cocci, 1 to 2 μm in diameter, arranged in short chains in clinical specimens and longer chains when grown in liquid media (Figure 12-1). Growth is optimal on enriched-blood agar media but is inhibited if the medium contains a high concentration of glucose. After 24 hours of incubation, 1- to 2-mm white colonies with large zones of β-hemolysis are observed (Figure 12-2).

The basic structural framework of the cell wall is the peptidoglycan layer. Within the cell wall are group-specific and type-specific antigens. The **group-specific carbohydrate** that constitutes approximately 10% of the dry weight of the cell (**Lancefield group A antigen**) is a dimer of *N*-acetylglucosamine and rhamnose. This antigen is used to classify group A streptococci and distinguish them from other strep-

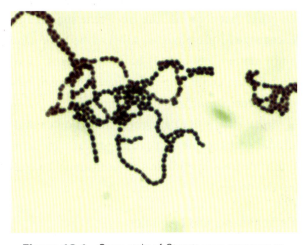

Figure 12-1 Gram stain of *Streptococcus pyogenes*.

tococcal groups. **M protein** is the major type-specific protein associated with virulent strains. The protein is anchored in the cytoplasmic membrane, extends through the cell wall, and protrudes above the cell surface. M proteins are subdivided into class I and class II molecules. The class I M proteins share exposed antigens, whereas the class II M proteins do not have exposed shared antigens. Although strains with both classes of antigens can cause suppurative infections and glomerulonephritis, only bacteria with

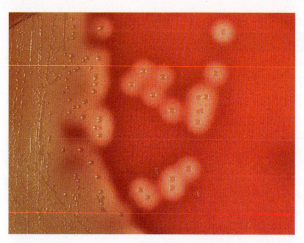

Figure 12-2 *Streptococcus pyogenes* (group A) typically appear as small colonies with a large zone of hemolysis.

control. These proteins interfere with phagocytosis by binding either the Fc fragment of antibodies or fibronectin, which blocks activation of complement by the alternate pathway and reduces the amount of bound C3b. Finally, all strains of *S. pyogenes* have **C5a peptidase** on their surface. This serine protease inactivates C5a and protects the bacteria from early clearance from infected tissues.

More than 10 different bacterial antigens have been demonstrated to mediate **adherence to host cells,** with lipoteichoic acid, M proteins, and F protein the most important. *S. pyogenes* can **invade into epithelial cells,** a process that is mediated by **M protein** and **F protein** and other bacterial antigens.

Toxins and Enzymes

The **streptococcal pyrogenic exotoxins (Spe),** originally called *erythrogenic toxins,* are produced by lysogenic strains of streptococci and are similar to the toxin produced in *Corynebacterium diphtheriae.* Four immunologically distinct heat-labile toxins (SpeA, SpeB, SpeC, and SpeF) have been described in *S. pyogenes* and in rare strains of groups C and G streptococci. The toxins act as superantigens, interacting with both macrophages and helper T cells. This family of exotoxins is believed responsible for many of the clinical manifestations of severe streptococcal diseases, including necrotizing fasciitis and streptococcal toxic shock syndrome, as well as the rash observed in patients with scarlet fever.

Streptolysin S is an oxygen-stable, nonimmunogenic, cell-bound hemolysin that can lyse erythrocytes, leukocytes, and platelets. It can also stimulate the release of lysosomal contents after engulfment, with subsequent death of the phagocytic cell. Streptolysin S is produced in the presence of serum (the S indicates serum stable) and is responsible for the characteristic β-hemolysis seen on blood agar media.

Streptolysin O is an oxygen-labile hemolysin capable of lysing erythrocytes, leukocytes, platelets, and cultured cells. Antibodies are readily formed against streptolysin O (**antistreptolysin O [ASO] antibodies**), are useful for documenting recent group A streptococcal infection (anti-ASO test). Streptoly-

class I (exposed shared antigen) M proteins cause rheumatic fever. The epidemiologic classification of *S. pyogenes* is based on sequence analysis of the *emm* gene that encodes the M proteins.

Other important components in the cell wall of *S. pyogenes* include **M-like surface proteins, lipoteichoic acid,** and **F protein.** A complex of more than 20 genes that comprise the *emm* gene superfamily encode the M-like proteins as well as the M proteins and immunoglobulin (Ig)-binding proteins. Lipoteichoic acid and F protein facilitate binding of host cells by complexing with fibronectin.

Some strains of *S. pyogenes* have an outer hyaluronic acid **capsule** that is antigenically indistinguishable from hyaluronic acid in mammalian connective tissues.

Pathogenesis and Immunity

The virulence of group A streptococci is determined by the ability of the bacteria to avoid opsonization and phagocytosis, adhere to and invade host cells, and produce a variety of toxins and enzymes.

Initial Host-Parasite Interactions

S. pyogenes has multiple mechanisms for **avoiding opsonization and phagocytosis.** The **hyaluronic acid capsule** is a poor immunogen and interferes with phagocytosis. The **M proteins** also interfere with phagocytosis. M-like proteins resemble M proteins in structure and are under the same regulatory sin O is irreversibly **inhibited by cholesterol** in skin lipids, so patients with cutaneous infections do not develop anti-ASO antibodies.

At least two forms of **streptokinase (A and B)** have been described. These enzymes can lyse blood clots and fibrin deposits and facilitate the rapid spread of *S. pyogenes* in infected tissues. Antibodies directed against these enzymes (**anti-streptokinase antibodies**) are a useful marker for infection.

Four immunologically distinct deoxyribonucleases (**DNases A to D**) have been identified. These enzymes are not cytolytic but can depolymerize free deoxyribonucleic acid (DNA) present in pus. Antibodies developed against DNase B are an important marker of *S. pyogenes* infections (**anti-DNase B test**), particularly for patients with cutaneous infections.

Clinical Diseases

Suppurative Streptococcal Disease

Pharyngitis

Pharyngitis generally develops 2 to 4 days after exposure to the pathogen, with an abrupt onset of sore throat, fever, malaise, and headache. The posterior pharynx can appear erythematous, with an exudate, and cervical lymphadenopathy can be prominent. An accurate diagnosis can be made only with specific laboratory tests.

Scarlet fever is a complication of streptococcal pharyngitis that occurs when the infecting strain is lysogenized by a bacteriophage that mediates production of a pyrogenic exotoxin. Within 1 to 2 days after the initial clinical symptoms of pharyngitis develop, a diffuse erythematous rash initially appears on the upper chest and then spreads to the extremities. The area around the mouth is generally spared (**circumoral pallor**), as are the palms and soles. A yellowish-white coating initially covers the tongue and is later shed, revealing a red, raw surface beneath (**"strawberry tongue"**). The rash, which blanches when pressed, is best seen on the abdomen and in skin folds (**Pastia lines**). The rash disappears over the next 5 to 7 days and is followed by desquamation of the superficial skin layer.

Pyoderma

Pyoderma (**impetigo**) is a confined, purulent (*"pyo"*) infection of the skin (*"derma"*) that primarily affects exposed areas (i.e., face, arms, legs). Infection begins when the skin is colonized with *S. pyogenes*. The organism is introduced into the subcutaneous tissues through a break in the skin (e.g., scratch, insect bite). Vesicles develop, progressing to pustules (pus-filled vesicles), and then rupture and crust over. The regional lymph nodes can become enlarged. Secondary dermal spread of the infection caused by scratching is typical.

Pyoderma is seen primarily during the warm, moist months, in young children with poor personal hygiene. Although *S. pyogenes* is responsible for most streptococcal skin infections, groups C and G streptococci have also been implicated. *Staphylococcus aureus* is also commonly present in the lesions.

Erysipelas

Erysipelas (*erythros*, "red"; *pella*, "skin") is an acute infection of the skin. Patients experience localized pain, inflammation (erythema, warmth), lymph node enlargement, and systemic signs (chills, fever, leukocytosis). The involved skin area is typically raised and distinctly differentiated from the uninvolved skin (Figure 12-3). Erysipelas occurs most commonly in young children or older adults, historically on the face but now more commonly on the legs, and usually is preceded by infections of the respiratory tract or skin with *S. pyogenes* (less commonly with group C or G streptococci).

Cellulitis

Unlike erysipelas, **cellulitis** typically involves both the skin and deeper subcutaneous tissues, and the distinction between infected and noninfected skin is not as clear. As in erysipelas, local inflammation and systemic signs are observed. Precise identification of the offending organism is necessary because many different organisms can cause cellulitis.

Necrotizing Fasciitis

Necrotizing fasciitis (also called *streptococcal gangrene*) is an infection that occurs deep in the subcutaneous tissue, spreads along the fascial planes, and is

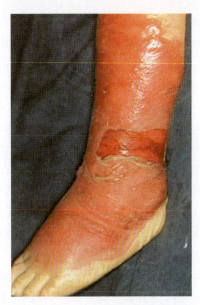

Figure 12-3 Acute stage of erysipelas of the leg. Note the erythema in the involved area and bullae formation. (From Emond RTD, Rowland HAK: *A color atlas of infectious diseases*, ed 2, London, 1989, Wolfe.)

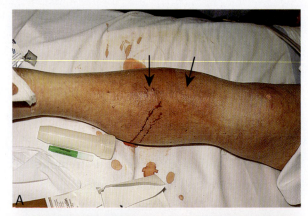

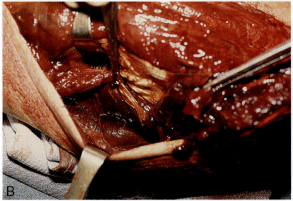

Figure 12-4 Necrotizing fasciitis caused by *Streptococcus pyogenes*. The patient presented with a 3-day history of malaise, diffuse myalgia, and low-grade fever. Over 3 hours, the pain became excruciating and was localized to the calf. **A,** Note the two small, purple bullae over the calf *(arrows).* **B,** Extensive necrotizing fasciitis was present on surgical exploration. The patient died despite aggressive surgical and medical management. (From Cohen J, Powderly W: *Infectious diseases*, ed 2, St Louis, 2004, Mosby.)

characterized by an extensive destruction of muscle and fat (Figure 12-4). The organism (referred to by the news media as "flesh-eating bacteria") is introduced into the tissue through a break in the skin (e.g., minor cut or trauma, vesicular viral infection, burn, surgery). Toxicity, multiorgan failure, and death are the hallmarks of this disease; thus prompt medical intervention is necessary to save the patient. Unlike cellulitis, which can be treated with antibiotic therapy, fasciitis must also be treated aggressively with the surgical debridement of infected tissue.

Streptococcal Toxic Shock Syndrome

Patients with this syndrome initially experience soft-tissue inflammation at the site of the infection, pain, and nonspecific symptoms, such as fever, chills, malaise, nausea, vomiting, and diarrhea. The pain intensifies as the disease progresses to shock and organ failure (e.g., kidney, lungs, liver, heart). However, in contrast with staphylococcal disease, most patients with streptococcal disease are bacteremic, and many have necrotizing fasciitis.

The strains of *S. pyogenes* responsible for this syndrome differ from the strains causing pharyngitis, in that most of the former are M serotypes 1 or 3 and many have prominent mucopolysaccharide hyal-

uronic acid capsules (mucoid strains). The production of pyrogenic exotoxins, particularly SpeA and SpeC, is also a prominent feature of these organisms.

Nonsuppurative Streptococcal Disease

Rheumatic Fever

Rheumatic fever is a nonsuppurative complication of *S. pyogenes* pharyngitis. It is characterized by inflammatory changes involving the heart, joints, blood vessels, and subcutaneous tissues. Involvement of the heart manifests as a pancarditis (endocarditis, pericarditis, myocarditis) and is often associated with subcutaneous nodules. Joint manifestations can range from arthralgias to frank arthritis, with multiple joints involved in a migratory pattern (i.e., involvement shifts from one joint to another).

It is most common in young school-age children, with no male or female predilection, and occurs primarily during the cooler months of the fall or winter. The disease occurs most commonly in patients with severe streptococcal pharyngitis; however, as many as one third of patients have asymptomatic or mild infection. Rheumatic fever can recur with a subsequent streptococcal infection if antibiotic prophylaxis is not used. The risk for recurrence decreases with time.

Because no specific diagnostic test can identify patients with rheumatic fever, the diagnosis is made on the basis of clinical findings and documented evidence of a recent *S. pyogenes* infection, such as (1) positive throat culture or specific nucleic acid based test, (2) detection of the group A antigen in a throat swab, or (3) an elevation of anti-ASO, anti-DNase B, or anti-hyaluronidase antibodies. The absence of an elevated or rising antibody titer would be strong evidence against rheumatic fever.

Acute Glomerulonephritis

The second nonsuppurative complication of streptococcal disease is **glomerulonephritis**, which is characterized by acute inflammation of the renal glomeruli with edema, hypertension, hematuria, and proteinuria. Specific nephritogenic strains of group A streptococci are associated with this disease. In contrast with rheumatic fever, acute glomerulonephritis is a sequela of both pharyngeal and pyodermal streptococcal infections; however, the nephrogenic M serotypes differ for the two primary diseases. Diagnosis is determined on the basis of the clinical presentation and the finding of evidence of a recent *S. pyogenes* infection.

Epidemiology

Group A streptococci can colonize the oropharynx of healthy children and young adults in the absence of clinical disease. However, isolation of *S. pyogenes* in a patient with pharyngitis is generally considered significant. Untreated patients produce antibodies against the specific bacterial M protein that can result in long-lived immunity; however, this antibody response is diminished in treated patients.

In general, *S. pyogenes* disease is caused by recently acquired strains that can establish an infection of the pharynx or skin before specific antibodies are produced or competitive organisms are able to proliferate. Pharyngitis caused by *S. pyogenes* is primarily a disease of children between the ages of 5 and 15 years, but infants and adults are also susceptible. The pathogen is spread from person to person through respiratory droplets. Soft-tissue infections (i.e., pyoderma, erysipelas, cellulitis, fasciitis) are typically preceded by initial skin colonization with group A streptococci, after which the organisms are introduced into the superficial or deep tissues through a break in the skin.

Laboratory Diagnosis

Microscopy

Gram stains of samples of affected tissue can be used to make a rapid, preliminary diagnosis of *S. pyogenes* soft-tissue infections or pyoderma. Because streptococci are not observed in Gram stains of uninfected skin, the finding of gram-positive cocci in pairs and chains in association with leukocytes is important. Observation of streptococci in a respiratory specimen from a patient with pharyngitis has no diagnostic significance.

Antigen Detection

A variety of immunologic tests using antibodies that react with the group-specific carbohydrate in the bacterial cell wall can be used to detect group A streptococci directly in throat swabs. All negative results must be confirmed by an alternative test. Antigen tests are not used for cutaneous or nonsuppurative diseases.

Nucleic Acid-Based Tests

Commercial nucleic acid probe assay and nucleic acid amplification assays are available for the detection of *S. pyogenes* in pharyngeal specimens. Probe assays are less sensitive than culture, but amplification assays are as sensitive as culture, and confirmatory tests are not needed for negative reactions.

Culture

Despite the difficulty of collecting throat swab specimens from children, specimens must be obtained from the posterior oropharynx (e.g., tonsils). The recovery of *S. pyogenes* from patients with impetigo is not a problem. The crusted top of the lesion is raised, and the purulent material and base of the lesion are cultured. Culture specimens should not be obtained from open, draining skin pustules because they might be superinfected with staphylococci. Organisms are readily recovered in the tissues and blood cultures obtained from patients with necrotizing fasciitis; however, relatively few organisms may be present in the skin of patients with erysipelas or cellulitis. The growth of *S. pyogenes* on the plates may be delayed, so prolonged incubation (2 to 3 days) should be used before a culture is considered negative.

Identification

Group A streptococci are identified definitively through the demonstration of the **group-specific carbohydrate**. Differentiation of *S. pyogenes* from other species of streptococci with the group-specific A antigen can be determined by their susceptibility to **bacitracin** or the presence of the enzyme L-**pyrrolidonyl arylamidase (PYR)**. The PYR test measures hydrolysis L-pyrrolindonyl-β-naphthylamide, releasing β-naphthylamine, which, in the presence of p-dimethylaminocinnamaldehyde, forms a red compound. The advantage of this specific test is that it takes less than 1 minute to determine whether the reaction is positive *(S. pyogenes)* or negative *(all other streptococci)*.

Antibody Detection

Patients with *S. pyogenes* disease produce antibodies to specific streptococcal enzymes. The measurement of antibodies against streptolysin O (**ASO test**) is useful for confirming rheumatic fever or acute glomerulonephritis resulting from a recent streptococcal pharyngeal infection. These antibodies appear 3 to 4 weeks after the initial exposure to the organism and then persist. An elevated ASO titer is not observed in patients with streptococcal pyoderma. The production of antibodies against other streptococcal enzymes, particularly DNase B, has been documented in patients with either streptococcal pyoderma or pharyngitis. The **anti-DNase B test** should be performed if streptococcal glomerulonephritis is suspected.

Treatment, Prevention, and Control

S. pyogenes is very sensitive to penicillin, so oral penicillin V or amoxicillin can be used to treat streptococcal pharyngitis. For penicillin-allergic patients, an oral cephalosporin or macrolide may be used. The combined use of intravenous penicillin with a protein-synthesis-inhibiting antibiotic (e.g., clindamycin) is recommended for severe, systemic infections. Drainage and aggressive surgical debridement must be promptly initiated in patients with serious soft-tissue infections.

Persistent oropharyngeal carriage of *S. pyogenes* can occur after a complete course of therapy. Because penicillin resistance has not been observed in patients with oropharyngeal carriage, penicillin can be given for an additional course of treatment. If carriage persists, re-treatment is not indicated because prolonged antibiotic therapy can disrupt the normal bacterial flora. Antibiotic therapy in patients with pharyngitis speeds the relief of symptoms and, if initiated within 10 days of the initial clinical disease, prevents rheumatic fever. Antibiotic therapy does not appear to influence the progression to acute glomerulonephritis.

Patients with a history of rheumatic fever require long-term **antibiotic prophylaxis** to prevent recurrence of the disease. Because damage to the heart valve predisposes these patients to endocarditis, they also require antibiotic prophylaxis before they undergo procedures that can induce transient bacteremias (e.g., dental procedures).

STREPTOCOCCUS AGALACTIAE

Physiology and Structure

Group B streptococci are gram-positive cocci (0.6 to 1.2 μm) that form short chains in clinical specimens and longer chains in culture, features that make them indistinguishable on Gram stain from *S. pyogenes.* They grow well on nutritionally enriched media, and in contrast with the colonies of *S. pyogenes*, the colonies of *S. agalactiae* are large with a narrow zone of β-hemolysis. Some strains (1% to 2%) are nonhemolytic. Strains of *S. agalactiae* can be characterized on the basis of three serologic markers: (1) the **group-specific cell wall polysaccharide B antigen** (Lancefield grouping antigen, composed of rhamnose, *N*-acetylglucosamine, and galactose); (2) nine **type-specific capsular polysaccharides** (Ia, Ib, and II to VIII); and (3) **surface proteins** (the most common is the **c antigen**). The type-specific polysaccharides are important epidemiologic markers, with serotypes Ia, III, and V most commonly associated with colonization and disease.

Pathogenesis and Immunity

The most important virulence factor of *S. agalactiae* is the **polysaccharide capsule**, which interferes with phagocytosis until the patient develops type-specific antibodies. Genital colonization with group B streptococci has been associated with increased risk of premature delivery, and premature infants are at greater risk of disease. There is a greater likelihood of systemic spread of the organism in colonized premature infants with physiologically **low complement levels** or for infants in whom the receptors for complement, or for the Fc fragment of IgG antibodies, are not exposed on neutrophils. It has also been found that the type-specific capsular polysaccharides of types Ia, Ib, and II streptococci have a terminal residue of sialic acid. **Sialic acid** can interfere with the phagocytosis of these strains of group B streptococci.

Clinical Diseases

Early-Onset Neonatal Disease

Clinical symptoms of group B streptococcal disease acquired in utero or at birth develop during the first week of life. Early-onset disease, characterized by **bacteremia, pneumonia,** or **meningitis,** is indistinguishable from sepsis caused by other organisms. Because pulmonary involvement is observed in most infants, and meningeal involvement may be initially inapparent, examination of cerebrospinal fluid is required for all infected children.

Late-Onset Neonatal Disease

Late-onset disease is acquired from an exogenous source (e.g., mother, another infant) and develops between 1 week and 3 months of age. The predominant manifestation is **bacteremia with meningitis,** which resembles disease caused by other bacteria.

Infections in Pregnant Women

Postpartum endometritis, wound infection, and **urinary tract infections** occur in women during and immediately after pregnancy. Because childbearing women are generally in good health, the prognosis is excellent for those who receive appropriate therapy.

Infections in Men and Nonpregnant Women

Compared with pregnant women who acquire group B streptococcal infection, men and nonpregnant women with group B streptococcal infections are generally older and have debilitating underlying conditions. The most common presentations are **bacteremia, pneumonia, bone and joint infections,** and **skin and soft-tissue infections.** Because these patients often have compromised immunity, mortality is higher in this population.

Epidemiology

Group B streptococci colonize the lower gastrointestinal tract and the genitourinary tract. Transient vaginal carriage has been observed in 10% to 30% of pregnant women. A similar incidence has been observed in women who are not pregnant.

The likelihood of colonization at birth is higher when the mother is colonized with large numbers of bacteria. Other risk factors for neonatal colonization are premature delivery, prolonged membrane rupture, and intrapartum fever. Disease in infants younger than 7 days of age is called **early-onset disease**; disease appearing between 1 week and 3 months of life is considered **late-onset disease**. The serotypes most commonly associated with early-onset disease are Ⅰa (35% to 40%), Ⅲ (30%), and Ⅴ (15%). Serotype Ⅲ is responsible for most late-onset disease. Serotypes Ⅰa and Ⅴ are the most common in adult disease.

S. agalactiae is the most common cause of septicemia and meningitis in newborns. There are more group B streptococcal infections in adults than in neonates, but the overall incidence is higher in neonates. The risk of disease is greater in pregnant women than in men and nonpregnant women. Urinary tract infections, amnionitis, endometritis, and wound infections are the most common manifestations in pregnant women. Infections in men and nonpregnant women are primarily skin and soft-tissue infections, bacteremia, urosepsis (urinary tract infection with bacteremia), and pneumonia.

Laboratory Diagnosis

Antigen Detection

Tests for the direct detection of group B streptococci in urogenital specimens are available but are too insensitive to be used to screen mothers and predict which newborns are at increased risk for acquiring neonatal disease. Likewise, the antigen tests are too insensitive (<30%) to be used with cerebrospinal fluid (CSF). A Gram stain of CSF has much better sensitivity and should be used.

Nucleic Acid-Based Tests

A polymerase chain reaction (PCR)-based nucleic acid amplifcation assay is sensitive and specific comparable to culture and the results are available within one hour, this assay is an alternative to standard culture for group B *Streptococcus*.

Culture

Group B streptococci readily grow on a nutritionally enriched medium. β-Hemolysis may be difficult to detect or absent, posing a problem in the detection of the organism when other organisms are present in the culture (e.g., vaginal culture). Thus a selective broth medium with antibiotics added to suppress the growth of other organisms (e.g., LIM broth with colistin and nalidixic acid) is currently recommended for the detection of group B streptococci in women between weeks 35 and 37 of pregnancy.

Identification

Isolates of S. agalactiae are identified definitively by the demonstration of the group-specific cell wall carbohydrate.

Treatment, Prevention, and Control

Group B streptococci are susceptible to **penicillin**, which is the drug of choice. Because other bacteria can be responsible for neonatal disease (e.g., S. pneumoniae, Listeria, gram-negative rods), broad-spectrum therapy should be selected for empiric therapy. A cephalosporin or vancomycin can be used in penicillin-allergic patients.

A pregnant woman is considered to be at high risk to give birth to a baby with invasive group B disease if she has previously given birth to an infant with the disease or risk factors for the disease are present at birth. These risk factors are (1) intrapartum temperature of at least 38℃, (2) membrane rupture at least 18 hours before delivery, and (3) vaginal or rectal culture positive for organisms at 35 to 37 weeks of gestation. Intravenous penicillin G administered at least 4 hours before delivery is recommended; cefazolin is used for penicillin-allergic women or clindamycin (if susceptible) or vancomycin for mothers at high risk for anaphylaxis.

OTHER β-HEMOLYTIC STREPTOCOCCI

Among the other β-hemolytic streptococci, groups C, F, and G are most commonly associated with human disease. Organisms of particular importance are the *Streptococcus anginosus* group (includes *S. anginosus*, *Streptococcus constellatus*, and *Streptococcus intermedius*) and *Streptococcus dysgalactiae*. β-Hemolytic members of the *S. anginosus* group can possess the group A, C, F, or G polysaccharide antigen (or not have any group-specific antigen), and *S. dysgalactiae* can have either the group C or G antigen. It should be noted that an individual isolate possesses only one group antigen. Isolates of the *S. anginosus* group grow as small colonies (requiring 2 days of incubation) with a narrow zone of β-hemolysis (Figure 12-5A). These species are primarily associated with abscess formation and not pharyngitis, in contrast with the other group A *Streptococcus*, *S. pyogenes*. *S. dysgalactiae* produces large colonies with a large zone of β-hemolysis on blood agar media (Figure 12-5B), a behavior similar to that of *S. pyogenes*. Similar to *S. pyogenes*, *S. dysgalactiae* causes pharyngitis, which is sometimes complicated by acute glomerulonephritis but never rheumatic fever.

many of these bacteria produce a green pigment on blood agar media (Figure 12-6). More than 30 species and subspecies have been identified, and most are classified into five subgroups. Many of the species in the five subgroups are responsible for specific diseases (see Table 12-3). Some members of the viridans streptococci (e.g., *S. anginosus* group) can have β-hemolytic strains with the group-specific cell wall polysaccharides (thus contributing to the confusing taxonomy of this genus). Because *S. pneumoniae* is the most virulent member of the viridans group, it is discussed separately.

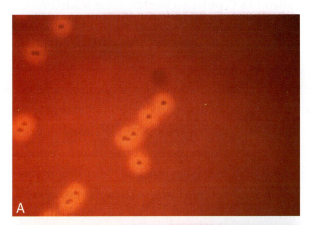
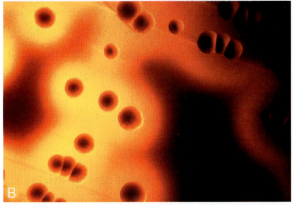

Figure 12-5 Group C *Streptococcus*. **A,** *S. anginosus*, small-colony species. **B,** *S. dysgalactiae*, large-colony species.

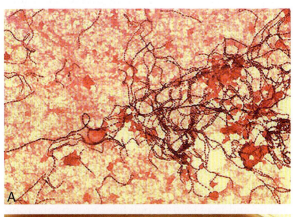
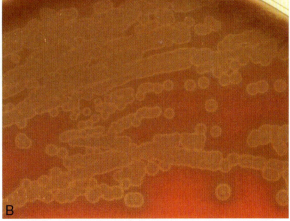

Figure 12-6 *Streptococcus mitis*. **A,** Gram stain from blood culture. **B,** α-Hemolytic colonies.

VIRIDANS STREPTOCOCCI

The viridans group of streptococci is a heterogeneous collection of α-hemolytic and nonhemolytic streptococci. Their group name is derived from *viridis* (Latin for "green"), a reflection of the fact that

The viridans streptococci colonize the oropharynx, gastrointestinal tract, and genitourinary tract. Similar to most other streptococci, viridans species are nutritionally fastidious, requiring complex media supplemented with blood products and, frequently, an inc ubation atmosphere augmented with 5% to 10% carbon dioxide.

In the past, most strains of viridans streptococci

were highly susceptible to penicillin. However, moderately resistant (penicillin MIC of 0.2 to 2 μg/ml) and highly resistant (MIC >2 μg/ml) streptococci have become common in the *S. mitis* group, which includes *S. pneumoniae*.

STREPTOCOCCUS PNEUMONIAE

Physiology and Structure

The pneumococcus is an **encapsulated**, gram-positive coccus. The cells are 0.5 to 1.2μm in diameter, oval, and arranged in pairs (**diplococci**) or short chains (Figure 12-7). Older cells decolorize readily and can stain gram-negative. Colonial morphology varies with colonies of encapsulated strains generally large (1 to 3 mm in diameter on blood agar; smaller on chocolatized or heated blood agar), round, and mucoid, and colonies of nonencapsulated strains are smaller and flat. All colonies undergo autolysis with aging–that is, the central portion of the colony dissolves, leaving a dimpled appearance. Colonies appear α-hemolytic on blood agar if incubated aerobically and may be β-hemolytic if grown anaerobically. The α-hemolytic appearance results from production of **pneumolysin**, an enzyme that degrades hemoglobin, producing a green product.

The organism has fastidious nutritional requirements and can grow only on enriched media supplemented with blood products. *S. pneumoniae* can ferment carbohydrates, producing lactic acid, the organism lacks catalase.

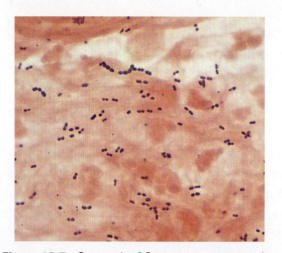

Figure 12-7   Gram stain of *Streptococcus pneumoniae*.

Virulent strains of *S. pneumoniae* are covered with a complex **polysaccharide capsule**. The capsular polysaccharides have been used for the serologic classification of strains; currently, 90 serotypes are recognized. Purified capsular polysaccharides from the most commonly isolated serotypes are used in a **polyvalent vaccine**.

The peptidoglycan layer of the cell wall of the pneumococcus is typical of gram-positive cocci. The other major component of the cell wall is teichoic acid. Two forms of teichoic acid exist in the pneumococcal cell wall, one exposed on the cell surface and a similar structure covalently bound to the plasma membrane lipids. This species-specific structure, called the **C polysaccharide**, is unrelated to the group-specific carbohydrate observed by Lancefield in β-hemolytic streptococci. The C polysaccharide precipitates a serum globulin fraction (**C-reactive protein [CRP]**) in the presence of calcium. CRP is present in low concentrations in healthy people but in elevated concentrations in patients with acute inflammatory diseases (hence, monitoring levels of CRP is used to predict inflammation). The teichoic acid bound to lipids in the bacterial cytoplasmic membrane is called the **F antigen**. Both forms of teichoic acid are associated with phosphorylcholine residues. **Phosphorylcholine** is unique to the cell wall of *S. pneumoniae* and plays an important regulatory role in cell wall hydrolysis. Phosphorylcholine must be present for activity of the pneumococcal autolysin, **amidase**, during cell division.

Pathogenesis and Immunity

The manifestations of pneumococcal disease are caused primarily by the host response to infection rather than the production of organism-specific toxic factors. However, an understanding of how *S. pneumoniae* colonizes the oropharynx, spreads into normally sterile tissues, stimulates a localized inflammatory response, and evades being killed by phagocytic cells is crucial.

Colonization and Migration

S. pneumoniae is a human pathogen that colonizes

the oropharynx and then, in specific situations, is able to spread to the lungs, paranasal sinuses, or middle ear. It can also be transported in the blood to distal sites such as the brain. The initial colonization of the oropharynx is mediated by the binding of the bacteria to epithelial cells by means of **surface protein adhesins**. Subsequent migration of the organism to the lower respiratory tract can be prevented if the bacteria are enveloped in mucus and removed from the airways by the action of ciliated epithelial cells. The bacteria counteract this envelopment by producing **secretory IgA protease** and **pneumolysin**. Secretory IgA traps bacteria in mucus by binding the bacteria to mucin with the Fc region of the antibody. The bacterial IgA protease prevents this interaction. **Pneumolysin,** a cytotoxin similar to the streptolysin O in *S. pyogenes*, binds cholesterol in the host cell membrane and creates pores. This activity can destroy the ciliated epithelial cells and phagocytic cells.

Tissue Destruction

A characteristic of pneumococcal infections is the mobilization of inflammatory cells to the focus of infection. Pneumococcal teichoic acid, peptidoglycan fragments, and pneumolysin mediate the process. The production of **hydrogen peroxide** by *S. pneumoniae* can also lead to tissue damage. Finally, **phosphorylcholine** present in the bacterial cell wall can bind to receptors for platelet-activating factor that are expressed on the surface of endothelial cells, leukocytes, platelets, and tissue cells.

Phagocytic Survival

S. pneumoniae survives phagocytosis because of the antiphagocytic protection afforded by its **capsule** and the pneumolysin-mediated suppression of the phagocytic cell oxidative burst. The virulence of *S. pneumoniae* is a direct result of this capsule. Encapsulated (smooth) strains can cause disease in humans and experimental animals, whereas nonencapsulated (rough) strains are avirulent. The capsular polysaccharides are soluble and have been called **specific soluble substances**. Free polysaccharides can protect viable organisms from phagocytosis by binding with opsonic antibodies.

Clinical Diseases

Pneumonia

Pneumococcal **pneumonia** develops when the bacteria multiply in the alveolar spaces. After aspiration, the bacteria grow rapidly in the nutrient-rich edema fluid. Erythrocytes, leaking from congested capillaries, accumulate in the alveoli, followed by the neutrophils, then the alveolar macrophages. Resolution occurs when specific anticapsular antibodies develop, facilitating phagocytosis of the organism and microbial killing.

The onset of the clinical manifestations of pneumococcal pneumonia is abrupt, consisting of a severe shaking chill and sustained fever of 39℃ to 41℃. The patient often has symptoms of a viral respiratory tract infection 1 to 3 days before the onset. Most patients have a productive cough with blood-tinged sputum, and they commonly have chest pain (pleurisy). Because the disease is associated with aspiration, it is generally localized in the lower lobes of the lungs (hence the name **lobar pneumonia**; Figure 12-8). However, children and the elderly can have a more generalized bronchopneumonia. Patients usually recover rapidly after the initiation of appropriate

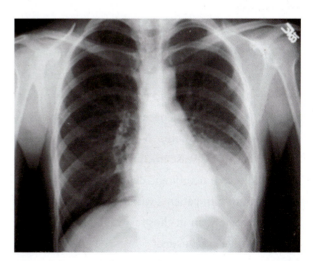

Figure 12-8 Dense consolidation of left lower lobe in patient with pneumonia caused by *Streptococcus pneumoniae.* (From Mandell G, Bennett J, Dolin R: *Principles and practice of infectious diseases*, ed 6, Philadelphia, 2005, Elsevier.)

antimicrobial therapy, with complete radiologic resolution in 2 to 3 weeks.

The mortality rate is considerably higher in patients with disease caused by *S. pneumoniae* type 3, as well as in elderly patients and patients with documented bacteremia. Patients with splenic dysfunction or splenectomy can also have severe pneumococcal disease, because of decreased bacterial clearance from the blood and the defective production of early antibodies. In these patients, disease can be associated with a fulminant course and high mortality rate.

Abscesses do not commonly form in patients with pneumococcal pneumonia, except in those infected with specific serotypes (e.g., serotype 3). Pleural effusions are seen in approximately 25% of patients with pneumococcal pneumonia and empyema (purulent effusion) is a rare complication.

Sinusitis and Otitis Media

S. pneumoniae is a common cause of acute infections of the paranasal sinuses and ear. The disease is usually preceded by a viral infection of the upper respiratory tract, after which polymorphonuclear neutrophils (leukocytes) (PMNs) infiltrate and obstruct the sinuses and ear canal. Middle ear infection (**otitis media**) is primarily seen in young children, but bacterial **sinusitis** can occur in patients of all ages.

Meningitis

S. pneumoniae can spread into the central nervous system after bacteremia, infections of the ear or sinuses, or head trauma that causes a communication between the subarachnoid space and the nasopharynx. Although **pneumococcal meningitis** is relatively uncommon in neonates, *S. pneumoniae* is now a leading cause of disease in children and adults. Mortality and severe neurologic deficits are 4 to 20 times more common in patients with meningitis caused by *S. pneumoniae* than in those with meningitis resulting from other organisms.

Bacteremia

Bacteremia occurs in 25% to 30% of patients with pneumococcal pneumonia and in more than 80%

of patients with meningitis. In contrast, bacteria are generally not present in the blood of patients with sinusitis or otitis media. Endocarditis can occur in patients with normal or previously damaged heart valves. Destruction of valve tissue is common.

Epidemiology

S. pneumoniae is a common inhabitant of the throat and nasopharynx in healthy people, with colonization more common in children than in adults and more common in adults living in a household with children. Colonization initially occurs at approximately 6 months of age. Subsequently, the child is transiently colonized with other serotypes of the organism. The duration of carriage decreases with each successive serotype carried, in part because of the development of serotype-specific immunity. Although new serotypes are acquired throughout the year, the incidence of carriage and associated disease is highest during the cool months. The strains of pneumococci that cause disease are the same as those associated with carriage.

Pneumococcal disease occurs when organisms colonizing the nasopharynx and oropharynx spread to the lungs (pneumonia), paranasal sinuses (sinusitis), ears (otitis media), or meninges (meningitis). Spread of *S. pneumoniae* in blood to other body sites can occur with all of these diseases. The organism is a common cause of bacterial pneumonia acquired outside the hospital, meningitis, otitis media and sinusitis, and bacteremia. Disease is most common in children and the elderly; both populations have low levels of protective antibodies directed against the pneumococcal capsular polysaccharides.

Pneumonia occurs when the endogenous oral organisms are aspirated into the lower airways. Although strains can spread on airborne droplets from one person to another in a closed population, epidemics are rare. Pneumococcal disease is most commonly associated with an antecedent viral respiratory disease, such as influenza, or with other conditions that interfere with bacterial clearance, such as chronic pulmonary disease, alcoholism, congestive heart failure, diabetes mellitus, chronic renal disease, and splenic dysfunction or splenectomy.

Laboratory Diagnosis

Microscopy

Gram stain of sputum specimens is a rapid way to diagnose pneumococcal pneumonia and meningitis. The organisms characteristically appear as enlongated, pairs of gram-positive cocci surrounded by an unstained capsule; however, they may also appear to be gram negative because they tend not to stain well (particularly in older cultures). In addition, their morphology may be distorted in a patient receiving antibiotic therapy. A Gram stain consistent with *S. pneumoniae* can be confirmed with the **quellung** (German for "swelling") reaction. In this test, polyvalent anticapsular antibodies are mixed with the bacteria, and then the mixture is examined microscopically. A greater refractiveness around the bacteria is a positive reaction for *S. pneumoniae*.

Antigen Detection

Pneumococcal C polysaccharide is excreted in urine and can be detected using a commercially prepared immunoassay. Maximum sensitivity requires that the urine be concentrated by ultrafiltration before it is assayed. Sensitivity has been reported to be 70% in patients with bacteremic pneumococcal pneumonia; however, specificity can be low, particularly in pediatric patients. For this reason, the test is not recommended for children with suspected infections. The test has a sensitivity approaching 100% for patients with pneumococcal meningitis if CSF is tested; however, the test has poor sensitivity and specificity if urine is tested in these patients.

Nucleic Acid-Based Tests

Nucleic acid probes and PCR assays have been developed for identification of *S. pneumoniae* isolates in culture but are not currently used for detection of bacteria in clinical specimens such as respiratory secretions or CSF.

Culture

Sputum specimens should be inoculated onto an enriched nutrient medium supplemented with blood.

S. pneumoniae is recovered in the sputum cultures from only half of the patients who have pneumonia because the organism has fastidious nutritional requirements and is rapidly overgrown by contaminating oral bacteria. Selective media have been used with some success to isolate the organism from sputum specimens, but it takes some technical skill to distinguish *S. pneumoniae* from the other α-hemolytic streptococci that are often present in the specimen. An aspirate must be obtained from the sinus or middle ear for the organism responsible for sinusitis or otitis to be diagnosed definitively. Specimens taken from the nasopharynx or outer ear should not be cultured. It is not difficult to isolate *S. pneumoniae* from specimens of cerebrospinal fluid if antibiotic therapy has not been initiated before the specimen is collected; however, as many as half of infected patients who have received even a single dose of antibiotics will have negative cultures.

Identification

Isolates of *S. pneumoniae* are lysed rapidly when the autolysins are activated after exposure to bile (**bile solubility test**). Thus the organism can be identified by placing a drop of bile on an isolated colony. Most colonies of *S. pneumoniae* are dissolved within a few minutes, whereas other α-hemolytic streptococci remain unchanged. *S. pneumoniae* can also be identified by its susceptibility to **optochin** (ethylhydrocupreine dihydrochloride). The isolate is streaked onto a blood agar plate and a disk saturated with optochin is placed in the middle of the inoculum. A zone of inhibited bacterial growth is seen around the disk after overnight incubation. Additional biochemical, serologic, or molecular diagnostic tests can be performed for a definitive identification.

Treatment, Prevention, and Control

Now resistance to penicillin is observed for as many as half of the strains isolated in the United States and in other countries. Resistance to penicillins is associated with a decreased affinity of the antibiotic for the penicillin-binding proteins present in the bacterial cell wall, and patients infected with resistant bacteria have an increased risk of an adverse outcome. Resistance to macrolides (e.g., erythromycin), tetracyclines, and, to a lesser extent, cephalosporins (e.g., ceftriaxone) has also become commonplace. Thus, for serious pneumococcal infections, treatment with a combination of antibiotics is recommended until in vitro susceptibility results are available. **Vancomycin** combined with **ceftriazone** is used commonly for empiric treatment, followed by monotherapy with an effective cephalosporin, fluoroquinolone or vancomycin. Efforts to prevent or control the disease have focused on the development of effective anticapsular vaccines. The effectiveness of these vaccines is determined by the prevalent serotypes of *S. pneumoniae* responsible for invasive disease in the population.

SUMMARY

Streptococcus pyogenes (Group A)

The bacteria are rapidly growing gram-positive cocci arranged in chains. Virulence is determined by ability to avoid phagocytosis (mediated primarily by capsule, M and M-like proteins, C5a peptidase), adhere to and invade host cells (M protein, lipoteichoic acid, F protein), and produce toxins (streptococcal pyrogenic exotoxins, streptolysin S, streptolysin O, streptokinase, DNases).

The **Streptococcus pyogenes** *can cause a range of suppurative infections, including pharyngitis, scarlet fever, pyoderma, erysipelas, cellulitis, necrotizing fasciitis, streptococcal toxic shock syndrome, and other suppurative diseases. The bacteria can also cause nonsuppurative infections, including rheumatic fever and acute glomerulonephritis. Pharyngitis and soft-tissue infections typically are caused by strains with different M proteins.*

Microscopy is useful in soft-tissue infections but not pharyngitis or nonsuppurative complications. Direct tests for the group A antigen are useful for the diagnosis of streptococcal pharyngitis, but negative results must be confirmed by culture or molecular assays.

Isolates can be identified by catalase (negative), positive PYR (*L*-pyrrolidonyl arylamidase) reaction,

susceptibility to bacitracin, and presence of group-specific antigen (group A antigen).

Antistreptolysin O test is useful for confirming rheumatic fever or glomerulonephritis associated with streptococcal pharyngitis. Anti-DNase B test should be performed for glomerulonephritis associated with pharyngitis or soft-tissue infections.

Penicillin V or amoxicillin is used to treat pharyngitis. Oral cephalosporin or macrolide is used for penicillin-allergic patients; intravenous penicillin plus clindamycin are used for systemic infections.

Streptococcus agalactiae (Group B)

The bacteria are responsible for neonatal disease (early-onset and late-onset disease with meningitis, pneumonia, bacteremia), infections in pregnant women (endometritis, wound infections, urinary tract infections), and other adults (bacteremia, pneumonia, bone and joint infections, skin and soft-tissue infections).

Streptococcus pneumoniae

The bacteria are elongated gram-positive cocci arranged in pairs (diplococci) and short chains. The bacterial virulence is determined by ability to colonize oropharynx (surface protein adhesions), spread into normally sterile tissues pneumolysin, IgA protease), stimulate local inflammatory response (teichoic acid, peptidoglycan fragments, pneumolysin), and evade phagocytic killing (**polysaccharide capsule**). The bacteria are responsible for pneumonia, sinusitis and otitis media, meningitis, and bacteremia.

KEYWORDS

English	Chinese
Streptococcus	链球菌属
Streptococcus pyogenes	化脓性链球菌
Streptococcal pyrogenic exotoxins	链球菌致热外毒素
Streptolysin	链球菌素
Streptokinase	链激酶
Scarlet fever	猩红热
Streptococcal toxic shock syndrome	链球菌毒素休克综合征
Rheumatic Fever	风湿热

Acute Glomerulonephritis	急性肾小球肾炎
Streptococcus agalactiae	无乳链球菌
Streptococcus pneumoniae	肺炎链球菌
Pneumolysin	肺炎链球菌溶素
Lobar pneumonia	大叶性肺炎
Bile solubility test	胆汁溶菌试验

BIBLIOGRAPHY

1. Ahn S-Y, Ingulli E: Acute poststreptococcal glomerulone-phritis: an update, Curr Opin Pediatr 20: 157-162, 2008.

2. Centers for Disease Control and Prevention: Prevention of perinatal group B streptococcal disease, MMWR 59(RR-10): 1-32, 2010.

3. Greene CM, et al: Preventability of invasive pneumococcal disease and assessment of current polysaccharide vaccine recommendations for adults: United States, 2001-2003, Clin Infect Dis 43: 141-150, 2006.

4. Harboe Z, et al: Pneumococcal serotypes and mortality following invasive pneumococcal disease: a population-based cohort study, PLoS Med 6: e1000081, 2009.

5. Johansson L, et al: Getting under the skin: the immuno-pathogenesis of *Streptococcus pyogenes* deep tissue infec-tions, Clin Infect Dis 51: 58-65, 2010.

6. Johnson D, et al: A comparison of group A streptococci from invasive and uncomplicated infections: are virulent clones responsible for serious streptococcal infections? J Infect Dis 185: 1586-1595, 2002.

Enterococcus and Other Gram-Positive Cocci

The number of genera of catalase-negative, gram-positive cocci that are recognized as human pathogens continues to increase; however, *Streptococcus* (see Chapter 12) and *Enterococcus* (Table 13-1) are the genera most frequently isolated and most commonly responsible for human disease (Tables 13-2 and 13-3). The other genera are relatively uncommon and are discussed only briefly here.

Table 13-1   Important Enterococci

Organism	Historical Derivation
Enterococcus	*enteron*, intestine; *coccus*, berry (intestinal coccus)
E. faecalis	*faecalis*, relating to feces
E. faecium	*faecium*, of feces
E. gallinarum	*gallinarum*, of hens (original source was intestines of domestic fowl)
E. casseliflavus	*casseli*, Kassel's; *flavus*, yellow (Kassel's yellow)

Table 13-2   Frequency of Human Colonization and Disease Caused by Some Catalase-Negative, Gram-Positive Cocci

Genus	Human Colonization	Human Disease
Enterococcus	Common	Common
Streptococcus	Common	Common
Abiotrophia	Uncommon	Uncommon
Granulicatella	Uncommon	Uncommon
Leuconostoc	Uncommon	Uncommon
Pediococcus	Uncommon	Rare
Lactococcus	Uncommon	Rare
Aerococcus	Uncommon	Rare

Table 13-3   Catalase-Negative, Gram-Positive Cocci and Their Diseases

Organism	Diseases
Abiotrophia	Bacteremia, endocarditis (native and prosthetic valves), nosocomial brain abscesses and meningitis, eye infections
Aerococcus	Bacteremia, endocarditis, urinary tract infections
Enterococcus	Bacteremia, endocarditis, urinary tract infections, peritonitis, wound infections
Granulicatella	Bacteremia, endocarditis (native and prosthetic valves), eye infections
Lactococcus	Bacteremia in immunocompromised patients, endocarditis (native and prosthetic valves), urinary tract infections, osteomyelitis
Leuconostoc	Opportunistic infections, including bacteremia, wound infections, central nervous system infections, and peritonitis
Pediococcus	Opportunistic infections, including bacteremia in severely immunocompromised patients
Streptococcus	Refer to Chapter 12

ENTEROCOCCUS

The enterococci ("enteric cocci") were previously classified as **group D streptococci** because they share the **group D cell wall antigen**, a glycerol teichoic acid, with other streptococci. In 1984, the enterococci were reclassified into the new genus *Enterococcus*, and there are currently 40 species in this genus. The most commonly isolated and clinically important species are ***Enterococcus faecalis*** and ***Enterococcus faecium. Enterococcus gallinarum*** and ***Enterococ-***

cus casseliflavus are also common colonizers of the human intestinal tract and are important because these species are inherently vancomycin-resistant.

Physiology and Structure

The enterococci are gram-positive cocci, typically arranged in **pairs and short chains** (Figure 13-1). The microscopic morphology of these isolates cannot be differentiated reliably from that of *Streptococcus pneumoniae*. The cocci grow both aerobically and anaerobically in a broad temperature range (10℃ to 45℃), in a wide pH range (4.6 to 9.9), and in the presence of high concentrations of sodium chloride (**NaCl**) and **bile salts**. Glucose is fermented with L-lactic acid as the predominant end product. These basic properties can be used to distinguish enterococci from most other catalase-negative, gram-positive cocci. After 24 hours of incubation, colonies on enriched sheep blood agar are large and can appear nonhemolytic, α-hemolytic, or, rarely, β-hemolytic.

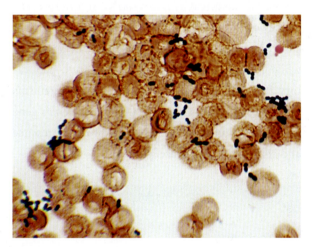

Figure 13-1 Gram stain of blood culture with *Enterococcus faecalis*.

Pathogenesis and Immunity

Although enterococci do not possess the broad range of virulence factors, life-threatening disease with antibiotic-resistant strains has become a serious problem in hospitalized patients. Virulence is mediated by two general properties: (1) ability to adhere to tissues and form biofilms and (2) antibiotic resistance. A number of factors have been described that mediate adherence and biofilm formation, including surface proteins, membrane glycolipids, gelatinase, and pili. In addition, the enterococci either are **inherently resistant to many commonly used antibiotics** (e.g., oxacillin, cephalosporins) or have acquired resistance genes (e.g., to aminoglycosides, vancomycin). Clearance of enterococci from blood and tissues is mediated by the rapid influx of neutrophils and opsonization of the bacteria.

Clinical Diseases

Enterococci are important pathogens, particularly in hospitalized patients; indeed, enterococci are one of the most common causes of infections acquired in the hospital (**nosocomial infection**). The urinary tract is the most common site of enterococcal infections, and infections are frequently associated with urinary catheterization or instrumentation. Peritoneal infections are typically polymicrobic and associated with leakage of intestinal bacteria either from trauma or due to disease that compromises the intestinal lining. Enterococci recovered in the blood may either be dissemination from a localized infection of the urinary tract, peritoneum or a wound, or represent primary infection of the endocardium (endocarditis). Endocarditis is a particularly serious infection because many enterococci are resistant to most commonly used antibiotics.

Epidemiology

As their name implies, enterococci are enteric bacteria that are commonly recovered in feces collected from humans and from a variety of animals. Significant risk factors for enterococcal infections include use of urinary or intravascular catheters, prolonged hospitalization, and use of **broad-spectrum antibiotics**, particularly antibiotics that are inherently inactive against enterococci (e.g., nafcillin, oxacillin, cephalosporins).

Laboratory Diagnosis

Although enterococci may resemble *S. pneumoniae* on Gram-stained specimens, the organisms can be readily differentiated on the basis of simple biochemical reactions. For example, enterococci are resistant to optochin (*S. pneumoniae* is susceptible), do not dissolve when exposed to bile (*S. pneumoniae* is dissolved), and produces *L*-pyrrolidonyl arylamidase (PYR) (the only *Streptococcus* that is PYR positive is *Streptococcus pyogenes*). Catalase-negative, PYR-positive cocci arranged in pairs and short chains can be presumptively identified as enterococci. Phenotypic properties (e.g., pigment production, motility), biochemical tests, and nucleic acid sequencing are necessary to differentiate among *E. faecalis*, *E. faecium*, and the other *Enterococcus* species, but this topic is beyond the scope of this text.

Treatment, Prevention, and Control

Antimicrobial therapy for enterococcal infections is complicated because most antibiotics are not bactericidal at clinically relevant concentrations. Therapy for serious infections has traditionally consisted of the synergistic **combination of an aminoglycoside and a cell wall-active antibiotic** (e.g., ampicillin, vancomycin); however, some cell wall antibiotics have no activity against enterococci (e.g., nafcillin, oxacillin, cephalosporins), ampicillin and penicillin are generally ineffective against *E. faecium*, and vancomycin resistance (particularly in *E. faecium*) is commonplace. In addition, more than 25% of enterococci are resistant to the aminoglycosides, and resistance to aminoglycosides and vancomycin is particularly troublesome because it is mediated by plasmids and can be transferred to other bacteria.

Newer antibiotics have been developed that can treat enterococci resistant to ampicillin, vancomycin, or the aminoglycosides. They include linezolid, daptomycin, tigecycline, and quinupristin/dalfopristin. Unfortunately, resistance to linezolid is steadily increasing, and quinupristin/dalfopristin is not active against *E. faecalis* (the most commonly isolated enterococcal species).

It is difficult to prevent and control enterococcal infections. Careful restriction of antibiotic usage and the implementation of appropriate infection-control practices (e.g., isolation of infected patients, use of gowns and gloves by anyone in contact with patients) can reduce the risk of colonization with these bacteria, but the complete elimination of infections is unlikely.

OTHER CATALASE-NEGATIVE, GRAM-POSITIVE COCCI

Other catalase-negative, gram-positive cocci associated with human disease are *Abiotrophia*, *Granulicatella*, *Leuconostoc*, *Lactococcus*, *Pediococcus*, *Aerococcus*, and other less commonly isolated genera. All are **opportunistic pathogens**.

Abiotrophia and *Granulicatella*, formerly called **nutritionally deficient streptococci**, are problematic because they will initially grow in blood culture broths or in mixed cultures but do not grow when subcultured onto sheep blood agar media unless the medium is supplemented with pyrodoxal (vitamin B_6). *Leuconostoc* and *Pediococcus* can resemble streptococci but are **resistant to vancomycin**, a trait that has not been seen in streptococci. *Lactococcus* can be misidentified as *Enterococcus*, and *Aerococcus* ("air coccus") is typically an airborne organism that can contaminate the patient's skin or the specimen while it is being collected or processed in the laboratory. It is difficult to identify most of these organisms precisely without using molecular tools such as gene sequencing, but having knowledge of their presence and clinical features is useful.

SUMMARY

Enterococcus

The bacteria are gram-positive cocci arranged in pairs and short chains. Bacterial virulence is mediated by ability to adhere to host surfaces and form biofilms and by antibiotic resistance. The bacteria can cause urinary tract infections, peritonitis (usually polymicrobic), wound infections, and bacteremia with or without endocarditis. Dysuria and pyuria are most commonly in hospitalized patients with an indwelling urinary catheter and receiving broad-spectrum cephalosporin antibiotics. Antibiotic resistance to each of these drugs is becoming increasingly common, and infections with many isolates (particularly *Enterococcus faecium*) are not treatable with any antibiotics.

KEYWORDS

English	Chinese
Enterococcus	肠球菌属
Enterococcus faecalis	粪肠球菌
Enterococcus faecium	屎肠球菌
Nosocomial infection	院内感染

BIBLIOGRAPHY

1. Arias C, Contreras G, Murray B: Management of multidrug-resistant enterococcal infections, Clin Microbiol Infect 16: 555-562, 2010.

2. Facklam R, Elliott JA: Identification, classification, and clinical relevance of catalase-negative, gram-positive cocci, excluding the streptococci and enterococci, Clin Microbiol Rev 8: 479-495, 1995.

3. Fisher K, Phillips C: The ecology, epidemiology and virulence of *Enterococcus*, Microbiol 155: 1749-1757, 2009.

4. Garbutt JM, et al: Association between resistance to vancomycin and death in cases of *Enterococcus faecium* bacteremia, Clin Infec Dis 30: 466-472, 2000.

5. Handwerger S, et al: Infection due to *Leuconostoc* species: six cases and review, Rev Infect Dis 12: 602-610, 1990.

6. Hegstad K, et al: Mobile genetic elements and their contribution to the emergence of antimicrobial resistant *Enterococcus faecalis* and *Enterococcus faecium*, Clin Microbiol Infect 16: 541-554, 2010.

7. Murray BE: Vancomycin-resistant enterococci, Am J Med 101: 284-293, 1997.

8. Sava I, et al: Pathogenesis and immunity in enterococcal infections, Clin Microbiol Infect 16: 533-540, 2010.

Bacillus

The family Bacillaceae consists of a diverse collection of bacteria, including organisms that grow only aerobically or only anaerobically, organisms shaped as cocci or rods, and organisms that stain gram-positive or gram-negative. The one feature this diverse group of bacteria all share is the ability to form endospores (Figure 14-1). Despite the dozens of genera in this family, students need to know only two clinically important genera: *Bacillus* (the aerobic and facultative anaerobic spore formers; Table 14-1) and *Clostridium* (the strict, anaerobic spore formers; see Chapter 29).

Almost 250 species are in the genus *Bacillus*. Fortunately, the species that are of medical interest are relatively limited. *Bacillus anthracis*, the organism responsible for anthrax, is the most important member of this genus. The other clinically important species in this genus is *Bacillus cereus*, an organism responsible for gastroenteritis, traumatic eye infections, catheter-associated sepsis, and, rarely, severe pneumonia.

BACILLUS ANTHRACIS

Physiology and Structure

B. anthracis is a large (1 × 3 to 8 μm) organism arranged as single or paired rods (Figure 14-2) or as long, serpentine chains. Although spores are readily observed in 2- to 3-day-old cultures, they are not seen in clinical specimens.

Table 14-1   Important *Bacillus* Species

Organism	Historical Derivation
Bacillus	*bacillum*, a small rod
B. anthracis	*anthrax*, charcoal, a carbuncle (refers to the black, necrotic wound associated with cutaneous anthrax)
B. cereus	*cereus*, waxen, wax-colored (refers to colonies with a typical dull or frosted-glass surface)

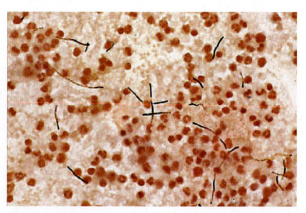

Figure 14-2   *Bacillus anthracis* in the blood of a patient with inhalation anthrax.

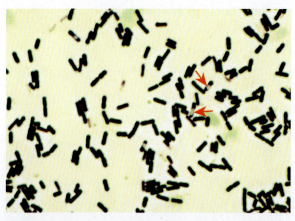

Figure 14-1   *Bacillus cereus*. The clear areas in the gram-positive rods are unstained spores *(arrows)*.

Virulent *B. anthracis* carries genes for three toxin protein components on a large plasmid, pXO1. The individual proteins, **protective antigen (PA), edema factor (EF),** and **lethal factor (LF),** are nontoxic individually but form important toxins when combined: PA plus EF forms **edema toxin,** and PA plus LF forms **lethal toxin.** After PA binds to its receptor, host proteases cleave PA, releasing a small fragment and retaining the 63-kDa fragment (PA_{63}) on the cell surface. The PA_{63} fragments self-associate on the cell surface, forming a ring-shaped complex of seven fragments (pore precursor or "prepore"). This heptameric complex can then bind up to three molecules of LF and/or EF. **LF is a zinc-dependent protease** that is capable of cleaving mitogen-activated protein (MAP) kinase, leading to cell death by incompletely understood mechanisms. **EF is a calmodulin-dependent adenylate cyclase** that increases the intracellular cyclic adenosine monophosphate (cAMP) levels, resulting in edema.

A second, important virulence factor carried by *B. anthracis* is a prominent polypeptide **capsule** (consisting of poly-D-glutamic acid). The capsule is observed in clinical specimens but is not produced in vitro unless special growth conditions are used. Three genes (*capA*, *capB*, and *capC*) are responsible for synthesis of this capsule and are carried on a second plasmid (pXO2). Only one serotype of capsule has been identified, presumably because the capsule is composed of only glutamic acid.

Pathogenesis and Immunity

The major factors responsible for the virulence of *B. anthracis* are the capsule, edema toxin, and lethal toxin. The capsule inhibits phagocytosis of replicating cells. The adenylate cyclase activity of edema toxin is responsible for the fluid accumulation observed in anthrax. The zinc metalloprotease activity of lethal toxin stimulates macrophages to release tumor necrosis factor-α (TNF-α), interleukin-1β (IL-1β), and other proinflammatory cytokines. This toxin also mediates lysis of macrophages in selected cell cultures. Of the major proteins of *B. anthracis*, PA is the most immunogenic (hence the name). Both LF and EF inhibit the host's innate immune system.

Clinical Diseases

Typically, **cutaneous anthrax** starts with the development of a painless papule, at the site of inoculation, that rapidly progresses to an ulcer surrounded by vesicles, then to a necrotic eschar (Figure 14-3). Systemic signs, painful lymphadenopathy, and massive edema may develop. The mortality rate in patients with untreated cutaneous anthrax is 20%.

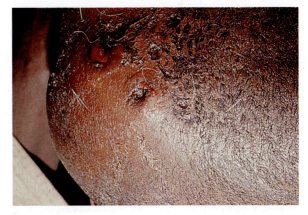

Figure 14-3 Cutaneous anthrax demonstrating marked erythema, edema, and vesicle rupture. (From Cohen J, Powderly WG: *Infectious diseases*, ed 2, St Louis, 2004, Mosby.)

Clinical symptoms of **gastrointestinal anthrax** are determined by the site of the infection. If organisms invade the upper intestinal tract, ulcers form in the mouth or esophagus, leading to regional lymphadenopathy, edema, and sepsis. If the organism invades the cecum or terminal ileum, the patient presents with nausea, vomiting, and malaise, which rapidly progress to systemic disease. The mortality associated with gastrointestinal anthrax is believed to approach 100%.

Unlike the other two forms of anthrax, **inhalation anthrax** can be associated with a prolonged latent period (2 months or more), during which the infected patient remains asymptomatic. The initial clinical symptoms of disease are nonspecific–fever, myalgias, nonproductive cough, and malaise. The second stage of disease is more dramatic, with a rapidly worsening course of fever, edema, massive enlargement of the mediastinal lymph nodes (this is responsible for the widened mediastinum observed on chest radiography [Figure 14-4]), respiratory failure, and sepsis. Although the route of infection is by inhalation, pneumonia rarely develops. Meningeal symptoms are seen in half of patients with inhalation anthrax. Almost all cases progress to shock and death within 3 days of initial symptoms, unless anthrax is suspected and treatment is initiated immediately. Serologic evidence indicates that a subclinical or asymptomatic form of inhalation anthrax does not exist. Virtually all patients who develop disease progress to a fatal outcome, unless there is immediate medical intervention.

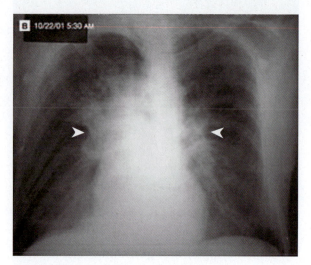

Figure 14-4   Inhalation anthrax demonstrating enlarged mediastinal lymph nodes *(arrowheads).*

Epidemiology

Anthrax is primarily a disease of herbivores; humans are infected through exposure to contaminated animals or animal products. The disease is a serious problem in countries where animal vaccination is not practiced or is impractical (e.g., disease established in African wildlife). Human *B. anthracis* disease is acquired by one of the following three routes: **inoculation, ingestion,** and **inhalation.** Approximately 95% of anthrax infections in humans result from the inoculation of *Bacillus* spores through exposed skin from either contaminated soil or infected animal products, such as hides, goat hair, and wool.

Ingestion anthrax is very rare in humans, but ingestion is a common route of infection in herbivores. Because the organism can form resilient spores, contaminated soil or animal products can remain infectious for many years.

Inhalation anthrax was historically called **wool-sorters' disease** because most human infections

resulted from the inhalation of *B. anthracis* spores during the processing of goat hair. Inhalation is the most likely route of infection with biologic weapons, and the infectious dose of the organism is believed to be low. Person-to-person transmission does not occur because bacterial replication occurs in the mediastinal lymph nodes rather than the bronchopulmonary tree.

Laboratory Diagnosis

Anthrax is one of the few bacterial diseases were organisms can be seen when peripheral blood is Gram stained (see Figure 14-2). Therefore the detection of organisms by microscopy and culture is not a problem. The diagnostic difficulty is distinguishing *B. anthracis* from other members of the taxonomically related *B. cereus* group. A preliminary identification of *B. anthracis* is based on microscopic and colonial morphology. Spores are not observed in clinical specimens but only in cultures incubated in a low carbon dioxide (CO_2) atmosphere and can be best seen with the use of a special spore stain (e.g., malachite green stain; Figure 14-5). The **capsule** of *B. anthracis* is produced in vivo but is not typically observed in culture. The capsule can be observed with a contrasting stain, such as India ink (the ink particles are excluded by the capsule so that the background, but not the area around bacteria, appears black), M'Fadyean methylene blue stain, or a direct fluorescent antibody (DFA) test developed against the capsular polypeptide. Colonies cultured on sheep blood agar are large, nonpigmented, and have a dry "ground-glass" surface and irregular edges with projections along the lines, where the specimen was inoculated onto the agar plate (referred to as "Medusa head" morphology). The colonies are quite sticky and adherent to the agar, and, if the edge is lifted with a bacteriologic loop, it will remain standing like beaten egg whites. Colonies are **not hemolytic.** *B. anthracis* will appear **nonmotile** in motility tests. The definitive identification of nonmotile, nonhemolytic organisms resembling *B. anthracis* is made in a public health reference laboratory. This is accomplished by demonstrating capsule production (by microscopy or DFA) and either lysis of the bacteria with gamma phage or a positive DFA test for a specific *B. anthracis* cell wall polysaccharide. In addition, nucleic acid amplification tests (e.g., polymerase chain reaction [PCR]) have been developed and are performed in reference laboratories. The PCR tests are also commercially available.

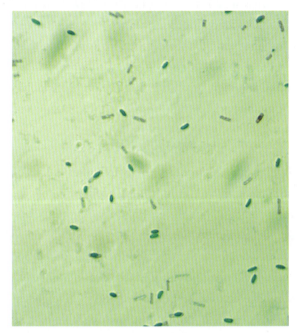

Figure 14-5   *Bacillus cereus.* Spores retain the malachite green dye in this special spore stain, and the vegetative cells are gray or colorless.

Treatment, Prevention, and Control

The current empiric treatment recommendation is use of **ciprofloxacin** or **doxycycline** combined with one or two additional antibiotics (e.g., rifampin, vancomycin, penicillin, imipenem, clindamycin, clarithromycin). Although penicillin resistance is observe for naturally acquired anthrax, oral penicillin (**amoxicillin**) is still recommended for naturally acquired cutaneous anthrax.

The control of naturally acquired human disease requires the control of animal disease, which involves the **vaccination of animal herds** in endemic regions and the burning or burial of animals that die of anthrax.

Vaccination has also been used to protect (1) people who live in areas where the disease is endemic, (2) people who work with animal products imported from countries with endemic anthrax, and (3) mili-

tary personnel. Although the current vaccine appears to be effective, research to develop a less toxic vaccine is underway. Alternative approaches to inactivating anthrax toxins have focused on PA and its receptor target. How these alternative approaches can be used to treat human disease remains to be demonstrated.

BACILLUS CEREUS

Bacillus species other than *B. anthracis* are primarily opportunistic pathogens that have relatively low capacities for virulence. Although most of these species have been found to cause disease, *B. cereus* is clearly the most important pathogen, with gastroenteritis, ocular infections, and intravenous catheter-related sepsis being the diseases most commonly observed, as well as rare cases of severe pneumonia.

Pathogenesis

Gastroenteritis caused by *B. cereus* is mediated by one of **two enterotoxins** (Table 14-2). The **heat-stable**, proteolysis-resistant enterotoxin causes the **emetic form** of the disease, and the **heat-labile** enterotoxin causes the **diarrheal form** of the disease.

Table 14-2   *Bacillus cereus* Food Poisoning

	Emetic Form	Diarrheal Form
Implicated food	Rice	Meat, vegetables
Incubation period (hours)	<6 (mean, 2)	>6 (mean, 9)
Symptoms	Vomiting, nausea, abdominal cramps	Diarrhea, nausea, abdominal cramps
Duration (hours)	8-10 (mean, 9)	20-36 (mean, 24)
Enterotoxin	Heat stable	Heat labile

The pathogenesis of *B. cereus* ocular infections is also incompletely defined. At least three toxins have been implicated; they are **necrotic toxin** (a heat-labile enterotoxin), **cereolysin** (a potent hemolysin named after the species), and **phospholipase C** (a potent lecithinase). It is likely that the rapid destruction of the eye that is characteristic of *B. cereus* infections results from the interaction of these toxins and other unidentified factors.

Bacillus species can colonize skin transiently and

can be recovered as insignificant contaminants in blood cultures. In the presence of an intravascular foreign body, however, these organisms can be responsible for persistent bacteremia and signs of sepsis (i.e., fever, chills, hypotension, shock).

Epidemiology

B. cereus and other *Bacillus* species are ubiquitous organisms, present in virtually all environments. Virtually all infections originate from an environmental source (e.g., contaminated soil). Isolation of bacteria from clinical specimens in the absence of characteristic disease usually represents insignificant contamination.

Clinical Diseases

B. cereus is responsible for two forms of food poisoning: **vomiting disease (emetic form)** and **diarrheal disease (diarrheal form)**. In most patients, the emetic form of disease results from the consumption of **contaminated rice**. Symptoms consist of vomiting, nausea, and abdominal cramps. Fever and diarrhea are generally absent. Fulminant liver failure has also been associated with consumption of food contaminated with large amounts of emetic toxin, which impairs mitochondrial fatty acid metabolism. Fortunately, this is a rare complication.

The diarrheal form of *B. cereus* food poisoning is a true infection, resulting from ingestion of the bacteria in contaminated meat, vegetables, or sauces. There is a longer incubation period. This enterotoxin is responsible for the diarrhea, nausea, and abdominal cramps that develop. This form of disease generally lasts 1 day or longer.

B. cereus **ocular infections** usually occur after traumatic, penetrating injuries of the eye with a soil-contaminated object. *Bacillus* panophthalmitis is a rapidly progressive disease that almost universally results in the complete loss of light perception within 48 hours of the injury. Disseminated infections with ocular manifestations can also develop in intravenous drug abusers.

Other common infections with *B. cereus* and other *Bacillus* species are intravenous catheter and central nervous system shunt infections and endocarditis (most common in drug abusers), as well as pneumonitis, bacteremia, and meningitis in severely immunosuppressed patients.

One rare disease of *B. cereus* deserves special attention—**severe pneumonia mimicking anthrax in immunocompetent patients.** Four patients with this disease, all metal workers residing in Texas or Louisiana, have been described in the literature. Most interesting is that the strains contained the ***B. anthracis* pXO1 toxin genes** and all were **encapsulated**, although this was not the *B. anthracis* poly-γ-D-glutamic acid capsule.

Laboratory Diagnosis

Similar to *B. anthracis*, *B. cereus* and other species can be readily cultured from clinical specimens collected from patients with the emetic form of food poisoning. Because individuals can be transiently colonized with *B. cereus*, the implicated food (e.g., rice, meat, vegetables) must be cultured for confirmation of the existence of foodborne disease. In practice, neither cultures nor tests to detect the heat-stable or heat-labile enterotoxins are commonly performed, so most cases of *B. cereus* gastroenteritis are diagnosed by epidemiologic criteria. *Bacillus* organisms grow rapidly and are readily detected with the Gram stain and culture of specimens collected from infected eyes, intravenous culture sites, and other locations.

Treatment, Prevention, and Control

Because the course of *B. cereus* gastroenteritis is short and uncomplicated, symptomatic treatment is adequate. The treatment of other *Bacillus* infections is complicated because they have a rapid and progressive course and a high incidence of multiple-drug resistance (e.g., *B. cereus* carries genes for resistance to penicillins and cephalosporins). **Vancomycin, clindamycin, ciprofloxacin,** and **gentamicin** can be used to treat infections. Penicillins and cephalosporins are ineffective. Eye infections must be treated rapidly. Rapid consumption of foods after cooking and proper refrigeration of uneaten foods can prevent food poisoning.

SUMMARY

Bacillus anthracis

The bacteria are spore-forming, nonmotile, non-hemolytic gram-positive rods. Polypeptide capsule consisting of poly-ᴅ-glutamic acid is observed in clinical specimens. Virulent strains also produce three exotoxins that combine to form edema toxin (combination of protective antigen and edema factor) and lethal toxin (protective antigen with lethal factor). *B. anthracis* primarily infects herbivores, with humans as accidental hosts. *B. anthracis* is rarely isolated in developed countries but is prevalent in impoverished areas where vaccination of animals is not practiced. The greatest danger of anthrax in industrial countries is the use of *B. anthracis* as an agent of bioterrorism. Three forms of anthrax are recognized: cutaneous (most common in humans), gastrointestinal (most common in herbivores), and inhalation (bioterrorism).

Inhalation or gastrointestinal anthrax or bioterrorism-associated anthrax should be treated with ciprofloxacin or doxycycline, combined with one or two additional antibiotics (e.g., rifampin, vancomycin, penicillin, imipenem, clindamycin, clarithromycin). Naturally acquired cutaneous anthrax can be treated with amoxicillin. Vaccination of animal herds and people in endemic areas can control disease, but spores are difficult to eliminate from contaminated soils. Animal vaccination is effective, but human vaccines have limited usefulness.

Bacillus cereus

The bacteria are spore-forming, motile gram-positive rods and they can produce heat-stable and heat-labile enterotoxin. People at risk include those who consume food contaminated with the bacterium (e.g., rice, meat, vegetables, sauces), those with penetrating injuries (e.g., to eye), those who receive intravenous injections, and immunocompromised patients exposed to *B. cereus*. The bacteria are capable of causing an anthrax-like disease in immunocompetent patients.

KEYWORDS

English	Chinese
Bacillus	芽胞杆菌属
Bacillus anthracis	炭疽芽胞杆菌
Bacillus cereus	蜡样芽胞杆菌
Protective antigen (PA)	保护性抗原
Edema factor (EF)	水肿因子
Lethal factor (LF)	致死因子
Cutaneous anthrax	皮肤炭疽
Gastrointestinal anthrax	肠炭疽
Inhalation anthrax	肺炭疽

BIBLIOGRAPHY

1. Avashia S, et al: Fatal pneumonia among metal workers due to inhalation exposure to *Bacillus cereus* containing *Bacillus anthracis* toxin genes, Clin Infect Dis 44: 414-416, 2006.

2. Baggett HC, et al: No evidence of a mild form of inhalational *Bacillus anthracis* infection during a bioterrorism-related inhalational anthrax outbreak in Washington, D.C., in 2001, Clin Infect Dis 41: 991-997, 2005.

3. Basha S, et al: Polyvalent inhibitors of anthrax toxin that target host receptors, Proc Natl Acad Sci U S A 103: 13509-13513, 2006.

4. BellCA, et al: Detection of *Bacillus anthracis* DNA by LightCycler PCR, J Clin Microbiol 40: 2897-2902, 2002.

5. Bottone E: *Bacillus cereus*, a volatile human pathogen, Clin Microbiol Rev 23: 382-398, 2010.

6. Collier RJ, Young JAT: Anthrax toxin, Annu Rev Cell Dev Biol 19: 45-70, 2003.

7. Doganay M, Metan G, Alp E: A review of cutaneous anthrax and its outcome, J Infect Public Health 3: 98-105, 2010.

8. Hoffmaster A, et al: Characterization of *Bacillus cereus* isolates associated with fatal pneumonias: strains are closely related to *Bacillus anthracis* and harbor *B. anthracis* virulence genes, J Clin Microbiol 44: 3352-3360, 2006.

9. Krantz BA, et al: A phenylalanine clamp catalyzes protein translocation through the anthrax toxin pore, Science 309: 777-781, 2005.

10. Mahtab M, Leppla SH: The roles of anthrax toxin in pathogenesis, Curr Opin Microbiol 7: 19-24, 2004.

11. Melnyk RA, et al: Structural determinants for the binding of anthrax lethal factor to oligomeric protective antigen, J

Biol Chem 281: 1630-1635, 2006.

12. PickeringAK, Merkel TJ: Macrophages release tumor necrosis factor alpha and interleukin-12 in response to intracellular *Bacillus anthracis* spores, Infect Immun 72: 3096-3072, 2004.

13. Saleeby CM, et al: Association between tea ingestion and invasive *Bacillus cereus* infection among children with cancer, Clin Infect Dis 39: 1536-1539, 2004.

14. Subramanian GM, et al: A Phase 1 study of PAmAb, a fully human monoclonal antibody against *Bacillus anthracis* protective antigen, in healthy volunteers, Clin Infect Dis 41: 12-20, 2005.

15. Turnbull, PC: Introduction: anthrax history, disease and ecology, Curr Top Microbiol Immunol 271: 1-19, 2002.

Chapter 15

Listeria

Listeria is a genus of gram-positive, asporogenous, aerobic/facultatively anaerobic bacteria. They are rods or coccobacilli (0.5 × 0.5 to 2 μm), occurring singly or in small groups ('Chinese letter' arrangements), palisades or filaments. Optimum temperature range from 25℃ to 37℃, and growth occurs slowly even at 4℃. Most strains are catalase-positive, oxidase negative and indole negative. Sugars are fermented to acid but no gas produces. The bacteria are generally motile.

Listeria currently includes 15 recognized species. *Listeria* spp occur (apparently as saprotrophs) e.g. in soil, decaying plant matter, silage, etc., and have been isolated from e.g. faeces of healthy humans and animals. Some haemolytic strains of *Listeria* can be pathogenic in man (only *Listeriamonocytogenes*) and also in animals (listeriosis and meningitis).

LISTERIA MONOCYTOGENES

Physiology and Structure

L. monocytogenes is a short (0.4 to 0.5 × 0.5 to 2 μm), nonbranching, gram-positive, facultatively anaerobic rod capable of growth at a broad temperature range (1℃ to 45℃) and in a high concentration of salt. The **short rods** appear singly, in pairs, or in short chains (Figure 15-1) and can be mistaken for *Streptococcus pneumoniae* or *Enterococcus*. This is important because both *S. pneumoniae* and *L. monocytogenes* can cause meningitis. The organisms are motile with peritrichous flagellation that are quite active at room temperature (20℃) but less so at 37℃, and exhibit a characteristic end-over-end tumbling motion when a drop of broth is examined microscopically. The

colonies are grey, translucent, about 1 mm in diameter after 24-48 hours with a characteristic bluish colour in obliquely transmitted light. *L. monocytogenes* may exhibit clear **β-hemolysis** when grown on sheep blood agar plates. These differential characteristics (i.e., Gram-stain morphology, motility, and β-hemolysis) are useful for the preliminary identification of *Listeria*.

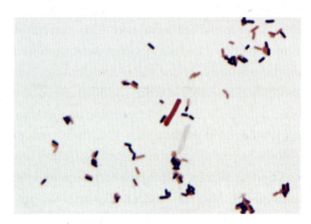

Figure 15-1 Gram stain of *Listeria monocytogenes* in culture. *Listeria* appear as small gram-positive rods; some readily decolorize and appear gram-negative. The much larger gram-negative rod in the center of the photograph is *Escherichia coli*.

Although the bacteria are widely distributed in nature, human disease is uncommon (opportunistic) and is restricted primarily to several well-defined populations: neonates, the elderly, pregnant women, and patients with defective cellular immunity.

Pathogenesis and Immunity

As the only human infective Listeriae, *L. monocytogenes* is a **foodborne facultative intracellular pathogen.** Following ingestion in contaminated food (10^6-10^9), *L. monocytogenes* is able to survive exposure to proteolytic enzymes, stomach acid, and bile salts through the protective action of stress-response genes. The bacteria are then able to **adhere to host cells** (macrophages and a broad range of non-phagocytic cells, including epithelial cells, hepatocytes, fibroblasts, and cells of the endothelium and nervous tissue) via the interaction of proteins on the surface of the bacteria (i.e., internalin A [InlA]) with glycoprotein receptors on the host cell surface (e.g., epithelial cadherin [E-cadherin]). Other internalins (e.g., InlB) can recognize receptors on a wider range of host cells. Studies with animal models have shown that infection is initiated in the enterocytes or M cells in Peyer patches. After penetration into the cells, the acid pH of the phagolysosome that surrounds the bacteria activates a bacterial pore-forming cytolysin (**listeriolysin O**) and two different **phospholipase C** enzymes, leading to release of the bacteria into the cell cytosol. The bacteria proceed to replicate and then move to the cell membrane. This movement is mediated by a bacterial protein, **ActA** (localized on the cell surface at one end of a bacterium), that coordinates **assembly of actin.** The distal ends of the actin tail remain fixed while assembly occurs adjacent to the end of the bacterium. Thus the bacterium is pushed to the cell membrane and a protrusion (listeriopod) is formed, pushing the bacterium into the adjacent cell. After the adjacent cell ingests the bacterium, the process of **phagolysosome lysis, bacterial replication,** and **directional movement** repeats. Entry into macrophages after passage through the intestinal lining carries the bacteria to the liver and spleen, leading to disseminated disease. The genes responsible for membrane lysis, intracellular replication, and directional movement are clustered together and regulated by a single gene, *prfA* or the "positive regulatory factor" gene.

Humoral immunity is relatively unimportant for management of infections with *L. monocytogenes*. These bacteria can replicate in macrophages and move within cells, thus avoiding antibody-mediated clearance. For this reason, patients with defects in **cellular immunity**, but not in humoral immunity, are particularly susceptible to severe infections.

Clinical Diseases

Neonatal Disease

Two forms of neonatal disease have been described: (1) early-onset disease, acquired transplacentally in utero, and (2) late-onset disease, acquired at or soon after birth. Early-onset disease can result in abortion, stillbirth, or premature birth. **Granulomatosis infantiseptica** is a severe form of early-onset listeriosis, characterized by the formation of abscesses and granulomas in multiple organs and a high mortality rate unless treated promptly.

Late-onset disease occurs 2 to 3 weeks after birth, in the form of meningitis or meningoencephalitis with septicemia. The clinical signs and symptoms are not unique; thus other causes of neonatal central nervous system disease, such as group B streptococcal disease, must be excluded.

Infections in Pregnant Women

Most infections in pregnant women occur during the third trimester when cellular immunity is most impaired. Infected women typically develop nonspecific influenza-like symptoms that may resolve without treatment. Unless blood cultures are collected in pregnant febrile women without another source of infection (e.g., urinary tract infection), listeria bacteremia and the associated neonatal risk may be unappreciated.

Disease in Healthy Adults

Most *Listeria* infections in healthy adults are asymptomatic or occur in the form of a mild influenza-like illness. An acute, self-limited gastronenteritis develops in some patients, characterized by a 1-day incubation period, followed by 2 days of symptoms, including watery diarrhea, fever, nausea, headache, myalgias, and arthralgias. In contrast to these self-limited illnesses, listeriosis in elderly patients and those with compromised cellular immunity is more severe.

Meningitis in Adults

Meningitis is the most common form of disseminated *Listeria* infection in adults. Although the clinical signs and symptoms of meningitis caused by this organism are not specific, *Listeria* should always be suspected in patients with organ transplants or cancer and in pregnant women in whom meningitis develops. Disease is associated with a high mortality (20% to 50%) and significant neurologic sequelae among the survivors.

Primary Bacteremia

Patients with bacteremia may have an unremarkable history of chills and fever (commonly observed in pregnant women) or a more acute presentation with high-grade fever and hypotension. Only severely immunocompromised patients and the infants of pregnant women with sepsis appear to be at risk of death.

Epidemiology

L. monocytogenes is isolated from a variety of environmental sources and from the feces of mammals, birds, fish, and other animals. The primary source of infection with this organism is consumption of contaminated food; however, human to human transmission can occur primarily from mother to child in utero or at birth. Fecal carriage is estimated to occur in 1% to 5% of healthy people. Because the organism is ubiquitous, exposure and transient colonization are likely to occur in most individuals. Large outbreaks associated with **contaminated food products** are well documented. Many people were exposed to the bacteria before the recall could be accomplished. The incidence of disease is also disproportionate in **high-risk populations**, such as neonates, the elderly, pregnant women, and patients with severe defects in cell-mediated immunity (e.g., transplants, lymphomas, acquired immunodeficiency syndrome [AIDS]).

Human listeriosis is a sporadic disease seen throughout the year, with focal epidemics and sporadic cases of listeriosis associated with consumption of undercooked processed meat (e.g., turkey franks, cold cuts), unpasteurized or contaminated milk or cheese, unwashed raw vegetables, including cabbage. Because *Listeria* can grow in a wide pH range

and at cold temperatures ("cold enrichment"), foods with small numbers of organisms can become heavily contaminated during prolonged refrigeration. Disease can occur if the food is uncooked or inadequately cooked (e.g., microwaved beef and turkey franks) before consumption.

Laboratory Diagnosis

Microscopy

Gram-stain preparations of cerebrospinal fluid (CSF) typically show no organisms because the bacteria are generally present in concentrations below the limit of detection (e.g., 10^4 bacteria per milliliter CSF or less). This is in contrast with most other bacterial pathogens of the central nervous system, which are present in concentrations of 100-fold to 1000-fold higher. If the Gram stain shows organisms, they are intracellular and extracellular gram-positive coccobacilli. Care must be used to distinguish them from other bacteria, such as *S. pneumoniae*, *Enterococcus*, and *Corynebacterium*.

Culture

Listeria grows on most conventional laboratory media, with small, round colonies observed on agar media after incubation for 1 to 2 days. It may be necessary to use selective media and cold enrichment (storage of the specimen in the refrigerator for a prolonged period) to detect listeriae in specimens contaminated with rapidly growing bacteria. *β*-Hemolysis on sheep blood agar media can serve to distinguish *Listeria* from morphologically similar bacteria; however, hemolysis is generally weak and may not be observed initially. Hemolysis is enhanced when the organisms are grown next to *β*-hemolytic *Staphylococcus aureus*. This enhanced hemolysis is referred to as a positive CAMP (Christie, Atkins, Munch-Petersen) test. The characteristic motility of the organism in a liquid medium or semisolid agar is also helpful for the preliminary identification of listeriae. All gram-positive rods isolated from blood and CSF should be identified to distinguish between *Corynebacterium* (presumably a contaminant) and *Listeria*.

Identification

Selected biochemical tests are used to identify the pathogen definitively, which is important because *L. monocytogenes*, the only species responsible for human disease, must be differentiated from other *Listeria* species that may contaminate food products. Serologic and molecular typing methods are used for epidemiologic investigations. A total of 13 serotypes have been described; however, serotypes 1/2a, 1/2b, and 4b are responsible for most infections in neonates and adults, so serotyping is generally not useful in epidemiologic investigations. Pulsed-field gel electrophoresis (PFGE) is the most commonly used molecular method for epidemiologic investigations of suspected outbreaks.

Treatment, Prevention, and Control

Because most antibiotics are only bacteriostatic with *L. monocytogenes*, the combination of **gentamicin with either penicillin or ampicillin** is the treatment of choice for serious infections. Listeriae are naturally resistant to cephalosporins, and resistance to macrolides, fluoroquinolones, and tetracyclines has been observed, which can limit the utility of these drugs. Trimethoprim-sulfamethoxazole is bactericidal to *L. monocytogenes* and has been used successfully. Other antibiotics, such as linezolid, daptomycin, and tigecycline, have good in vitro activity but have not been used extensively to treat patients.

Because listeriae are ubiquitous and most infections are sporadic, prevention and control are difficult. People at high risk of infection should avoid eating raw or partially cooked foods of animal origin, soft cheeses, and unwashed raw vegetables. A vaccine is not available, and prophylactic antibiotic therapy for high-risk patients has not been evaluated.

SUMMARY

Listeria is gram-positive coccobacilli, often arranged in pairs resembling enterococci and *Streptococcus pneumoniae*. It is facultative intracellular pathogen that can avoid antibody-mediated clearance. Virulent strains produce cell attachment factors (internalins), hemolysins (listeriolysin O, two phospholipase C enzymes), and a protein that mediates actin-directed intracellular motility (ActA). *Listeria* has the ability to grow at 4℃, in a wide pH range, and in the presence of salt can lead to high concentrations of the bacteria in contaminated foods.

Neonates, elderly, pregnant women, and patients with defects in cellular immunity are at increased risk for disease.

KEYWORDS

English	Chinese
Listeria	李斯特菌属
Listeria monocytogenes	单核细胞增生李斯特菌
Facultative intracellular pathogen	兼性胞内寄生菌
Listeriolysin	李斯特菌溶素
Listeriosis	李斯特菌病

BIBLIOGRAPHY

1. Allerberger F, Wagner M: Listeriosis: a resurgent foodborne infection, Clin Microbiol Infect 16: 16-23, 2010.

2. Azizoglu R, Kathariou S. *Listeria*: Properties and Occurrences, In Encyclopedia of Food and Health, Academic Press, Oxford, 2016, 567-570.

3. Freitag N, Port G, Miner M: *Listeria monocytogenes*—from saprophyte to intracellular pathogen, Nat Rev Microbiol 7: 623-628, 2009.

4. Gray MJ, Freitag NE, Boor KJ: How the bacterial pathogen *Listeria monocytogenes* mediates the switch from environmental Dr. Jekyll to pathogenic Mr. Hyde, Infect Immun 74: 2505-2512, 2006.

5. de las Heras A, Cain RJ, Bielecka MK, Vázquez-Boland JA: Regulation of Listeria virulence: PrfA master and commander, Curr Opin Microbiol 14(2): 118-27, 2011.

6. Pamer EG: Immune responses to *Listeria monocytogenes*, Nat Rev Immunol 4: 812-823, 2004.

7. Liu D: Identification, subtyping and virulence determination of *Listeria monocytogenes*, an important foodborne pathogen, J Med Microbiol 55: 645-659, 2006.

Corynebacterium

The genus *Corynebacterium* is a large, heterogeneous collection of gram-positive rods (order *Actinomycetales*, wall type IV) loosely grouped on the basis of cell morphology, staining properties, and G+C% content. It is commonly referred to as coryneform ("club-shaped") (Figure 16-1) bacteria that include *Corynebacterium* and other genera (Table 16-1).

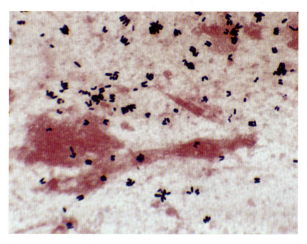

Figure 16-1 Gram stain of ***Corynebacterium*** species in sputum specimen.

Corynebacteria are aerobic or facultatively anaerobic, nonmotile, asporogenous, non-acid-fast, and catalase-positive. *Corynebacterium* spp exhibit certain features common to all nocardioform actinomycetes—e.g. the presence of cell wall **mycolic acids**. Most species ferment carbohydrates, producing lactic acid as a byproduct. Many species grow well on common culture media; however, some require supplementation of lipids for good growth.

Corynebacteria are ubiquitous in plants and animals, and also normally colonize on the skin, conjunctiva, upper respiratory tract, gastrointestinal tract, and urogenital tract in humans. Although all species of corynebacteria can function as opportunistic pathogens, relatively few are associated with human diseases (Table 16-2). The most famous of these is *Corynebacterium diphtheriae*, the etiologic agent of **diphtheria**.

Table 16-1 Important Coryneform Bacteria

Organism	Historical Derivation
Corynebacterium	*coryne*, a club; *bakterion*, a small rod (a small, club-shaped rod)
C. diphtheriae	*diphthera*, leather or skin (reference to the leathery membrane that forms initially on the pharynx)
C. jeikeium	*jeikeium* (species originally classified as group JK)
C. urealyticum	*urea*, urea; *lyticum*, lyse (capable of lysing urea; species rapidly hydrolyzes urea)
C. pseudotuberculosis	*pseudo*, like; *tuberculosis* (produces chronic purulent infections [e.g., tuberculosis] in sheep and other warm-blooded animals)
C. ulcerans	*ulcerans* (can produce pharyngeal ulcers like *C. diphtheriae*)
C. amycolatum	*a*, without; *mycolatum*, pertaining to mycolic acids (species does not have mycolic acids in the cell wall)

CORYNEBACTERIUM DIPHTHERIA

Toxinogenic strains of *C. diphtheriae* are the causal agents of **diphtheria**, an acute respiratory contagious infection with characteristic grey **pseudomembrane** on patients' pharynx. It can produce potent exotoxin and cause systemic toxic symptoms via toxaemia.

Table 16-2 *Corynebacterium* Species Associated with Human Diseases

Organism	Diseases
C. diphtheriae	Diphtheria (respiratory, cutaneous); pharyngitis and endocarditis (nontoxigenic strains)
C. jeikeium (group JK)	Septicemia, endocarditis, wound infections, foreign body (catheter, shunt, prosthesis) infections
C. urealyticum	Urinary tract infections (including pyelonephritis and alkaline-encrusted cystitis), septicemia, endocarditis, wound infections
C. pseudotuberculosis	Lymphadenitis, ulcerative lymphangitis, abscess formation, respiratory diphtheria
C. ulcerans	Respiratory diphtheria
C. amycolatum	Wound infections, foreign body infections, septicemia, urinary tract infections, respiratory tract infections

Physiology and Structure

C. diphtheriae is an irregularly staining, highly pleomorphic rod (0.3 to 0.8 × 1.0 to 8.0 μm) with no particular arrangement. Special stains, like Albert's stain using methylene blue, are used to demonstrate the diagnostic **metachromatic granules** in the polar regions, which are primarily composed of polyphosphates and RNA.

After overnight incubation, large (1 to 3 mm) colonies are observed on blood agar medium. This species is subdivided into four biotypes based on the cell and colonial morphology and biochemical properties: *belfanti*, *gravis*, *intermedius*, and *mitis*, with most disease caused by **biotype *mitis***. On blood-tellurite ($K_2TeO_2 \cdot 3H_2O$) media, *mitis* strains typically form shiny, greyish-black colonies at 24 hours when tellurite is reduced, and haemolysis is common.

Variationis often seen in *C. diphtheriae* in terms of cell and colonial morphology, and virulence. Diphtheria toxin is only produced by certain lysogenic strains of *C. diphtheriae* and responsible for the symptoms of diphtheria. *C. diphtheriae* is sensitive to disinfectants and sterilization, but resistant to sunlight, cold, and desiccation.

Pathogenesis and Immunity

Diphtheria toxin (DT) is the major virulence factor of *C. diphtheriae*. The *tox* gene encoding the exotoxin is introduced into strains of *C. diphtheriae* by a lysogenic bacteriophage, **β-phage**. Two processing steps are necessary for the active gene product to be secreted: (1) proteolytic cleavage of the leader sequence from the Tox protein during secretion from the bacterial cell, and (2) cleavage of the toxin molecule into two polypeptides (A and B) that remain attached by a disulfide bond. This 58,300-Da protein is an example of the classic **A-B exotoxin**.

Three functional regions exist on the toxin molecule: a **catalytic region** on the A subunit and a **receptor-binding region** and a **translocation region** on the B subunit. The receptor for the toxin is **heparin-binding epidermal growth factor**, present on the surface of many eukaryotic cells, particularly heart and nerve cells; its presence explains the cardiac and neurologic symptoms observed in severe diphtheria patients. After the toxin becomes attached to the host cell, the translocation region is inserted into the endosomal membrane, facilitating the movement of the catalytic region into the cytosol. The A subunit then terminates host cell protein synthesis by inactivating **elongation factor-2 (EF-2)**, a factor required for the movement of nascent peptide chains on ribosomes. Because the turnover of EF-2 is very slow and approximately only one molecule per ribosome is present in a cell, it has been estimated that one exotoxin molecule can inactivate the entire EF-2 content in a cell, completely terminating host cell protein synthesis. Toxin synthesis is regulated by a chromosomally encoded element, **diphtheria toxin repressor (DTxR)**. This protein, activated in the presence of high iron concentrations, can bind to the toxin gene operator and prevent toxin production.

Mycolic acids (6,6'-dimycolyl-α, α'-D-trehalose) from the cell wall may act as endotoxins by uncoupling mitochondrial electron transport and oxidative phosphorylation.

The protective immunity primarily relies on the neutralizing antibodies against DT B subunit through inhibiting toxin entry into cells. Children under 5-year old are most vulnerable as the passive humoral protection acquired through placenta and lactation during embryo and infancy fades away.

Clinical Diseases

The clinical manifestation of diphtheria is determined by (1) the site of infection, (2) the immune status of the patient, and (3) the virulence of the organism. Exposure to *C. diphtheriae* may result in asymptomatic colonization in fully immune people, mild respiratory disease in partially immune patients, or a fatal diphtheria in nonimmune patients. DT is produced at the site of the infection and then disseminates through the blood to produce the systemic signs of diphtheria without entering the blood of *C. diphtheriae* themselves.

Respiratory Diphtheria

The symptoms of diphtheria involving the respiratory tract develop after a 2- to 4-day incubation period. Organisms multiply locally on epithelial cells in the pharynx or adjacent surfaces and initially cause localized damage as a result of exotoxin activity. The onset is sudden, with malaise, sore throat, exudative pharyngitis, and a low-grade fever. The exudate evolves into a thick whitish or grey **pseudomembrane** composed of bacteria, lymphocytes, plasma cells, fibrin, and dead cells that can cover the tonsils, uvula, and palate and can extend up into the nasopharynx or down into the larynx (Figure 16-2). The pseudomembrane firmly adheres to the underlying tissue and is difficult to dislodge without making the tissue bleed (unique to diphtheria). As the patient recovers after 1-week course of the disease, the pseudomembrane dislodges and is expectorated. Systemic complications in severe patients primarily involve the heart and nervous system. **Myocarditis** can be detected in the majority of patients, typically developing 1-2 weeks into the illness and at a time when the pharyngeal symptoms are improving. Symptoms can present acutely or gradually, progressing to congestive heart failure, cardiac arrhythmias, and death in severe cases. **Neurotoxicity** is proportional to the severity of diphtheria,

which is influenced by the patient's immunity. The majority with severe disease develops neuropathy, initially localized to the soft palate and pharynx, later involving oculomotor and ciliary paralysis, with progression to peripheral neuritis.

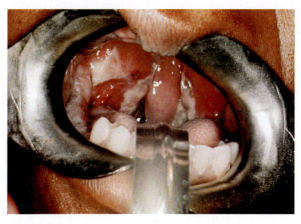

Figure 16-2 Pharynx of a 39-year-old woman with bacteriologically confirmed diphtheria. The photograph was taken 4 days after the onset of fever, malaise, and sore throat. Hemorrhage caused by removal of the membrane by swabbing appears as a dark area on the left. (From Mandell GL, Bennett JE, Dolin R: *Principles and practice of infectious diseases*, ed 7, Philadelphia, 2010, Elsevier Churchill Livingstone.)

Cutaneous Diphtheria

Cutaneous diphtheria is acquired through skin contact with other infected persons. The organism colonizes the skin and gains entry into the subcutaneous tissue through breaks in the skin. A papule develops first and then evolves into a **chronic, nonhealing ulcer,** sometimes covered with a grayish membrane. *Staphylococcus aureus* or *Streptococcus pyogenes* is also frequently present in the wound.

Epidemiology

Diphtheria is a disease worldwide, particularly in poor urban areas where people crowds and the protective level of vaccine-induced immunity are low. *C. diphtheriae* is maintained in the population by **asymptomatic carriage** in the oropharynx or on the skin of immune people. Respiratory droplets or skin contact transmits it from person to person. **Humans are the only known reservoir** for this organism.

Diphtheria has become uncommon in China

as the result of active immunization program, as shown by the fact that more than 167,000 cases were reported in 1960 but no cases have been reported since 1996. As primarily a pediatric disease, the highest incidence has shifted toward older age groups in areas where there are active immunization programs for children.

Laboratory Diagnosis

The initial treatment of a patient with diphtheria is instituted on the basis of the clinical diagnosis, not laboratory results, because definitive results are not available for days.

Culture

Specimens for the recovery of *C. diphtheriae* should be collected from both the nasopharynx and the throat and should be inoculated onto a nonselective, enriched blood agar plate and a selective medium, e.g., cysteine-tellurite blood agar, Tinsdale medium, colistin-nalidixic agar. Tellurite inhibits the growth of most upper respiratory tract bacteria and gram-negative rods, and is reduced by *C. diphtheriae*, producing characteristic gray to black color on agar. Degradation of cysteine by *C. diphtheriae* cysteinase activity produces a brown halo around the colonies. Regardless of the media that are used, all isolates resembling *C. diphtheriae* must be identified by biochemical testing and the presence of the diphtheria exotoxin confirmed because nontoxigenic strains occur as normal flora.

Microscopy

The results of microscopic examination of clinical materials are unreliable. Metachromatic granules in bacteria stained with methylene blue have been described, but this appearance is not specific to *C. diphtheriae*.

Identification

The presumptive identification of *C. diphtheriae* can be based on the presence of cystinase and absence of pyrazinamidase (two enzyme reactions that can be rapidly determined). More extensive biochemical

tests or nucleic acid sequencing of species-specific genes is required for identification at the species level.

Toxigenicity Testing

All isolates of *C. diphtheriae* should be tested for the production of exotoxin. The gold standard for DT detection is an *in vitro* immunodiffusion assay (**Elek test**). A plate of suitable medium is inoculated in a straight line with the strain under test, and the streak is then overlaid perpendicularly with a strip of paper impregnated with anti-DT antitoxin (1000 U/ml). After 24-48 hours incubation, toxin production is indicated by the development of lines of whitish precipitates which approximately bisect each of the four right angles formed by the paper strip and the line of microbial growth. The precipitates result from the combination of toxin and antitoxin following their diffusion from the line of growth and paper strip respectively. Known negative and positive strains must be used as controls. An *in vivo* DT detection may also be applied using guinea pigs. Cultures of suspected isolates are subcutaneously injected in animals with or without pre-administration of anti-DT antitoxin 500 U at 12-hour prior to injection. DT is produced if animals without antitoxin treatment die in 2-4 days.

The *tox* gene may be detected using a PCR-based amplification method in clinical isolates and directly in clinical specimens, e.g., swabs from the diphtheritic membrane or biopsy material. Although this test is rapid and specific, strains in which the *tox* gene is not expressed (presumably because the **DTxR** is expressed) can give a positive signal.

Treatment, Prevention, and Control

The most important aspect of the treatment for diphtheria is the early administration of **diphtheria antitoxin** to specifically neutralize the exotoxin before it is bound by the host cell. Once the cell internalizes the toxin, cell death is inevitable. Unfortunately, because diphtheria may not be suspected initially, significant progression of disease can occur before the antitoxin is administered. Antibiotic therapy with penicillin or erythromycin is also used to eliminate *C. diphtheriae* and terminate toxin production. Bed rest, isolation to prevent secondary spread, and maintenance of an open airway in patients with respiratory diphtheria are all important. After the patient has recovered, immunization with **toxoid** is required because most patients fail to develop protective antibodies after a natural infection.

Symptomatic diphtheria can be prevented by actively immunizing people with diphtheria toxoid. Initially, children are given five injections of toxoid preparation with pertussis and tetanus antigens (**DPT vaccine**) at ages of 3, 4, 5, 18-24 months, and 6 years. After that, it is recommended that booster vaccinations with diphtheria toxoid combined with tetanus toxoid be given every 10 years. The effectiveness of immunization is well documented, with disease restricted to nonimmune or incompletely immunized individuals.

People in close contact with patients who have documented diphtheria are at risk for acquiring the disease. Nasopharyngeal specimens for culture should be collected from all close contacts and antimicrobial prophylaxis with erythromycin or penicillin started immediately. Any contact who has not completed the series of diphtheria immunizations or who has not received a booster within the previous 5 years should receive a dose of toxoid. People exposed to cutaneous diphtheria should be managed in the same manner because it is reported that they are more contagious than patients with respiratory diphtheria. If the respiratory or cutaneous infection is caused by a nontoxigenic strain, it is unnecessary to institute prophylaxis in contacts.

OTHER *CORYNEBACTERIUM* SPECIES

A large number of other *Corynebacterium* species has been found as part of the human normal flora and are capable of causing opportunistic infections (see Table 16-2). So their isolation in clinical specimen may represent an important finding or simply represent contamination of the specimen.

Treatment of *Corynebacterium* infections can be problematic, because some species are resistant to most antibiotics. Hence, *in vitro* testing may be required before a treatment regimen is selected. Diphtheria caused by *C. ulcerans* and *C. pseudotuberculosis* should be managed in the same manner as disease caused by *C. diphtheriae*.

SUMMARY

***Corynebacterium diphtheriae* is** gram-positive pleomorphic rod. The major virulence factor is the diphtheria toxin which inhibits protein synthesis. The bacteria can cause respiratory and cutaneous diphtheria. Humans are the only known reservoir, with carriage in oropharynx or on skin surface. Microscopy is nonspecific; metachromatic granules are observed in *C. diphtheriae* and other corynebacteria. Culture should be performed on nonselective (blood agar) and selective (cysteine-tellurite agar, Tinsdale medium, colistin-nalidixic agar) media. Demonstration of exotoxin is performed by Elek test or PCR assay. Immunization of convalescing patients with diphtheria toxoid to stimulate protective antibodies. Diphtheria vaccine and booster shots are administrated to susceptible population.

KEYWORDS

English	Chinese
Corynebacterium	棒状杆菌属
Corynebacterium diphtheriae	白喉棒状杆菌
Diphtheria toxin	白喉毒素
Pseudomembrane	假膜（伪膜）
Metachromatic granule	异染颗粒
Elek test	埃莱克试验（白喉毒素-抗毒素琼脂免疫扩散反应）
DPT vaccine	百白破疫苗

BIBLIOGRAPHY

1. Coyle MA, Lipsky BA: Coryneform bacteria in infectious diseases: clinical and laboratory aspects, Clin Microbiol Rev 3: 227-246, 1990.
2. Funke G, et al: Clinical microbiology of coryneform bacteria, Clin Microbiol Rev 10: 125-159, 1997.
3. George MJ: Clinical significance and characterization of

Corynebacterium species, Clin Microbiol Newsletter 17: 177-180, 1995.

4. Bernard K: The genus *Corynebacterium* and other medically relevant coryneform-like bacteria, J Clin Microbiol 50(10): 3152-3158, 2012.

5. Pascual C, Lawson PA, Farrow JA, Gimenez MN, Collins MD: Phylogenetic analysis of the genus *Corynebacterium* based on 16S rRNA gene sequences, Int J Syst Bacteriol 45: 724-728, 1995.

6. Soriano F, Aguado JM, Ponte C, Fernández-Roblas R, Rodríguez-Tudela JL: Urinary tract infection caused by *Corynebacterium* group D2: report of 82 cases and review, Rev Infect Dis 12: 1019-1034, 1990.

Chapter 17

Actinomyces and *Nocardia*

The order *Actinomycetales* is a large group of phylogenetically related, filamentous, and often branching gram-positive rods in diversity. As a result of successful growth and branching, a ramifying network of filaments called a mycelium is formed. Although it is of bacterial dimensions, the mycelium is analogous to the mycelium formed by filamentous fungi. Here we focus on genera *Actinomyces* and *Nocardia*, the well-recognized opportunistic pathogens in this group.

ACTINOMYCES

Actinomyces is a genus of asporogenous gram-positive bacteria. Species occur in warm-blooded animals e.g. as part of the microflora of the mucous membranes (particularly in the mouth) and can act as opportunist pathogens.

Physiology and Structure

Actinomyces organisms are facultatively anaerobic or strictly anaerobic gram-positive rods. They are not acid-fast (in contrast to the morphologically similar *Nocardia* species), they grow slowly in culture, and they tend to produce **chronic, slowly developing infections.** They typically develop delicate filamentous forms, mycelium or hyphae (resembling fungi), in clinical specimens or when isolated in culture (Figure 17-1). However, these organisms are true bacteria in that they lack mitochondria and a nuclear membrane, reproduce by fission, and are inhibited by penicillin but not antifungal antibiotics. Numerous species have been described; *Actinomyces israelii, Actinomyces naeslundii, Actinomyces radingae,*

and *Actinomyces turicensis* are responsible for most human infections.

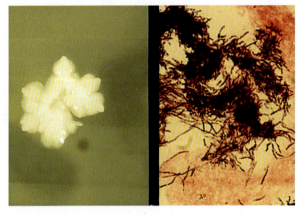

Figure 17-1 Macroscopic colony *(left)* and Gram stain *(right)* of ***Actinomyces***.

Pathogenesis and Immunity

Actinomyces organisms colonize the upper respiratory, gastrointestinal, and female genital tracts. These bacteria are not normally present on the skin surface. The organisms have a low virulence potential and cause disease only when the normal mucosal barriers are disrupted by trauma, surgery, or infection.

Classic disease caused by actinomyces is termed **actinomycosis** (in keeping with the original idea that these organisms were fungi or "mycoses"). Actinomycosis is characterized by the development of chronic granulomatous lesions that become suppurative and form abscesses connected by sinus tracts. Macroscopic colonies of organisms resembling grains of sand can frequently be seen in the abscesses and sinus tracts. These colonies, called **sulfur granules** because they appear yellow or orange, are masses of filamentous organisms bound together by calcium

143

phosphate (Figure 17-2). The areas of suppuration are surrounded by fibrosing granulation tissue, which gives the surface overlying the involved tissues a hard or woody consistency. Actinomycosis is now relatively uncommon. Currently, most infections involving actinomyces are polymicrobic, oral infections such as endodontic infections, odontogenic abscesses, and dental implant-associated infections.

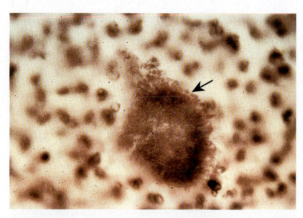

Figure 17-2   Sulfur granule collected from the sinus tract in a patient with actinomycosis. Delicate filamentous rods *(arrow)* are seen at the periphery of the crushed granule.

Clinical Diseases

Most actinomyces infections are the **cervicofacial** type (Figure 17-3). The disease may occur as an acute, pyogenic infection or as a slowly evolving, relatively painless process. The finding of tissue swelling with fibrosis and scarring, as well as draining sinus tracts along the angle of the jaw and neck, should alert the physician to the possibility of actinomycosis. Symptoms of **thoracic actinomycosis** are nonspecific. Abscesses may form in the lung tissue early in the disease and then spread into adjoining tissues as the disease progresses. **Abdominal actinomycosis** can spread throughout the abdomen, potentially involving virtually every organ system. **Pelvic actinomycosis** can occur as a relatively benign form of vaginitis or, more commonly, there can be extensive tissue destruction, including the development of tuboovarian abscesses or ureteral obstruction. The most common manifestation of **central nervous system actinomycosis** is a solitary brain abscess, but meningitis, subdural empyema, and epidural abscess

are also seen. Actinomycosis in patients with chronic granulomatous disease, presenting as a nonspecific febrile illness, has recently been described.

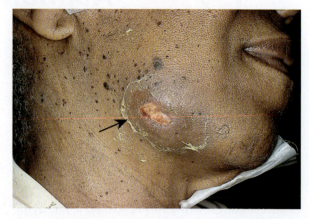

Figure 17-3   This patient is suffering from cervicofacial actinomycosis. Note the draining sinus tract *(arrow)*.

Epidemiology

Infections caused by actinomyces are **endogenous**, with no evidence of person-to-person spread or disease originating from an external source, such as soil or water. Cervicofacial infections are seen in patients who have poor oral hygiene or have undergone an invasive dental procedure or oral trauma. In these patients, the actinomyces that are present in the mouth invade into the diseased tissue and initiate the infectious process.

Patients with thoracic infections generally have a history of aspiration, with the disease becoming established in the lungs and then spreading to adjoining tissues. Abdominal infections most commonly occur in patients who have undergone gastrointestinal surgery or have suffered trauma to the bowel. Pelvic infection can be a secondary manifestation of abdominal actinomycosis or may be a primary infection in a woman with an intrauterine. Central nervous system infections usually represent hematogenous spread from another infected tissue, such as the lungs.

Laboratory Diagnosis

Laboratory confirmation of actinomycosis is often difficult. Care must be used during collection of clinical specimens that they not become contaminated with *Actinomyces* that are part of the normal bacterial population on mucosal surfaces. The significance of *Actinomyces* isolated from contaminated specimens cannot be determined. Because the organisms are concentrated in sulfur granules and are sparse in involved tissues, a large amount of tissue or pus should be collected. If sulfur granules are detected in a sinus tract or in tissue, the granule should be crushed between two glass slides, stained, and examined microscopically. Thin, gram-positive, branching rods can be seen along the periphery of the granules.

Actinomyces are fastidious and grow slowly under anaerobic conditions; it can take 2 weeks or more for the organisms to be isolated. Colonies appear white and have a domed surface that can become irregular after incubation for a week or more, resembling the top of a molar (Figure 17-4). The individual species of *Actinomyces* can be differentiated by biochemical tests; however, this process can be time consuming. In general, it is necessary to determine only that the isolate is a member of the genus *Actinomyces*.

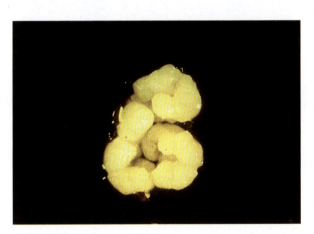

Figure 17-4 Molar tooth appearance of **Actinomyces israelii** after incubation for 1 week. This colonial morphology serves as a reminder that the bacteria are normally found in the mouth.

Recovery of *Actinomyces* in blood cultures should be evaluated carefully. Most isolates represent transient, insignificant bacteremia from the oropharynx or gastrointestinal tract. If the isolate is clinically significant, evidence of tissue pathology should be obtained.

Treatment, Prevention, and Control

Treatment for actinomycosis involves the combina-tion of drainage of a localized abscess or **surgical debridement** of the involved tissues and the prolonged administration of antibiotics. *Actinomyces* are uniformly susceptible to **penicillin** (considered the antibiotic of choice), carbapenems, macrolides, and clindamycin. Most species are resistant to metronidazole, and the tetracyclines have variable activity. An undrained focus should be suspected in patients with infections that do not appear to respond to prolonged therapy (e.g., 4 to 12 months). The clinical response is generally good even in patients who have suffered extensive tissue destruction. Maintenance of good oral hygiene and the use of appropriate antibiotic prophylaxis when the mouth or gastrointestinal tract is penetrated can lower the risk of these infections.

NOCARDIA

Nocardia is a genus of aerobic gram-positive rods that stain weakly acid-fast (i.e., resist decolorization with weak acid solutions) due to the **medium-length** chains of mycolic acids in their cell wall (Table 17-1). Acid-fast bacteria with **long-chain** mycolic acids in cell walls include the genus *Mycobacterium* and are discussed in the next chapter. *Nocardia* is the most medically important weak acid-fast organism, and the spectrum of the infections is extensive and includes insignificant colonization, cutaneous infections, pulmonary disease, systemic infections, and opportunistic infections (Table 17-2).

Table 17-1 Weakly Acid-Fast Gram-Positive Rods

Organism	Historical Derivation
Nocardia	Named after the French veterinarian Edmond Nocard
Rhodococcus	*rhodo*, rose or red colored; *coccus*, berry (red-colored coccus)
Gordonia	Named after the American microbiologist Ruth Gordon
Tsukamurella	Honoring the Japanese microbiologist, Michio Tsukamura, who first described the original isolate of this genus

Table 17-2 Diseases of Pathogenic *Nocardia*

Organism	Diseases	Frequency
Nocardia	Pulmonary diseases (bronchitis, pneumonia, lung abscesses); primary or secondary cutaneous infections (e.g., mycetoma, lymphocutaneous infections, cellulitis, subcutaneous abscesses); secondary central nervous system infections (e.g., meningitis, brain abscesses)	Common

Physiology and Structure

Nocardiae are strict aerobic rods that form branched filaments in tissues and culture. These filaments resemble the hyphae formed by molds, and, at one time, *Nocardia* was thought to be a fungus; however, the organisms have a gram-positive cell wall and other cellular structures that are characteristic of bacteria. Most isolates stain poorly with the Gram stain and appear to be gram-negative, with intracellular gram-positive beads (Figure 17-5). The reason for this staining property is that nocardiae have a cell wall structure similar to that of mycobacteria (see Chapter 18), with a number of branched-chain fatty acids (e.g., **tuberculostearic acid**, *meso*-diaminopimelic acid [*meso*-DAP], mycolic acids) present in the cell wall. The length of the mycolic acids in norcardiae (50 to 62 carbon atoms) is shorter than in mycobacteria (70 to 90 carbon atoms). This difference

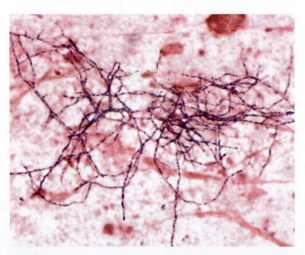

Figure 17-5 Gram stain of *Nocardia* in expectorated sputum. Note the delicate beaded filaments.

may explain why even though both genera stain acid-fast, *Nocardia* is described as **"weakly acid-fast"**; that is, a weak decolorizing solution of hydrochloric acid must be used to demonstrate the acid-fast property of nocardiae (Figure 17-6). This acid-fastness is also a helpful characteristic for distinguishing *Nocardia* organisms from morphologically similar organisms, such as *Actinomyces*. Most strains of *Nocardia* have trehalose linked to two molecules of mycolic acid (trehalose-6,6'-dimycolate; **cord factor**). Cord factor is an important virulence factor that facilitates intracellular survival (see Pathogenesis and Immunity section).

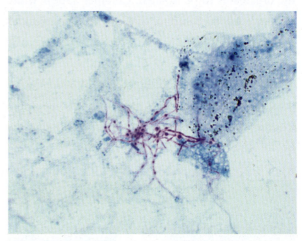

Figure 17-6 Acid-fast stain of *Nocardia* species in expectorated sputum. In contrast with the mycobacteria, members of the genus *Nocardia* do not uniformly retain the stain ("partially acid-fast").

Nocardia species are catalase-positive, use carbohydrates oxidatively, and can grow on most nonselective laboratory media used for the isolation of bacteria, mycobacteria, and fungi; however, their growth is **slow**, requiring 3 to 5 days of incubation before colonies may be observed on the culture plates, so the laboratory should be notified that the cultures should be incubated beyond the normal 1 to 2 days. The colonies initially appear white but can be quite variable (e.g., dry to waxy, white to orange; Figure 17-7). Aerial hyphae (hyphae that protrude upward from the surface of a colony) are usually observed when the colonies are viewed with a dissecting microscope (Figure 17-8). The combination of both **presence of aerial hyphae and acid-fastness** is unique to the genus *Nocardia* and can be used as a rapid test for the presumptive identification of the genus.

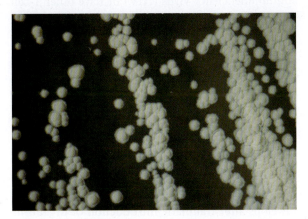

Figure 17-7   Colonies of *Nocardia*.

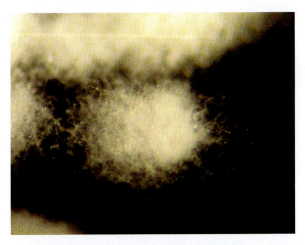

Figure 17-8   Aerial hyphae of *Nocardia*.

The taxonomic classification of this genus is—simply stated—a mess, with most of the organisms described in the literature now recognized as incorrectly identified. Historically, these organisms were classified by their ability to utilize carbohydrates and decompose a variety of substrates, as well as their antimicrobial susceptibility patterns. The true taxonomic relationships among the members of the genus were appreciated only recently through the use of gene sequencing. Currently, almost 100 species have been identified, far more than what can be identified by biochemical testing. Fortunately, most infections are caused by a relatively few species and identification of this group of organisms at the genus level combined with *in vitro* susceptibility testing is sufficient for the management of most patients.

Pathogenesis and Immunity

Although toxins and hemolysins have been described for nocardiae, the role these factors play in disease has not been defined. It would appear that the primary factor associated with virulence is the ability of pathogenic strains to **avoid phagocytic killing**. When phagocytes contact microbes, an oxidative burst occurs, with release of toxic oxygen metabolites (i.e., hydrogen peroxide, superoxide). Pathogenic strains of nocardiae are protected from these metabolites by their secretion of **catalase** and **superoxide dismutase**. Surface-associated superoxide dismutase also protects the bacteria. Nocardiae are also able to survive and **replicate in macrophages** by (1) preventing fusion of the phagosome-lysosome (mediated by **cord factor**), (2) preventing acidification of the phagosome, and (3) avoiding acid phosphatase-mediated killing by metabolic utilization of the enzyme as a carbon source.

Clinical Diseases

Bronchopulmonary disease caused by *Nocardia* species cannot be distinguished from infections caused by other pyogenic organisms, although *Nocardia* infections tend to develop more slowly, and primary pulmonary disease caused by *Nocardia* occurs almost always in immunocompromised patients. Signs such as cough, dyspnea, and fever are usually present but are not diagnostic. Cavitation and spread into the pleura are common. Although the clinical picture is not specific for *Nocardia*, these organisms should be considered when immunocompromised patients experience pneumonia with cavitation, particularly if there is evidence of dissemination to the central nervous system or subcutaneous tissues. If a pulmonary or disseminated *Nocardia* infection is diagnosed in an individual with no underlying disease, then a comprehensive immunologic workup is indicated.

Cutaneous infections may be primary infections (e.g., mycetoma, lymphocutaneous infections, cellulitis, subcutaneous abscesses) or from the result of the secondary spread of organisms from a primary pulmonary infection. **Mycetoma** is a painless, chronic infection primarily of the feet, characterized by localized subcutaneous swelling with involvement of the underlying tissues, muscle, and bone; suppuration; and the formation of multiple sinus tracts (narrow path from the focus of infection to the skin surface). A variety of organisms can cause mycetoma, although *Nocardia brasiliensis* is the most common cause in North America, Central America, and South America. **Lymphocutaneous infections** can manifest as cutaneous nodules and ulcerations along the lymphatics and regional lymph node involvement. These infections resemble cutaneous infections caused by some species of mycobacteria and by the fungus *Sporothrix schenckii*. *Nocardia* can also cause **chronic ulcerative lesions, subcutaneous abscesses,** and **cellulitis** (Figure 17-9).

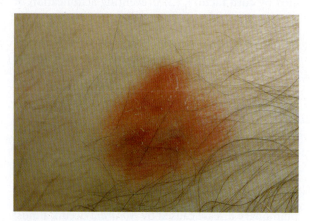

Figure 17-9 Cutaneous lesion caused by *Nocardia*. (From Sorrell TC, et al: *Nocardia* species. In Mandell GL, Bennett JE, Dolin R, editors: *Principles and practices of infectious diseases,* ed 6, Philadelphia, 2004, Elsevier Churchill Livingstone.)

As many as one third of all patients with *Nocardia* infections have dissemination to the brain, most commonly involving the formation of single or multiple **brain abscesses**. The disease can present initially as chronic meningitis.

Epidemiology

Nocardia infections are **exogenous** (i.e., caused by organisms not normally part of the normal human flora). The ubiquitous presence of the organism in soil rich with organic matter and the increasing numbers of immunocompromised individuals living in communities have led to dramatic increases in disease

caused by this organism. The increase is particularly noticeable in high-risk populations, such as ambulatory patients who are infected with human immunodeficiency virus (HIV) or have other T-cell deficiencies, patients receiving immunosuppressive therapy for bone marrow or solid organ transplants, and immunocompetent patients with pulmonary function compromised by bronchitis, emphysema, asthma, bronchiectasis, and alveolar proteinosis. Bronchopulmonary disease develops after the initial colonization of the upper respiratory tract by inhalation and then aspiration of oral secretions into the lower airways. Primary cutaneous nocardiosis develops after traumatic introduction of organisms into subcutaneous tissues, and secondary cutaneous involvement typically follows dissemination from a pulmonary site.

Laboratory Diagnosis

Multiple sputum specimens should be collected from patients with pulmonary disease. Because nocardiae are usually distributed throughout the tissue and abscess material, it is relatively easy to detect them by microscopy and to recover them in culture of specimens from patients with pulmonary, cutaneous, or CNS disease. The delicate hyphae of *Nocardia* in tissues resemble *Actinomyces* organisms; however, in contrast with *Actinomyces*, nocardiae are typically weakly acid-fast (see Figure 17-6).

The organisms grow on most laboratory media incubated in an atmosphere of 5% to 10% carbon dioxide, but the presence of these slow-growing organisms may be obscured by more rapidly growing commensal bacteria. If a specimen is potentially contaminated with other bacteria (e.g., oral bacteria in sputum), selective media should be inoculated. Success has been achieved with the medium used for the *Legionella* isolation (**buffered charcoal yeast extract [BCYE] agar**), as this medium can recover both *Nocardia* and *Legionella* from pulmonary specimens. *Nocardia* occasionally grows on media used for the isolation of mycobacteria and fungi; however, this method is less reliable than the use of special bacterial media. It is important to notify the laboratory that nocardiosis is suspected because most laboratories do not routinely use special culture media or incubate clinical specimens for more than 1 to 2 days. It takes more time (i.e., as long as a week) for *Nocardia* species to be detected in culture.

The preliminary identification of *Nocardia* is uncomplicated. Members of the genus can be classified initially on the basis of the presence of **filamentous, weakly acid-fast bacilli** and **aerial hyphae** on the colony surface. Definitive identification at the species level is more difficult because most species cannot be identified accurately by biochemical tests, although many laboratories continue to use these tests. The accurate identification of most species requires molecular analysis of RNA genes and "housekeeping" genes (e.g., heat shock protein gene). Alternatively, *Nocardia*, as well as other bacteria and fungi, can be identified rapidly and accurately at the species level by protein analysis using mass spectrometry. Although this approach to organism identification has only recently been introduced into diagnostic laboratories, this will likely become the method of choice within the next few years.

Treatment, Prevention, and Control

Antibiotics with activity against *Nocardia* include trimethoprim-sulfamethoxazole (TMP-SMX), amikacin, imipenem, and broad-spectrum cephalosporins (e.g., ceftriaxone, cefotaxime). Because antibiotic susceptibility can vary among individual isolates, antimicrobial susceptibility tests should be performed to guide specific therapy. TMP-SMX can be used as initial empiric therapy for cutaneous infections in immunocompetent patients. Antibiotic therapy for severe infections and cutaneous infections in immunocompromised patients should include two or three antibiotics, such as TMP-SMX plus amikacin for pulmonary or cutaneous infections and TMP-SMX plus imipenem or a cephalosporin for CNS infections. Because *Nocardia* grows slowly and is associated with therapeutic relapses, prolonged treatment (up to 12 months) is recommended. Whereas the clinical response is favorable in patients with localized infections, the prognosis is poor for immunocompro-

mised patients with disseminated disease.

Nocardiae are ubiquitous, so it is impossible to avoid exposure to them. However, bronchopulmonary disease caused by nocardiae is uncommon in immunocompetent persons, and primary cutaneous infections can be prevented with proper wound care. The complications associated with disseminated disease can be minimized if nocardiosis is considered in the differential diagnosis for immunocompromised patients with cavitary pulmonary disease and promptly treated.

SUMMARY

Actinomyces

Actinomyces are gram-positive, asporogenous, nonmotile rods; not acid-fast; facultatively anaerobic or strictly anaerobic, slow growth in culture (a week or more), mycelium. Low virulence, patients are only infected when the normal mucosal barriers are disrupted. Suppurative infection (actinomycosis): cervicofacial, thoracic, abdominal, pelvic, or brain type can be observed. Endogenous infection, no person-to-person spread, is not common in healthy population. *Actinomyces* are difficult to confirm because of clinical specimen contamination. Laboratory confirmation includes fastidious and slow growth in anaerobic culture, white colonies (molar tooth); sulfur granules in specimens, gram-positive branching rods.

Nocardia

Nocardia are gram-positive, partially acid-fast, filamentous rods, have cell wall with mycolic acid. The primary factor associated with virulence is the ability of pathogenic strains to **avoid phagocytic killing**.

Catalase and superoxide dismutase inactivate toxic oxygen metabolites (e.g., hydrogen peroxide, superoxide). Cord factor prevents intracellular killing in phagocytes by interfering with fusion of phagosomes with lysosomes. Primary disease is most commonly bronchopulmonary (e.g., cavitary disease) or primary cutaneous infections (e.g., mycetoma, lymphocutaneous infection, cellulitis, subcutaneous abscesses). ***Nocardia*** are most commonly disseminated to central nervous system (e.g., brain abscesses) or skin.

KEYWORDS

English	Chinese
Actinomyces	放线菌属
Mycelium	菌丝
Sulfur granule	硫磺样颗粒
Actinomycosis	放线菌病
Nocardia	诺卡菌属
Nocardiosis	诺卡菌病
Aerial hyphae	气生菌丝

BIBLIOGRAPHY

1. Boyanova L, et al. Actinomycosis: a frequently forgotten disease, Future Microbiol 10(4): 613-628, 2015

2. Reichenbach J, et al: Actinomyces in chronic granulomatous disease: an emerging and unanticipated pathogen, Clin Infect Dis 49: 1703-1710, 2009.

3. Ambrosioni J, Lew D, Garbino J: Nocardiosis: updated clinical review and experience at a tertiary center, Infection 38: 89-97, 2010.

4. Beaman B, Beaman L: Nocardia species: host-parasite relationships, Clin Microbiol Rev 7: 213-264, 1994.

5. Dodiuk-Gad R, Cohen E, Ziv M, Goldstein LH, Chazan B, Shafer J, Sprecher H, Elias M, Keness Y, Rozenman D: Cutaneous nocardiosis: report of two cases and review of the literature, Internatl J Derm 49: 1380-1385, 2010.

6. Martinez R, Reyes S, Menendez R: Pulmonary nocardiosis: risk factors, clinical features, diagnosis and prognosis, Curr Opin Pulm Med 14: 219-227, 2008.

7. Steingrube VA, Wilson RW, Brown BA, Jost KC Jr, Blacklock Z, Gibson JL, Wallace RJ Jr: Rapid identification of clinically significant species and taxa of aerobic actinomycetes, including Actinomadura, Gordona, Nocardia, Rhodococcus, Streptomyces, and Tsukamurella isolates, by DNA amplification and restriction endonuclease analysis, J Clin Microbiol 35: 817-822, 1997.

Chapter 18

Mycobacterium

The genus *Mycobacterium* consists of nonmotile, non-spore-forming, aerobic rods that are 0.2 to 0.6 × 1 to 10 μm in size. The rods occasionally form branched filaments, but these can be readily disrupted. The cell wall is rich in lipids, making the surface hydrophobic and the mycobacteria resistant to many disinfectants and common laboratory stains. Once stained, the rods also cannot be decolorized with acid solutions; hence the name **acid-fast** bacteria. Most mycobacteria divide slowly, and cultures require incubation for up to 8 weeks before growth is detected because the structure of the cell wall is complex and the organisms have fastidious growth requirements.

Mycobacteria are a significant cause of morbidity and mortality, particularly in countries with limited medical resources. Currently, more than 150 species of mycobacteria have been described, many of which are associated with human disease (Table 18-1). Despite the abundance of mycobacterial species, the following few species or groups cause most human infections: *M. tuberculosis*, *M. leprae*, *M. avium* complex, *M. kansasii*, *M. fortuitum*, *M. chelonae*, and *M. abscessus*.

PHYSIOLOGY AND STRUCTURE OF MYCOBACTERIA

Bacteria are classified in the genus *Mycobacterium* on the basis of (1) their acid-fastness, (2) the presence of **mycolic acids** containing 70 to 90 carbons, and (3) a high (61% to 71 mol%) guanine plus cytosine (G+C) content in their deoxyribonucleic acid (DNA). Although other species of bacteria can be acid-fast

Table 18-1 Classification of Selected Mycobacteria Pathogenic for Humans

Organism	Pathogenicity	Frequency in United States
Mycobacterium tuberculosis Complex		
M. tuberculosis	Strictly pathogenic	Common
M. leprae	Strictly pathogenic	Uncommon
M. africanum	Strictly pathogenic	Rare
M. bovis	Strictly pathogenic	Rare
M. bovis BCG (bacille Calmette-Guérin strain)	Sometimes pathogenic	Rare
Slow-Growing Nontuberculous Mycobacteria		
M. leprae	Strictly pathogenic	Common
M. avium complex	Usually pathogenic	Common
M. kansasii	Usually pathogenic	Uncommon
M. marinum	Usually pathogenic	Uncommon
M. simiae	Usually pathogenic	Uncommon
M. szulgai	Usually pathogenic	Uncommon
M. genavense	Usually pathogenic	Uncommon
M. haemophilum	Usually pathogenic	Uncommon
M. malmoense	Usually pathogenic	Uncommon
M. ulcerans	Usually pathogenic	Uncommon
M. scrofulaceum	Sometimes pathogenic	Uncommon
M. xenopi	Sometimes pathogenic	Uncommon
Rapidly Growing Nontuberculous Mycobacteria		
M. abscessus	Sometimes pathogenic	Common
M. chelonae	Sometimes pathogenic	Common
M. fortuitum	Sometimes pathogenic	Common
M. mucogenicum	Sometimes pathogenic	Common

(i.e., *Nocardia, Rhodococcus, Tsukamurella, Gordonia*), they stain less intensely (**partially acid-fast**) and their mycolic acids chains are shorter.

Mycobacteria possess a complex, **lipid-rich cell**

wall (Figure 18-1). This cell wall is responsible for many of the characteristic properties of the bacteria (e.g., acid-fastness; slow growth; resistance to detergents, common antibacterial antibiotics, and the host immune response; antigenicity). The basic structure of the cell wall consists of peptidoglycan, arabinogalactan, and mycolic acids. Anchored in the plasma membrane are proteins, phosphatidylinositol mannosides, and **lipoarabinomannan (LAM)**. Additional lipids, glycolipids, and peptidoglycolipids are also present. The lipid components comprise 60% of the cell wall weight. Transport proteins and porins are interspersed throughout the cell wall layers, and these constitute 15% of the cell wall weight. The proteins are biologically important antigens, stimulating the patient's cellular immune response. Extracted and partially purified preparations of these protein derivatives (**purified protein derivatives [PPDs]**) are used as skin test reagents to measure exposure to *M. tuberculosis*. Similar preparations from other mycobacteria have been used as species-specific skin test reagents.

Growth properties and colonial morphology are used for the preliminary classification of mycobacteria. As noted earlier, *M. tuberculosis* and closely related species in the *M. tuberculosis* complex are slow-growing bacteria. The colonies of these mycobacteria are either nonpigmented or a light tan color (Figure 18-2). The other mycobacteria, now referred to as "nontuberculous mycobacteria" (NTM), were classified originally by Runyon by their rate of growth and pigmentation (see Table 18-1). The pigmented mycobacteria produce intensely **yellow carotenoids**, which may be stimulated by exposure to light (photochromogenic organisms Figure 18-3) or produced in the absence of light (scotochromogenic organisms). The **Runyon classification** scheme of NTM consists of four groups: slow-growing photochromogens (e.g., *M. kansasii, M. marinum*), slow-growing scotochromogens (e.g., *M. gordonae*– a commonly isolated nonpathogen), slow-growing nonpigmented mycobacteria (e.g., *M. avium, M. intracellulare*), and rapidly growing mycobacteria (e.g., *M. fortuitum, M. chelonae, M. abscessus*).

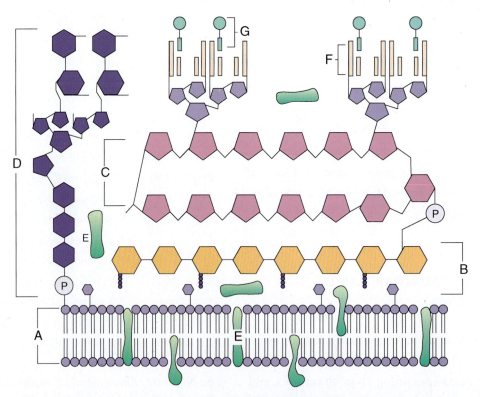

Figure 18-1 Mycobacterial cell wall structure. The components include the *(A)* plasma membrane, *(B)* peptidoglycans, *(C)* arabinogalactan, *(D)* mannose-capped lipoarabinomannan, *(E)* plasma-associated and cell wall-associated proteins, *(F)* mycolic acids, and *(G)* glycolipid surface molecules associated with the mycolic acids. (Modified from Karakousis, et al: *Mycobacterium tuberculosis* cell wall lipids and the host immune response, *Cell Microbiol* 6: 105-116, 2004.)

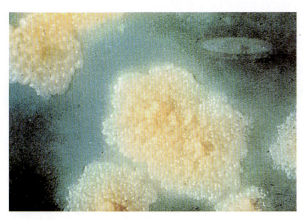

Figure 18-2 *Mycobacterium tuberculosis* colonies on Löwenstein-Jensen agar after 8 weeks of incubation. (From Baron EJ, Peterson LR, Finegold SM: *Bailey and Scott's diagnostic microbiology*, ed 9, St Louis, 1994, Mosby.)

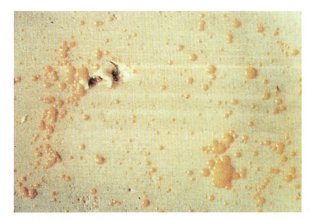

Figure 18-3 *Mycobacterium kansasii* colonies on Middlebrook agar; pigment develops after brief exposure to light.

MYCOBACTERIUM TUBERCULOSIS

Pathogenesis and Immunity

M. tube rculosis is an intracellular pathogen that is able to establish lifelong infection. At the time of exposure, *M. tuberculosis* enters the respiratory airways and infectious particles penetrate to the alveoli where they are phagocytized by alveolar macrophages. In contrast with most phagocytized bacteria, *M. tuberculosis* **prevents fusion of the phagosome with lysosomes**. Phagocytized bacteria are able to evade macrophage killing mediated by reactive nitrogen intermediates formed between nitric oxide and superoxide anions by catalytically catabolizing the oxidants that are formed.

In response to infection with *M. tuberculosis*, macrophages secrete **interleukin-12 (IL-12)** and **tumor necrosis factor-α (TNF-α)**. These cytokines increase localized inflammation with the recruitment of T cells and natural killer (NK) cells into the area of the infected macrophages, inducing T-cell differentiation into **TH1 cells** (**T-helper cells**), with subsequent secretion of **interferon-γ (IFN-γ)**. In the presence of IFN-γ, the infected macrophages are activated, leading to increased phagosome-lysosome fusion and intracellular killing. In addition, TNF-α stimulates production of nitric oxide and related reactive nitrogen intermediates, leading to enhanced intracellular killing. Patients with decreased production of IFN-γ or TNF-α, or who have defects in the receptors for these cytokines, are at increased risk for severe mycobacterial infections.

Alveolar macrophages, epithelioid cells, and **Langhans giant cells** (fused epithelioid cells) with intracellular mycobacteria form the central core of a necrotic mass that is surrounded by a dense wall of macrophages and CD4, CD8, and NK T cells. This structure, a **granuloma**, prevents further spread of the bacteria. If a small antigenic burden is present at the time the macrophages are stimulated, the granuloma is small and the bacteria are destroyed with minimal tissue damage; however, if many bacteria are present, the large necrotic or caseous granulomas become encapsulated with fibrin that effectively protects the bacteria from macrophage killing. The bacteria can remain dormant in this stage or can be reactivated years later when the patient's immunologic responsiveness wanes as the result of old age or immunosuppressive disease or therapy. This process is the reason that disease may not develop until late in life in patients exposed to *M. tuberculosis*.

Epidemiology

Although tuberculosis can be established in primates and laboratory animals, such as guinea pigs, **humans are the only natural reservoir**. The disease is spread by close person-to-person contact through the inhalation of infectious aerosols. Large particles are trapped on mucosal surfaces and removed by the ciliary action of the respiratory tree. However, small particles containing one to three tubercle bacilli can reach the alveolar spaces and establish infection.

The World Health Organization (WHO) estimates that one third of the world's population is infected with *M. tuberculosis.* Currently there are almost 9 million new cases and 2 million deaths caused by *M. tuberculosis* annually (that is, one death every 20 seconds). Regions with the highest incidence of disease are sub-Saharan Africa, Southeast Asia, and Eastern Europe. People co-infected with the human immunodeficiency virus (HIV) and drug-resistant *M. tuberculosis* poses a significant public health problem. In 1990, the first outbreaks of **multidrug-resistant *M. tuberculosis* (MDR TB;** resistant to at least isoniazid and rifampin) were observed in patients with AIDS and in homeless persons in New York City and Miami. They are increasing dramatically in prevalence in developing countries since then. In addition, new strains of resistant *M. tuberculosis,* called **extensively drug-resistant (XDR) TB**, have emerged in most regions of the world. These strains, defined as MDR TB that are resistant to fluoroquinolones and at least one of the second-line drugs (e.g., kanamycin, amikacin, capreomycin), are potentially untreatable.

Clinical Diseases

Although tuberculosis can involve any organ, most infections in immunocompetent patients are restricted to the lungs. The initial pulmonary focus is the middle or lower lung fields, where the tubercle bacilli can multiply freely. The patient's cellular immunity is activated, and mycobacterial replication ceases in most patients within 3 to 6 weeks after exposure to the organism. Approximately 5% of patients exposed to *M. tuberculosis* progress to having active disease within 2 years, and another 5% to 10% experience disease sometime later in life.

The likelihood that infection will progress to active disease is a function of both the infectious dose and the patient's immune competence. For example, active disease develops within 1 year of exposure in approximately 10% of patients who are infected with HIV and have a low CD4 T-cell count, compared with a 10% risk of disease during the lifetime of patients without HIV infection. In patients with HIV infection, disease usually appears before the onset of other opportunistic infections, is twice as likely to spread to extrapulmonary sites, and can progress rapidly to death.

The clinical signs and symptoms of tuberculosis reflect the site of infection, with primary disease usually restricted to the lower respiratory tract. The disease is insidious at onset. Patients typically have nonspecific complaints of malaise, weight loss, cough, and night sweats. Sputum may be scant or bloody and purulent. Sputum production with hemoptysis is associated with tissue destruction (e.g., **cavitary disease**). The clinical diagnosis is supported by (1) radiographic evidence of pulmonary disease (Figure 18-4), (2) positive skin test reactivity, and (3) the laboratory detection of mycobacteria, either with microscopy or in cultures. One or both upper lobes of the lungs are usually involved in patients with active disease that includes pneumonitis or abscess formation and cavitation.

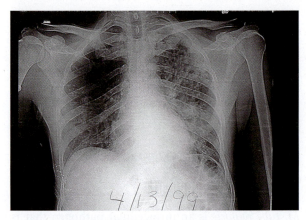

Figure 18-4   Pulmonary tuberculosis.

Extrapulmonary tuberculosis can occur as the result of the hematogenous spread of the bacilli during the initial phase of multiplication. There may be no evidence of pulmonary disease in patients with **disseminated tuberculosis**.

MYCOBACTERIUM LEPRAE

Pathogenesis and Immunity

Leprosy (also called **Hansen disease**) is caused by *M. leprae.* Because the bacteria multiply very slowly, the incubation period is prolonged, with symptoms developing as long as 20 years after infection. As with *M. tuberculosis* infections, the clinical manifestations of leprosy depend on the patient's immune reaction to the bacteria. The clinical presentation of leprosy ranges from the tuberculoid form to the lepromatous form. Patients with **tuberculoid leprosy** (also called **paucibacillary Hansen disease**) have a strong cellular immune reaction with many lymphocytes and granulomas present in the tissues and relatively few bacteria (Table 18-2). As in *M. tuberculosis* infections in immunocompetent patients, the bacteria induce cytokine production that mediates macrophage activation, phagocytosis, and bacillary clearance.

Patients with **lepromatous leprosy (multibacillary Hansen disease)** have a strong antibody response but a specific defect in the cellular response to *M. leprae* antigens. Thus an abundance of bacteria are typically observed in dermal macrophages and the Schwann cells of the peripheral nerves. As would be expected, this is the most infectious form of leprosy.

Epidemiology

Leprosy was first described in 600 BC and was recognized in the ancient civilizations of China, Egypt, and India. The global **prevalence of leprosy has fallen dramatically** with the widespread use of effective therapy. More than 5 million cases were documented in 1985 and fewer than 300,000 cases 20 years later. Currently, 90% of the cases are in Brazil, Madagascar, Mozambique, Tanzania, and Nepal. In the China, leprosy is uncommon, approximately 400new cases reported annually. Most cases occur in the Provinces of Yunnan, Guizhou, and Sichuan.

Leprosy is spread by person-to-person contact. Although the most important route of infection is unknown, it is believed that *M. leprae* is spread either through the inhalation of infectious aerosols or through skin contact with respiratory secretions and wound exudates. Numerous *M. leprae* are found in the nasal secretions of patients with lepromatous leprosy.

***M. leprae* cannot grow in cell-free cultures.** Thus laboratory confirmation of leprosy requires histopathologic findings consistent with the clinical disease and either **skin test reactivity to lepromin in tuberculoid leprosy** or observation of **acid-fast bacteria in the lesions of patients with lepromatous leprosy.**

Clinical Diseases

Leprosy is a chronic infection that affects the skin and peripheral nerves. The spectrum of tissue involvement is influenced by the patient's immune status, as noted earlier (see Table 18-2). The tuberculoid form (Figure 18-5) is milder and is characterized by hypopigmented skin macules. The lepromatous form (Figure 18-6) is associated with disfiguring skin lesions, nodules, plaques, thickened dermis, and involvement of the nasal mucosa.

Table 18-2 Clinical and Immunologic Manifestations of Leprosy

Features	Tuberculoid Leprosy	Lepromatous Leprosy
Skin lesions	Few erythematous or hypopigmented plaques with flat centers and raised, demarcated borders; peripheral nerve damage with complete sensory loss; visible enlargement of nerves	Many erythematous macules, papules, or nodules extensive tissue destruction (e.g., nasal cartilage, bones, ears); diffuse nerve involvement with patchy sensory loss; lack of nerve enlargement
Histopathology	Infiltration of lymphocytes around center of epithelial cells; presence of Langhans cells; few or no acid-fast rods observed	Predominantly "foamy" macrophages with few lymphocytes; lack of Langhans cells; numerous acid-fast rods in skin lesions and internal organs
Infectivity	Low	High
Immune response	Delayed hypersensitivity reactivity to lepromin	Nonreactivity to lepromin
Immunoglobulin levels	Normal	Hypergammaglobulinemia
Erythema nodosum	Absent	Usually present

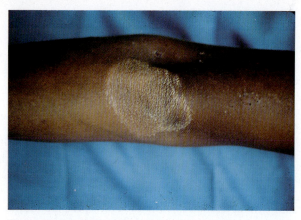

Figure 18-5 Tuberculoid leprosy. Early tuberculoid lesions are characterized by anesthetic macules with hypopigmentation. (From Cohen J, Powderly WB: *Infectious diseases*, ed 2, St Louis, 2004, Mosby.)

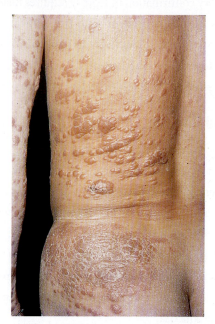

Figure 18-6 Lepromatous leprosy. Diffuse infiltration of the skin by multiple nodules of varying size, each with many bacteria. (From Cohen J, Powderly WB: *Infectious diseases*, ed 2, St Louis, 2004, Mosby.)

MYCOBACTERIUM AVIUM COMPLEX

The classification of mycobacteria in the *M. avium* complex has been defined recently by genomic-based studies. Two species, *M. avium* and *M. intracellulare*, and four subspecies are recognized currently (Table 18-3).

Both species in the *M. avium* complex (MAC) produce disease in immunocompetent patients, whereas disease in HIV-infected patients is primarily caused by *M. avium*. Before the HIV epidemic, recovery of the organisms in clinical specimens typically

Table 18-3 *Mycobacterium avium* Complex

Species	Disease
M. avium subsp. Avium	Avian tuberculosis
M. avium subsp. Hominissuis	Disease in humans and pigs; disseminated disease in HIV-infected patients; cervical lymphadenitis in children; chronic pulmonary disease in adolescents with cystic fibrosis and older adults with underlying pulmonary disease
M. avium subsp. Silvaticum	Disease in wood pigeons
M. avium subsp. Paratuberculosis	Chronic granulomatous enteric disease in ruminants (Johne disease) and possibly in humans (Crohn disease)
M. intracellulare	Pulmonary disease in immunocompetent patients

represented transient colonization or, less commonly, chronic pulmonary disease. Pulmonary disease in immunocompetent patients presents in one of three forms. Most commonly, disease is seen in middle-age or older men with a history of smoking and **underlying pulmonary disease**. These patients typically have a slowly evolving cavitary disease that resembles tuberculosis on chest radiography. The second form of MAC infection is observed in elderly, female nonsmokers. These patients have lingular or middle lobe infiltrates with a patchy, nodular appearance on radiography and associated bronchiectasis (chronically dilated bronchi). This form of disease is indolent and has been associated with significant morbidity and mortality. This specific disease has been called **Lady Windermere syndrome**, the name of the principle character in an Oscar Wilde play. The third form of MAC disease is formation of a **solitary pulmonary nodule**. *M. avium* complex is the most common mycobacterial species that causes solitary the pulmonary nodules.

Although some patients with **acquired immunodeficiency syndrome** (AIDS) develop *M. avium* disease after pulmonary exposure (e.g., infectious aerosols of contaminated water), most infections are believed to develop after ingestion of the bacteria. Person-to-person transmission has not been demonstrated. After exposure to the mycobacteria, replication is initiated in localized lymph nodes followed by systemic spread. The clinical manifestations of disease are not observed until the mass of replicating bacteria impairs normal organ function.

OTHER SLOW-GROWING MYCOBACTERIA

Many other slow-growing mycobacteria can cause human disease, and new species continue to be reported as better diagnostic test methods are developed. The spectrum of diseases produced by these mycobacteria also continues to expand, in large part because diseases such as AIDS, malignancies, and organ transplantation with concomitant use of immunosuppressive drugs have created a population of patients who are highly susceptible to organisms with relatively low virulence potential. Some mycobacteria produce disease identical to pulmonary tuberculosis (e.g., *Mycobacterium bovis, M. kansasii*), other species commonly cause infections localized to lymphatic tissue (*Mycobacterium scrofulaceum*), and others that grow optimally at cool temperatures primarily produce cutaneous infections (*Mycobacterium ulcerans, M. marinum, Mycobacterium haemophilum*). However, disseminated disease can be observed in patients with AIDS who are infected with these same species, as well as with relatively uncommon mycobacteria (e.g., *Mycobacterium genavense, Mycobacterium simiae*).

Most of these mycobacteria have been isolated in water and soil and occasionally from infected animals (e.g., *M. bovis* causes bovine tuberculosis). Often the isolation of these mycobacteria in clinical specimens simply represents transient colonization with organisms that the patient ingested. With the exception of *M. bovis* and other mycobacteria closely related to *M. tuberculosis*, person-to-person spread of these mycobacteria does not occur.

RAPIDLY GROWING MYCOBACTERIA

As discussed previously, NTM can be subdivided into slow-growing species and rapidly growing species (growth in less than 7 days). This distinction is important because the rapidly growing species have a relatively low virulence potential, stain irregularly with traditional mycobacterial stains, and are more susceptible to "conventional" antibacterial antibiotics than to drugs used to treat other mycobacterial infections. The most common species associated with disease are *M. fortuitum, M. chelonae, M. abscessus,* and *M. mucogenicum.*

The rapidly growing mycobacteria rarely cause disseminated infections. Rather, they are most commonly associated with disease occurring after bacteria are introduced into the deep subcutaneous tissues by **trauma or iatrogenic infections** (e.g., infections associated with an intravenous catheter, contaminated wound dressing, prosthetic device such as a heart valve, peritoneal dialysis, or bronchoscopy). Unfortunately, the incidence of infections with these organisms is increasing as more invasive procedures are performed in hospitalized patients and advanced medical care lengthens the life expectancy of immunocompromised patients. Opportunistic infections in immunocompetent patients are becoming commonplace.

LABORATORY DIAGNOSIS

Mycobacteria that cause pulmonary disease, particularly in patients with evidence of cavitation, are abundant in the respiratory secretions (e.g., 10^8 bacilli per milliliter or more). Recovery of the organisms is virtually assured in patients from whom early morning respiratory specimens are collected for 3 consecutive days; however, it is more difficult to isolate *M. tuberculosis* and NTM species from other sites in patients with disseminated disease (e.g., genitourinary tract, tissues, cerebrospinal fluid). In such cases, additional specimens must be collected for cultures, and a large volume of fluid or tissue must be processed. The following laboratory tests are routinely used in the diagnosis of infections caused by mycobacteria.

Immunodiagnosis

The traditional test to assess the patient's response to exposure to *M. tuberculosis* is the **tuberculin skin test.** Reactivity to an intradermal injection of mycobacterial antigens can differentiate between infected and noninfected people, with a positive PPD reaction usually developing 3 to 4 weeks after exposure to *M. tuberculosis*. The only evidence of infection with mycobacteria in most patients is a lifelong positive skin test reaction and radiographic evidence of calcification of granulomas in the lungs or other organs.

The currently recommended tuberculin antigen is a **PPD** from the mycobacterial cell wall. In this test, a specific amount of the antigen (5 tuberculin units of PPD) is inoculated into the intradermal layer of the patient's skin. Skin test reactivity (defined by the diameter of the area of induration) is measured 48 hours later. Patients infected with *M. tuberculosis* may not show a response to the tuberculin skin test if they are anergic (nonreactive to antigens; particularly true of HIV-infected patients). Additionally, individuals from countries where vaccination with attenuated *M. bovis* (**bacille Calmette-Guérin [BCG]**) is widespread will have a positive skin test reaction.

In recent years, **in vitro IFN-γ release assays** have been introduced as an alternative to the PPD skin test. The tests use immunoassays to measure IFN-γ produced by sensitized T cells stimulated by *M. tuberculosis* specific antigens (i.e., **early secreted antigenic target-6 [ESAT-6], culture filtrate protein-10 [CFP-10]**). If an individual was previously infected with *M. tuberculosis*, exposure of sensitized T cells present in whole blood to *M. tuberculosis*-specific antigens results in IFN-γ production. The assays can be used to discriminate between infections with *M. tuberculosis* and BCG vaccination. Although the tests are sensitive and highly specific, the technical complexity of the assays currently limits their use.

Reactivity to **lepromin**, which is prepared from inactivated *M. leprae*, is valuable for confirming the clinical diagnosis of tuberculoid leprosy. Papular induration develops 3 to 4 days after the intradermal injection of the antigen. This test is not useful for identifying patients with lepromatous leprosy because such patients are anergic to the antigen.

Microscopy

The microscopic detection of acid-fast bacteria in clinical specimens is the most rapid way to confirm mycobacterial disease. The clinical specimen is stained with carbolfuchsin (**Ziehl-Neelsen** or **Kinyoun** methods) or fluorescent auramine-rhodamine dyes (**Truant fluorochrome** method), decolorized with an acid-alcohol solution, and then counterstained. The specimens are examined with a light microscope or, if fluorescent dyes are used, a fluorescent microscope (Figure 18-7). The sensitivity of this test is high for respiratory specimens (particularly from patients with radiographic evidence of cavitation). Thus a positive acid-fast stain reaction corresponds to higher infectivity.

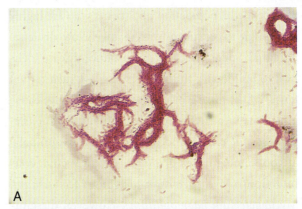
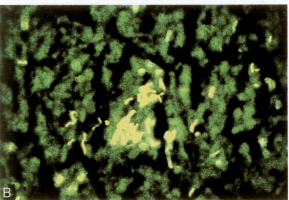

Figure 18-7   Acid-fast stains of *Mycobacterium tuberculosis*. A, Stained with carbolfuchsin using the Kinyoun method. B, Stained with the fluorescent dyes auramine and rhodamine using the Truant fluorochrome method.

Nucleic Acid-Based Tests

A gene encoding a secretory protein, *secA* gene, has been demonstrated to be a useful target for identifying all species of mycobacteria directly in clinical specimens. The gene can be amplified by polymerase chain reaction (PCR), and then the species-specific portion of the gene can be sequenced to determine the identity of the isolate. The test is highly sensitive with acid-fast smear-positive specimens and specific, but it is relatively insensitive in smear-negative specimens. A commercial, 1-hour PCR amplification assay named Xpert MTB/RIF was introduced in 2010; it can detect *M. tuberculosis* in clinical specimens and also determine susceptibility to rifampin, a surrogate marker for multidrug-resistant strains.

Culture

The in vitro growth of mycobacteria is complicated by the fact that most isolates grow slowly and can be obscured by the rapidly growing bacteria that normally colonize people. Thus specimens such as sputum are initially treated with a **decontaminating reagent** (e.g., 2% sodium hydroxide) to eliminate organisms that could confound results. Mycobacteria can tolerate brief alkali treatment that kills the rapidly growing bacteria and permits the selective isolation of mycobacteria.

Formerly, when specimens were inoculated onto egg-based (e.g., **Löwenstein-Jensen**) and agar-based (e.g., **Middlebrook**) media, it generally took 4 to 8 weeks for *M. tuberculosis*, *M. avium* complex, and other important slow-growing mycobacteria to be detected. However, this time has been shortened through the use of specially formulated **broth cultures** that support the rapid growth of most mycobacteria. Thus the average time to grow mycobacteria has been decreased from 10 to 21 days.

The ability of *M. tuberculosis* to grow rapidly in broth cultures has been used for performing rapid susceptibility tests. The technique, **MODS** or *microscopic observation drug susceptibility assay*, uses an inverted light microscope to examine 24-well plates inoculated with Middlebrook broth and decontaminated sputum. *M. tuberculosis* growth can be detected as tangles or cords of growth in the broth, generally after 1 week of incubation. Incorporation of antimycobacterial drugs in the broth enables rapid, direct susceptibility testing with clinical specimens.

Some mycobacterial species (e.g., *M. marinum*, *M. haemophilum*, *M. malmoense*) require a lower **incubation temperature** than that used for most cultures (30℃ versus 37℃). In addition, *M. haemophilum* requires supplementation of media with hemin or ferric ammonium citrate for growth. Because infections with these organisms characteristically involve the skin, laboratories should culture superficial specimens (e.g., skin biopsies and lesions) at both 30℃ and 37℃ and on at least one medium supplemented with hemin.

Identification

Growth properties and colonial morphology can be used for the preliminary identification of the most common species of mycobacteria. The definitive identification of mycobacteria can made using a variety of techniques. Biochemical tests were the standard method for identifying mycobacteria; however, the results are not available for at least 3 weeks or more, and many species cannot be differentiated by this approach. **Species-specific molecular probes** are the most useful means of identifying commonly isolated mycobacteria (e.g., *M. tuberculosis*, *M. avium*, *M. kansasii*), and, because many organisms are present in the culture at the time of initial detection, it is not necessary to amplify the target genomic sequence. The commercially prepared probe identification systems currently used are rapid (test time, 2 hours), sensitive, and specific. Mycobacterial species for which probes are not available can be identified by amplifying species-specific gene sequences (e.g., hypervariable regions of the 16S rRNA gene or *secA* gene), followed by sequence analysis to identify the species. This method is rapid (1 to 2 days), is not limited by the availability of specific probes, and is likely to replace the alternative identification methods.

TREATMENT, PREVENTION, AND CONTROL

Treatment

The number of treatment regimens that have been developed for drug-susceptible and drug-resistant tuberculosis is too complex to review here comprehensively (refer to the Centers for Disease Control and Prevention [CDC] website, www.cdc.gov/tb/).

Most treatment regimens begin with 2 months of isoniazid (isonicotinyl-hydrazine [INH]), ethambutol, pyrazinamide, and rifampin, followed by 4 to 6 months of INH and rifampin or alternative combination drugs. Modifications to this treatment scheme are dictated by the drug susceptibility of the isolate and the patient population.

The treatment regimens advanced by the WHO (http://WHO.int/lep) have distinguished between patients with the tuberculoid (paucibacillary) form and the lepromatous (multibacillary) form. The paucibacillary form should be treated with rifampicin and dapsone for a minimum of 6 months, whereas the multibacillary form should have clofazimine added to the regimen, and treatment should be extended to 12 months.

M. avium complex and many other slow-growing mycobacteria are resistant to common antimycobacterial agents. One regimen recommended currently for MAC infections is clarithromycin or azithromycin, combined with ethambutol and rifampin. The American Thoracic Society has recommended that *M. kansasii* infections be treated with INH, rifampin, and ethambutol. Unlike the slow-growing mycobacteria, the rapidly growing species are resistant to most commonly used antimycobacterial agents but are susceptible to antibiotics such as clarithromycin, imipenem, amikacin, cefoxitin, and the sulfonamides. The specific activity of these agents must be determined with in vitro tests. Because infections with these mycobacteria are generally confined to the skin or are associated with prosthetic devices, surgical debridement or removal of the prosthesis is also necessary.

Chemoprophylaxis

The prophylactic regimens that have been recommended for use in patients (HIV positive and HIV negative) exposed to *M. tuberculosis*, include daily or twice weekly INH for 6 to 9 months, or daily rifampin for 4 months. Patients who have been exposed to drug-resistant *M. tuberculosis* should receive prophylaxis with pyrazinamide and either ethambutol or levofloxacin for 6 to 12 months. For patients with other mycobacterial infections, chemoprophylaxis is unnecessary.

Immunoprophylaxis

Vaccination with attenuated *M. bovis* (**BCG**) is commonly used in countries where tuberculosis is endemic and is responsible for significant morbidity and mortality. This practice can lead to a significant reduction in the incidence of tuberculosis if BCG is administered to people when they are young (it is less effective in adults). Unfortunately, BCG immunization cannot be used in immunocompromised patients (e.g., those with HIV infection).

Control

Because one third of the world's population is infected with *M. tuberculosis*, the elimination of this disease is highly unlikely. Disease can be controlled, however, with a combination of active surveillance, prophylactic and therapeutic intervention, and careful case monitoring.

SUMMARY

Mycobacterium tuberculosis

Mycobacterium tuberculosis is weakly gram-positive, strongly acid-fast, aerobic rods. The lipid-rich cell wall makes the organism resistant to disinfectants, detergents, common antibacterial antibiotics, host immune response, and traditional stains. The bacteria are capable of intracellular growth in alveolar macrophages. Disease results primarily from host response to infection, and the primary infection is pulmonary while dissemination to any body site occurs most commonly in immunocompromised patients. One third of the world's population is infected with this organism. Populations at greatest risk for disease are immunocompromised patients, drug or alcohol abusers, homeless persons, and individuals exposed to diseased patients. Humans are the only natural reservoir. Tuberculin skin test and interferon-γ release tests are sensitive markers for exposure to organism. Microscopy and culture are sensitive and specific. Direct detection by molecular probes is relatively insensitive except for acid-fast smear-positive specimens. Identification most commonly made using species-specific molecular probes. Prolonged treatment with multiple drugs is required to prevent development of drug-resistant strains.

Prophylaxis for exposure to tuberculosis can include INH for 6 to 9 months or rifampin for 4 months; pyrazinamide and ethambutol or levofloxacin are used for 6 to 12 months after exposure to drug-resistant *M. tuberculosis*. Immunoprophylaxis with bacille Calmette-Guérin in endemic countries

Mycobacterium leprae

The *Mycobacterium leprae* is unable to be cultured on artificial media. The tuberculoid (paucibacillary) and lepromatous (multibacillary) are the forms of leprosy.

Mycobacterium avium Complex

Disease includes asymptomatic colonization, chronic localized pulmonary disease, solitary nodule, or disseminated disease, particularly in patients with acquired immunodeficiency syndrome (AIDS). Despite worldwide distribution, the disease is most commonly seen in countries where tuberculosis is less common.

KEYWORDS

English	Chinese
Mycobacterium	分枝杆菌属
Mycobacterium tuberculosis	结核分枝杆菌
Mycobacterium tuberculosis complex	结核分枝杆菌复合群
Mycobacterium leprae	麻风分枝杆菌
Nontuberculous mycobacteria	非结核分枝杆菌
Acid-fast	抗酸的
Mycobacterium avium Complex	鸟分枝杆菌复合群
Tuberculin skin test	结核菌素皮肤试验
Slow-Growing Mycobacteria	缓慢生长分枝杆菌
Granuloma	肉芽肿
Pulmonary tuberculosis	肺结核
Extrapulmonary tuberculosis	肺外结核
Löwenstein-Jensen media	罗氏培养基
Leprosy	麻风病
Tuberculoid leprosy	结核样型麻风病
Lepromatous leprosy	瘤型麻风病

BIBLIOGRAPHY

1. Appelberg R: Pathogenesis of *Mycobacterium avium* infection, Immunol Res 35: 179-190, 2006.

2. De Groote M, Huitt G: Infections due to rapidly growing mycobacteria, Clin Infect Dis 42: 1756-1763, 2006.

3. Drobniewski F, et al: Antimicrobial susceptibility testing of *Mycobacterium tuberculosis*, Clin Microbiol Infect 13: 1144-1156, 2007.

4. Flynn JL, Chan J: Immune evasion by *Mycobacterium tuberculosis*: living with the enemy, Curr Opin Immunol 15: 450-455, 2003.

5. Griffith D, et al: An official ATS/IDSA statement: diagnosis, treatment, and prevention of nontuberculous mycobacterial diseases, Am J Respir Crit Care Med 175: 367-416, 2007.

6. Karakousis PC, Bishai WR, Dorman SE: Microreview: *Mycobacterium tuberculosis* cell envelope lipids and the host immune response, Cell Microbiol 6: 105-116, 2004.

7. Mazurek G, et al: Updated guidelines for using interferon gamma release assays to detect *Mycobacterium tuberculosis* infection—United States, 2010, MMWR Recomm Rep 59(RR-5): 1-24, 2010.

8. Smith I: *Mycobacterium tuberculosis* pathogenesis and molecular determinants of virulence, Clin Microbiol Rev 16: 463-496, 2003.

9. Turenne C, et al: *Mycobacterium avium* in the postgenomic era, Clin Microbiol Rev 20: 205-229, 2007.

10. Ulrichs T, Kaufmann S: New insights into the function of granulomas in human tuberculosis, J Pathol 208: 261-269, 2006.

11. Wells C, et al: HIV infection and multidrug-resistant tuberculosis—the perfect storm, J Infect Dis 196: S86-S107, 2007.

Neisseria and Related Genera

Three genera of medically important bacteria are in the family Neisseriaceae: *Neisseria, Eikenella,* and *Kingella.* The genus *Neisseria* consists of 28 species, with 10 species found in humans and two species, *Neisseria gonorrhoeae* and *Neisseria meningitidis,* strictly human pathogens. The remaining species are commonly present on mucosal surfaces of the oropharynx and nasopharynx and occasionally colonize the anogenital mucosal membranes. Diseases caused by *N. gonorrhoeae* and *N. meningitidis* are well known, and the other *Neisseria* species have limited virulence and generally produce opportunistic infections. *Eikenella corrodens* and *Kingella kingae* colonize the human oropharynx and are also opportunistic pathogens.

NEISSERIA GONORRHOEAE AND NEISSERIA MENINGITIDIS

Infections caused by *N. gonorrhoeae,* particularly the **sexually transmitted disease gonorrhea,** have been recognized for centuries. Despite effective antibiotic therapy, gonorrhea is still one of the most common sexually transmitted diseases in China. The presence of *N. gonorrhoeae* in a clinical specimen is always considered significant. In contrast, strains of *N. meningitidis* can colonize the nasopharynx of healthy people without producing disease or can cause community-acquired meningitis, overwhelming and rapidly fatal sepsis, or bronchopneumonia.

Physiology and Structure

Neisseria species are aerobic, **gram-negative** bacteria, typically coccoid shaped (0.6 to 1.0 μm in diameter)

and arranged in pairs (**diplococci**) with adjacent sides flattened together (resembling coffee beans; Figure 19-1). All species are oxidase positive and most produce catalase, properties that combined with the Gram-stain morphology allow a rapid, presumptive identification of a clinical isolate. Acid is produced by oxidation of carbohydrates (not by fermentation). *N. gonorrhoeae* strains produce acid by oxidizing glucose, and *N. meningitidis* strains oxidize both glucose and maltose. Other carbohydrates are not oxidized by these species, and this pattern of carbohydrate utilization is useful for differentiating these pathogenic strains from other *Neisseria* species.

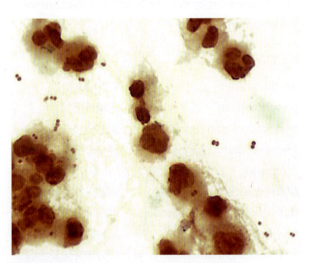

Figure 19-1 *Neisseria menigitidis* in cerebrospinal fluid. Note the spatial arrangement of the pairs of cocci with sides pressed together, which is characteristic of this genus.

Nonpathogenic species of *Neisseria* can grow on blood agar and nutrient agar (general purpose medium for nonfastidious bacteria) incubated at 35℃ to 37℃. In contrast, *N. meningitidis* has variable growth on nutrient agar, and *N. gonorrhoeae* cannot grow on this medium because it has complex nutritional requirements. All strains of *N. gonorrhoeae* require cystine and an energy source (e.g., glucose, pyruvate, lactate) for growth, and many strains require supplementation of media with amino acids, purines, pyrimidines, and vitamins. Soluble starch is added to the media to neutralize the toxic effect of the fatty acids. Thus *N. gonorrhoeae* does not grow on blood agar but does grow on **chocolate agar** and other enriched supplemented media. The optimum growth temperature is 35℃ to 37℃, with poor survival of the organism at cooler temperatures. A humid atmosphere supplemented with **5% carbon dioxide** is either required or enhances growth of *N. gonorrhoeae*. Although the fastidious nature of this organism makes recovery from clinical specimens difficult, it is nevertheless easy for the organism to be transmitted sexually from person to person.

The cell wall structure of *N. gonorrhoeae* and *N. meningitidis* is typical of gram-negative bacteria, with the thin peptidoglycan layer sandwiched between the inner cytoplasmic membrane and the outer membrane. The major virulence factor for *N. meningitidis* is the polysaccharide capsule, while the outer surface of *N. gonorrhoeae* is not covered with a true carbohydrate capsule. Antigenic differences in the **polysaccharide capsule** of *N. meningitidis* are the basis for serogrouping these bacteria in vitro and play a prominent role in determining if an individual strain will cause disease. Thirteen serogroups are currently recognized, with most infections caused by serogroups A, B, C, Y, and W135.

Pathogenic and nonpathogenic strains of *Neisseria* have **pili** that extend from the cytoplasmic membrane through the outer membrane. The pili are composed of repeating protein subunits (**pilins**), whose expression is controlled by the *pil* gene complex. Pili expression is associated with virulence, in part because the pili mediate attachment to nonciliated epithelial cells and provide resistance to killing by neutrophils. Pilin proteins have a conserved region at the amino terminal end and a highly variable region at the exposed carboxyl terminus. The carboxyl terminal portion of the pilin protein can

be phosphorylated and glycosylated and is associated with a second protein, **PilC,** which contributes to its antigenity diversity. The lack of immunity to reinfection with *N. gonorrhoeae* results partially from the antigenic variation among the pilin proteins and partially from the phase variation in pilin expression; these factors complicate attempts to develop effective vaccines for gonorrhea.

Other prominent families of proteins are present in the outer membrane. The **porin proteins** are integral outer membrane proteins that form pores or channels for nutrients to pass into the cell and waste products to exit. *N. gonorrhoeae* and *N. meningitidis* have two porin genes, *porA* and *porB*. The gene products, **PorA and PorB proteins,** are both expressed in *N. meningitidis*, but the *porA* gene is silent in *N. gonorrhoeae*. Thus, not only is PorB the major outer membrane protein in *N. gonorrhoeae* (an estimated 60% of the gonococcal outer membrane proteins), but it must also be functionally active for *N. gonorrhoeae* to survive. PorB is expressed as two distinct classes of antigens, PorB1A and PorB1B, with many distinct serological variants. PorB is important for the virulence of *N. gonorrhoeae* because these proteins can interfere with degranulation of neutrophils (i.e., phagolysosome fusion that would lead to killing of intracellular bacteria) and presumably protect the bacteria from the host's inflammatory response. Additionally, PorB with other adhesins facilitates the bacterial invasion into epithelial cells. Finally, expression of some PorB antigens makes the bacteria resistant to complement-mediated serum killing.

Opa proteins (opacity proteins) are a family of membrane proteins that mediate intimate binding to epithelial and phagocytic cells and are important for cell-to-cell signaling. *N. gonorrhoeae* expressing the Opa proteins appear opaque when grown in culture (thus the source of the name). Opaque colonies are recovered most commonly in patients with localized disease (i.e., endocervicitis, urethritis, pharyngitis, proctitis), and transparent colonies are more commonly associated with pelvic inflammatory disease and disseminated infections.

The third group of proteins in the outer membrane is the highly conserved **Rmp proteins** (reduction-modifiable proteins). These proteins stimulate blocking antibodies that interfere with the serum bactericidal activity against pathogenic neisseriae.

Iron is essential for the growth and metabolism of *N. gonorrhoeae* and *N. meningitidis*. These pathogenic neisseriae are able to compete with their human hosts for iron by **binding host cell transferrin** to specific bacterial surface receptors. The specificity of this binding for human transferrin is likely the reason these bacteria are strict human pathogens. The presence of this receptor is fundamentally different from most bacteria that synthesize siderophores to scavenge iron. The gonococci also have a variety of additional surface receptors for other host iron complexes, such as lactoferrin and hemoglobin.

Another major antigen in the cell wall is **lipooligosaccharide (LOS)**. This antigen is composed of lipid A and a core oligosaccharide but lack the O-antigen polysaccharide found in lipopolysaccharide (LPS) in most gram-negative rods. The lipid A moiety possesses endotoxin activity. Both *N. gonorrhoeae* and *N. meningitidis* spontaneously release **outer membrane blebs** during rapid cell growth. These blebs contain LOS and surface proteins and may act to both enhance endotoxin-mediated toxicity and protect replicating bacteria by binding protein-directed antibodies.

N. gonorrhoeae and *N. meningitidis* produce **immu-noglobulin (Ig) A1 protease**, which cleaves the hinge region in IgA1. Some strains of *N. gonorrhoeae* also produce **β-lactamases** that can degrade penicillin.

Pathogenesis and Immunity (Table 19-1)

Gonococci attach to mucosal cells, penetrate into the cells and multiply, and then pass through the cells into the subepithelial space where infection is established. Pili, PorB, and Opa proteins mediate attachment and penetration into host cells. The gonococcal LOS stimulates release of the proinflammatory cytokine **tumor necrosis factor-α (TNF-α)**, which causes most of the symptoms associated with gonococcal disease.

IgG_3 is the predominant IgG antibody formed in response to gonococcal infection. Although the antibody response to PorB is minimal, serum antibodies to pilin, Opa protein, and LOS are readily detected. Antibodies to LOS can activate complement, releasing complement component C5a, which has a chemotactic effect on neutrophils; however, IgG and secretory IgA1 antibodies directed against Rmp protein can block this bactericidal antibody response.

Meningococci attach selectively to specific receptors for meningococcal type IV pili on nonciliated columnar cells of the nasopharynx. Meningococci without pili are less able to bind to these cells. Following attachment, meningococci are able to multiply, forming large aggregates of bacteria anchored to

Table 19-1   Virulence Factors in *Neisseria gonorrhoeae*

Virulence Factor	Biologic Effect
Pilin	Protein that mediates initial attachment to nonciliated human cells (e.g., epithelium of vagina, fallopian tube, and buccal cavity); interferes with neutrophil killing
Por protein (protein I)	Porin protein: promotes intracellular survival by preventing phagolysosome fusion in neutrophils
Opa protein (protein II)	Opacity protein: mediates firm attachment to eukaryotic cells
Rmp protein (protein III)	Reduction-modifiable protein: protects other surface antigens (Por protein, lipooligosaccharide) from bactericidal antibodies
Transferrin-binding proteins	Mediate acquisition of iron for bacterial metabolism
Lactoferrin-binding proteins	Mediate acquisition of iron for bacterial metabolism
Hemoglobin-binding proteins	Mediate acquisition of iron for bacterial metabolism
LOS	Lipooligosaccharide: has endotoxin activity
IgA1 protease	Destroys immunoglobulin A1 (role in virulence is unknown)
β-Lactamase	Hydrolyzes the β-lactam ring in penicillin

the host cells. Within a few hours of attachment, the pili undergo posttranslational modification, leading to destabilization of the aggregates. This results in the enhanced ability of the bacteria to both penetrate into the host cells and release into the airways, and thus person-to-person spread is potentially increased.

Meningococcal disease occurs in patients who lack specific antibodies directed against the polysaccharide capsule and other expressed bacterial antigens. Infants are initially afforded protection by the passive transfer of maternal antibodies. When the infant has reached age 6 months, however, this protective immunity has waned, a finding that is consistent with the observation that the incidence of disease is greatest in children younger than 2 years. Immunity can be stimulated by colonization with *N. meningitidis* or other bacteria with cross-reactive antigens (e.g., colonization with nonencapsulated *Neisseria* species; exposure to *Escherichia coli* K1 antigen that cross-reacts with the group B capsular polysaccharide). Bactericidal activity also requires the existence of complement. Patients with **deficiencies in C5, C6, C7, or C8** of the complement system are estimated to be at a 6000-fold greater risk for meningococcal disease. Although immunity is mediated primarily by the humoral immune response, lymphocyte responsiveness to meningococcal antigens is markedly depressed in patients with acute disease.

Similar to *N. gonorrhoeae*, meningococci are internalized into phagocytic vacuoles and are able to avoid intracellular death, replicate, and then migrate to the subepithelial spaces. The polysaccharide capsule protects *N. meningitidis* from phagocytic destruction. The diffuse vascular damage associated with meningococcal infections (e.g., endothelial damage, inflammation of vessel walls, thrombosis, disseminated intravascular coagulation) is largely attributed to the action of the **LOS endotoxin** present in the outer membrane.

Epidemiology

Gonorrhea occurs naturally only in humans; it has no other known reservoir. It is second only to syphilis as the most commonly reported sexually transmitted disease in China. Infection rates are higher in males than in females, and are highest in the Yangtze River Delta region (i.e, Zhejiang, Shanghai, Jiangsu Provinces). The peak incidence of the disease is in the age group 25 to 29 years. The incidence of disease generally has decreased since 2000. In 2015, only 100,245 new infections were reported in China.

N. gonorrhoeae is transmitted primarily by sexual contact. Women have a 50% risk of acquiring the infection as the result of a single exposure to an infected man, whereas men have a risk of approximately 20% as the result of a single exposure to an infected woman. The risk of infection rises as the person has more sexual encounters with infected partners.

The major reservoir for gonococci is the asymptomatically infected person. Asymptomatic carriage is more common in women than in men. As many as half of all infected women have mild or asymptomatic infections, whereas most men are initially symptomatic. The symptoms generally clear within a few weeks in individuals with untreated disease, and asymptomatic carriage may then become established. The site of infection also determines whether carriage occurs, with rectal and pharyngeal infections more commonly asymptomatic than genital infections.

Endemic meningococcal disease occurs worldwide, and epidemics are common in developing countries. Epidemic spread of disease results from the introduction of a new, virulent strain into an immunologically naïve population. Pandemics of disease have been uncommon in developed countries since World War II. Of the 13 serogroups, almost all infections are caused by serogroups A, B, C, Y, and W135. In Europe and the Americas, serogroups B, C, and Y predominate in meningitis or meningococcemia; serogroups A and W135 predominate in developing countries. Serogroups Y and W135 are most commonly associated with meningococcal pneumonia. In 2015, only 106 new cases and 13 deaths were reported in China, mainly caused by serogroups A and C. *N. meningitidis* is transmitted by respiratory droplets among people in prolonged close contact, such as family members living in the same household and soldiers living together in military barracks. Classmates in schools and hospital employees are not considered close contacts and are not at significantly higher risk of acquiring the disease, unless they are in direct contact with the respiratory secretions of an infected person.

Humans are the only natural carriers for *N. meningitidis*. Studies of the asymptomatic carriage of *N. meningitidis* have shown that there is a tremendous variation in its prevalence, from less than 1% to almost 40%. The oral and nasopharyngeal carriage rates are highest for school-age children and young adults, are higher in lower socioeconomic populations (caused by person-to-person spread in crowded areas), and do not vary with the seasons, even though disease is most common during the dry, cold months of the year. Carriage is typically transient, with clearance occurring after specific antibodies develop. Endemic disease is most common in children younger than 5 years, particularly infants, and teenagers and young adults. People who are immunocompromised, the elderly, or those who live in closed populations (e.g., military barracks, prisons) are prone to infection during epidemics.

NEISSERIA GONORRHOEAE

Clinical Diseases

Gonorrhea

Genital infection in men is primarily restricted to the **urethra**. A purulent urethral discharge (Figure 19-2) and dysuria develop after a 2- to 5-day incubation period. Approximately 95% of all infected men have acute symptoms. Although complications are rare, epididymitis, prostatitis, and periurethral abscesses may occur. The primary site of infection in women is the cervix because the bacteria infect the endocervical columnar epithelial cells. The organism cannot infect the squamous epithelial cells that line the vagina of postpubescent women. Symptomatic patients commonly experience vaginal discharge, dysuria, and abdominal pain. Ascending genital infections, including salpingitis, tuboovarian abscesses, and pelvic inflammatory disease, are observed in 10% to 20% of women.

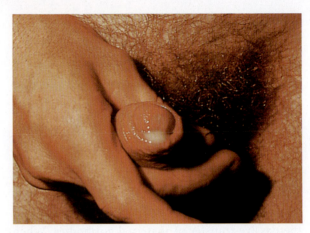

Figure 19-2   Purulent urethral discharge in man with urethritis. (From Morse S, et al: *Atlas of sexually transmitted diseases and AIDS*, ed 3, St Louis, 2003, Mosby.)

Gonococcemia

Disseminated infections with **septicemia** and **infection of skin and joints** occur in 1% to 3% of infected women and in a much lower percentage of infected men. The greater proportion of disseminated infections in women is caused by the numerous untreated asymptomatic infections in this population. The clinical manifestations of disseminated disease include fever; migratory arthralgias; suppurative arthritis in the wrists, knees, and ankles; and a pustular rash on an erythematous base (Figure 19-3) over the extremities but not on the head and trunk. *N. gonorrhoeae* is a leading cause of **purulent arthritis** in adults.

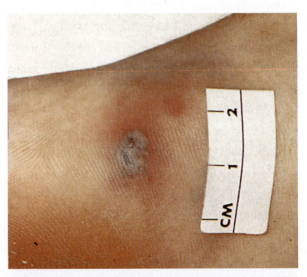

Figure 19-3   Skin lesions of disseminated gonococcal infection. Classic large lesions with a necrotic, grayish central lesion on an erythematous base. (From Morse S, et al: *Atlas of sexually transmitted diseases and AIDS*, ed 3, St Louis, 2003, Mosby.)

Other N. gonorrhoeae Syndromes

Other diseases associated with *N. gonorrhoeae* are perihepatitis (**Fitz-Hugh-Curtis syndrome**); purulent conjunctivitis (Figure 19-4), particularly in newborns infected during vaginal delivery (ophthalmia neonatorum); anorectal gonorrhea in homosexual men; and pharyngitis.

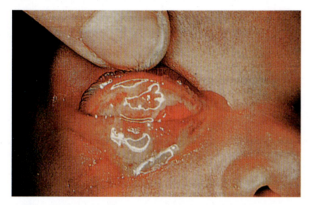

Figure 19-4   Gonococcal ophthalmia neonatorum. Lid edema, erythema, and marked purulent discharge are seen. A Gram-stained smear would reveal abundant organisms and inflammatory cells. (From Morse S, et al: *Atlas of sexually transmitted diseases and AIDS*, ed 3, St Louis, 2003, Mosby.)

NEISSERIA MENINGITIDIS

Clinical Diseases

Meningitis

Most of meningococcal diseases were meningitis. The disease usually begins abruptly with headache, meningeal signs, and fever. However, very young children may have only nonspecific signs, such as fever and vomiting. Mortality approaches 100% in untreated patients but is less than 10% in patients in whom appropriate antibiotic therapy is instituted promptly. The incidence of neurologic sequelae is low, with hearing deficits and arthritis most commonly reported.

Meningococcemia

Septicemia (meningococcemia) with or without meningitis is a life-threatening disease. Thrombosis of small blood vessels and multiorgan involvement are the characteristic clinical features. Small, pete-chial skin lesions on the trunk and lower extremities are common and may coalesce to form larger hemorrhagic lesions (Figure 19-5). Overwhelming disseminated_intravascular coagulation with shock, together with the bilateral destruction of the adrenal glands (**Waterhouse-Friderichsen syndrome**), may ensue. A milder, chronic septicemia has also been observed. Bacteremia can persist for days or weeks, and the only signs of infection are a low-grade fever, arthritis, and petechial skin lesions. The response to antibiotic therapy in patients with this form of the disease is generally excellent.

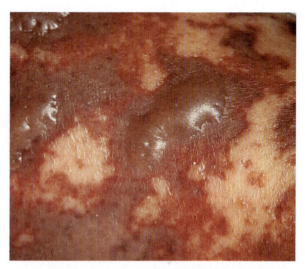

Figure 19-5   Skin lesions in a patient with meningococcemia. Note that the petechial lesions have coalesced and formed hemorrhagic bullae.

Other N. meningitidis Syndromes

Additional infections caused by *N. meningitidis* are pneumonia, arthritis, and urethritis. Meningococcal pneumonia is usually preceded by a respiratory tract infection. Symptoms include cough, chest pain, rales, fever, and chills. Evidence of pharyngitis is observed in most affected patients. The prognosis in patients with meningococcal pneumonia is good.

Laboratory Diagnosis

Microscopy

Gram stain can be reliably used to diagnose infections in men with purulent urethritis and women with cervicitis, but all negative results in women and asymptomatic men must be confirmed. A positive result is considered reliable when an experienced microscopist sees gram-negative diplococci within polymorphonuclear leukocytes.

N. meningitidis can be readily seen in the cerebrospinal fluid (CSF) of patients with meningitis (see Figure 19-1), unless the patient has received prior antimicrobial therapy. Patients with overwhelming meningococcal disease commonly have large numbers of organisms in their blood, which can be seen when the peripheral blood leukocytes are Gram stained.

Antigen Detection

Antigen testing for the detection of *N. gonorrhoeae* is less sensitive than culture or nucleic acid amplification tests and is not recommended, unless confirmatory tests are performed on negative specimens. Commercial tests to detect *N. meningitidis* capsular antigens in CSF, blood, and urine (where the antigens are excreted) were widely used in the past but have fallen into disfavor in recent years because the tests are less sensitive than the Gram stain, and false-positive reactions, particularly with urine specimens, can occur.

Nucleic Acid-Based Tests

Nucleic acid amplification (NAA) assays specific for *N. gonorrhoeae* have been developed for the direct detection of bacteria in clinical specimens. Tests using these assays are sensitive, specific, and rapid (results are available in 1 to 2 hours). Combination NAA assays for both *N. gonorrhoeae* and *Chlamydia* organisms are available and have replaced culture or other diagnostic tests in most laboratories. The primary problem with this approach is that it cannot be used to monitor antibiotic resistance of the identified pathogens.

Culture

The gonococci die rapidly if specimens are allowed to dry. Therefore drying and cold temperatures should be avoided by directly inoculating the specimen onto prewarmed media at the time of collection.

The endocervix must be properly exposed to ensure that an adequate specimen is collected. Although the endocervix is the most common site of infection in women, rectal cultures may be the only positive specimens in women who have asymptomatic infections, as well as in homosexual and bisexual men. Blood culture results are generally positive for gonococci only during the first week of the infection in patients with disseminated disease. In addition, special handling of blood specimens is required to ensure the adequate recovery of gonococci because supplements present in the blood culture media can be toxic to *Neisseria*. Cultures of specimens from infected joints are positive for the organism if the specimens are collected at the time the arthritis develops, but cultures of skin specimens are usually negative.

N. meningitidis is generally present in large numbers in CSF, blood, and sputum. Care should be used in processing CSF and blood specimens because bacterial strains responsible for disseminated disease are more virulent and pose a safety risk for the laboratory technologists.

Identification

Pathogenic *Neisseria* species are identified preliminarily on the basis of the isolation of oxidase-positive, gram-negative diplococci that grow on chocolate blood agar or on media that are selective for pathogenic *Neisseria* species. Definitive identification is guided by the pattern of oxidation of carbohydrates and other select tests.

Treatment, Prevention, and Control

Penicillin was historically the antibiotic of choice for treatment of gonorrhea; however, penicillin is not used today because the concentration of drug required to kill "susceptible" strains has steadily increased, and frank resistance, because of β-lactamase production (plasmid mediated) or chromosomally mediated changes in penicillin-binding proteins and in cell wall permeability, has become common. Resistance to tetracyclines, erythromycin, and fluoroquinolones, such as ciprofloxacin, has also become prevalent. Currently, **ceftriaxone** should be used as initial empiric therapy. If *Chlamydia trachomatis* infection has not been excluded, treatment should be combined with either a single dose of azithromycin or a 1-week course of doxycycline.

Major efforts to stem the epidemic of gonorrhea encompass education, aggressive detection, and follow-up screening of sexual contacts. It is important to realize that gonorrhea is a significant disease. Chronic infections can lead to sterility, and asymptomatic infections perpetuate the reservoir of disease and lead to a higher incidence of disseminated infections. Chemoprophylaxis with 1% silver nitrate, 1% tetracycline, or 0.5% erythromycin eye ointments are routinely used to protect newborns against gonococcal eye infections (ophthalmia neonatorum); however, the prophylactic use of antibiotics to prevent genital disease is ineffective and not recommended. An **effective vaccine** against **N. gonorrhoeae is not yet available.**

Cefotaxime or ceftriaxone should be used initially to treat *N. meningitidis* infections. If the organism is demonstrated to be penicillin susceptible, treatment can be changed to penicillin G. Chemoprophylaxis is recommended for contacts with significant exposure to patients with meningococcal disease (defined as individuals with direct exposure to respiratory secretions or greater than 8 hours of close contact to the patient). Currently, rifampin, ciprofloxacin, or ceftriaxone are recommended for prophylaxis.

Antibiotic eradication of *N. meningitidis* in healthy carriers is ineffective, so prevention of disease has focused on the enhancement of immunity through the use of vaccines directed against the serogroups most commonly associated with disease. **Two tetravalent vaccines effective against serogroups A, C, Y, and W135 are currently available**–a polysaccharide vaccine and a polysaccharide-protein conjugate vaccine.

OTHER *NEISSERIA* SPECIES

Neisseria species such as *Neisseria sicca* and *Neisseria mucosa* are commensal organisms in the oropharynx. These organisms have been implicated in isolated cases of meningitis, osteomyelitis, endocarditis, bronchopulmonary infections, acute otitis media, and acute sinusitis. The true incidence of respiratory tract infections caused by these organisms is not known because most specimens are contaminated with oral secretions. However, the observation of many gram-negative diplococci associated with inflammatory cells in a well-collected respiratory specimen would support the etiologic role of these organisms. Most isolates of *N. sicca* and *N. mucosa* are susceptible to penicillin, although low-level resistance caused by altered penicillin-binding protein (i.e., PBP2) has been observed.

EIKENELLA CORRODENS

E. corrodens is a moderate-sized (0.2 by 2.0 μm), nonmotile, non-spore-forming, facultatively anaerobic, gram-negative rod. The organism is named after Eiken, who characterized the bacterium and observed the ability of the organism to pit or "corrode" agar (from its ability to split polygalacturonic acid). *E. corrodens* is a normal inhabitant of the human upper respiratory tract, but because of its fastidious growth requirements, it is difficult to detect unless specific selective culture media are used. It is an opportunistic pathogen that causes infections in patients who are immunocompromised or have diseases or trauma of the oral cavity. *E. corrodens* is most commonly isolated in the settings of a **human bite wound** or fistfight injury. Other infections are endocarditis, sinusitis, meningitis, brain abscesses, pneumonia, and lung abscesses.

E. corrodens is susceptible to penicillin (unusual for a gram-negative bacterium), ampicillin, extended-spectrum cephalosporins, tetracyclines, and fluoroquinolone but is resistant to oxacillin, first-generation cephalosporins, clindamycin, erythromycin, and the aminoglycosides. Thus *E. corrodens* is resistant to many antibiotics that are selected empirically to treat bite-wound infections.

KINGELLA KINGAE

Kingella species are small, gram-negative coccobacilli

that morphologically resemble *Neisseria* species and reside in the human oropharynx. The bacteria are facultatively anaerobic, ferment carbohydrates, and have fastidious growth requirements. *K. kingae*, the most commonly isolated species, has been primarily responsible for septic arthritis in children and endocarditis in patients of all ages. Because the organism grows slowly, it may take 3 or more days of incubation for the organism to be detected in clinical specimens. Most strains are susceptible to β-lactam antibiotics, including penicillin, tetracyclines, erythromycin, fluoroquinolones, and aminoglycosides.

SUMMARY

Neisseria gonorrhoeae

Neisseria gonorrhoeae *is* gram-negative diplococci with fastidious growth requirements, growth best at 35℃ to 37℃ in a humid atmosphere supplemented with CO_2. Oxidase and catalase are positive in ***Neisseria gonorrhoeae***. There are multiple antigens located in the outer surface: pili protein; Por proteins; Opa proteins; Rmp protein; protein receptors for transferrin, lactoferrin, and hemoglobin; lipooligosaccharide; immunoglobulin protease; β-lactamase. Humans are the only natural hosts. Transmission is primarily by sexual contact. **Gonorrhea** is characterized by purulent discharge for involved site (e.g., urethra, cervix, epididymis, prostate, anus) after 2- to 5-day incubation period. **Disseminated infections** are the spread of infection from genitourinary tract through blood to skin or joints; characterized by pustular rash with erythematous base and suppurative arthritis in involved joints. **Ophthalmia neonatorum** is acquired by neonate at birth.

Neisseria meningitidis

Neisseria meningitidis is gram-negative diplococci with fastidious growth requirements. Oxidase and catalase are positive in the bacteria. Outer surface antigens include polysaccharide capsule, pili, and lipooligosaccharides. Bacteria can survive intracellular killing in the absence of humoral immunity. Humans are the only natural hosts. Meningitis and meningococcemia are most commonly caused by serogroups B, C, and Y; pneumonia is most commonly caused by serogroups Y and W135; serogroups A and W135 are associated with disease in underdeveloped countries. **Meningitis** is the purulent inflammation of meninges associated with headache, meningeal signs, and fever; it has high mortality rate unless it is promptly treated with effective antibiotics. Gram stain of cerebrospinal fluid is sensitive and specific but is of limited value for blood specimens. For immunoprophylaxis, vaccination is an adjunct to chemoprophylaxis; it is used only for serogroups A, C, Y, and W135; no effective vaccine is available for serogroup B.

KEYWORDS

English	Chinese
Neisseria	奈瑟菌属
Chocolate agar	巧克力(色)血琼脂平板
Neisseria gonorrhoeae	淋病奈瑟菌
Neisseria meningitides	脑膜炎奈瑟菌
Lipooligosaccharide, LOS	脂寡糖
Gonorrhea	淋病
Ophthalmia neonatorum	新生儿淋球菌性结膜炎
Endemic meningococcal disease	流行性脑膜炎奈瑟菌病
Meningitis	脑膜炎
Meningococcemia	脑膜炎奈瑟菌病败血症

BIBLIOGRAPHY

1. Gardner P: Clinical practice: prevention of meningococcal disease, N Engl J Med 355: 1466-1473, 2006.

2. Glikman D, et al: Pneumonia and empyema caused by penicillin-resistant *Neisseria meningitidis*: a case report and literature review, Pediatrics 117: 1061-1066, 2007.

3. Milonovich L: Meningococcemia: epidemiology, pathophysiology, and management, J Pediatr Health Care 21: 75-80, 2007.

4. Quagliarella V: Dissemination of *Neisseria meningitidis*, N Engl J Med 364: 1573-1575, 2011.

5. Schielke S, Frosch M, Kurzai O: Virulence determinants involved in differential host niche adaptation of *Neisseria meningitidis* and *Neisseria gonorrhoeae*, Med Microbiol Immunol 199: 185-196, 2010.

6. Stephens D: Conquering the meningococcus, FEMS Microbiol Rev 31: 3-14, 2007.

7. Tan L, Carlone G, Borrow R: Advances in the development of vaccines against *Neisseria meningitidis*, N Engl J Med 362: 1511-1520, 2010.

8. Whiley D, et al: Nucleic acid amplification testing for *Neisseria gonorrhoeae*: an ongoing challenge, J Mol Diagn 8: 3-15, 2006.

9. Winstead JM, et al: Meningococcal pneumonia: characterization and review of cases seen over the past 25 years, Clin Infect Dis 30: 87-94, 2000.

Enterobacteriaceae

The family Enterobacteriaceae is the largest, most heterogeneous collection of medically important **gram-negative rods**. Fifty genera and hundreds of species and subspecies have been described. These genera have been classified based on biochemical properties, antigenic structure, DNA-DNA hybridization, and 16S rRNA sequencing. Despite the complexity of this family, most human infections are caused by relatively few species.

Enterobacteriaceae are **ubiquitous** organisms, found worldwide in soil, water, and vegetation and are part of the normal intestinal flora of most animals, including humans. These bacteria cause a variety of human diseases, including one third of all bacteremias, more than 70% of urinary tract infections (UTIs), and many intestinal infections. Some organisms (e.g., *Salmonella* serotype Typhi, *Shigella* species, *Yersinia pestis*) are **always associated with human disease**, whereas others (e.g., *Escherichia coli*, *Klebsiella pneumoniae*, *Proteus mirabilis*) are members of the normal commensal flora that can cause **opportunistic infections**. A third group of Enterobacteriaceae exists—those normally commensal organisms that become pathogenic when they acquire virulence genes present on plasmids, bacteriophages, or pathogenicity islands. Infections with the Enterobacteriaceae can originate from an animal reservoir (e.g., most *Salmonella* species, *Yersinia* species), from a human carrier (e.g., *Shigella* species, *Salmonella* serotype Typhi), or through the endogenous spread of organisms (e.g., spread of *E. coli* from the intestine to the peritoneal cavity following perforation of the intestine) (Figure 20-1).

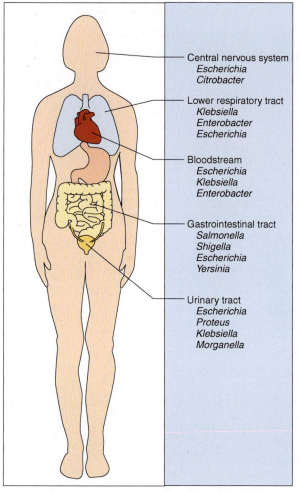

Figure 20-1   Sites of infections with common members of the Enterobacteriaceae listed in order of prevalence.

PHYSIOLOGY AND STRUCTURE

Members of the Enterobacteriaceae family are moderately sized (0.3 to 1.0 × 1.0 to 6.0 µm) gram-negative rods (Figure 20-2). They share a common antigen (**enterobacterial common antigen**), are either motile with peritrichous flagella (uniformly distributed over the cell) or nonmotile, and do not form spores. All members can grow rapidly, aerobically and anaerobically (**facultative anaerobes**), on a variety of nonselective (e.g., blood agar) and selective (e.g., MacConkey agar) media. The Enterobacteriaceae have simple nutritional requirements, ferment glucose, reduce nitrate, and are catalase positive and oxidase negative. The absence of cytochrome oxidase activity is an important characteristic because it can be measured rapidly with a simple test and is used to distinguish the Enterobacteriaceae from many other fermentative and nonfermentative gram-negative rods (e.g., *Vibrio*, *Pseudomonas*).

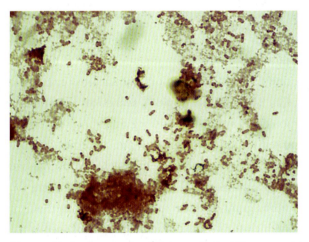

Figure 20-2 Gram stain of *Salmonella Typhi* from a positive blood culture. Note the intense staining at the ends of the bacteria. This "bipolar staining" is characteristic of the Enterobacteriaceae.

The appearance of the bacteria on culture media has been used to differentiate common members of the Enterobacteriaceae. For example, the ability to **ferment lactose** (detected by color changes in lactose-containing media, such as the commonly used MacConkey agar) has been used to differentiate lactose-fermenting strains (e.g., *Escherichia*, *Klebsiella*, *Enterobacter*, *Citrobacter*, and *Serratia*; pink-purple colonies on MacConkey agar) from strains that do not ferment lactose or do so slowly (e.g., *Proteus*, *Salmonella*, *Shigella*, and *Yersinia* spp.; colorless colonies on MacConkey agar). **Resistance to bile salts** in some selective media has been used to separate enteric pathogens (e.g., *Shigella*, *Salmonella*) from commensal organisms that are inhibited by bile

salts (e.g., gram-positive and some gram-negative bacteria present in the gastrointestinal tract). Some Enterobacteriaceae appear mucoid (wet, heaped, viscous colonies) have prominent **capsules** (e.g., most *Klebsiella*, some *Enterobacter* and *Escherichia* strains), whereas a loose-fitting, diffusible slime layer surrounds other strains.

The heat-stable **lipopolysaccharide (LPS)** is the major cell wall antigen and consists of three components: the outermost somatic **O polysaccharide**, a **core polysaccharide** common to all Enterobacteriaceae (enterobacterial common antigen mentioned earlier), and **lipid A** (Figure 20-3). The core polysaccharide is important for classifying an organism as a member of the Enterobacteriaceae, the O polysaccharide is important for the epidemiologic classification of strains within a species, and the lipid A component of LPS is responsible for endotoxin activity, an important virulence factor.

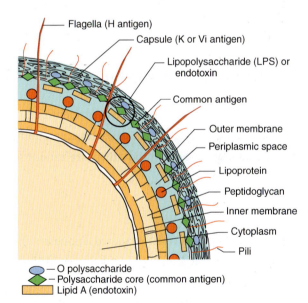

Figure 20-3 Antigenic structure of Enterobacteriaceae.

The epidemiologic (serologic) classification of the Enterobacteriaceae is based on three major groups of antigens: **somatic O polysaccharides, K antigens** in the capsule (type-specific polysaccharides), and the **H proteins** in the bacterial flagella. Strain-specific O antigens are present in each genus and species, although cross-reactions between closely related genera are common (e.g., *Salmonella* with *Citrobacter*, *Escherichia* with *Shigella*). The antigens are detected by agglutination with specific antibodies. The K antigens are not commonly used for strain typing but are important because they may interfere with detection of the O antigens (i.e., a problem with some strains of *Salmonella*). Boiling the organism to remove the heat-labile K antigen and expose the heat-stable O antigen circumvents this problem. The H antigens are heat-labile flagellin proteins. They may be absent from a cell, or they may undergo antigenic variation and be present in two phases.

Most Enterobacteriaceae are motile, with the exception of some common genera (e.g., *Klebsiella, Shigella*). The motile strains are surrounded with **flagella** (peritrichous). Many Enterobacteriaceae also possess fimbriae (also referred to as *pili*), which have been subdivided into two general classes: chromosomally mediated common fimbriae and sex pili that are encoded on conjugative plasmids. The **common fimbriae** are important for the ability of bacteria to adhere to specific host cell receptors, whereas the **sex** or **conjugative pili** facilitate genetic transfer between bacteria.

PATHOGENESIS AND IMMUNITY

Numerous virulence factors have been identified in the members of the family Enterobacteriaceae. Some are common to all genera, and others are unique to specific virulent strains.

Endotoxin

Endotoxin is a virulence factor shared among aerobic and some anaerobic gram-negative bacteria. Many of the systemic manifestations of gram-negative bacterial infections are initiated by endotoxin—activation of complement, release of cytokines, leukocytosis, thrombocytopenia, disseminated intravascular coagulation, fever, decreased peripheral circulation, shock, and death.

Capsule

Encapsulated Enterobacteriaceae are protected from phagocytosis by the hydrophilic capsular antigens, which repel the hydrophobic phagocytic cell surface. These antigens interfere with the binding of anti-

bodies to the bacteria and are poor immunogens or activators of complement. The protective role of the capsule is diminished, however, if the patient develops specific anticapsular antibodies.

Antigenic Phase Variation

The expression of the somatic O antigens, capsular K antigens and flagellar H antigens is under the genetic control of the organism. Each of these antigens can be alternately expressed or not expressed (phase variation), a feature that protects the bacteria from antibody-mediated cell death.

Type III Secretion Systems

A variety of bacteria (e.g., *Yersinia, Salmonella, Shigella*, enteropathogenic *Escherichia, Pseudomonas, Chlamydia*) have a common effector system for delivering their virulence factors into targeted eukaryotic cells. Think of the **type III secretion system** as a molecular syringe consisting of approximately 20 proteins that facilitate transfer of bacterial virulence factors into the targeted host cells. Although the virulence factors and their effects differ among the various gram-negative rods, the general mechanism by which the virulence factors are introduced is the same. In the absence of the type III secretion system, the bacteria have diminished virulence.

Sequestration of Growth Factors

Nutrients are provided to the organisms in enriched culture media, but the bacteria must become nutritional scavengers when growing in vivo. Iron is an important growth factor required by bacteria, but it is bound in **heme proteins** (e.g., hemoglobin, myoglobin) or in **iron-chelating proteins** (e.g., transferrin, lactoferrin). The bacteria counteract the binding by producing their own competitive **siderophores** or iron-chelating compounds (e.g., **enterobactin, aerobactin**). Iron can also be released from host cells by hemolysins produced by the bacteria.

Resistance to Serum Killing

Whereas many bacteria can be rapidly cleared from blood, virulent organisms capable of producing systemic infections are often resistant to serum killing. The bacterial capsule can protect the organism from serum killing as well as other factors that prevent the binding of complement components to the bacteria and subsequent complement-mediated clearance.

Antimicrobial Resistance

As rapidly as new antibiotics are introduced, organisms can develop resistance to them. This resistance can be encoded on transferable plasmids and exchanged among species, genera, and even families of bacteria.

ESCHERICHIA COLI

E. coli is the most common and important member of the genus *Escherichia*. This organism is associated with a variety of diseases, including gastroenteritis and extraintestinal infections, such as UTIs, meningitis, and sepsis. A multitude of strains are capable of causing disease, with some serotypes associated with greater virulence (e.g., *E. coli* O157 is the most common cause of hemorrhagic colitis and hemolytic uremic syndrome).

Pathogenesis and Immunity

E. coli possesses a broad range of virulence factors (Table 20-1). In addition to the general factors possessed by all members of the family Enterobacteriaceae, *Escherichia* strains possess specialized virulence factors that can be placed into two general categories: adhesins and exotoxins. The function of these factors will be discussed in greater detail in the following sections.

Epidemiology

Large numbers of *E. coli* are present in the gastrointestinal tract. Although these organisms can be opportunistic pathogens when the intestines are perforated and the bacteria enter the peritoneal cavity, most *E. coli* that cause gastrointestinal and extraintestinal disease do so because they have acquired specific virulence factors encoded on plasmids or in bacteriophage DNA. The effectiveness of *E. coli* as a pathogen is illustrated by the fact the bacteria are (1) the most common gram-negative rods isolated from patients with sepsis (Figure 20-4); (2) responsible for causing more than 80% of all community-acquired UTIs, as well as many hospital-acquired infections; and (3) a prominent cause of gastroenteritis. Most infections (with the exception of neonatal meningitis and gastroenteritis) are endogenous; that is, the *E. coli* that are part of the patient's normal microbial flora are able to establish infection when the patient's defenses are compromised (e.g., through trauma or immune suppression).

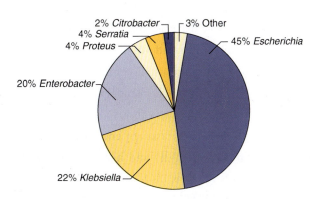

Figure 20-4   Incidence of Enterobacteriaceae associated with bacteremia.

Table 20-1   Specialized Virulence Factors Associated with *Escherichia coli*

Bacteria	Adhesins	Exotoxins
ETEC	Colonization factor antigens (CFA/I, CFA/II, CFA/III)	Heat labile toxin (LT-1); heat stable toxin (STa)
EPEC	BFP; intimin	
EAEC	Aggregative adherence fimbriae (AAF/I, AAF/II, AAF/III)	Enteroaggregative heat stable toxin; plasmid-encoded toxin
EHEC	BFP; intimin	Shiga toxins (Stx-1, Stx-2)
EIEC	Invasive plasmid antigen	Hemolysin (HlyA)
Uropathogens	P pili; Dr fimbriae	

BFP, Bundle-forming pili; *EAEC,* enteroaggregative *E. coli; EHEC,* enterohemorrhagic *E. coli; EIEC,* enteroinvasive *E. coli; EPEC,* enteropathogenic *E. coli; ETEC,* enterotoxigenic *E. coli.*

Clinical Diseases

Gastroenteritis

The strains of *E. coli* that cause gastroenteritis are subdivided into five major groups: enterotoxigenic, enteropathogenic, enteroaggregative, enterohemorrhagic, and enteroinvasive *E. coli* (Table 20-2). The first three groups primarily cause a secretory diarrhea involving the small intestine, while the last two groups primarily involve the large intestine.

Enterotoxigenic *E. coli*

Disease caused by **enterotoxigenic *E. coli* (ETEC)** is seen most commonly in developing countries (an estimated 650 million cases per year). Infections are observed most commonly in either young children in developing countries or travelers to these areas. The inoculum for disease is high, so infections are primarily **acquired through consumption of fecally contaminated food or water.** Person-to-person spread does not occur. **Secretory diarrhea** caused by ETEC develops after a 1- to 2-day incubation period and persists for an average of 3 to 5 days. The symptoms (watery diarrhea and abdominal cramps; less commonly nausea and vomiting) are similar to those of cholera but are usually milder, particularly in adults. Neither histologic changes of the intestinal mucosa nor inflammation is observed.

ETEC produce two classes of enterotoxins: **heat-labile toxins (LT-I, LT-II)** and **heat-stable toxins (STa and STb).** Whereas LT-II is not associated with human disease, LT-I is functionally and structurally similar to cholera toxin (see Chapter 28) and is associated with human disease. This toxin consists of one A subunit and five identical B subunits. The B subunits bind to the same receptor as cholera toxin (GM_1 gangliosides), as well as other surface glycoproteins on epithelial cells in the small intestine.

After endocytosis, the A subunit of LT-I moves across the membrane of the vacuole and interacts with a membrane protein (Gs) that regulates adenylate cyclase. The net effect of this interaction is an **increase in cyclic adenosine monophosphate (cAMP)** levels, resulting in enhanced secretion of chloride and a decreased absorption of sodium and chloride. These changes are manifested in a watery diarrhea. Exposure to the toxin also stimulates prostaglandin secretion and production of inflammatory cytokines, resulting in further fluid loss.

The heat-stable toxin STa, but not STb, is also associated with human disease. STa is a small, monomeric peptide that binds to the transmembrane guanylate cyclase receptor, leading to an **increase in cyclic guanosine monophosphate (cGMP)** and subsequent hypersecretion of fluids. Genes for LT-I and STa are present on a **transferable plasmid**, which can also carry the genes for **colonization factor adhesins (CFA/I, CFA/II, CFA/III).** The colonization factors are fimbriae that recognize specific host glycoprotein receptors (this defines the host specificity). Both the toxin and colonization factors are required for disease to develop. Disease mediated by STa is indistinguishable from that mediated by LT-I.

Enteropathogenic *E. coli*

Enteropathogenic *E. coli* (EPEC) was the first *E. coli* associated with diarrheal disease and remains a **major cause of infant diarrhea in impoverished countries.** Disease is uncommon in developed countries, except in rare outbreaks in daycare nurseries, and is rare in older children and adults, presumably because they have developed protective immunity. In contrast with ETEC disease, **person-to-person spread** occurs with EPEC, so the infectious dose is likely to be low. Disease is characterized by **watery diarrhea** that may be severe and protracted. Fever and vomiting may also be present.

Infection is initiated by bacterial attachment to epithelial cells of the small intestine, with subsequent effacement (destruction) of the microvillus (**attachment/effacement [A/E] histopathology**). The initial aggregation of the bacteria, leading to the formation of microcolonies on the epithelial cell surface, is mediated by plasmid-encoded **bundle-forming pili (BFP).** The subsequent stages of attachment are regulated by genes encoded on the **"locus of enterocyte effacement" pathogenicity island.** This island of more than 40 genes is responsible for attachment

Table 20-2 Gastroenteritis Caused by *Escherichia coli*

Organism	Site of Action	Disease	Pathogenesis	Diagnosis
Enterotoxigenic *E. coli* (ETEC)	Small intestine	Traveler's diarrhea; infant diarrhea in developing countries; watery diarrhea, vomiting, cramps, nausea, low-grade fever	Plasmid-mediated, heat-stable and/or heat-labile enterotoxins that stimulate hyper-secretion of fluids and electrolytes	Most U.S. outbreaks caused by ST producing strains; two commercial immunoassays available for detecting ST in broth cultures; molecular probes for ST and LT from cultured bacteria available in research laboratories; PCR assays used with clinical specimens
Enteropathogenic *E. coli* (EPEC)	Small intestine	Infant diarrhea in developing countries; watery diarrhea and vomiting, nonbloody stools; believed to be rare in United States	Plasmid-mediated A/E histopathology, with disruption of normal microvillus structure resulting in malabsorption and diarrhea	Characteristic adherence to HEp-2 or HeLa cells; probes and amplification assays developed for the plasmid-encoded bundle-forming pili and gene targets on the "locus of enterocyte effacement" pathogenicity island
Enteroaggregative *E. coli* (EAEC)	Small intestine	Infant diarrhea in developing and probably developed countries; traveler's diarrhea; persistent watery diarrhea with vomiting, dehydration, and low-grade fever	Plasmid-mediated aggregative adherence of rods ("stacked bricks") with shortening of microvilli, mononuclear infiltration, and hemorrhage; decreased fluid absorption	Characteristic adherence to HEp-2 cells; DNA probe and amplification assays developed for conserved plasmid
Enterohemorrhagic *E. coli* (EHEC)	Large intestine	Initial watery diarrhea, followed by grossly bloody diarrhea (hemorrhagic colitis) with abdominal cramps; little or no fever; may progress to hemolytic uremic syndrome	EHEC evolved from EPEC; A/E lesions with destruction of intestinal microvilli resulting in decreased absorption; pathology mediated by cytotoxic Shiga toxins (Stx-1, Stx-2), which disrupt protein synthesis	Screen for O157:H7 with sorbitol-MacConkey agar; confirm by serotyping; immunoassays (ELISA, latex agglutination) for detection of the Stx toxins in stool specimens and cultured bacteria; DNA probes and amplification assays developed for Stx toxins
Enteroinvasive *E. coli* (EIEC)	Large intestine	Rare in developing and developed countries; fever, cramping, watery diarrhea; may progress to dysentery with scant, bloody stools	Plasmid-mediated invasion and destruction of epithelial cells lining colon	Sereny (guinea pig kerato-conjunctivitis) test; plaque assay in HeLa cells; probes and amplification assays for genes regulating invasion (cannot discriminate between EIEC and *Shigella*)

A/E, Attachment/effacement; *DNA,* deoxyribonucleic acid; *ELISA,* enzyme-linked immunosorbent assay; *LT,* labile toxin; *PCR,* polymerase chain reaction; *ST,* stable toxin.

and destruction of the host cell surface. Following the loose attachment mediated by BFP, active secretion of proteins into the host epithelial cell occurs by the bacterial type III secretion system. One protein, **translocated intimin receptor (Tir),** is inserted into the epithelial cell membrane and functions as a receptor for an outer membrane bacterial adhesin, **intimin.** Binding of intimin to Tir results in polymerization of actin and accumulation of cytoskeletal elements beneath the attached bacteria, loss of cell surface integrity, and cell death.

Enteroaggregative *E. coli*

Enteroaggregative *E. coli* (EAEC) strains have been implicated as a cause of persistent, watery diarrhea with dehydration in infants in developing countries and in travelers to these countries. Outbreaks of gastroenteritis caused by EAEC have also been reported in the United States, Europe, and Japan and are likely an important caused of childhood diarrhea in developed countries. This is one of the few bacteria associated with **chronic diarrhea and growth retardation** in children.

The bacteria are characterized by their autoagglutination in a "stacked-brick" arrangement. This process is mediated by **aggregative adherence fimbriae I (AAF1),** adhesins that are similar to the BFP responsible for microcolony formation of EPEC. Other aggregative adherence fimbriae (AAF/II, AAF/III) have also been described. After EAEC adhere to the surface of the intestine, mucus secretion is stimulated leading to the formation of a thick biofilm. This protects the aggregated bacteria from antibiotics and phagocytic cells. In addition, two groups of toxins are associated with EAEC: **enteroaggregative heat stable toxin** that is antigenically related to the heat-stable toxin of ETEC and **plasmid-encoded toxin.** Both toxins induce fluid secretion.

Enterohemorrhagic *E. coli*

Enterohemorrhagic *E. coli* (EHEC) are the most common strains producing disease in developed countries. EHEC disease is most common in the warm months, and the highest incidence is in children younger than 5 years. Most infections are attributed to the consumption of undercooked ground beef or other meat products, water, unpasteurized milk or fruit juices (e.g., cider made from apples contaminated with feces from cattle), uncooked vegetables such as spinach, and fruits. The **ingestion of fewer than 100 bacteria can produce disease,** and person-to-person spread occurs.

Disease caused by EHEC ranges from mild, uncom-plicated diarrhea to **hemorrhagic colitis** with severe abdominal pain and bloody diarrhea. Initially, diarrhea with abdominal pain develops in patients after 3 to 4 days of incubation. Vomiting is observed in approximately half the patients, but a high fever is generally absent. Within 2 days of onset, disease in 30% to 65% of patients progresses to a bloody diarrhea with severe abdominal pain. Complete resolution of symptoms typically occurs after 4 to 10 days in most untreated patients. **Hemolytic uremic syndrome (HUS),** a disorder characterized by acute renal failure, thrombocytopenia, and microangiopathic hemolytic anemia, is a complication in 5% to 10% of infected children younger than 10 years. Resolution of symptoms occurs in uncomplicated disease after 4 to 10 days in most untreated patients; however, death can occur in 3% to 5% of patients with HUS and severe sequelae (e.g., renal impairment, hypertension, central nervous system [CNS] manifestations) can occur in as many as 30% of HUS patients.

The most common strain of EHEC is serotype O157:H7, although disease has been associated with other serotypes, including *E. coli* O104:H4, which was responsible for a 2011 outbreak in Germany that infected more than 3000 persons and produced more than 800 cases of HUS and 35 deaths. These strains represent clones that evolved from EPEC and express **attaching and effacing activity.** In addition, these strains have acquired **Shiga toxin** (i.e., Stx-1, Stx-2, or both). Stx-1 is essentially identical to the Shiga toxin produced by *Shigella dysenteriae* (thus the source of the name); Stx-2 has 60% homology. Both toxins are acquired by lysogenic bacteriophages. Both have one A subunit and five B subunits, with the B subunits binding to a specific glycolipid on the host cell (globotriaosylceramide [Gb3]). A high concentration of Gb3 receptors is found in the intestinal villi and renal endothelial cells. After the A subunit is internalized, it is cleaved into two molecules, and the A_1 fragment binds to 28S rRNA and causes a cessation of protein synthesis. EHEC strains with both Shiga toxins and attaching and effacing activity are more pathogenic than strains producing only one Shiga toxin.

HUS has been preferentially associated with the

production of Stx-2, which has been shown to destroy glomerular endothelial cells. Damage to the endothelial cells leads to platelet activation and thrombin deposition, which, in turn, results in decreased glomerular filtration and acute renal failure. The Shiga toxins also stimulate expression of inflammatory cytokines (e.g., tumor necrosis factor-γ [TNF]-γ, interleukin-6 [IL]-6), which, among other effects, enhance expression of Gb3.

Enteroinvasive *E. coli*

Enteroinvasive *E. coli* (EIEC) strains are rare in both developed and developing countries. Pathogenic strains are primarily associated with a few restricted O serotypes: O124, O143, and O164. The strains are closely related by phenotypic and pathogenic properties to *Shigella*. The bacteria are able to invade and destroy the colonic epithelium, producing a disease characterized initially by **watery diarrhea**. A minority of patients progress to the dysenteric form of disease, consisting of fever, abdominal cramps, and blood and leukocytes in stool specimens.

A series of genes on a plasmid mediate bacterial invasion (***pInv* genes**) into the colonic epithelium. The bacteria then lyse the phagocytic vacuole and replicate in the cell cytoplasm. Movement within the cytoplasm and into adjacent epithelial cells is regulated by formation of actin tails (similar to that observed with *Listeria*). This process of epithelial cell destruction with inflammatory infiltration can progress to colonic ulceration.

Extraintestinal Infections

Urinary Tract Infection

Most gram-negative rods that produce UTIs originate in the colon, contaminate the urethra, ascend into the bladder, and may migrate to the kidney or prostate. Although most strains of *E. coli* can produce UTIs, disease is more common with certain specific serogroups. These bacteria are particularly virulent because of their ability to produce **adhesins** (primarily P pili, AAF/I, AAF/III, and Dr) that bind to cells lining the bladder and upper urinary tract (preventing the elimination of the bacteria in voided

urine) and **hemolysin HlyA** that lyses erythrocytes and other cell types (leading to cytokine release and stimulation of an inflammatory response).

Neonatal Meningitis

E. coli and group B streptococci cause the majority of CNS infections in infants younger than 1 month. Approximately 75% of the *E. coli* strains possess the **K1 capsular antigen.** This serogroup is also commonly present in the gastrointestinal tracts of pregnant women and newborn infants. However, the reason this serogroup has a predilection for causing disease in newborns is not understood.

Septicemia

Typically, septicemia caused by gram-negative rods, such as *E. coli*, originates from infections in the urinary or gastrointestinal tract (e.g., intestinal leakage leading to an intraabdominal infection). The mortality associated with *E. coli* septicemia is high for patients in whom immunity is compromised or the primary infection is in the abdomen or CNS.

SALMONELLA

The taxonomic classification of the genus *Salmonella* is problematic. DNA homology studies have revealed that most clinically significant isolates belong to the species *Salmonella enterica*. More than 2500 unique serotypes have been described for this single species; however, these serotypes are commonly listed as individual species (e.g., *Salmonella typhi*, *Salmonella choleraesuis*, *Salmonella typhimurium*, *Salmonella enteritidis*). These designations are incorrect—for example, the correct nomenclature is *Salmonella enterica*, serovar. Typhi. In an effort to prevent confusion and still retain the historical terms, individual serotypes are now commonly written with the serotype name capitalized and not in italics. For example, *Salmonella enterica*, serovar. Typhi is commonly designated as *Salmonella Typhi*. For the sake of consistency, this nomenclature will be used in this chapter.

Pathogenesis and Immunity

After ingestion and passage through the stomach,

salmonellae attach to the mucosa of the **small intestine** and invade into the **M (microfold) cells** located in Peyer patches, as well as into enterocytes. The bacteria remain in endocytic vacuoles, where they replicate. The bacteria can also be transported across the cytoplasm and released into the blood or lymphatic circulation. Regulation of the attachment, engulfment, and replication is controlled primarily by two large clusters of genes (**pathogenicity island I and II**) on the bacterial chromosome. Pathogenicity island I encodes **salmonella-secreted invasion proteins (Ssps)** and a **type III secretion system** that injects the proteins into the host cell. Pathogenicity island II contains genes that allow the bacteria to evade the host's immune response and a second type III secretion system for this function. The inflammatory response confines the infection to the gastrointestinal tract, mediates the release of prostaglandins, and stimulates cAMP and active fluid secretion.

Epidemiology

Salmonella can colonize virtually all animals, including poultry, reptiles, livestock, rodents, domestic animals, birds, and humans. Animal-to-animal spread and the use of *Salmonella*-contaminated animal feeds maintain an **animal reservoir.** Serotypes such as *Salmonella Typhi* and *Salmonella Paratyphi* are highly **adapted to humans** and do not cause disease in nonhuman hosts. Other *Salmonella* serotypes (e.g., *Salmonella* Choleraesuis) are adapted to animals and, when they infect humans, can cause severe disease. In addition, in contrast with other *Salmonella* serotypes, strains that are highly adapted to humans (i.e., *Salmonella Typhi, Salmonella Paratyphi*) can survive in the gallbladder and establish chronic carriage. Finally, many *Salmonella* strains have no host specificity and cause disease in both human and nonhuman hosts.

Most infections result from the **ingestion** of contaminated food products and, in children, from direct fecal-oral spread. The incidence of disease is greatest in children younger than 5 years and adults older than 60 years who are infected during the summer and autumn months, when contaminated foods are consumed at outdoor social gatherings. The most common sources of human infections are **poultry, eggs, dairy products,** and foods prepared on contaminated work surfaces (e.g., cutting boards where uncooked poultry was prepared). *Salmonella Typhi* infections occur when food or water contaminated by infected food handlers is ingested. There is no animal reservoir. It is estimated that 21 million *Salmonella Typhi* infections and 200,000 deaths occur each year worldwide. The risk of disease is highest in children living in poverty in a developing country.

The infectious dose for *Salmonella Typhi* infections is low, so person-to-person spread is common. In contrast, a large inoculum (e.g., 10^6 to 10^8 bacteria) is required for symptomatic disease to develop with most other *Salmonella* serotypes. The organisms can multiply to this high density if contaminated food products are improperly stored (e.g., left at room temperature). The infectious dose is lower for people at high risk for disease because of age, immunosuppression or underlying disease (leukemia, lymphoma, sickle cell disease), or reduced gastric acidity.

Clinical Diseases

The following four forms of *Salmonella* infection exist: gastroenteritis, septicemia, enteric fever, and asymptomatic colonization.

Gastroenteritis

Gastroenteritis is the **most common form of salmonellosis** in the United States. Symptoms generally appear 6 to 48 hours after the consumption of contaminated food or water, with the initial presentation consisting of **nausea, vomiting, and nonbloody diarrhea.** Fever, abdominal cramps, myalgias, and headache are also common. Colonic involvement can be demonstrated in the acute form of the disease. Symptoms can persist from 2 to 7 days before spontaneous resolution.

Septicemia

All *Salmonella* species can cause bacteremia, although infections with *Salmonella Typhi, Salmonella Paratyphi,* and *Salmonella* Choleraesuis more commonly lead to a bacteremic phase. The risk for *Salmonella* bacteremia is higher in pediatric and geriatric patients and in immunocompromised patients (HIV infections, sickle-cell disease, congenital immunodeficiencies). The clinical presentation of *Salmonella* bacteremia is like that of other gram-negative bacteremias; however, localized suppurative infections (e.g., osteomyelitis, endocarditis, arthritis) can occur in as many as 10% of patients.

Enteric Fever

Salmonella typhi produces a febrile illness called **typhoid fever.** A milder form of this disease, referred to as **paratyphoid fever,** is produced by *Salmonella paratyphi* A, *Salmonella* Schottmuelleri (formerly *Salmonella paratyphi* B), and *Salmonella* Hirschfeldii (formerly *Salmonella paratyphi* C). Other *Salmonella* serotypes can rarely produce a similar syndrome. The bacteria responsible for enteric fever pass through the cells lining the intestines and are engulfed by macrophages. They replicate after being transported to the liver, spleen, and bone marrow. Ten to 14 days after ingestion of the bacteria, patients experience gradually increasing fever, with nonspecific complaints of headache, myalgias, malaise, and anorexia. These symptoms persist for 1 week or longer and are followed by gastrointestinal symptoms. This cycle corresponds to an initial bacteremic phase that is followed by colonization of the gallbladder and then reinfection of the intestines. Enteric fever is a serious clinical disease and must be suspected in febrile patients who have recently traveled to developing countries where disease is endemic.

Asymptomatic Colonization

The strains of *Salmonella* responsible for causing typhoid and paratyphoid fevers are maintained by human colonization. **Chronic colonization** for more than 1 year after symptomatic disease develops in 1% to 5% of patients, the gallbladder being the reservoir in most patients. Chronic colonization with other species of *Salmonella* occurs in less than 1% of patients and does not represent an important source of human infection.

SHIGELLA

The commonly used taxonomic classification of *Shigella* is simple, although technically incorrect. Four species consisting of almost 50 O-antigen-based serogroups have been described: *S. dysenteriae*, *Shigella flexneri*, *Shigella boydii*, and *Shigella sonnei*. However, analysis of DNA has determined that these four species are actually biogroups within the species *E. coli*. Because it would be confusing to refer to these bacteria as *E. coli*, their historical names have been retained.

Pathogenesis and Immunity

Shigellae cause disease by invading and replicating in cells lining the **colon.** Structural gene proteins mediate the adherence of the organisms to the cells, as well as their invasion, intracellular replication, and cell-to-cell spread. These genes are carried on a large virulence plasmid but are regulated by chromosomal genes. Thus the presence of the plasmid does not ensure functional gene activity.

Shigella species appear unable to attach to differentiated mucosal cells; rather, they first attach to and invade the M cells located in Peyer patches. The **type III secretion system** mediates secretion of four proteins (**IpaA, IpaB, IpaC, IpaD**) into epithelial cells and macrophages. These proteins induce membrane ruffling on the target cell, leading to engulfment of the bacteria. Shigellae lyse the phagocytic vacuole and replicate in the host cell cytoplasm (unlike *Salmonella*, which replicate in the vacuole). With the rearrangement of actin filaments in the host cells, the bacteria are propelled through the cytoplasm to adjacent cells, where **cell-to-cell passage** occurs. In this way, *Shigella* organisms are protected from immune-mediated clearance. Shigellae survive phagocytosis by inducing programmed cell death (**apoptosis**). This process also leads to the release of IL-1β, resulting in the attraction of polymorphonuclear leukocytes into the infected tissues. This, in turn, destabilizes the integrity of the intestinal wall and allows the bacteria to reach the deeper epithelial cells.

S. dysenteriae strains produce an exotoxin, **Shiga**

toxin. Similar to Shiga toxin produced by EHEC, this toxin has one A subunit and five B subunits. The B subunits bind to a host cell glycolipid (Gb3) and facilitate transfer of the A subunit into the cell. The A subunit cleaves the 28S rRNA in the 60S ribosomal subunit, thereby preventing the binding of amino-acyl-transfer RNA and disrupting protein synthesis. The primary manifestation of toxin activity is damage to the intestinal epithelium; however, in a small subset of patients, the Shiga toxin can mediate damage to the glomerular endothelial cells, resulting in renal failure (HUS).

Epidemiology

Humans are the only reservoir for *Shigella*. It is estimated that 150 million cases of *Shigella* infections occur each year worldwide. **S. sonnei** is responsible for almost 85% of the U.S. infections, while **S. flexneri** predominates in developing countries. Epidemics of **S. dysenteriae,** a particularly virulent species, occur in Africa and Central America with case fatality rates of 5% to 15%.

Shigellosis is primarily a pediatric disease with 60% of all infections in children younger than 10 years. Endemic disease in adults is common in male homosexuals and in household contacts of infected children. Epidemic outbreaks of disease occur in daycare centers, nurseries, and custodial institutions. Shigellosis is **transmitted person-to-person** by the fecal-oral route, primarily by people with contaminated hands and less commonly in water or food. Because as few as 100 to 200 bacteria can establish disease, shigellosis spreads rapidly in communities where sanitary standards and the level of personal hygiene are low.

Clinical Diseases

Shigellosis is characterized by **abdominal cramps, diarrhea, fever,** and **bloody stools.** The clinical signs and symptoms of the disease appear 1 to 3 days after the bacteria are ingested. Shigellae initially colonize the small intestine and begin to multiply within the first 12 hours. The first sign of infection (profuse, watery diarrhea without histologic evidence of mucosal invasion) is mediated by an enterotoxin. However, the cardinal feature of shigellosis is lower abdominal cramps and tenesmus (straining to defecate), with abundant pus and blood in the stool. It results from invasion of the colonic mucosa by the bacteria. Abundant neutrophils, erythrocytes, and mucus are found in the stool. Infection is generally self-limited, although antibiotic treatment is recommended to reduce the risk of secondary spread to family members and other contacts. Asymptomatic colonization of the organism in the colon develops in a small number of patients and represents a persistent reservoir for infection.

OTHER ENTEROBACTERIACEAE

Klebsiella

Members of the genus *Klebsiella* have a prominent capsule that is responsible for the mucoid appearance of isolated colonies and the enhanced virulence of the organisms in vivo. The most commonly isolated members of this genus are **K. pneumoniae** and **Klebsiella oxytoca,** which can cause community- or hospital-acquired primary **lobar pneumonia.** Pneumonia caused by *Klebsiella* species frequently involves the necrotic destruction of alveolar spaces, formation of cavities, and the production of blood-tinged sputum. These bacteria also cause wound, soft-tissue, and UTIs.

The organism formerly called *Donovania granulomatis* and then *Calymmatobacterium granulomatis* has been reclassified as **Klebsiella granulomatis.** *K. granulomatis* is the etiologic agent of **granuloma inguinale,** a granulomatous disease affecting the genitalia and inguinal area. Unfortunately, this disease is commonly called **donovanosis** in reference to the historical origin of the genus name. Granuloma inguinale is a rare disease in the United States but is endemic in parts of Papua New Guinea, the Caribbean, South America, India, southern Africa, Vietnam, and Australia. It can be transmitted after repeated exposure through sexual intercourse or nonsexual trauma to the genitalia. After a prolonged incubation of weeks to months, subcutaneous nodules appear on the genitalia or in the inguinal area. The nodules subsequently break down, revealing one or more painless granulomatous lesions that can extend and coalesce into ulcers resembling syphilitic lesions.

Two other *Klebsiella* species of clinical importance are **Klebsiella rhinoscleromatis,** cause of a granulomatous disease of the nose, and **Klebsiella ozaenae,** cause of chronic atrophic rhinitis. Both diseases are relatively uncommon in the United States.

Proteus

P. mirabilis, the most common member of this genus, primarily produces infections of the urinary tract (e.g., bladder infection or cystitis; kidney infection or pyelonephritis). *P. mirabilis* produces large quantities of urease, which splits urea into carbon dioxide and ammonia. This process raises the urine pH, precipitating magnesium and calcium in the form of struvite and apatite crystals, respectively, and results in the formation of **renal (kidney) stones.** The increased alkalinity of the urine is also toxic to the uroepithelium.

Enterobacter, Citrobacter, Morganella, and Serratia

Primary infections caused by *Enterobacter, Citrobacter, Morganella,* and *Serratia* are rare in immunocompetent patients. They are more common causes of hospital-acquired infections in neonates and immunocompromised patients. For example, **Citrobacter koseri** has been recognized to have a predilection for causing meningitis and brain abscesses in neonates. Antibiotic therapy for these genera can be ineffective because the organisms are frequently resistant to multiple antibiotics. Resistance is a particularly serious problem with **Enterobacter** species.

LABORATORY DIAGNOSIS

Culture

Members of the family Enterobacteriaceae grow readily on culture media. Specimens of normally sterile material, such as spinal fluid and tissue collected at surgery, can be inoculated onto nonselective blood agar media. Selective media (e.g., MacConkey agar, eosin-methylene blue [EMB] agar) are used for the culture of specimens normally contaminated with other organisms (e.g., sputum, feces). Use of these selective differential agars enables the separation of lactose-fermenting Enterobacteriaceae from nonfermenting strains, thereby providing information that can be used to guide empiric antimicrobial therapy.

Diagnosis of *E. coli* strains responsible for gastroenteritis is most commonly performed by reference laboratories. The exception is detection of EHEC. Two approaches have been used: culture and toxin detection. In contrast with most *E. coli*, many strains of EHEC do not ferment sorbitol. Thus **sorbitol-containing Mac Conkey agar** (S-MAC) has been used to screen stool specimens for sorbitol-negative (colorless), gram-negative bacteria that are then confirmed by serogrouping and biochemical tests to be *E. coli* O157, the most common serotype of EHEC. The limitation to this approach is that some strains of O157 and many other EHEC serotypes ferment sorbitol and would be missed by this screening approach. The preferred method to detect EHEC is to test stool specimens directly for the presence of toxin by use of commercial immunoassays. These tests are rapid and sensitive.

Highly selective or organism-specific media are useful for the recovery of organisms such as *Salmonella* and *Shigella* in stool specimens, where an abundance of normal flora can obscure the presence of these important pathogens.

Biochemical Identification

There are many diverse species in the family Enterobacteriaceae. The citations listed in the bibliography at the end of this chapter provide additional information about their biochemical identification. Biochemical test systems have become increasingly sophisticated, and the most common members of the family can be identified accurately in less than 24 hours with one of the many commercially available identification systems. Sequencing of species-specific genes (e.g., 16S rRNA gene) or detection of characteristic protein profiles by mass spectrometry is used to identify the less common species.

Serologic Classification

Serologic testing is very useful for determining the clinical significance of an isolate (e.g., serotyping specific pathogenic strains, such as *E. coli* O157 or *Y. enterocolitica* O8) and for classifying isolates for epidemiologic purposes. The usefulness of this procedure is limited, however, by cross-reactions with antigenically related Enterobacteriaceae and with organisms from other bacterial families.

TREATMENT, PREVENTION, AND CONTROL

Antibiotic therapy for infections with Enterobacteriaceae must be guided by in vitro susceptibility test results and clinical experience. Some organisms, such as *E. coli* and *P. mirabilis*, are susceptible to many antibiotics, but others can be highly resistant. Whereas use of carbapenems (e.g., imipenem, meropenem, ertapenem) was once a mainstay of treatment, the recent recovery of carbapenemase-producing bacteria has limited the empiric use of this class of antibiotics for some regions of the country. Furthermore, susceptible organisms exposed to sub-therapeutic concentrations of antibiotics in a hospital setting can rapidly develop resistance. In general, **antibiotic resistance** is more common in hospital-acquired infections than in community-acquired infections. Antibiotic therapy is not recommended for some infections. For example, symptomatic relief but not antibiotic treatment is usually recommended for patients with enterohemorrhagic *E. coli* and *Salmonella* gastroenteritis because antibiotics can prolong the fecal carriage of these organisms or increase the risk of secondary complications (e.g., HUS with EHEC infections in children). Treatment of *Salmonella typhi* infections or other systemic *Salmonella* infections is indicated; however, increasing resistance to antibiotics, such as the fluoroquinolones, has complicated therapy.

It is difficult to prevent infections with Enterobacteriaceae because these organisms are a major part of the endogenous microbial population. However, some risk factors for the infections should be avoided. These include the unrestricted use of antibiotics that can select for resistant bacteria; the performance of procedures that traumatize mucosal barriers without prophylactic antibiotic coverage; and the use of urinary catheters. Unfortunately, many of these factors are present in patients at greatest risk for infection (e.g., immunocompromised patients confined to the hospital for extended periods).

Exogenous infection with Enterobacteriaceae is theoretically easier to control. For example, the source of infections with organisms such as *Salmonella* is well defined. However, these bacteria are ubiquitous in poultry and eggs. Unless care is taken in the preparation and refrigeration of such foods, little can be done to control these infections. *Shigella* organisms are predominantly transmitted in young children, but it is difficult to interrupt the fecal-hand-mouth transmission responsible for spreading the infection in this population. Outbreaks of these infections can be effectively prevented and controlled only through education and the introduction of appropriate infection-control procedures (e.g., hand washing, proper disposal of soiled diapers and linens) in the settings where these infections typically occur.

SUMMARY

The family Enterobacteriaceae is the largest, most heterogeneous collection of medically important **gram-negative rods**. Some organisms (e.g., *Salmonella* serotype Typhi, *Shigella* species, *Yersinia pestis*) are **always associated with human disease**, whereas others (e.g., *Escherichia coli*, *Klebsiella pneumoniae*, *Proteus mirabilis*) are members of the normal commensal flora that can cause **opportunistic infections**.

Escherichia coli

Most infections are endogenous (patient's microbial flora), although strains causing gastroenteritis are generally acquired exogenously. At least five different pathogenic groups cause gastroenteritis (EPEC, ETEC, EHEC, EIEC, EAEC); most cause diseases in developing countries, EHEC is an important cause of hemorrhagic colitis and hemolytic uremic syndrome. Extraintestinal disease include bacteremia, neonatal meningitis, urinary tract infections, and intraabdominal infections.

Salmonella

More than 2500 O serotypes are included in the genera of *Salmonella*, which can survive in macrophages and spread from the intestine to other body sites. *Salmonella* is the cause of enteritis (fever, nausea, vomiting, bloody or nonbloody diarrhea, abdominal cramps); enteric fever (typhoid fever, paratyphoid fever); bacteremia (most commonly seen with *Salmonella typhi*, *Salmonella paratyphi*, *Salmonella choleraesuis*); asymptomatic colonization (primarily with *Salmonella typhi and Salmonella paratyphi)*. Most infections are acquired by eating contaminated food products (poultry, eggs, and dairy products are the most common sources of infection). Infections with *Salmonella typhi* and *Salmonella paratyphi* or disseminated infections with other organisms should be treated with an effective antibiotic. Carriers of *Salmonella typhi* and *Salmonella paratyphi* should be identified and treated.

Shigella

Four species are recognized: *S. sonnei* responsible for most infections in developed countries; *S. flexneri* for infections in developing countries; *S. dysenteriae* for the most severe infections; and *S. boydii* not commonly isolated. Most common form of disease is gastroenteritis (shigellosis). Humans are the only reservoir for these bacteria.

KEYWORDS

English	Chinese
Enterobacteriaceae	肠杆菌科
Escherichia	埃希菌属
Escherichia	大肠埃希菌
EPEC	肠致病型大肠埃希菌
ETEC	肠产毒型大肠埃希菌
EAEC	肠聚集型大肠埃希菌
EIEC	肠侵袭型大肠埃希菌
EHEC	肠出血型大肠埃希菌
Shigella	志贺菌属
Tenesmus	里急后重
Salmonella	沙门菌属
Enteric fever	肠热症

BIBLIOGRAPHY

1. Abbott S: *Klebsiella, Enterobacter, Citrobacter, Serratia, Plesiomonas,* and other Enterobacteriaceae. In Murray PR, et al, editors: Manual of clinical microbiology, ed 9, Washington, DC, 2007, American Society of Microbiology Press.

2. Ackers ML, et al: Laboratory-based surveillance of *Salmonella* serotype *typhi* infections in the United States: antimicrobial resistance on the rise, JAMA 283: 2668-2673, 2000.

3. Darwin KH, Miller VL: Molecular basis of the interaction of *Salmonella* with the intestinal mucosa, Clin Microbiol Rev 12: 405-428, 1999.

4. Farmer JJ, et al: Enterobacteriaceae: introduction and identification. In Murray PR, et al, editors: Manual of clinical microbiology, ed 9, Washington, DC, 2007, American Society of Microbiology Press.

5. Nataro J, et al: *Escherichia, Shigella,* and *Salmonella.* In Murray PR, et al, editors: Manual of clinical microbiology, ed 9, Washington, DC, 2007, American Society of Microbiology Press.

6. Qadri F, et al: Enterotoxigenic *Escherichia coli* in developing countries: epidemiology, microbiology, clinical features, treatment, and prevention, Clin Microbiol Rev 18: 465-483, 2005.

7. Su C, Brandt LJ: *Escherichia coli* O157:H7 infection in humans, Ann Intern Med 123: 698-714, 1995.

8. Wanger A: *Yersinia.* In Murray PR, et al, editors: Manual of clinical microbiology, ed 9, Washington, DC, 2007, American Society of Microbiology Press.

9. Wong CS, et al: The risk of the hemolytic-uremic syndrome after antibiotic treatment of *Escherichia coli* O157:H7 infections, N Engl J Med 342: 1930-1936, 2000.

10. Zaharik ML, et al: Delivery of dangerous goods: type III secretion in enteric pathogens, Int J Med Microbiol 291: 593-603, 2002.

Vibrio and *Aeromonas*

The second major group of **gram-negative, facultatively anaerobic, fermentative rods** are the genera *Vibrio* and *Aeromonas*. These organisms were at one time classified together in the family Vibrionaceae and were separated from the Enterobacteriaceae on the basis of a **positive oxidase reaction** and the presence of **polar flagella**. These organisms were also classified together because they are primarily found in water and are able to cause gastrointestinal disease. However, molecular biology techniques have established that these genera are only distantly related and belong in separate families: *Vibrio* and *Aeromonas* are now classified in the families Vibrionaceae and Aeromonadaceae, respectively (Table 21-1). Despite this taxonomic reorganization, it is appropriate to consider these bacteria together because their epidemiology and range of diseases are similar.

VIBRIO

The genus *Vibrio* has undergone numerous changes in recent years, with a number of less common species described or reclassified. Currently, the genus is composed of more than 100 species of **curved rods**. A number of species are associated with human disease, but three species are particularly important human pathogens (Table 21-2): ***Vibrio cholerae***, ***Vibrio parahaemolyticus***, and ***Vibrio vulnificus***.

Physiology and Structure

Vibrio species can grow on a variety of simple media within a broad temperature range (from 14°C to 40°C). All species of ***Vibrio* require sodium chloride (NaCl)** for growth. *V. cholerae* can grow on most media without added salt, but most other species

Table 21-1 Important *Vibrio* and *Aeromonas* Species

Organism	Historical Derivation
Vibrio	*vibrio*, move rapidly or vibrate (rapid movement caused by polar flagellae)
V. cholerae	*cholera*, cholera or an intestinal disease
V. parahaemolyticus	*para*, by the side of; *haema*, blood; *lyticus*, dissolving (dissolving blood; Kanagawa toxin-positive strains are hemolytic)
V. vulnificus	*vulnificus*, inflicting wounds (associated with prominent wound infections)
Aeromonas	*aero*, gas or air; *monas*, unit or monad (gas-producing bacteria)
A. caviae	*cavia*, guinea pig (first isolated in guinea pigs)
A. hydrophila	*hydro*, water; *phila*, loving (water loving)
A. veronii	*veron*, named after the bacteriologist Veron

Table 21-2 *Vibrio* Species Associated with Human Disease

Species	Source of Infection	Clinical Disease
V. cholerae	Water, food	Gastroenteritis, bacteremia
V. parahaemolyticus	Shellfish, seawater	Gastroenteritis, wound infection, bacteremia
V. vulnificus	Shellfish, seawater	Bacteremia, wound infection

(halophilic species) require the addition of NaCl. Vibrios tolerate a wide range of pH (e.g., pH of 6.5 to 9.0) but are **susceptible to stomach acids.** If gastric acid production is reduced or neutralized, patients are more susceptible to *Vibrio* infections.

Most vibrios have **polar flagella** (important for motility), as well as various pili that are important for virulence. For example, epidemic strains of *V. cholerae*, the etiologic agent of cholera, have the **toxin co-regulated pilus** (see the next section). The cell wall structure of vibrios is also important. All strains possess **lipopolysaccharides** consisting of lipid A (endotoxin), core polysaccharide, and an O polysaccharide side chain. The O polysaccharide is used to subdivide *Vibrio* species into **serogroups:** There are 200 serogroups of *V. cholerae* plus multiple serogroups of *V. vulnificus* plus *V. parahaemolyticus.* The interest in this classification scheme is more than academic—***V. cholerae* O1 and O139** produce **cholera toxin** and are associated with epidemics of cholera. Other strains of *V. cholerae* generally do not produce cholera toxin and do not cause epidemic disease. *V. cholerae* serogroup O1 is further subdivided into serotypes and biotypes. Three **serotypes** are recognized: **Inaba, Ogawa,** and **Hikojima.** Strains can shift between serotype Inaba and serotype Ogawa, with Hikojima a transitional state in which both Inaba and Ogawa antigens are expressed. Two **biotypes** of *V. cholerae* O1 are recognized: **Classical** and **El Tor.** These biotypes are subdivided by differ-ences in phenotypic and morphologic properties. Seven worldwide pandemics of *V. cholerae* infections have been documented. *V. cholerae* strains responsible for the sixth worldwide pandemic of cholera were of the Classical biotype, whereas most strains responsible for the current seventh pandemic are the El Tor biotype.

V. vulnificus and non-O1 *V. cholerae* produce acidic **polysaccharide capsules** that are important for disseminated infections. *V. cholerae* O1 does not produce a capsule, so infections with this organism do not spread beyond the confines of the intestine.

V. cholerae and *V. parahaemolyticus* possess two circular chromosomes, each of which carry essential genes for these bacteria. It is not known if other *Vibrio* species have a similar genomic structure. Plasmids, including those encoding antimicrobial resistance, are also commonly found in *Vibrio* species.

Pathogenesis and Immunity (Table 21-3)

The **bacteriophage CTXΦ** encodes the genes for the two subunits of **cholera toxin** (*ctxA* and *ctxB*). This bacteriophage binds to the **toxin co-regulated pilus (TCP)** and moves into the bacterial cell, where it becomes integrated into the *V. cholerae* genome. The lysogenic bacteriophage chromosomal locus also contains other virulence factors: the *ace* gene for **accessory cholera enterotoxin,** *zot* gene for the **zonnula occludens toxin,** and the *cep* gene for **chemotaxis proteins.** Multiple copies of these genes are found

Table 21-3 Virulence Factors of *Vibrio* species

Species	Virulence Factor	Biologic Effect
V. cholerae	Cholera toxin	Hypersecretion of electrolytes and water
	Toxin co-regulated pilus	Binding site for CTXΦ; mediates adherence to intestinal mucosal cells
	Chemotaxis protein	Adhesin factor
	Accessory cholera enterotoxin	Increases intestinal fluid secretion
	Zonula occludens toxin	Increases intestinal permeability
	Neuraminidase	Modifies cell surface to increases GM_1 binding sites for cholera toxin
V. parahaemolyticus	Kanagawa hemolysin	Enterotoxin that induces chloride ion secretion (watery diarrhea)
V. vulnificus	Polysaccharide capsule	Antiphagocytic
	Cytolysins, proteases, collagenase	Mediates tissue destruction

in *V. cholerae* O1 and O139, and their expression is coordinated by regulatory genes.

The cholera toxin is a **complex A-B toxin** that is structurally and functionally similar to the heat-labile enterotoxin of *Escherichia coli.* A ring of five identical B subunits of cholera toxin binds to the ganglioside GM_1 receptors on the intestinal epithelial cells. The active portion of the A subunit is internalized, interacts with G proteins that control adenylate cyclase, leading to the catabolic conversion of adenosine triphosphate (ATP) to cyclic adenosine monophosphate (cAMP). This results in a hypersecretion of water and electrolytes. Severely infected patients can lose as much as 1 liter of fluid per hour during the height of the disease. Such a tremendous loss of fluid would normally flush the organisms out of the gastrointestinal tract; however, *V. cholerae* are able to **adhere to the mucosal cell layer** by means of (1) the **TCP** encoded by the *tcp* gene complex and (2) **chemotaxis proteins** encoded by the *cep* genes. Thus the TCP is important both as a receptor for the cholera toxin carrying phage and for adherence to the mucosa lining the intestines. Nonadherent strains are unable to establish infection.

In the absence of cholera toxin, *V. cholerae* O1 can still produce significant diarrhea through the action of the **zonula occludens toxin** and **accessory cholera enterotoxin.** As the name implies, the zonula occludens toxin loosens the tight junctions (zonula occludens) of the small intestine mucosa, leading to increased intestinal permeability, and the enterotoxin produces increased fluid secretion.

Unlike other non-O1 serotypes, *V. cholerae* O139 possesses the same virulence complex as that of the O1 strains. Thus the ability of the O139 strains to adhere to the intestinal mucosa and produce cholera toxin is the reason these strains can produce a watery diarrhea similar to cholera.

The means by which other *Vibrio* species cause disease is less clearly understood, although a variety of potential virulence factors have been identified. Most virulent strains of *V. parahaemolyticus* produce a thermostable direct hemolysin (TDH; also called **Kanagawa hemolysin**). TDH is an enterotoxin that

induces chloride ion secretion in epithelial cells by increasing intracellular calcium. An important method for classifying virulent strains of *V. parahaemolyticus* is detection of this hemolysin, which produces β-hemolytic colonies on agar media with human blood but not sheep blood. These virulent strains are referred to as **Kanagawa positive.** In the presence of gastric acids, *V. vulnificus* rapidly degrades lysine, producing alkaline byproducts. In addition, the bacteria are able to evade the host immune response by inducing macrophage apoptosis and to avoid phagocytosis by expression of a polysaccharide capsule. *V. vulnificus* also possesses surface proteins that mediate attachment to host cells and secretes cytolytic toxins leading to tissue necrosis.

Epidemiology

Vibrio species, including *V. cholerae*, grow naturally in **estuarine and marine environments** worldwide. All *Vibrio* species are able to survive and replicate in contaminated waters with increased salinity. Pathogenic vibrios can also flourish in waters with chitinous **shellfish** (e.g., oxysters, clams, mussels)—hence the association between *Vibrio* infections and the consumption of shellfish. Asymptomatically infected humans can also be an important reservoir for this organism in areas where *V. cholerae* disease is endemic.

Seven major pandemics of cholera have occurred since 1816, resulting in thousands of deaths and major socioeconomic changes. Sporadic disease and epidemics occurred before this time, but worldwide spread of the disease became possible with intercontinental travel resulting from increased commerce and wars.

It is estimated that 3 to 5 million cases of cholera and 100,000 deaths occur worldwide each year. The most recent epidemics occurred in 2004 in Bangladesh following flooding, in 2008 to 2009 in Zimbabwe, and in 2010 in Haiti following the devastating earthquake. Cholera is spread by **contaminated water and food** rather than direct person-to-person spread because a high inoculum (e.g., more than 10^8 organisms) is required to establish infection in a person with normal gastric acidity. In a person with achlorhydria or hypochlorhydria, the infectious dose can be as low as 10^3 to 10^5 organisms. Cholera is usually seen in communities with **poor sanitation.** Indeed, one outcome from the cholera pandemics was recognition of the role of contaminated water in the spread of disease and the need to improve community sanitation systems so that the disease could be controlled. Thus it is not surprising to observe cholera outbreaks when natural disasters, such as the earthquake in Haiti, compromise the control of sanitary wastes.

Infections caused by *V. parahaemolyticus, V. vulnificus,* and other pathogenic vibrios result from the consumption of improperly cooked seafood, particularly oysters, or exposure to contaminated seawater. *V. parahaemolyticus* is the most common cause of bacterial gastroenteritis in Japan and Southeast Asia and is the most common *Vibrio* species responsible for gastroenteritis in the United States. *V. vulnificus* is not frequently isolated but is responsible for severe wound infections and a high incidence of fatal outcomes. *V. vulnificus* is the most common cause of *Vibrio* septicemia. Gastroenteritis caused by vibrios occurs throughout the year because oysters are typically contaminated with abundant organisms year-round. In contrast, septicemia and wound infections with *Vibrio* occur during the warm months, when the organisms in seawater can multiply to high numbers.

Clinical Diseases

Vibrio cholerae

The majority of individuals exposed to toxigenic *V. cholerae* O1 have asymptomatic infections or self-limited diarrhea; however, some individuals develop severe, rapidly fatal diarrhea. The clinical manifestations of cholera begin an average of 2 to 3 days after ingestion of the bacteria, with the abrupt onset of watery diarrhea and vomiting. As more fluid is lost, the feces-streaked stool specimens become colorless and odorless, free of protein, and speckled with mucus (**"rice-water" stools**). The resulting severe fluid and electrolyte loss can lead to dehydration, painful muscle cramps, metabolic acidosis (bicarbonate loss), and hypokalemia and hypovolemic shock (potassium loss), with cardiac arrhythmia and renal failure. The mortality rate is 60% in untreated patients but less than 1% in patients who are promptly treated with replacement of lost fluids and electrolytes. Disease caused by **V. cholerae** O139 can be as severe as disease caused by *V. cholerae* O1. Other serotypes of *V. cholerae* (commonly called **V. cholerae non-O1**) do not produce cholera toxin and are usually responsible for mild watery diarrhea. These strains can also cause extraintestinal infections, such as septicemia, particularly in patients with liver disease or hematologic malignancies.

Vibrio parahaemolyticus

The severity of gastroenteritis caused by *V. parahaemolyticus* can range from a self-limited diarrhea to a mild, cholera-like illness. In general, the disease develops after a 5- to 72-hour incubation period (mean, 24 hours), with explosive, **watery diarrhea.** No grossly evident blood or mucus is found in stool specimens except in severe cases. Headache, abdominal cramps, nausea, vomiting, and low-grade fever may persist for 72 hours or more. The patient usually experiences an uneventful recovery. Wound infections with this organism can occur in people exposed to contaminated seawater.

Vibrio vulnificus

V. vulnificus is a particularly virulent species of *Vibrio* responsible for more than 90% of the *Vibrio*-related deaths in the United States. The most common presentations are **primary septicemia** after consumption of contaminated raw oysters or rapidly progressive **wound infection** after exposure to contaminated seawater. Patients with primary septicemia present with a sudden onset of fever and chills, vomiting, diarrhea, and abdominal pain. Secondary skin lesions with tissue necrosis are often present. The mortality in patients with *V. vulnificus* septicemia can be as high as 50%. The wound infections are characterized by initial swelling, erythema, and pain at the wound site, followed by the development of vesicles or bullae and eventual tissue necrosis together with systemic signs of fever and chills. Mortality associated with wound infections ranges from 20% to 30%. *V. vulnificus* infections are most severe in patients with hepatic disease, hematopoietic disease, or chronic renal failure and in those receiving immunosuppressive drugs.

Laboratory Diagnosis

Microscopy

Vibrio species are small (0.5 to 1.5 to 3 μm), curved, gram-negative rods. Large numbers of organisms are typically present in the stools of patients with cholera, so the direct microscopic examination of stool specimens can provide a rapid, presumptive diagnosis in endemic cholera outbreaks. Examination of Gram-stained wound specimens may also be useful in a setting suggestive of *V. vulnificus* infection (e.g., exposure of susceptible individual to seafood or seawater).

Culture

Vibrio organisms survive poorly in an acidic or dry environment. Specimens must be collected early in the disease and inoculated promptly onto culture media. If culture will be delayed, the specimen should be mixed in a Cary-Blair transport medium and refrigerated. Vibrios have low survival rates in buffered glycerol-saline, the transport medium used for most enteric pathogens.

Vibrios grow on most media used in clinical laboratories for stool and wound cultures, including blood agar and MacConkey agar. Special selective agar for vibrios (e.g., thiosulfate citrate bile salts sucrose [**TCBS**] agar), as well as an enrichment broth (e.g., **alkaline peptone broth**; pH 8.6), can also be used to recover vibrios in specimens with a mixture of organisms (e.g., stools). Isolates are identified with selective biochemical tests and serotyped using polyvalent antisera. In tests performed to identify halophilic vibrios, the media for biochemical testing must be supplemented with 1% NaCl.

Treatment, Prevention, and Control

Patients with cholera must be promptly treated with **fluid and electrolyte replacement** before the resultant massive fluid loss leads to hypovolemic shock. Antibiotic therapy, although of secondary value, can reduce toxin production and clinical symptoms, as well as decrease transmission by the more rapid elimination of the organism. A single dose of **azithromycin** is currently the drug of choice for children and adults because macrolide resistance is relatively uncommon. A single dose of doxycycline or ciprofloxacin in nonpregnant adults can be used as alternative therapy if demonstrated to be active in vitro; however, resistance to the tetracycline and fluoroquinolones is relatively common.

V. parahaemolyticus gastroenteritis is usually a self-limited disease, although antibiotic therapy can be used in addition to fluid and electrolyte therapy in patients with severe infections. *V. vulnificus* wound infections and septicemia must be promptly treated with antibiotic therapy. The combination of minocycline or doxycycline combined with ceftriaxone or cefotaxime appears to be the most effective treatment.

People infected with *V. cholerae* can shed bacteria for the first few days of acute illness and represent important sources of new infections. Although long-term carriage of *V. cholerae* does not occur, vibrios are free living in estuarine and marine reservoirs. Only improvements in sanitation can lead to effective control of the disease. This involves adequate sewage management, the use of purification systems to eliminate contamination of the water supply, and the implementation of appropriate steps to prevent contamination of food.

Although no oral cholera vaccine is available in the United States, a variety of killed, oral **vaccines** are available outside the United States; however, none of the vaccines provide long-term protection. A killed vaccine consisting of whole cells of *V. cholerae* O1 plus recombinant cholera toxin B subunit or a bivalent killed vaccine of whole cells of *V. cholerae* O1 and O139 is recommended for short-term protection of travelers in high-risk settings (e.g., exposure to untreated water or care of ill patients) to endemic regions of the world. Antibiotic prophylaxis of contacts to household patients with cholera can limit the spread but is generally ineffective in communities where disease occurs.

AEROMONAS

Aeromonas is a **gram-negative, facultative anaerobic fermentative rod** that morphologically resembles members of the family Enterobacteriaceae. As with *Vibrio*, extensive reorganization of the taxonomy of these bacteria has occurred. Thirty species and 12 subspecies of *Aeromonas* have been described, many of which are associated with human disease. The most important pathogens are **Aeromonas hydrophila, Aeromonas caviae,** and **Aeromonas veronii** biovar sobria. The organisms are ubiquitous in fresh and brackish water.

Aeromonas species cause three forms of disease: (1) **diarrheal disease** in otherwise healthy people, (2) **wound infections**, and (3) **opportunistic systemic disease** in immunocompromised patients (particularly those with hepatobiliary disease or an underlying malignancy). Intestinal disease can present as acute watery diarrhea, dysenteric diarrhea characterized by severe abdominal pain and blood and leukocytes in the stools, or a chronic illness with intermittent diarrhea. Gastrointestinal carriage has been observed in individuals with the highest carriage in the warm months. Thus the significance of isolating *Aeromonas* in enteric specimens must be determined by the clinical presentation of the patient. Gastroenteritis typically occurs after the ingestion of contaminated water or food (e.g., fresh produce, meats, dairy products), whereas wound infections most commonly result from a traumatic injury associated with exposure to contaminated water. One unusual form of *Aeromonas* wound infections is associated with the use of medicinal leeches, whose gut is colonized with *A. veronii* biovar. sobria.

Although numerous potential virulence factors (e.g., endotoxin, hemolysins, heat-labile and heat-stable enterotoxins) have been identified for *Aeromonas*, their precise role in disease is unknown.

Acute diarrheal disease is self-limited, and only supportive care is indicated in affected patients. Antimicrobial therapy is necessary in patients with chronic diarrheal disease, wound infections, or systemic disease. *Aeromonas* species are resistant to penicillins, most cephalosporins, and erythromycin. Fluoroquinolones (e.g., levofloxacin, ciprofloxacin) are almost uniformly active against *Aeromonas* strains isolated in the United States and Europe; however, resistance has been reported in strains recovered in Asia. Thus the long-term effectiveness of fluoroquinolones remains to be seen. A fluoroquinolone can be used initially for empiric therapy, but activity should be confirmed with in vitro susceptibility tests.

SUMMARY

Vibrio cholerae

The strains of **Vibrio cholerae** can be subdivided into more than 200 serogroups (O-cell wall antigens), *V. cholerae* serogroup O1 is further subdivided into serotypes (Inaba, Ogawa, Hikojima) and biotypes (Classical, El Tor). The disease is mediated by cholera toxin (complex A-B toxin) and toxin co-regulated pilus. Infection can range from asymptomatic colonization or mild diarrhea to severe, rapidly fatal diarrhea. The **cholera** begins with an abrupt onset of watery diarrhea and vomiting and can progress to severe dehydration, metabolic acidosis and hypokalemia, and hypovolemic shock. **Gastroenteritis** is the milder forms of diarrheal disease can occur in toxin-negative strains of *V. cholerae* O1 and in non-O1 serotypes. Serotype O1 is responsible for major pandemics (worldwide epidemics), with significant mortality in developing countries; O139 can cause similar diseases. Organism can be found in estuarine and marine environments worldwide and spread by consumption of contaminated food or water. For treatment, fluid and electrolyte replacement are crucial. Antibiotics (e.g., azithromycin) reduce the bacterial burden and exotoxin production, as well as duration of diarrhea. Improved hygiene is critical for control.

Vibrio parahaemolyticus

The infection is associated with consumption of contaminated raw shellfish. Gastroenteritis is the main form of the disease, generally self-limited, with an explosive onset of watery diarrhea and nausea, vomiting, abdominal cramps, headache, and low-grade fever. **Wound infection** is associated with exposure to contaminated water.

Vibrio vulnificus

Wound infection is a kind of severe, potentially fatal infections characterized by erythema, pain, bullae formation, tissue necrosis, and septicemia caused by **Vibrio vulnificus.** Life-threatening illnesses must be promptly treated with antibiotics.

Aeromonas

Aeromonas species cause three forms of disease: (1) **diarrheal disease** in otherwise healthy people, (2) **wound infections**, and (3) **opportunistic systemic disease** in immunocompromised patients (particularly those with hepatobiliary disease or an underlying malignancy).

KEYWORDS

English	Chinese
Vibrio	弧菌属
Vibrio cholerae	霍乱弧菌
Cholera toxin	霍乱毒素
Vibrio parahaemolyticus	副溶血性弧菌
Kanagawa hemolysin	神奈川溶血素
Vibrio vulnificus	创伤弧菌
Aeromonas	气单胞菌属

BIBLIOGRAPHY

1. Albert MJ, Nair GB: *Vibrio cholerae* O139-10 years on, Rev Med Microbiol 16: 135-143, 2005.

2. Ali M, et al: Herd immunity conferred by killed oral cholera vaccines in Bangladesh: a reanalysis, Lancet 366: 44-48, 2005.

3. Janda JM, Abbott S: The genus *Aeromonas*: taxonomy, pathogenicity, and infection, Clin Microbiol Rev 23: 35-73, 2010.

4. Jones M, Oliver J: *Vibrio vulnificus*: disease and pathogenesis, Infect Immun 77: 1723-1733, 2009.

5. Kitaoka M, et al: Antibiotic resistance mechanisms of *Vibrio cholerae*, J Med Microbiol 60: 397-407, 2011.

6. Klose KE: Regulation of virulence in *Vibrio cholerae*, Int J Med Microbiol 291: 81-88, 2001.

7. Parker J, Shaw J: *Aeromonas* spp. clinical microbiology and disease, J Infect 62: 109-118, 2011.

8. Snower DP, et al: *Aeromonas hydrophila* infection associated with the use of medicinal leeches, J Clin Microbiol 27: 1421-1422, 1989.

9. Yeung PSM, Boor KJ: Epidemiology, pathogenesis, and prevention of foodborne *Vibrio parahaemolyticus*, Foodborne Pathog Dis 1: 74-88, 2004.

Chapter 22

Helicobacter and *Campylobacter*

*C*ampylobacter and *Helicobacter* are now widely recognized as significant human pathogens; however, they were only discovered in the last 20 to 30 years.

The classification of *Campylobacter* and *Helicobacter* (Table 22-1) has undergone many changes since the bacteria were first discovered. *Campylobacter* and *Helicobacter* are the most important human pathogens and will be the focus of this chapter.

Table 22-1 Important *Campylobacter* and *Helicobacter* Species

Organism	Historical Derivation
Campylobacter	*kampylos*, curved; *bacter*, rod (a curved rod)
C. jejuni	*jejuni*, of the jejunum
C. coli	*coli*, of the colon
C. fetus	*fetus*, refers to the initial observation that these bacteria caused fetal infections
C. upsaliensis	*upsaliensis*, original isolates recovered from the feces of dogs at an animal clinic in Uppsala, Sweden
Helicobacter	*helix*, spiral; *bacter*, rod (a spiral rod)
H. pylori	*pylorus*, lower part of the stomach
H. cinaedi	*cinaedi*, of a homosexual (the organism was first isolated from homosexuals with gastroenteritis)
H. fennelliae	*fennelliae*, named after C. Fennell, who first isolated the organism

CAMPYLOBACTER

Only four species of *Campylobacter* including *Campylobacter jejuni*, *Campylobacter coli*, *Campylobacter fetus*, and *Campylobacter upsaliensis* are common human pathogens. The primary diseases caused by campylobacters are gastroenteritis and septicemia.

Physiology and Structure

The genus *Campylobacter* consists of small (0.2 to 0.5 μm wide and 0.5 to 5.0 μm long), **comma-shaped, gram-negative rods** (Figure 22-1) that are motile by means of a polar flagellum. Older cultures may appear coccoid.

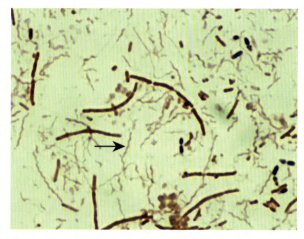

Figure 22-1 Mixed culture of bacteria from a fecal specimen. *Campylobacter jejuni* is the thin, curved, gram-negative bacteria *(arrow)*.

Campylobacters grow best in an atmosphere of reduced oxygen (5% to 7%) and increased carbon dioxide (5% to 10%). In addition, **C. jejuni grows better at 42℃** than at 37℃. These properties have been exploited for the selective isolation of pathogenic campylobacters in stool specimens. The **small size** of the organisms has also been used to recover the bacteria by filtration of stool specimens. Campylobacters pass through 0.45-μm filters, whereas other bacteria are retained. Campylobacters have a typical gram-negative cell wall structure. The major antigen of the genus is the lipopolysaccharide of the outer membrane.

Pathogenesis and Immunity

C. jejuni is the best-studied *Campylobacter* species. Specific role in disease of adhesins, cytotoxic enzymes, and enterotoxins of this species remains poorly defined. It is clear that the risk of disease is influenced by the infectious dose. The organisms are killed when exposed to gastric acids, so conditions that decrease or neutralize gastric acid secretion favor disease. The patient's immune status also affects the severity of disease.

C. jejuni gastrointestinal disease characteristically produces **histologic damage to the mucosal surfaces of the jejunum**, ileum, and colon. The mucosal surface appears ulcerated, edematous, and bloody, with crypt abscesses in the epithelial glands and infiltration of the lamina propria with neutrophils, mononuclear cells, and eosinophils. This inflammatory process is consistent with invasion of the organisms into the intestinal tissue.

C. jejuni and *C. upsaliensis* have been associated with **Guillain-Barré syndrome**, an autoimmune disorder of the peripheral nervous system. The syndrome has been associated with specific serotypes (primarily *C. jejuni* serotype O:19). It is believed that the pathogenesis of this disease is related to **antigenic cross-reactivity** between the surface lipopolysaccharides of some strains of *Campylobacter* and peripheral nerve gangliosides. Another immune-related late complication of campylobacter infections is **reactive arthritis**.

C. fetus has a propensity to spread from the gastrointestinal tract to the blood and distal foci. This spread is particularly common in debilitated and immunocompromised patients, such as those with liver disease, diabetes mellitus, chronic alcoholism, or malignancies. *C. fetus* is covered with a heat-stable, capsule-like protein (**S protein**) that prevents C3b binding to the bacteria and subsequent complement-mediated killing in serum.

Clinical Diseases

Gastrointestinal infections with *C. jejuni*, *C. coli*, and *C. upsaliensis* present most commonly as **acute enteri-**tis with diarrhea, fever, and severe abdominal pain. Affected patients can have 10 or more bowel movements per day during the peak of disease, and stools may be bloody on gross examination. The disease is generally self-limited, although symptoms may last for a week or longer. The range of clinical manifestations includes colitis, **abdominal pain mimicking acute appendicitis,** and bacteremia. Chronic enteric infections may develop in immunocompromised patients and be difficult to treat. **Guillain-Barré syndrome** and **reactive arthritis** are well-recognized complications of *Campylobacter* infections. *C. fetus* differs from other *Campylobacter* species in that this species is primarily responsible for **intravascular** (e.g., septicemia, endocarditis, septic thrombophlebitis) and **extraintestinal** (e.g., meningoencephalitis, abscesses) **infections**.

Epidemiology

Campylobacter infections are **zoonotic**, with a variety of animals serving as reservoirs. Humans acquire the infections with *C. jejuni* and *C. coli* after consumption of contaminated food, milk, or water; **contaminated poultry** are responsible for more than half of the *Campylobacter* infections in developed countries. Fecal-oral transmission from person-to-person contact may also occur, but it is **uncommon for the disease to be transmitted by food handlers.**

Disease occurs sporadically through the year, with a peak incidence during the summer months. Disease is most commonly observed in **infants and young children**, with a second peak of disease in 20- to 40-year-old adults. The incidence of disease is higher in developing countries, with symptomatic disease in infants and young children and asymptomatic carriage frequently observed in adults.

Laboratory Diagnosis

Microscopy

Observation of the characteristic **thin, "S-shaped" organisms** in a stool specimen (see Figure 22-1) is useful for a presumptive confirmation of *Campylobacter* infection.

Antigen Detection

A commercial immunoassay for detection of *C. jejuni* and *C. coli* is available. When compared with culture, the test has a sensitivity of 80% to 90% and a specificity of greater than 95%.

Culture and Identification

C. jejuni, *C. coli*, and *C. upsaliensis* isolation requires growth in a **microaerophilic atmosphere** (i.e., 5% to 7% oxygen, 5% to 10% carbon dioxide, and the balance nitrogen), at an **elevated incubation temperature** (i.e., 42°C), and on selective agar media. The selective media must contain blood or charcoal to remove toxic oxygen radicals, and antibiotics are added to inhibit the growth of contaminating organisms. Campylobacters are **slow-growing** organisms, usually requiring incubation for 48 to 72 hours or longer.

A presumptive identification of isolates is based on growth under selective conditions, typical microscopic morphology, and positive oxidase and catalase tests.

Antibody Detection

Serologic testing for immunoglobin (Ig) M and IgG is useful for epidemiologic surveys but is not used for diagnosis in an individual patient.

Treatment, Prevention, and Control

Campylobacter gastroenteritis is typically a self-limited infection managed by the replacement of lost fluids and electrolytes. Antibiotic therapy may be used in patients with severe infections or septicemia. Campylobacters are susceptible to a variety of antibiotics, including macrolides, tetracyclines, aminoglycosides, chloramphenicol, fluoroquinolones, clindamycin, amoxicillin/clavulanic acid, and imipenem. Most isolates are resistant to penicillins, cephalosporins, and sulfonamide antibiotics. **Erythromycin** or **azithromycin** are the antibiotics of choice for the treatment of enteritis, with tetracycline or fluoroquinolones used as secondary antibiotics. Amoxicillin/clavulanic acid can be used in place of tetracycline, which is contraindicated in young children. Systemic infections are treated with an aminoglycoside, chloramphenicol, or imipenem.

Exposure to enteric campylobacters is prevented by the proper preparation of food (particularly poultry), avoidance of unpasteurized dairy products, and the implementation of safeguards to prevent the contamination of water supplies.

HELICOBACTER

In 1983, **spiral, gram-negative rods** resembling campylobacters were found in patients with type B gastritis. The organisms were originally classified as *Campylobacter* but were subsequently reclassified as a new genus, *Helicobacter*. Helicobacters were subsequently subdivided into species that primarily colonize the stomach (**gastric helicobacters**) and those that colonize the intestines (**enterohepatic helicobacters**). The most important helicobacter species is ***Helicobacter pylori***, a gastric helicobacter associated with **gastritis, peptic ulcers, gastric adenocarcinoma,** and **gastric mucosa-associated lymphoid tissue (MALT) B-cell lymphomas** (Table 22-2). The most important enterohepatic helicobacters associated with human disease are ***Helicobacter cinaedi*** and ***Helicobacter fennelliae***, which have been isolated from homosexual men with proctitis, proctocolitis, or enteritis. Most of the discussion in this chapter will be restricted to the gastric helicobacter, *H. pylori*.

Table 22-2 *Helicobacter* Species Associated with Human Disease

Species	Common Reservoir Hosts	Human Disease
H. pylori	**Humans**, primates, pigs	**Gastritis, peptic ulcers, gastric adenocarcinoma,** mucosa-associated lymphoid tissue B-cell lymphomas
H. cinaedi	**Humans**, hamster	**Gastroenteritis,** septicemia, proctocolitis
H. fenneliae	**Humans**	**Gastroenteritis,** septicemia, proctocolitis

Bold type signifies the most common hosts and diseases.

Physiology and Structure

Helicobacters have a bacillary or **spiral shape** in young cultures (0.5 to1.0 μm wide by 2 to 4 μm long) and can assume coccoid forms in older cultures (Figure 22-2).

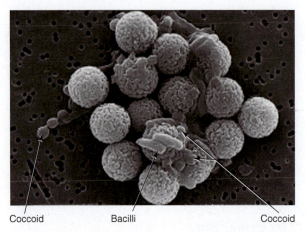

Coccoid   Bacilli   Coccoid

Figure 22-2 Scanning electron micrograph of *Helicobacter pylori* in a 7-day culture. Bacillary and coccoid forms *(arrows)* are bound to paramagnetic beads used in immunomagnetic separation. (Courtesy Dr. L. Engstrand, Uppsala, Sweden.)

All gastric helicobacters are highly **motile** (corkscrew motility) via polar flagella and produce an abundance of **urease.** These properties are believed to be important for survival in gastric acids and rapid movement through the viscous mucus layer toward a neutral pH environment.

H. pylori lipid A in lipopolysaccharide (LPS) has low endotoxin activity compared with other gram-negative bacteria, and the O side chain is antigenically similar to the Lewis blood group antigens, which may protect the bacteria from immune clearance.

Growth of *H. pylori* and other helicobacters requires a complex medium supplemented with blood, serum, charcoal, starch, or egg yolk, in microaerophilic conditions (decreased oxygen and increased carbon dioxide), and in a temperature range between 30°C and 37°C.

H. pylori is catalase- and oxidase-positive and does not ferment or oxidize carbohydrates.

Pathogenesis and Immunity

H. pylori is a remarkable bacterium in its ability to establish lifelong colonization in the stomach of untreated humans. Multiple factors contribute to the gastric colonization, inflammation, alteration of gastric acid production, and tissue destruction that are characteristic of *H. pylori* disease. Initial colonization is facilitated by (1) blockage of acid production by a bacterial acid-inhibitory protein and (2) neutralization of gastric acids with the ammonia produced by bacterial urease activity. The actively motile helicobacters can then pass through the gastric mucus and adhere to the gastric epithelial cells by multiple surface adhesion proteins. Surface proteins can also bind host proteins and help the bacteria evade immune detection. Localized tissue damage is mediated by urease byproducts, **mucinase, phospholipases,** and the activity of the **vacuolating cytotoxin A (VacA),** a protein that, after endocytosis by epithelial cells, damages the cells by producing vacuoles. Another important virulence factor of *H. pylori* is the **cytotoxin-associated gene (cagA)** that resides on a pathogenicity island containing approximately 30 genes. These genes encode a structure (type VI secretion system) that acts like a syringe to inject the CagA protein into the host epithelial cells, which interferes with the normal cytoskeletal structure of the epithelial cells. The *cag p*hosphoribosylanthranilate *i*somerase (PAI) genes also induce **interleukin-8 (IL-8) production,** which attracts neutrophils. Release of proteases and reactive oxygen molecules by the neutrophils is believed to contribute to gastritis and gastric ulcers.

Clinical Diseases

Colonization with *H. pylori* invariably leads to histologic evidence of **gastritis.** The acute phase of gastritis is characterized by a feeling of fullness, nausea, vomiting, and hypochlorhydria. This can evolve into chronic gastritis with disease confined to the gastric antrum in individuals with normal acid secretion or involve the entire stomach (pangastritis) if acid secretion is suppressed. Approximately 10% to 15% of patients with chronic gastritis will progress to develop peptic ulcers. The ulcers develop at the sites of intense inflammation, commonly involving the junction between the corpus and antrum (**gastric ulcer**) or the proximal duodenum (**duodenal ulcer).**

H. pylori is responsible for 85% of the gastric ulcers and 95% of the duodenal ulcers. Recognition of the role of *H. pylori* has dramatically changed the treatment and prognosis of peptic ulcer disease.

Chronic gastritis eventually leads to replacement of the normal gastric mucosa with fibrosis and proliferation of intestinal-type epithelium. This process increases the patient's risk for **gastric cancer** by almost 100-fold. This risk is influenced by the strain of *H. pylori* and the host's response (*cagA*-positive strains and high levels of IL-1 production are associated with a higher risk for cancer). Infection with *H. pylori* is also associated with infiltration of lymphoid tissue into the gastric mucosa. In a small number of patients, a monoclonal population of B cells may develop and evolve into a **MALT lymphoma.**

H. cinaedi and *H. fennelliae* can cause **gastroenteritis** and **bacteremia,** most commonly in immunocompromised patients.

Epidemiology

The highest incidence of *H. pylori* carriage is found in developing countries, where 70% to 90% of the population is colonized, most before the age of 10 years. The prevalence of *H. pylori* in industrial countries, such as the United States, is less than 40% and is decreasing because of improved hygiene and active treatment of colonized individuals. 70% to 100% of patients with gastritis, gastric ulcers, or duodenal ulcers are infected with *H. pylori*. **Humans are the primary reservoir for *H. pylori*,** and colonization is believed to persist for life unless the host is specifically treated. Transmission is most likely via the **fecal-oral route.**

An interesting observation about *H. pylori* colonization has been made. This organism is clearly associated with diseases such as gastritis, gastric ulcers, gastric adenocarcinoma, and gastric MALT lymphomas. It is anticipated that treatment of colonized or infected individuals will lead to a reduction of these diseases. However, colonization with *H. pylori* appears to offer protection from gastroesophageal reflux disease and adenocarcinomas of the lower esophagus and gastric cardia. Thus it may be unwise to eliminate *H. pylori* in patients without symptomatic disease. Certainly, the complex relationship between *H. pylori* and its host remains to be defined.

Laboratory Diagnosis

Microscopy

H. pylori is detected by histologic examination of gastric biopsy specimens. Although the organism can be seen in specimens stained with hematoxylin-eosin or Gram stain, the Warthin-Starry silver stain is the most sensitive. Because this is an invasive test, alternative test procedures are preferred for routine diagnosis.

Urease Related Detection

Biopsy specimens can also be tested for the presence of bacterial urease activity. The abundance of urease produced by *H. pylori* permits detection of the alkaline byproduct in less than 2 hours. The sensitivity of the direct test with biopsy specimens varies from 75% to 95%; however, the specificity approaches 100%. Noninvasive urease testing of human breath (urea breath test), following consumption of an isotopically labeled urea solution, has excellent sensitivity and specificity.

Culture and Identification

H. pylori can be isolated in culture if the specimen is inoculated onto enriched medium supplemented with blood, hemin, or charcoal and incubated in a microaerophilic atmosphere for up to 2 weeks.

Presumptive identification of isolates is based on their growth characteristics under selective conditions, typical microscopic morphologic findings, and detection of oxidase, catalase, and urease activity.

Antigen Detection

A number of polyclonal and monoclonal immunoassays for *H. pylori* antigens excreted in stool have been develop and demonstrated to have sensitivities and specificities exceeding 95%. These assays are now widely recommended for both detection of *H. pylori* infections and confirmation of cure after antibiotic treatment.

Nucleic Acid-Based Tests

Currently, nucleic acid-based amplification tests for *H. pylori* are restricted to research laboratories and not used in clinical laboratories.

Antibody Detection

Serology is an important screening test for the diagnosis of *H. pylori*. Because the **antibody titers persist** for many years, the test cannot be used to discriminate between past and current infection. However, the tests are useful for documenting exposure to the bacteria, either for epidemiologic studies or for the initial evaluation of a symptomatic patient.

Treatment, Prevention, and Control

Use of a single antibiotic or an antibiotic combined with bismuth is ineffective. The greatest success in curing gastritis or peptic ulcer disease has been accomplished with the combination of a **proton pump inhibitor** (e.g., omeprazole), a **macrolide** (e.g., clarithromycin), and a β-**lactam** (e.g., amoxicillin), with administration for 7 to 10 days initially. Treatment failure is most commonly associated with clarithromycin resistance. Susceptibility testing should be performed if the patient does not respond to therapy. Metronidazole can also be used in combination therapy, but resistance is commonplace.

Use of *H. pylori* antigens in combination with mucosal adjuvants that induce a Th$_2$ cell-response is protective in an animal model and can eradicate existing infections. The effectiveness of these vaccines in humans remains to be demonstrated.

SUMMARY

Campylobacter

Campylobacter is commonly thin, curved, gram-negative rods. Enteric infections caused by *Campylobacter* are worldwide distributed. Most of common diseases caused by *Campylobacter* are acute enteritis with diarrhea, malaise, fever, and abdominal pain. Guillain-Barré syndrome is believed to be an autoimmune disease caused by antigenic cross-reactivity between oligosaccharides in *Campylobacter* capsule and glycosphingolipids on surface of neural tissues

Helicobacter pylori

H. pylori is curved, gram-negative rods. The typical characteristic of *H. pylori* is urease production at very high levels. *H. pylori* is an important cause of acute and chronic gastritis, peptic ulcers, gastric adenocarcinoma, and mucosa-associated lymphoid tissue lymphoma.

Histologic examination of biopsy specimens and antigen test of *H. pylori* in stool specimens is sensitive and specific. Urease test is also relatively sensitive and highly specific; urea breath test is a noninvasive test. Serology test is useful for demonstrating exposure to *H. pylori*. Combined therapy with a proton pump inhibitor, a macrolide and a β-lactam for 2 weeks has a high success rate. Prophylactic treatment of colonized individuals has not been useful and has potentially adverse effects, such as predisposing patients to adenocarcinomas of the lower esophagus.

KEYWORDS

English	Chinese
Campylobacter	弯曲菌属
Campylobacter jejuni	空肠弯曲菌
Cytotoxin-associated gene	细胞毒素相关基因
Duodenal ulcer	十二指肠溃疡
Gastric cancer	胃癌
Gastric ulcer	胃溃疡
Gastritis	胃炎
Gastroenteritis	胃肠炎
Guillain-Barré syndrome	格林 - 巴利综合征
Helicobacter	螺杆菌属
Helicobacter pylori	幽门螺杆菌
MALT lymphoma	MALT 淋巴瘤
Reactive arthritis	反应性关节炎
Vacuolating cytotoxin A	空泡细胞毒素 A

BIBLIOGRAPHY

1. Algood H, Cover T: *Helicobacter pylori* persistence: an overview of interactions between *H. pylori* and host immune defenses, Clin Microbiol Rev 19: 597-613, 2006.

2. Farinha P, Gascoyne R: *Helicobacter pylori* and MALT lymphoma, Gastroenterology 128: 1579-1605, 2005.

3. Friedman L: *Helicobacter pylori* and nonulcer dyspepsia (editorial), N Engl J Med 339: 1928-1930, 1998.

4. Kabir S: The current status of *Helicobacter pylori* vaccines: a review, Helicobacter 12: 89-102, 2007.

5. Kusters JG, van Vliet A, Kuipers EJ: Pathogenesis of *Helicobacter pylori* infection, Clin Microbiol Rev 19: 449-490, 2006.

6. Lastovica A: Emerging *Campylobacter* spp.: the tip of the iceberg, Clin Microbiol Newslett 28: 49-55, 2006.

7. Marshall B: *Helicobacter pylori*: 20 years on, Clin Med 2: 147-152, 2002.

8. Nachamkin I, et al: *Campylobacter* species and Guillain-Barré syndrome, Clin Microbiol Rev 11: 555-567, 1998.

9. Passaro D, Chosy EJ, Parsonnet J: *Helicobacter pylori*: consensus and controversy, Clin Infect Dis 35: 298-304, 2002.

10. Samuel MC, et al: Epidemiology of sporadic *Campylobacter* infection in the United States and declining trend in incidence, FoodNet 1996-1999, Clin Infect Dis 38: S165-S174, 2004.

11. Solnick J: Clinical significance of *Helicobacter* species other than *Helicobacter pylori*, Clin Infect Dis 36: 348-354, 2003.

Pseudomonas and Related Bacteria

Pseudomonas and related nonfermentative rods are opportunistic pathogens of plants, animals, and humans. Despite the many genera, most clinically significant isolates are members of five genera: *Pseudomonas, Burkholderia, Stenotrophomonas, Acinetobacter,* and *Moraxella* (Table 23-1). These organisms will be the focus of this chapter.

PSEUDOMONAS

The genus *Pseudomonas* consisted of almost 200 species. They were referred to as pseudomonads because they are commonly arranged in pairs of cells that resemble a single cell (Figure 23-1). **Pseudomonas aeruginosa** is the most important species and the one discussed here.

Members of the genus are found in soil, decaying organic matter, vegetation, and water. Unfortunately, they are also found throughout the hospital environment in moist reservoirs, such as food, cut flowers, sinks, toilets, floor mops, respiratory therapy and dialysis equipment, and even in disinfectant solutions.

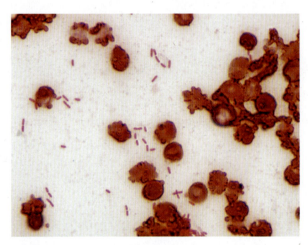

Figure 23-1 Gram stain of *Pseudomonas aeruginosa* with cells arranged singly and in pairs.

Table 23-1 Important Nonfermentative Gram-Negative Rods

Organism	Historical Derivation
Acinetobacter	*akinetos*, unable to move; *bactrum*, rod (nonmotile rods)
A. baumannii	*baumannii*, named after the microbiologist Baumann
Burkholderia	*Burkholderia*, named after the microbiologist Burkholder
B. cepacia	*cepacia*, like an onion (original strains isolated from rotten onions)
B. pseudomallei	*pseudes*, false; *mallei* (refers to the fact this species closely resembles *B. mallei*)
Moraxella	*Moraxella*, named after the Swiss ophthalmologist Morax, who first recognized the species
M. catarrhalis	*catarrhus*, downflowing or catarrh (refers to inflammation of the respiratory tract mucus membranes)
Pseudomonas	*pseudes*, false; *monas*, a unit (refers to Gram-stain appearance of pairs of organisms that resemble a single cell)
P. aeruginosa	*aeruginosa*, full of copper rust or green (refers to blue and yellow pigments produced by this species that appear green)
Stenotrophomonas	*Stenos*, narrow; *trophos*, one who feeds; *monas*, unit (refers to observation that these are narrow bacteria that require few substrates for growth)
S. maltophilia	*malt*, malt; *philia*, friend (friend of malt)

The broad environmental distribution of *Pseudomonas* is made possible by their simple growth requirements and nutritional versatility. They are capable of using many organic compounds as sources of carbon and nitrogen, and some strains can even grow in distilled water by using trace nutrients. These organisms also possess many structural factors, enzymes, and toxins that enhance their virulence and render them resistant to most commonly used antibiotics. Fortunately, *Pseudomonas* infections are **primarily opportunistic** (i.e., restricted to patients receiving broad-spectrum antibiotics that suppress the normal intestinal bacterial population or patients with compromised host defenses).

Physiology and Structure

Pseudomonas species are usually motile, straight or slightly curved, gram-negative rods (0.5 to 1.0 by 1.5 to 5.0 µm) typically **arranged in pairs** (see Figure 23-1). The organisms utilize carbohydrates through **aerobic respiration**, with oxygen the terminal electron acceptor. They can also grow anaerobically using nitrate or arginine as an alternate electron acceptor. The presence of **cytochrome oxidase** in *Pseudomonas* species is used to differentiate them from the Enterobacteriaceae and *Stenotrophomonas*. Some strains appear **mucoid** because of the abundance of a polysaccharide capsule (Figure 23-2); these strains are particularly common in patients with cystic fibrosis (CF).

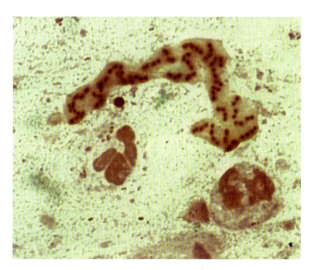

Figure 23-2   Gram stain of *Pseudomonas aeruginosa* surrounded by mucoid capsular material in cystic fibrosis patient.

Some species produce **diffusible pigments** (e.g., pyocyanin [blue], pyoverdin [yellow-green], pyorubin [reddish-brown]) that give them a characteristic appearance in culture and simplify the preliminary identification.

P. aeruginosa is inherently **resistant to many antibiotics** and can mutate to even more resistant strains during therapy. The **mutation of porin proteins** constitutes the major mechanism of resistance. Penetration of antibiotics into the pseudomonad cell is primarily through pores in the outer membrane. If the proteins forming the walls of these pores (porins) are altered to restrict flow into the cell, resistance to many classes of antibiotics can develop simultaneously. *P. aeruginosa* also produces a number of different β-lactamases that can inactivate many β-lactam antibiotics.

Pathogenesis and Immunity

P. aeruginosa has many virulence factors, including adhesins, toxins, and enzymes. In addition, the delivery system used by *Pseudomonas*, the type III secretion system, is particularly effective in injecting toxins into the host cell. The multiple factors must work together for *P. aeruginosa* to cause disease.

Adhesins

At least four surface components of *P. aeruginosa* facilitate adherence: (1) flagella, (2) pili, (3) lipopolysaccharide (LPS), and (4) alginate. Flagella and pili also mediate motility in *P. aeruginosa*, and the lipid A component of LPS is responsible for endotoxin activity. Alginate is a mucoid exopolysaccharide that forms a prominent **capsule** on the bacterial surface and protects the organism from phagocytosis and antibiotic killing. The genes controlling production of the alginate polysaccharide can be activated in patients, such as those with CF or other chronic respiratory diseases, who are predisposed to long-term colonization with these mucoid strains of *P. aeruginosa*.

Secreted Toxins and Enzymes

Exotoxin A (ETA) disrupts protein synthesis by blocking peptide chain elongation in eukaryotic cells. ETA most likely contributes to the dermatonecrosis that occurs in burn wounds, corneal damage in ocular infections, and tissue damage in chronic pulmonary infections.

A blue pigment, **pyocyanin,** produced by *P. aeruginosa* catalyzes the production of superoxide and hydrogen peroxide, toxic forms of oxygen. This pigment also stimulates interleukin-8 (IL-8) release, leading to enhanced attraction of neutrophils. A yellow-green pigment, **pyoverdin,** is a siderophore that binds iron for use in metabolism. This pigment also regulates secretion of other virulence factors including ETA.

Two elastases, LasA (**serine protease**) and LasB (**zinc metalloprotease**), act synergistically to degrade elastin, resulting in damage to elastin-containing tissues and producing the lung parenchymal damage and hemorrhagic lesions (**ecthyma gangrenosum**) associated with disseminated *P. aeruginosa* infections. These enzymes can also degrade complement components and inhibit neutrophil chemotaxis and function, leading to further spread and tissue damage in acute infections. Chronic *Pseudomonas* infections are characterized by the formation of antibodies to LasA and LasB, with the deposition of immune complexes in the infected tissues. Similar to the elastases, **alkaline protease** contributes to tissue destruction and spread of *P. aeruginosa*. It also interferes with the host immune response.

Phospholipase C is a heat-labile hemolysin that breaks down lipids and lecithin, facilitating tissue destruction.

Exoenzymes S and **T** are extracellular toxins produced by *P. aeruginosa*. When the type III secretion system introduces the proteins into their target eukaryotic cells, epithelial cell damage occurs, facilitating bacterial spread, tissue invasion, and necrosis.

Clinical Diseases

Pulmonary Infections

P. aeruginosa infections of the lower respiratory tract can range in severity from **asymptomatic colonization** or benign inflammation of the bronchials (**tracheobronchitis**) to severe **necrotizing bronchopneumonia.** Colonization is seen in patients with CF, other chronic lung diseases, or neutropenia. Infections in patients with CF have been associated with exacerbation of the underlying disease and invasive pulmonary disease. Mucoid strains are commonly isolated from these patients and are difficult to eradicate because chronic infections with these bacteria are associated with progressive increase in antibiotic resistance.

Conditions that predispose immunocompromised patients to infections with *Pseudomonas* include (1) previous therapy with broad-spectrum antibiotics that eliminate the normal, protective bacterial population and (2) use of mechanical ventilation equipment, which may introduce the organism to the lower airways.

Primary Skin and Soft-Tissue Infections

P. aeruginosa can cause a variety of primary skin infections. The most recognized are infections of **burn wounds** (Figure 23-3). Colonization of a burn wound, followed by localized vascular damage, tissue necrosis, and ultimately bacteremia, is common in patients with severe burns. The moist surface of the burn and inability of neutrophils to penetrate into the wounds predispose patients to such infections.

Folliculitis (Figure 23-4) is another common infection caused by *Pseudomonas*, resulting from immersion in contaminated water. Secondary infections with *Pseudomonas* also occur in people who

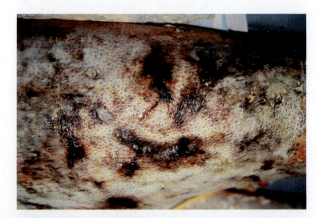

Figure 23-3 *Pseudomonas* infection of burn wound. (From Cohen J, Powderly WB: *Infectious diseases*, ed 2, St Louis, 2004, Mosby.)

have acne or who depilate their legs. Finally, *P. aeruginosa* can cause fingernail infections in people whose hands are frequently exposed to water or frequent "nail salons."

P. aeruginosa is also the most common cause of **osteochondritis** of the foot after a penetrating injury.

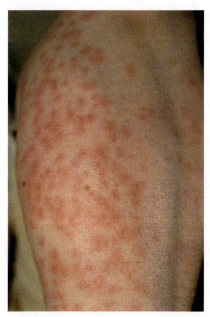

Figure 23-4 *Pseudomonas* folliculitis. (From Cohen J, Powderly WB: *Infectious diseases*, ed 2, St Louis, 2004, Mosby.)

Urinary Tract Infections

Infection of the urinary tract is seen primarily in patients with long-term **indwelling urinary catheters.**

Ear Infections

External otitis is frequently caused by *P. aeruginosa*, with swimming an important risk factor (**"swimmer's ear"**). This localized infection can be managed with topical antibiotics and drying agents. **Malignant external otitis** is a virulent form of disease seen primarily in persons with diabetes and elderly patients. It can invade the underlying tissues, can damage the cranial nerves and bones, and can be life threatening. *P. aeruginosa* is also associated with **chronic otitis media.**

Eye Infections

Infections of the eye occur after initial trauma to the cornea and then exposure to *P. aeruginosa* in contaminated water. **Corneal ulcers** develop and can

progress to rapidly progressive, eye-threatening disease unless prompt treatment is instituted.

Bacteremia and Endocarditis

Bacteremia caused by *P. aeruginosa* is clinically indistinguishable from that caused by other gram-negative bacteria. However, the mortality rate in affected patients is higher with *P. aeruginosa* bacteremia because of (1) the predilection of the organism for immunocompromised patients, (2) difficulty in treating antibiotic-resistant strains, and (3) the inherent virulence of *Pseudomonas*. Bacteremia occurs most often in patients with neutropenia, diabetes mellitus, extensive burns, and hematologic malignancies. Most bacteremias originate from infections of the lower respiratory tract, urinary tract, and skin and soft tissue (particularly burn wound infections).

Pseudomonas **endocarditis** is uncommon, primarily seen in intravenous drug abusers. These patients acquire the infection from the use of drug paraphernalia contaminated with the waterborne organisms.

Other Infections

P. aeruginosa is also the cause of a variety of other infections, including those localized in the gastrointestinal tract, central nervous system, and musculoskeletal system.

Epidemiology

Pseudomonas is an opportunistic pathogen present in a variety of environments. Indeed the recovery of *Pseudomonas* from an environmental source (e.g., hospital sink or floor) means very little unless there is epidemiologic evidence that the contaminated site is a reservoir for infection.

Furthermore, isolation of *Pseudomonas* from a hospitalized patient is worrisome but does not normally justify therapeutic intervention unless there is evidence of disease. The recovery of *Pseudomonas*, particularly species other than *P. aeruginosa*, from a clinical specimen may represent simple transient colonization of the patient or environmental contamination of the specimen during collection or laboratory processing.

Laboratory Diagnosis

Microscopy

Observation of thin, gram-negative rods arranged singly and in pairs is suggestive of *Pseudomonas* but not pathognomonic—*Burkholderia*, *Stenotrophomonas*, and other pseudomonads have a similar morphology.

Culture and Identification

Pseudomonas are readily recovered on common isolation media such as blood agar and MacConkey agar. Their growth in broth is generally confined to the broth-air interface.

The colonial morphology (e.g., colony size, hemolytic activity, pigmentation, odor; Figure 23-5) and the results of selected rapid biochemical tests (e.g., positive **oxidase** reaction) are sufficient for the preliminary identification of these isolates. For example, *P. aeruginosa* grows rapidly and has flat colonies with a spreading border, **β-hemolysis,** a **green pigmentation** caused by the production of the blue (pyocyanin) and yellow-green (pyoverdin) pigments, and a characteristic sweet, **grapelike odor.**

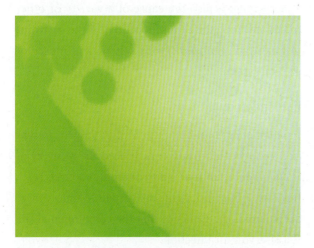

Figure 23-5 Colonial morphology of *Pseudomonas aeruginosa*; note the green pigmentation that results from the production of two water-soluble dyes: blue pyocyanin and yellow fluorescein.

Treatment, Prevention, and Control

The antimicrobial therapy for *Pseudomonas* infections is frustrating because (1) the bacteria are typically resistant to most antibiotics and (2) the infected patient with compromised host defenses cannot augment the antibiotic activity. A **combination of active antibiotics** is generally required for therapy to be successful in patients with serious infections.

Effective infection-control practices should concentrate on **preventing the contamination of sterile equipment,** such as mechanical ventilation equipment and dialysis machines, and the cross-contamination of patients by medical personnel. The inappropriate use of broad-spectrum antibiotics should also be avoided.

BURKHOLDERIA

In 1992, seven species formerly classified as *Pseudomonas* were reclassified as members of the new genus *Burkholderia*. **B. cepacia complex, *Burkholderia gladioli*,** and ***Burkholderia pseudomallei*** are important human pathogens in this genus.

Burkholderia species can colonize a variety of moist environmental surfaces and are **opportunistic pathogens.** Patients particularly susceptible to pulmonary infections with *B. cepacia* complex and *B. gladioli* are those with CF or chronic granulomatous disease. Colonization of the respiratory tract of CF patients with *B. cepacia* complex has such a poor prognosis that this is a contraindication for lung transplantation. *B. cepacia* complex is also responsible for urinary tract infections (UTIs) in catheterized patients, septicemia, and other opportunistic infections. With the exception of pulmonary infections, infections with *B. cepacia* complex do not commonly result in death.

B. pseudomallei is a saprophyte found in soil, water, and vegetation. It is endemic in Southeast Asia, India, Africa, and Australia. Infections are acquired by either inhalation or less commonly by percutaneous inoculation. Most persons exposed to *B. pseudomallei* remain asymptomatic; however, alcoholics, diabetics, and individuals with chronic renal or lung disease are susceptible to opportunistic infections cause by this organism. Infections are called **melioidosis.** Exposure by the percutaneous route presents as a localized, suppurative **cutaneous infection** accompanied by regional lymphadenitis, fever, and malaise. This form of disease can resolve without incident or can progress rapidly to overwhelming sepsis. **Pulmonary disease** that develops after respiratory exposure may range in severity from a mild bronchitis to necrotizing pneumonia. Cavitation progressing to overwhelming sepsis and death can develop if appropriate antimicrobial therapy is not instituted. *B. pseudomallei* has been used in biologic weapons programs, so work with this organism is restricted to appropriately licensed laboratories. Isolation of *B. pseudomallei* for diagnostic purposes should be approached carefully because the organism is highly infectious.

Burkholderia species are susceptible to **trimethoprim-sulfamethoxazole,** which distinguishes them from *P. aeruginosa*, which is uniformly resistant.

STENOTROPHOMONAS MALTOPHILIA

S. maltophilia was classified in the genus *Stenotrophomonas*. The clinical importance of this opportunistic pathogen is well known. It is responsible for infections in debilitated patients with impaired host-defense mechanisms. Also, because *S. maltophilia* is resistant to most commonly used *β*-lactam and aminoglycoside antibiotics, patients receiving long-term antibiotic therapy with these drugs are particularly at risk for acquiring infections.

The most common nosocomial infections caused *S. maltophilia* are bacteremia and pneumonia, with both associated with a high incidence of complications and death. Hospital infections with this organism have been traced to contaminated intravenous catheters, disinfectant solutions, mechanical ventilation equipment, and ice machines.

Antimicrobial therapy is complicated because the organism is resistant to many commonly used drugs. *Stenotrophomonas* is uniformly **resistant to carbapenems** (e.g., imipenem, meropenem, ergapenem) and susceptible to **trimethoprim-sulfamethoxazole.**

ACINETOBACTER

Acinetobacters are strictly aerobic, oxidase-negative, plump gram-negative coccobacilli (Figure 23-6).

They are **ubiquitous** saprophytes, recovered in nature and in the hospital and able to survive on both moist surfaces, such as mechanical ventilation equipment, and on dry surfaces, such as human skin. These bacteria are also part of the normal oropharyngeal flora of a small number of healthy people and can proliferate to large numbers during hospitalization. Most human infections are caused by *A. baumannii*.

Acinetobacters are **opportunistic pathogens** that cause infections in the respiratory tract, urinary tract, and wounds; they also cause septicemia. Patients at risk for *Acinetobacter* infections are those receiving broad-spectrum antibiotics, recovering from surgery, or on respiratory ventilation. Nosocomial wound and pulmonary infections in hospitalized patients have become a significant problem because many of the infections are caused by strains resistant to most antibiotics including the carbapenems. Specific therapy must be guided by in vitro susceptibility tests.

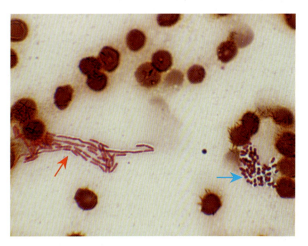

Figure 23-6 Gram stain of *Acinetobacter baumannii* (*blue arrow*) and *Pseudomonas aeruginosa* (*red arrow*).

MORAXELLA

The genus *Moraxella* was reorganized on the basis of nucleic acid analysis. *M. catarrhalis* is the most important pathogen. **M. catarrhalis** is a strictly aerobic, oxidase-positive, gram-negative diplococci (Figure 23-7). This organism is a common cause of bronchitis and bronchopneumonia (in elderly patients with chronic pulmonary disease), sinusitis, and otitis. The latter two infections occur most commonly in previously healthy people. Most isolates produce β-lactamases and are **resistant to penicillins**; however, these bacteria are uniformly susceptible to most other antibiotics, including cephalosporins, erythromycin, tetracycline, trimethoprim-sulfamethoxazole, and the combination of penicillins with a β-lactamase inhibitor (e.g., clavulanic acid).

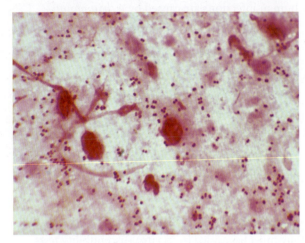

Figure 23-7 Gram stain of *Moraxella catarrhalis.*

SUMMARY

Pseudomonas aeruginosa is a group of small, gram-negative rods typically arranged in pairs, and is obligate aerobe, glucose oxidizer and simple nutritional requirements. In addition, other phenotypic feature is its mucoid polysaccharide capsule. P. aeruginesa is commonly ubiquitous in nature and moist environmental hospital sites and also transiently colonizes the respiratory and gastrointestinal tracts of hospitalized patients, particularly those treated with broad-spectrum antibiotics, exposed to respiratory therapy equipment, or hospitalized for extended periods. Diseases include pulmonary infections, skin infections, Urinary tract infections, Ear infections, Eye infections, as well as bacteremia and endocarditis.

KEYWORDS

English	Chinese
Acinetobacter	不动杆菌属
Acinetobacter baumannii	鲍曼不动杆菌
Cystic fibrosis (CF)	囊性纤维化
Cytochrome oxidase	细胞色素氧化酶
Exotoxin A (ETA)	外毒素 A
Moraxella	莫拉菌属
Moraxella catarrhalis	卡他莫拉菌
Nonfermentative rods	非发酵杆菌
Pseudomonas	假单胞菌属
Pseudomonas aeruginosa	铜绿假单胞菌
Stenotrophomonas	窄食单胞菌属
Stenotrophomonas maltophilia	嗜麦芽窄食单胞菌

BIBLIOGRAPHY

1. Broides A, et al: Acute otitis media caused by *Moraxella catarrhalis*: epidemiology and clinical characteristics, Clin Infect Dis 49: 1641-1647, 2009.

2. Dijkshoorn L, Nemec A, Seifert H: An increasing threat in hospitals: multidrug-resistant *Acinetobacter baumannii*, Nature Rev Microbiol 5: 939-951, 2007.

3. Hauser A: The type III secretion system of *Pseudomonas aeruginosa*: infection by injection, Nature Rev Microbiol 7: 654-665, 2009.

4. Ikonomidis A, et al: Heteroresistance to meropenem in carbapenem-susceptible *Acinetobacter baumannii*, J Clin Microbiol 47: 4055-4059, 2009.

5. Kipnis E, et al: Targeting mechanisms of *Pseudomonas aeruginosa* pathogenesis, Med Malad Infect 36: 78-91, 2006.

6. Looney WJ, Narita M, Muhlemann K: *Stenotrophomonas maltophilia*: an emerging opportunist human pathogen, Lancet Infect Dis 9: 312-323, 2009.

7. Mahenthiralingam E, et al: The multifarious, multireplicon *Burkholderia cepacia* complex, Nat Rev Microbiol 3: 144-156, 2005.

8. McGregor K, et al: *Moraxella catarrhalis*: clinical significance, antimicrobial susceptibility and BRO beta-lactamases, Eur J Clin Microbiol Infect Dis 17: 219-234, 1998.

9. Peleg A, Seifert H, Paterson D: *Acinetobacter baumannii*: emergence of a successful pathogen, Clin Microbiol Rev 21: 538-582, 2008.

10. Sadikot R, et al: Pathogen-host interactions in *Pseudomonas aeruginosa* pneumonia, Am J Respir Crit Care Med 171: 1209-1223, 2005.

11. Yates S, et al: Stealth and mimicry by deadly bacterial toxins, Trends Biochem Sci 31: 123-133, 2006.

Haemophilus and Related Bacteria

The four most important genera in the family Pasteurellaceae are **Haemophilus, Actinobacillus, Aggregatibacter,** and **Pasteurella** (Table 24-1). The members of this family are small (0.2 to 0.3 by 1.0 to 2.0 μm), facultative anaerobic, gram-negative rods. Members of the genus *Haemophilus* are the most commonly isolated and significant human pathogens and will be the main focus of this chapter (Table 24-2).

HAEMOPHILUS

Haemophilae are small, sometimes pleomorphic, gram-negative rods present on the mucous membranes of humans (Figure 24-1). **Haemophilus influenzae** is the species most commonly associated with disease, although introduction of the *H. influenzae* type b vaccine has dramatically reduced

Table 24-1 Important Pasteurellaceae

Organism	Historical Derivation
Haemophilus	*haemo*, blood; *hilos*, lover ("blood lover;" requires blood for growth on agar media)
H. influenzae	Originally thought to be the cause of influenza
H. aegyptius	*aegyptius*, Egyptian (observed by Robert Koch in 1883 in exudates from Egyptians with conjunctivitis)
H. ducreyi	Named after the bacteriologist Ducrey, who first isolated this organism
Actinobacillus	*actinis*, ray; *bacillus*, small staff or rod ("ray bacillus;" refers to the growth of filamentous forms [rays])
Aggregatibacter	*aggregare*, to come together; *bacter*, bacterial rod; rod-shaped bacteria that aggregate or clump together
A. actinomycetemcomitans	*comitans*, accompanying ("accompanying an actinomycetes;" isolates are frequently associated with *Actinomyces*)
A. aphrophilus	*aphros*, foam; *philos*, loving ("foam loving")
Pasteurella	Named after Louis Pasteur
P. multocida	*multus*, many; *cidus*, to kill ("many-killing"; pathogenic for many species of animals)
P. canis	*canis*, dogs (isolated from the mouths of dogs)

Table 24-2 *Haemophilus* Species Associated with Human Disease

Species	Primary Diseases	Frequency
H. influenzae	Pneumonia, sinusitis, otitis, meningitis, epiglottitis, cellulitis, bacteremia	Common worldwide;
H. aegyptius	Conjunctivitis	Uncommon
H. ducreyi	Chancroid	An important pathogen in Africa and Asia
H. parainfluenzae	Bacteremia, endocarditis, opportunistic infections	Rare
H. haemolyticus	Opportunistic infections	Rare
H. parahaemolyticus	Opportunistic infections	Rare

the incidence of disease particularly in the pediatric population. ***Haemophilus aegyptius*** is an important cause of acute, purulent conjunctivitis. ***Haemophilus ducreyi*** is well recognized as the etiologic agent of the sexually transmitted disease **soft chancre, or chancroid.** The other members of the genus are rarely pathogenic, being responsible primarily for opportunistic infections.

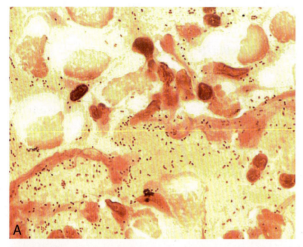

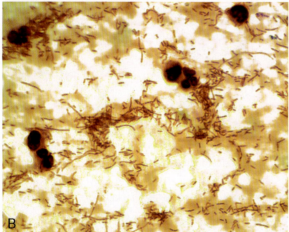

Figure 24-1 Gram stains of *Haemophilus influenzae.* **A,** Small coccobacilli forms seen in sputum from patient with pneumonia. **B,** Thin, pleomorphic forms seen in a 1-year-old unvaccinated child in Africa with overwhelming meningitis.

Physiology and Structure

The growth of most species of *Haemophilus* requires supplementation of media with one or both of the following growth-stimulating factors: (1) **hemin** (also called **X factor** for "unknown factor") and (2) **nicotinamide adenine dinucleotide** (**NAD;** also called **V factor** for "vitamin"). Although both factors are present in blood-enriched media, sheep blood agar must

be gently heated to destroy the inhibitors of V factor. For this reason, heated blood ("chocolate") agar is used for the in vitro isolation of *Haemophilus.*

The cell wall structure of *Haemophilus* is typical of other gram-negative rods. Lipopolysaccharide with endotoxin activity is present in the cell wall. The surface of many, but not all, strains of *H. influenzae* is covered with a **polysaccharide capsule** and six antigenic **serotypes** (**a** through **f**) have been identified. Before the introduction of the *H. influenzae* type b vaccine, *H. influenzae* serotype b was responsible for more than 95% of all invasive *Haemophilus* infections.

In addition to the serologic differentiation of *H. influenzae*, the species is subdivided into eight **biotypes** (I through VIII) as determined by three biochemical reactions: indole production, urease activity, and ornithine decarboxylase activity. The separation of these biotypes is useful for epidemiologic purposes.

Pathogenesis and Immunity

Haemophilus species, particularly *H. parainfluenzae* and nonencapsulated *H. influenzae*, colonize the upper respiratory tract in virtually all people within the first few months of life. These organisms can spread locally and cause disease in the ears (otitis media), sinuses (sinusitis), and lower respiratory tract (bronchitis, pneumonia). Disseminated disease, however, is relatively uncommon. In contrast, encapsulated *H. influenzae* (particularly serotype b [biotype I]) is uncommon in the upper respiratory tract or is present in only very small numbers but is a common cause of **disease in unvaccinated children** (i.e., meningitis, epiglottitis [obstructive laryngitis], cellulitis). Pili and nonpilus adhesins mediate colonization of the oropharynx with *H. influenzae.* Cell wall components of the bacteria (e.g., lipopolysaccharide and a low-molecular-weight glycopeptide) impair ciliary function, leading to damage of the respiratory epithelium. The bacteria can then be translocated across both epithelial and endothelial cells and can enter the blood. In the absence of specific opsonic antibodies directed against the polysaccharide capsule, high-grade bacteremia can develop, with dissemination to the meninges or other distal foci.

The major virulence factor in *H. influenzae* type b is the antiphagocytic polysaccharide capsule, which contains ribose, ribitol, and phosphate (commonly referred to as **polyribitol phosphate [PRP]**). Antibodies directed against the capsule greatly stimulate bacterial phagocytosis and complement-mediated bactericidal activity. These antibodies develop because of natural infection, vaccination with purified PRP, or the passive transfer of maternal antibodies. The lipopolysaccharide **lipid A** component induces meningeal inflammation in an animal model and may be responsible for initiating this response in humans. **IgA1 proteases** are produced by *H. influenzae* (both encapsulated and nonencapsulated strains) and may facilitate colonization of the organisms on mucosal surfaces by interfering with humoral immunity.

Clinical Diseases

The clinical syndromes seen in patients with *H. influenzae* infections are represented in Figure 24-2. The diseases caused by all *Haemophilus* species are described in the following sections.

Meningitis

H. influenzae type b was the most common cause of pediatric meningitis, but this situation changed rapidly when the conjugated vaccines became widely used. The peak incidence of meningitis was seen in children 3 to 18 months of age. Disease in nonimmune patients results from the bacteremic spread of the organisms from the nasopharynx and cannot be differentiated clinically from other causes of bacterial meningitis. The initial presentation is a 1- to 3-day history of mild upper respiratory disease, after which the typical signs and symptoms of meningitis appear. Mortality is less than 10% in patients who receive prompt therapy, and carefully designed studies have documented a low incidence of serious neurologic sequelae. Person-to-person spread in a nonimmune population is well documented.

Epiglottitis

Epiglottitis, characterized by cellulitis and the swelling of the supraglottic tissues, represents a life-threat-

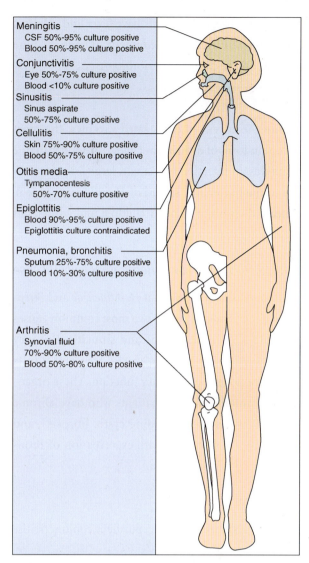

Figure 24-2 Infections caused by *Haemophilus influenzae*. With the advent of the conjugated vaccine, most infections in adults involve areas contiguous with the oropharynx (i.e., lower respiratory tract, sinuses, ears). Serious systemic infections (e.g., meningitis, epiglottitis) can occur in nonimmune patients. *CSF,* Cerebrospinal fluid.

Meningitis
CSF 50%-95% culture positive
Blood 50%-95% culture positive
Conjunctivitis
Eye 50%-75% culture positive
Blood <10% culture positive
Sinusitis
Sinus aspirate
50%-75% culture positive
Cellulitis
Skin 75%-90% culture positive
Blood 50%-75% culture positive
Otitis media
Tympanocentesis
50%-70% culture positive
Epiglottitis
Blood 90%-95% culture positive
Epiglottitis culture contraindicated
Pneumonia, bronchitis
Sputum 25%-75% culture positive
Blood 10%-30% culture positive
Arthritis
Synovial fluid
70%-90% culture positive
Blood 50%-80% culture positive

ening emergency. The peak incidence of this disease during the prevaccine era occurred in children 2 to 4 years of age. Children with epiglottitis have pharyngitis, fever, and difficulty breathing, which can progress rapidly to obstruction of the airway and death. Since the introduction of the vaccine, the incidence of this disease has also decreased dramatically in children and remains relatively rare in adults.

Cellulitis

Cellulitis is a pediatric disease caused by *H. influenzae* that has largely been eliminated by vaccination.

When it is observed, patients have fever and cellulitis characterized by the development of reddish-blue patches on the cheeks or periorbital areas.

Arthritis

Before the advent of conjugated vaccines, the most common form of arthritis in children younger than 2 years was an infection of a single, large joint secondary to the bacteremic spread of *H. influenzae* type b. Disease does occur in older children and adults, but it is very uncommon.

Otitis, Sinusitis, and Lower Respiratory Tract Disease

Most studies have shown that *H. influenzae* and *Streptococcus pneumoniae* are the two most common causes of acute and chronic otitis and sinusitis. Primary pneumonia is uncommon in children and adults who have normal pulmonary function. These organisms commonly colonize patients who have chronic pulmonary disease (including cystic fibrosis), and frequently are associated with exacerbation of bronchitis and frank pneumonia.

Conjunctivitis

H. aegyptius causes an acute, purulent conjunctivitis.

Chancroid

Chancroid is a sexually transmitted disease that is most commonly diagnosed in men, presumably because women can have asymptomatic or inapparent disease. Approximately 5 to 7 days after exposure, a tender papule with an erythematous base develops on the genitalia or perianal area. Within 2 days the lesion ulcerates and becomes **painful,** and inguinal **lymphadenopathy** is commonly present.

Other Infections

Other species of *Haemophilus* can cause opportunistic infections, such as otitis media, conjunctivitis, sinusitis, endocarditis, meningitis, and dental abscesses.

Epidemiology

Before the introduction of the *H. influenzae* vaccine, even though *H. influenzae* type b was the most com-

mon serotype that caused systemic disease, it was rarely isolated in healthy children. *H. influenzae* type b remains the most significant pediatric pathogen in many countries of the world. It is estimated that 3 million cases of serious disease and up to 700,000 fatalities occur in children each year worldwide, a tragedy considering that vaccination could eliminate virtually all disease. *H. influenzae* type b disease in children younger than 5 years was virtually eliminated in the United States by introduction of **conjugated *H. influenzae* type b vaccines**.

The epidemiology of disease caused by nonencapsulated *H. influenzae* and other *Haemophilus* species is distinct. Ear and sinus infections caused by these organisms are primarily pediatric diseases but can occur in adults. Pulmonary disease most commonly affects elderly people, particularly those with a history of underlying chronic obstructive pulmonary disease (COPD) or conditions predisposing to aspiration (e.g., alcoholism, altered mental state).

H. ducreyi is an important cause of genital ulcers (chancroid) in Africa and Asia but is less common in Europe and North America.

Laboratory Diagnosis

Specimen Collection

The specimen for detection *Haemophilus* infections include direct needle aspiration (sinusitis or otitis), sputum produced from the lower airways (pneumonia), blood (pneumonia, meningitis, epiglottitis, cellulitis, and arthritis), and cerebrospinal fluid (CSF) (meningitis).

Specimens for the detection of *H. ducreyi* should be collected with a moistened swab from the base or margin of the ulcer. Cultures of pus collected by aspiration from an enlarged lymph node can be performed but is generally less sensitive than culture of the ulcer.

Microscopy

Gram-negative rods ranging in shape from coccobacilli to long, pleomorphic filaments can be detected in more than 80% of CSF specimens from patients with untreated *Haemophilus* meningitis (see Figure 24-1). The microscopic examination of Gram-stained specimens is also useful for the rapid diagnosis of the organism in arthritis and lower respiratory tract disease.

Antigen Detection

The immunologic detection of *H. influenzae* antigen, specifically the PRP capsular antigen, is a rapid and sensitive way to diagnose *H. influenzae* type b disease. PRP can be detected with the particle agglutination test in CSF and urine (in which the antigen is eliminated intact).

Culture and Identification

Chocolate agar or Levinthal agar is used in most laboratories. The bacteria appear as 1- to 2-mm, smooth, opaque colonies after 24 hours of incubation. They can also be detected growing around colonies of *Staphylococcus aureus* on unheated blood agar (**satellite phenomenon; Figure 24-3**). The staphylococci provide the requisite growth factors by lysing the erythrocytes in the medium and releasing intracellular heme (X factor) and excreting NAD (V factor). The colonies of *H. influenzae* in these cultures are much smaller than they are on chocolate agar because the V factor inhibitors present in blood are not inactivated. Isolates of *H. influenzae* often grow better in anaerobically incubated blood cultures

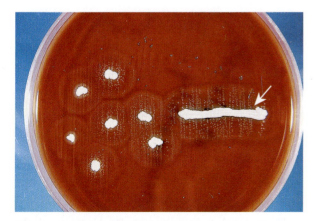

Figure 24-3 Satellite phenomenon. *Staphylococcus aureus* excretes nicotinamide adenine dinucleotide (NAD, or V factor) into the medium, providing a growth factor required for *Haemophilus influenzae* (small colonies surrounding *S. aureus* colonies [*arrow*]).

because, under these conditions, the organisms do not require X factor for growth.

H. aegyptius grows best on chocolate agar supplemented with 1% IsoVitaleX. Culture for *H. ducreyi* is relatively insensitive but reportedly is best on gonococcal (GC) agar supplemented with 1% to 2% hemoglobin, 5% fetal bovine serum, IsoViteleX enrichment, and vancomycin (3μg/ml).

A presumptive identification of *H. influenzae* can be made by the Gram-stain morphology and demonstration of a requirement for both X and V factors. Further subgrouping of *H. influenzae* can be done with biotyping, electrophoretic characterization of the membrane protein antigens, and analysis of the strain-specific nucleic acid sequences. Biochemical tests or nucleic acid analysis is used to identify other species in this genus.

Treatment, Prevention, and Control

Patients with systemic *H. influenzae* infections require prompt antimicrobial therapy because the mortality rate in patients with untreated meningitis or epiglottitis approaches 100%. Serious infections are treated with **broad-spectrum cephalosporins.** Less severe infections, such as sinusitis and otitis, can be treated with amoxicillin (if susceptible; approximately 30% of strains are resistant), an active cephalosporin, azithromycin, doxycycline or a fluoroquinolone. Most isolates of *H. ducreyi* are susceptible to **erythromycin,** the drug recommended for treatment.

The primary approach to preventing *H. influenzae* type b disease is through active immunization with purified capsular PRP. Currently, it is recommended that children receive three doses of vaccine against *H. influenzae* type b disease before the age of 6 months, followed by booster doses.

Antibiotic chemoprophylaxis is used to eliminate the carriage of *H. influenzae* type b in children at high risk for disease. Rifampin prophylaxis has been used in these settings.

ACTINOBACILLUS

Actinobacillus species are small, facultatively anaerobic, gram-negative rods that grow slowly (generally requiring 2 to 3 days of incubation). The members of the genus *Actinobacillus* colonize the oropharynx of humans and animals and are rare causes of periodontitis, endocarditis, bite wound infections, and opportunistic infections (Table 24-3).

Table 24-3 *Actinobacillus* Species Associated with Human Disease

Species	Primary Diseases	Frequency
A. equuli	Bite wound infections	Rare
A. hominis	Opportunistic infections (bacteremia, pneumonia)	Rare
A. lignieresii	Bite wound infections	Rare
A. ureae	Opportunistic infections (bacteremia, meningitis, pneumonia)	Rare

AGGREGATIBACTER

Two members of this genus are important human pathogens: **A. actinomycetemcomitans** and **A. aprophilus** (Table 24-4). Both species colonize the human mouth and can spread from the mouth into the blood and then stick to a previously damaged heart valve or artificial valve, leading to the development of endocarditis. The treatment of choice for endocarditis caused by these organisms is a cephalosporin such as ceftriaxone.

Table 24-4 *Aggregatibacter* Species Associated with Human Disease

Species	Primary Diseases	Frequency
A. actinomycetemcomitans	Periodontitis, endocarditis, bite wound infections	Common
A. aprophilus	Endocarditis, opportunistic infections	Uncommon

PASTEURELLA

Pasteurella are small, facultatively anaerobic, fermentative coccobacilli (Figure 24-4) commonly found as commensals in the oropharynx of healthy animals. Most human infections result from animal contact (e.g., animal bites, scratches, shared food). **Pasteu-**

rella multocida (the most common isolate) and **Pasteurella canis** are human pathogens; the other *Pasteurella* species are rarely associated with human infections (Table 24-5). The following three general forms of disease are reported: (1) localized **cellulitis** and **lymphadenitis** that occur after an animal bite or scratch, (2) an exacerbation of chronic **respiratory disease** in patients with underlying pulmonary dysfunction, and (3) a **systemic infection in immunocompromised patients,** particularly those with underlying hepatic disease.

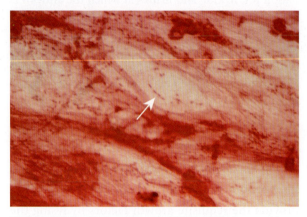

Figure 24-4 *Pasteurella multocida* in respiratory specimen from patient with pneumonia.

Table 24-5 *Pasteurella* Species Associated with Human Disease

Species	Primary Disease	Frequency
P. multocida	Bite wound infections, chronic pulmonary disease, bacteremia, meningitis	Common
P. canis	Bite wound infections	Uncommon
P. bettyae	Opportunistic infections (abscesses, bite wound infections, urogenital infections, bacteremia)	Rare
P. dagmatis	Bite wound infections	Rare
P. stomatis	Bite wound infections	Rare

P. multocida is susceptible to a variety of antibiotics. **Penicillin** is the antibiotic of choice and expanded-spectrum cephalosporins, macrolides, tetracyclines, or fluoroquinolones are acceptable alternatives. Semisynthetic penicillins (e.g., oxacillin), first-generation cephalosporins, and aminoglycosides have poor activity.

SUMMARY

Haemophilus species are commonly small, pleomorphic, gram-negative rods or coccobacilli, facultative anaerobes and fermentative. Most of species require X and/or V factor for growth. Diseases caused by *H. influenzae* infection include meningitis, epiglottitis, pneumonia, cellulitis, arthritis, otitis, and sinusitis. *H. aegyptius* causes **conjunctivitis**. *H. ducreyi* is an important cause of **chancroid**.

With the exception of *H. ducreyi*, which is spread by sexual contact, most *Haemophilus* infections are caused by the patient's oropharyngeal flora (endogenous infections).

KEYWORDS

English	Chinese
Actinobacillus	放线杆菌属
Chancroid	软下疳
Conjunctivitis	结膜炎
Haemophilus	嗜血杆菌属
Haemophilus aegyptius	埃及嗜血杆菌
Haemophilus ducreyi	杜克嗜血杆菌
Haemophilus influenzae	流感嗜血杆菌
Meningitis	脑膜炎
Pasteurella	巴斯德菌属
Pasteurella multocida	多杀巴斯德菌
Satellite phenomenon	卫星现象

BIBLIOGRAPHY

1. Chen HI, Hulten K, Clarridge JE: Taxonomic subgroups of *Pasteurella multocida* correlate with clinical presentation, J Clin Microbiol 40: 3438-3441, 2002.

2. Dworkin M, Park L, Borchardt S: The changing epidemiology of invasive *Haemophilus influenzae* disease, especially in persons >65 years old, Clin Infect Dis 44: 810-816, 2007.

3. Hallstrom T, Riesbeck K: *Haemophilus influenzae* and the complement system, Trends Microbiol 18: 258-265, 2010.

4. Holst E, et al: Characterization and distribution of *Pasteurella* species recovered from infected humans, J Clin Microbiol 30: 2984-2987, 1992.

5. Norskov-Lauritsen N, Kilian M: Reclassification of *Actinobacillus actinomycetemcomitans*, *Haemophilus aphrophilus*, *Haemophilus paraphrophilus*, and *Haemophilus segnis* as *Aggregatibacter actinomycetemcomitans*, *Aggregatibacter aphrophilus*, and *Aggregatibacter segnis*, respectively, and emended description of *Aggregatibacter aphrophilus* to include V factor-dependent and V factor-independent isolates, Intern J System Evol Microbiol 56: 2135-2146, 2006.

6. O'Loughlin R, et al: Methodology and measurement of the effectiveness of *Haemophilus influenzae* type b vaccine: systematic review, Vaccine 28: 6128-6136, 2010.

7. Peltola H: Worldwide *Haemophilus influenzae* type b disease at the beginning of the 21st century: global analysis of the disease burden 25 years after the use of the polysaccharide vaccine and a decade after the advent of conjugates, Clin Microbiol Rev 13: 302-317, 2000.

8. Trees D, Morse S: Chancroid and *Haemophilus ducreyi*: an update, Clin Microbiol Rev 8: 357-375, 1995.

9. Tristram S, Jacobs M, Appelbaum P: Antimicrobial resistance in *Haemophilus influenzae*, Clin Microbiol Rev 20: 368-389, 2007.

10. Tsang R, et al: Characterization if invasive *Haemophilus influenzae* disease in Manitoba, Canada, 2000-2006: invasive disease due to non-type B strains, Clin Infect Dis 44: 1611-1614, 2007.

11. Wang C, et al: Invasive infections of *Aggregatibacter actinomycetemcomitans*, J Microbiol Immunol Infect 43: 491-497, 2010.

Bordetella

*B*ordetella is an extremely **small** (0.2 to 0.5 × 1 μm in diameter), **strictly aerobic, gram-negative coccobacillus.** Four species including *Bordetella pertussis, Bordetella parapertussis, Bordetella bronchiseptica,* and *Bordetella holmesii* are responsible for human disease (Table 25-1).

Table 25-1 *Bordetella* Species Associated with Human Disease

Organism	Historical Derivation
Bordetella	Named after Jules Bordet, who first isolated the organism responsible for pertussis
B. pertussis	*per*, very or severe; *tussis*, cough (a severe cough)
B. parapertussis	*para*, resembling (resembling pertussis)
B. bronchiseptica	*bronchus*, the trachea; *septicus*, septic (an infected bronchus)
B. holmesii	Named after the microbiologist Barry Holmes

BORDETELLA PERTUSSIS

Physiology and Structure

Bordetella species have simple nutritional requirements, but some species are highly **susceptible to toxic substances and metabolites** in common laboratory media. These species (particularly *B. pertussis*) require media supplemented with charcoal, starch, blood, or albumin to absorb these toxic substances. The more fastidious species also grow slowly in culture. The organisms are nonmotile and oxidize amino acids, but they do not ferment carbohydrates.

Pathogenesis and Immunity

Infection with *B. pertussis* and the development of whooping cough require exposure to the organism, bacterial attachment to the ciliated epithelial cells of the respiratory tract, proliferation of the bacteria, and production of localized tissue damage and systemic toxicity. Attachment of the organisms to ciliated epithelial cells is mediated by protein adhesins (Table 25-2). **Pertactin** and **filamentous hemagglutinin** contain an Arg-Gly-Asp sequence (RGD motif) that promotes binding to sulfated glycoprotein integrins on the membranes of ciliated respiratory cells. These adhesins also bind to CR3, a glycoprotein receptor on the surface of macrophages. This interaction leads to phagocytosis of the bacteria without initiating an oxidative burst, which is important in the intracellular survival and replication of the bacteria. This also protects *B. pertussis* from humoral antibodies. **Pertussis toxin** is a classic A-B toxin consisting of a toxic subunit (S1) and five binding subunits (S2 to S5; two S4 subunits are present in each toxin molecule). The S2 subunit binds to lactosylceramide, a glycolipid presents on ciliated respiratory cells. The S3 subunit binds to receptors on phagocytic cells, leading to an increase in CR3 on the cell surface, which facilitates attachment mediated by pertactin and filamentous hemagglutinin and subsequent bacterial phagocytosis. Another adhesin, **fimbria,** has been identified in *B. pertussis* and has been demonstrated to mediate the binding to cultured mammalian cells. The role of fimbriae in the attachment to ciliated cells in vivo is unknown.

B. pertussis produces several toxins that mediate

Table 25-2 Virulence Factors Associated with *Bordetella pertussis*

Virulence Factor	Biologic Effect
Adhesins	
Filamentous hemagglutinin	Required for binding to sulfated glycoproteins on membranes of ciliated cells in trachea; highly immunogenic
Pertactin	As with filamentous hemagglutinin
Pertussis toxin	S2 subunit binds to glycolipid on surface of ciliated respiratory cells; S3 subunit binds to ganglioside on surface of phagocytic cells
Fimbriae	Bind to mammalian cells; role in disease is unknown but stimulate humoral immunity
Toxins	
Pertussis toxin	S1 subunit inactivates G1α, the membrane surface protein that controls adenylate cyclase activity; uncontrolled expression leads to increased cyclic adenoside monophosphate levels; toxin inhibits phagocytic killing and monocyte migration
Adenylate cyclase/hemolysin toxin	Increases intracellular level of adenylate cyclase; inhibits phagocytic killing and monocyte migration
Dermonecrotic toxin	Causes dose-dependent skin lesions or fatal reactions in experimental animal model; role in disease is unknown
Tracheal cytotoxin	A peptidoglycan fragment that kills ciliated respiratory cells and stimulates the release of interleukin-1 (fever)
Lipopolysaccharide	Two distinct lipopolysaccharide molecules with either lipid A or lipid X; activates alternate complement pathway and stimulates cytokine release; role in disease is unknown

the localized and systemic manifestations of disease. The S1 portion of **pertussis toxin** has adenosine diphosphate (ADP)-ribosylating activity for the membrane surface G proteins (guanine nucleotide-binding regulatory proteins). These proteins regulate adenylate cyclase activity. Pertussis toxin inactivates $G_i\alpha$, the inhibitory protein that controls adenylate cyclase activity. The uncontrolled expression of the enzyme leads to an increase in cyclic adenosine monophosphate (cAMP) levels and a subsequent increase in respiratory secretions and mucus production characteristic of the paroxysmal stage of pertussis.

Adenylate cyclase/hemolysin is a bifunctional toxin that is activated in the target mammalian cell by intracellular calmodulin and catalyzes the conversion of endogenous adenosine triphosphate (ATP) to cAMP in eukaryotic cells. Adenylate cyclase toxin also inhibits leukocyte chemotaxis, phagocytosis, and killing. This toxin may be important for the initial protection of the bacteria during the early stages of disease.

Dermonecrotic toxin is a heat-labile toxin. The toxin probably is responsible for the localized tissue destruction in human infections.

Tracheal cytotoxin is a low-molecular-weight cell wall peptidoglycan monomer that has a specific affinity for ciliated epithelial cells. Tracheal cytotoxin specifically interferes with deoxyribonucleic acid (DNA) synthesis, thereby impairing the regeneration of damaged cells. This process disrupts the normal clearance mechanisms in the respiratory tree and leads to the characteristic cough associated with pertussis. The toxin also stimulates the release of the cytokine interleukin-1 (IL-1), which leads to fever.

B. pertussis produces **lipopolysaccharides,** which can activate the alternate complement pathway and stimulate cytokine release.

Clinical Diseases

Infection is initiated when infectious aerosols are inhaled and the bacteria become attached to and proliferate on ciliated epithelial cells. After a 7- to 10-day incubation period, the classical presentation of pertussis proceeds through three stages (Figure 25-1). The first stage, the **catarrhal stage,** resembles a common cold, with serous rhinorrhea, sneezing, malaise, anorexia, and low-grade fever. Because the peak number of bacteria is produced during this stage and the cause of the disease is not yet recognized, patients in the catarrhal stage pose the highest risk to their contacts. After 1 to 2 weeks, the **paroxysmal stage** begins. During this time, ciliated epithelial cells are extruded from the respiratory tract, and the clearance of mucus is impaired. This stage is characterized by the **classic whooping cough paroxysms** (i.e., a series of repetitive coughs followed by an inspiratory whoop). Mucus production in the respiratory tract is common and is partially responsible for causing airway restriction. The paroxysms are frequently terminated with vomiting and exhaustion. A marked lymphocytosis is also prominent during this stage. Affected patients may experience as many as 40 to 50 paroxysms daily during the height of the illness. After 2 to 4 weeks, the disease enters the **convalescent stage**; at this time, the paroxysms diminish in number and severity, but secondary complications can occur. It is now appreciated that this classic presentation of pertussis may not be seen in patients with partial immunity or in adults. Such patients may have a history of a chronic persistent cough without whooping or vomiting.

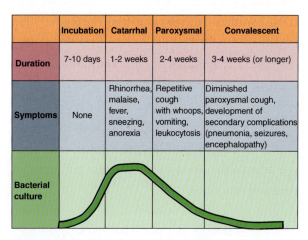

	Incubation	Catarrhal	Paroxysmal	Convalescent
Duration	7-10 days	1-2 weeks	2-4 weeks	3-4 weeks (or longer)
Symptoms	None	Rhinorrhea, malaise, fever, sneezing, anorexia	Repetitive cough with whoops, vomiting, leukocytosis	Diminished paroxysmal cough, development of secondary complications (pneumonia, seizures, encephalopathy)
Bacterial culture				

Figure 25-1   Clinical presentation of *Bordetella pertussis* disease.

Epidemiology

B. pertussis is a **human disease** with no other recognized animal or environmental reservoir. Although the incidence of pertussis, with its associated morbidity and mortality, was reduced considerably after the introduction of vaccines in 1949, the disease is still endemic worldwide, with an estimated 20 to 40 million infections and 200,000 to 400,000 deaths each year, primarily in unvaccinated children. Historically, pertussis was considered a pediatric disease, but now a significant proportion of infections are found in **adolescents and adults** (Figure 25-2). The recognition of milder forms of disease in older children and adults and improved diagnostic tests have contributed to the increase in reported disease.

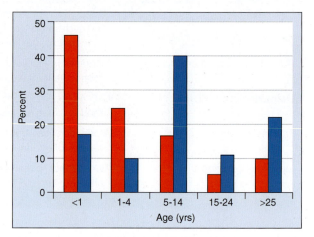

Figure 25-2   Age distribution for pertussis infections reported in 1988 *(red bars)* and 2005 *(blue bars)*.

Laboratory Diagnosis

Specimen Collection and Transport

B. pertussis organisms are extremely sensitive to drying and do not survive unless care is taken during the collection and transport of the specimen to the laboratory. The optimal diagnostic specimen is a nasopharyngeal aspirate. Oropharyngeal swabs should not be used because sufficient numbers of ciliated epithelial cells are not collected. Specimens for culture should be inoculated onto freshly prepared isolation media (e.g., Regan-Lowe agar) at the patient's bedside.

Microscopy

A direct fluorescent antibody procedure using either monoclonal or polyclonal antibodies can be used to examine specimens.

Nucleic Acid-Based Tests

PCR are the most sensitive diagnostic test available for pertussis. These methods have replaced microscopy and culture in most laboratories that offer laboratory testing.

Culture and Identification

The traditional use of **Bordet-Gengou** medium has been replaced by **Regan-Lowe charcoal medium** supplemented with glycerol, peptones, and horse blood. The media should be incubated in air at 35℃, in a humidified chamber, and for 7 to 12 days. Despite use of optimized culture conditions, fewer than half the infected patients have positive cultures.

B. pertussis organisms are identified by their characteristic microscopic and colonial morphology on selective media and their reactivity with a specific antiserum.

Antibody Detection

Enzyme-linked immunosorbent assay (ELISA) tests have been developed to detect immunoglobulin A (IgA), IgM, and IgG antibodies against pertussis toxin, filamentous hemagglutinin, pertactin, and fimbriae. Antibodies directed against pertussis toxin are specific for *B. pertussis*; however, antibodies to the other antigens may occur with infections caused by other *Bordetella* species and other bacteria.

Treatment, Prevention, and Control

Macrolides (i.e., erythromycin, azithromycin, clarithromycin) are effective in eradicating the organisms; however, this effect has limited value because the illness is usually unrecognized during the peak of contagiousness. Azithromycin and clarithromycin are generally better tolerated and the preferred macrolides. Trimethoprim-sulfamethoxazole or fluoroquinolones can be used in patients unable to tolerate macrolides.

Whole-cell, inactivated vaccines for pertussis have been associated with unacceptable levels of complications and have been replaced with acellular vaccines. Two **acellular vaccines** (one for children, one for adults) administered in combination with vaccines for tetanus and diphtheria are currently approved. Both vaccines contain inactivated pertussis toxin, filamentous hemagglutinin, and pertactin.

The pediatric vaccine is administered to children at the ages of 2, 4, 6, and 15 to 18 months, with the fifth dose between the ages of 4 and 6 years. The current recommendations for the adult vaccine is to administer it at 11 or 12 years of age, and then again to adults between the ages of 19 and 65.

Because pertussis is highly contagious in a susceptible population, and unrecognized infections in family members of a symptomatic patient can maintain disease in a community, azithromycin has been used for prophylaxis in select instances.

SUMMARY

Bordetella pertussis is a kind of very small gram-negative coccobacilli, non-fermentative but can oxidize amino acids as an energy source and strict aerobe. Growth in vitro requires prolonged incubation in media supplemented with charcoal, starch, blood, or albumin. Many virulence factors are responsible for adherence to eukaryotic cells and production of localized tissue destruction. Pertussis is a common infectious disease with worldwide distribution. Human is the only reservoir host of pertussis.

Children younger than 1 year and other nonvaccinated individuals are at greatest risk for pertussis infection. Disease spread route is person-to-person infectious aerosols. Pertussis is characterized by three stages: catarrhal, paroxysmal, and convalescent. Most of severe disease occur in nonvaccinated individuals, particularly infants and old people. Vaccines containing inactivated pertussis toxin, filamentous hemagglutinin, and pertactin are highly effective.

KEYWORDS

English	Chinese
Adenylate cyclase/hemolysin	腺苷酸环化酶 / 溶血素
Bordetella	鲍特菌属
Bordetella bronchiseptica	支气管败血鲍特菌
Bordetella holmesii	霍氏鲍特菌
Bordetella parapertussis	副百日咳鲍特菌
Bordetella pertussis	百日咳鲍特菌
Catarrhal stage	卡他期
Convalescent stage	恢复期

Dermonecrotic toxin	皮肤坏死毒素
Filamentous hemagglutinin	丝状血凝素
Paroxysmal stage	发作期
Pertactin	百日咳菌黏附素
Pertussis	百日咳
Pertussis toxin	百日咳毒素
Tracheal cytotoxin	气管细胞毒素

BIBLIOGRAPHY

1. Carbonetti N: Pertussis toxin and adenylate cyclase toxin: key virulence factors of *Bordetella pertussis* and cell biology tools, Future Microbiol 5: 455-469, 2010.

2. Cassiday P, et al: Polymorphism in *Bordetella pertussis* pertactin and pertussis toxin virulence factors in the United States, 1935-1999, J Infect Dis 182: 1402-1408, 2000.

3. Cherry J: Immunity to pertussis, Clin Infect Dis 44: 1278-1279, 2007.

4. De Gouw D, et al: Pertussis: a matter of immune modulation, FEMS Microbiol Rev 35: 441-474, 2011.

5. Edelman K, et al: Immunity to pertussis 5 years after booster immunization during adolescence, Clin Infect Dis 44: 1271-1277, 2007.

6. Guiso N: *Bordetella pertussis* and pertussis vaccines, Clin Infect Dis 49: 1565-1569, 2009.

7. Kirimanjeswara G, Mann P, Harvill E: Role of antibodies in immunity to *Bordetella* infections, Infect Immun 71: 1719-1724, 2003.

8. Mattoo S, Cherry J: Molecular pathogenesis, epidemiology, and clinical manifestations of respiratory infections due to *Bordetella pertussis* and other *Bordetella* subspecies, Clin Microbiol Rev 18: 326-382, 2005.

9. Preziosi M, Halloran M: Effects of pertussis vaccination on disease: vaccine efficacy in reducing clinical severity, Clin Infect Dis 37: 772-779, 2003.

10. Ward J, et al: *Bordetella pertussis* infections in vaccinated and unvaccinated adolescents and adults, as assessed in a national prospective randomized acellular pertussis vaccine trial (APERT), Clin Infect Dis 43: 151-157, 2006.

Chapter

26

Francisella and *Brucella*

Francisella and *Brucella* are important **zoonotic pathogens** that can cause significant human disease. These organisms have also gained notoriety as potential agents of bioterrorists. Although the organisms have some common properties (e.g., very **small coccobacilli**, fastidious and slow growth requirements, always pathogenic in humans), they are taxonomically unrelated.

FRANCISELLA TULARENSIS

Three species of the genus *Francisella* are associated with human disease, *Francisella tularensis*, *Francisella novicida*, and *Francisella philomiragia*. **F. tularensis** is the causative agent of **tularemia** (also called glandular fever, rabbit fever, tick fever, and deer fly fever) in animals and humans. *F. tularensis* is subdivided into three subspecies, based on their biochemical properties. Subspecies *tularensis* (type A) and subspecies *holarctica* (type B) are the most important, while *F. tularensis* subsp. *mediaasiatica* is rarely associated with human disease.

Physiology and Structure

F. tularensis is a very small (0.2 × 0.2 to 0.7 µm), faintly staining, gram-negative coccobacillus (Figure 26-1). The organism is nonmotile, has a thin lipid capsule, and has fastidious growth requirements (i.e., most strains require cysteine for growth). It is strictly aerobic and requires 3 or more days before growth is detected in culture.

Pathogenesis and Immunity

F. tularensis is an intracellular pathogen that can

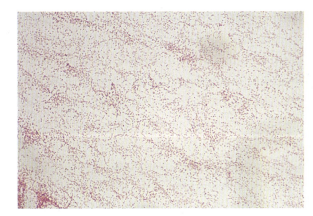

Figure 26-1 Gram stain of *Francisella tularensis* isolated in culture; note the extremely small, dotlike coccobacilli.

survive for prolonged periods in macrophages of the reticuloendothelial system because the organism inhibits phagosome-lysosome fusion through secretion of proteins that facilitate bacterial escape from the phagosome and subsequent replication in the macrophage cytosol. Pathogenic strains possess an anti-phagocytic, polysaccharide-rich capsule, and loss of the capsule is associated with decreased virulence. The capsule protects the bacteria from complement-mediated killing during the bacteremia phase of disease. Similar to all gram-negative rods, this organism has an endotoxin, but it is considerably less active than the endotoxin found in other gram-negative rods (e.g., *Escherichia coli*).

A strong, innate immune response with production of interferon-γ and tumor necrosis factor (TNF) is important for controlling bacterial replication in macrophages in the early phase of infection. Specific T-cell immunity is required for activation of macrophages for intracellular killing in the late stages of disease. B-cell-mediated immunity is less important for elimination of this facultative intracellular pathogen.

Epidemiology

F. tularensis subsp. *tularensis* (type A) is restricted to North America, while subsp. *holarctica* (type B) is endemic throughout the Northern Hemisphere. More than 200 species of mammals, as well as birds and blood-sucking arthropods, are infected naturally with *F. tularensis*. Type A infections are most commonly associated with exposure to lagomorphs (rabbits, hares) and cats; type B infections are associated with rodents and cats, but not lagomorphs. Infections caused by biting arthropods (e.g., hard ticks [*Ixodes, Dermacentor, Ambylomma* spp.], deer flies) are more common with type A than with type B strains.

The reported incidence of disease is low. In 2010, 124 cases were reported in the United States; however, the actual number of infections is likely to be much higher because tularemia is frequently unsuspected and is difficult to confirm by laboratory tests. Most of the infections occur during the summer (when exposure to infected ticks is greatest) and the winter (when hunters are exposed to infected rabbits). The incidence of disease increases dramatically when a relatively warm winter is followed by a wet summer, causing the tick population to proliferate. People at greatest risk for infection are hunters, laboratory personnel, and those exposed to ticks and other biting arthropods. In areas where the organism is endemic, it is said that if a rabbit is moving so slowly that it can be shot by a hunter or caught by a pet, the rabbit could be infected.

Clinical Diseases

Disease caused by *F. tularensis* is subdivided into several forms based on the clinical presentation:

Ulceroglandular tularemia is the most common manifestation. The skin lesion, which starts as a painful papule, develops at the site of the tick bite or direct inoculation of the organism into the skin (e.g., a laboratory accident). The papule then ulcerates and has a necrotic center and raised border. Localized lymph-

adenopathy and bacteremia are also typically present (although bacteremia may be difficult to document).

Oculoglandular tularemia (Figure 26-2) is a specialized form of the disease and results from direct contamination of the eye. The organism can be introduced into the eyes, for example, by contaminated fingers or through exposure to water or aerosols. Affected patients have a painful conjunctivitis and regional lymphadenopathy.

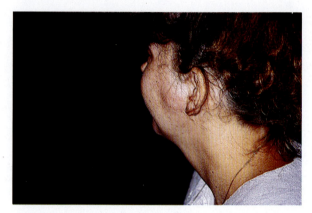

Figure 26-2 Patient with oculoglandular tularemia (note swelling beside the ear).

Pneumonic tularemia (Figure 26-3) results from inhalation of infectious aerosols and is associated with high morbidity and mortality unless the organism is recovered rapidly in blood cultures (it is generally difficult to detect in respiratory cultures). There is also concern that *F. tularensis* could be used as a biologic weapon. As such, creation of an infectious aerosol would be the most likely method of dispersal.

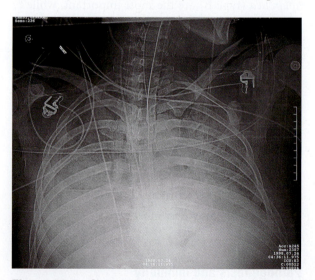

Figure 26-3 Chest radiograph of patient with pulmonary tularemia.

Laboratory Diagnosis

Detection of *F. tularensis* in Gram-stained aspirates from infected nodes or ulcers is almost always unsuccessful because the organism is extremely small and stains faintly (see Figure 26-1). A more sensitive and specific approach is direct staining of the clinical specimen with fluorescein-labeled antibodies directed against the organism. Antibody reagents against types A and B are available from the Centers for Disease Control and Prevention (CDC) and state public health facilities but are not available in most clinical laboratories.

F. tularensis can grow on chocolate agar or buffered charcoal yeast extract (BCYE) agar, media supplemented with cysteine that are used in most laboratories. Thus it is usually not necessary for a laboratory to use specialized media, such as cysteine blood agar or glucose cysteine agar. However, if infection with *F. tularensis* is suspected, the laboratory should be notified because *F. tularensis* grows slowly and may be overlooked if the cultures are not incubated for a prolonged period. In addition, because this organism is highly infectious, special care is required for microbiologic testing. Blood cultures are generally negative for the organism unless the cultures are incubated for a week or longer. Cultures of respiratory specimens will be positive if appropriate selective media are used to suppress the more rapidly growing bacteria from the upper respiratory tract. *F. tularensis* also grows on the selective media used for *Legionella* (e.g., BCYE agar). Aspirates of lymph nodes or draining sinuses are usually positive if the cultures are incubated for 3 days or longer.

Tularemia is diagnosed in most patients by the finding of a fourfold or greater increase in the titer of antibodies during the illness or a single titer of 1:160 or greater. However, antibodies (including IgG, IgM, and IgA) can persist for many years, making it difficult to differentiate between past and current disease. Reagents that are currently available react with subspecies *tularensis* and *holarctica* but not with *F. novicida* or *F. philomiragia*. Antibodies directed against *Brucella* can cross-react with *Francisella*. Therefore the diagnosis of tularemia should not be based solely on serologic tests.

Treatment, Prevention, and Control

Streptomycin was the traditional antibiotic of choice for the treatment of all forms of tularemia; however, this antibiotic is not readily available and is associated with a high level of toxicity. **Gentamicin** is now considered the antibiotic of choice. Doxycycline and ciprofloxacin can be used to treat mild infections. *F. tularensis* strains produce β-lactamase, which renders penicillins and cephalosporins ineffective. The mortality rate is less than 1% if patients are treated promptly but is much higher in untreated patients.

To prevent infection, people should avoid the reservoirs and vectors of infection (e.g., rabbits, ticks, biting insects), but this is often difficult. At a minimum, people should not handle ill-appearing rabbits and should wear gloves when skinning and eviscerating animals. Because the organism is present in the arthropod's feces and not saliva, the tick must feed for a prolonged time before the infection is transmitted. Prompt removal of the tick can therefore prevent infection. Wearing protective clothing and using insect repellents reduce the risk of exposure. Persons who have a high risk of exposure (e.g., exposure to an infectious aerosol) should be treated with prophylactic antibiotics. Interest in developing a live attenuated vaccine is motivated by fear of exposure to the bacteria as a bioterrorism agent; however, an effective vaccine is not currently available. Inactivated vaccines do not elicit protective cellular immunity.

BRUCELLA

Molecular studies of the genus *Brucella* demonstrate a close relationship among the strains and are consistent with a single genus; however, the genus has historically been subdivided into a number of species. Currently, there are 10 species of *Brucella*, with 4 species most commonly associated with human disease: *Brucella abortus*, *Brucella melitensis*, *Brucella suis*, and *Brucella canis*. The diseases caused by members of this genus are characterized by a number of names based on the original microbiologists who isolated and described the organisms (e.g., Sir David Bruce [brucellosis], Bernhard Bang [Bang disease]), its clinical presentation (undulant fever), and the sites of recognized outbreaks (e.g., Malta fever, Mediterranean remittent fever, rock fever of Gibraltar, county fever of Constantinople, fever of Crete). However, the most commonly used term is **brucellosis**, which will be used in this chapter.

Physiology and Structure

Brucellae are small (0.5 × 0.6 to 1.5 μm), nonmotile, nonencapsulated, gram-negative coccobacilli. The organism grows slowly in culture (taking a week or more) and generally requires complex growth media; is **strictly aerobic**, with some strains requiring supplemental carbon dioxide for growth; and does not ferment carbohydrates.

Colonies can assume both smooth (translucent, homogeneous) and rough (opaque, granular, or sticky) forms, as determined by the O antigen of the cell wall lipopolysaccharide (LPS). Antisera to one form (e.g., smooth) do not cross-react with the other form (e.g., rough). *Brucella* species can be further characterized by the relative proportion of antigenic epitopes, referred to as A and M antigens, that reside on the O polysaccharide chain of the smooth LPS.

Pathogenesis and Immunity

Brucella does not produce a detectable exotoxin, and the endotoxin is less toxic than that produced by other gram-negative rods. Reversion of smooth strains to the rough morphology is associated with greatly reduced virulence, so the O chain of the smooth LPS is an important marker for virulence. *Brucella* is also an intracellular parasite of the reticuloendothelial system. After the initial exposure, the organisms are phagocytosed by macrophages and monocytes. *Brucellae* survive and replicate in phagocytic cells by inhibiting phagosome-lysosome fusion, preventing release of toxic enzymes from intracellular granules, suppressing production of TNF-α, and inactivating hydrogen peroxide and superoxide by production of catalase and superoxide dismutase,

respectively. Phagocytosed bacteria are carried to the spleen, liver, bone marrow, lymph nodes, and kidneys. The bacteria secrete proteins that induce granuloma formation in these organs and destructive changes in these and other tissues occur in patients with advanced disease.

Epidemiology

Brucella infections have a worldwide distribution, with endemic disease most common in Latin America, Africa, the Mediterranean basin, the Middle East, and Western Asia. More than 500,000 documented cases are reported annually worldwide. Laboratory personnel are also at significant risk for infection through direct contact or inhalation of the organism. Disease in cattle, swine, sheep, and goats in the United States has been eliminated effectively through the destruction of infected animals and the vaccination of disease-free animals; thus infections in China are still very common. There are 56,989 reported infections in 2015.

Brucellosis in humans can be acquired by direct contact with the organism (e.g., a laboratory exposure), ingestion (e.g., consumption of contaminated food products), or inhalation. Of particular concern is the potential use of *Brucella* as a biologic weapon in which exposure would most likely be by inhalation.

Brucella causes mild or asymptomatic disease in the natural host: *B. abortus* infects cattle and American bison; *B. melitensis*, goats and sheep; *B. suis*, swine, reindeer, and caribou; and *B. canis*, dogs, foxes, and coyotes. The organism has a predilection for infecting organs rich in erythritol, a sugar metabolized by many *Brucella* strains in preference to glucose. Animal (but not human) tissues, including breast, uterus, placenta, and epididymis are rich in erythritol. The organisms thus localize in these tissues in nonhuman reservoirs and can cause sterility, abortions, or asymptomatic lifelong carriage. *Brucellae* are shed in high numbers in milk, urine, and birth products.

Clinical Diseases

The disease spectrum of brucellosis depends on the

infecting organism. *B. abortus* and *B. canis* tend to produce mild disease with rare suppurative complications. In contrast, *B. suis* causes the formation of destructive lesions and has a prolonged course. *B. melitensis* also causes severe disease with a high incidence of serious complications because the organisms can multiply to high concentrations in phagocytic cells.

Acute disease develops in approximately half of the patients infected with *Brucella*, with symptoms first appearing typically 1 to 3 weeks after exposure. Initial symptoms are nonspecific and consist of malaise, chills, sweats, fatigue, weakness, myalgias, weight loss, arthralgias, and nonproductive cough. Almost all patients have fever and this can be intermittent in untreated patients, hence the name undulant fever. Patients with advanced disease can have gastrointestinal tract symptoms (70% of patients), osteolytic lesions or joint effusions (20% to 60%), respiratory tract symptoms (25%), and less commonly, cutaneous, neurologic, or cardiovascular manifestations. Chronic infections can also develop in inadequately treated patients, with symptoms developing within 3 to 6 months after discontinuing antibiotic therapy. Relapses are associated with a persistent focus on infections (e.g., in bone, spleen, liver) and not with the development of antibiotic resistance.

Laboratory Diagnosis

Several blood samples should be collected for culture and serologic testing. Bone marrow cultures and cultures of infected tissues may also be useful.

Brucella organisms are readily stained using conventional techniques, but their intracellular location and small size make them difficult to detect in clinical specimens. Currently, specific immunofluorescent antibody tests are not available.

Brucella organisms grow slowly during primary isolation. The organisms can grow on most enriched blood agars and occasionally on MacConkey agar; however, incubation for 3 or more days may be required. **Blood cultures should be incubated for 2 weeks** before they are considered negative. More extended incubation of blood cultures is now unnec-essary with the use of automated culture systems.

Preliminary identification of *Brucella* is based on the isolate's microscopic and colonial morphology, positive oxidase and urease reactions, and reactivity with antibodies directed against *B. abortus* and *B. melitensis*. Identification at the genus level can also be accomplished by sequencing the 16S ribosomal ribonucleic acid (rRNA) gene.

Subclinical brucellosis and many cases of acute and chronic diseases are identified by a specific antibody response in the infected patient. Antibodies are detected in virtually all patients. IgM response is initially observed, after which both IgG and IgA antibodies are produced. Antibodies can persist for many months or years; thus a significant increase in the antibody titer is required to provide definitive serologic evidence of current disease. A presumptive diagnosis can be made if there is a fourfold increase in the titer or a single titer is greater than or equal to 1:160. High antibody titers (1:160 or more) are noted in 5% to 10% of the population living in endemic areas; thus serologic tests should be used to confirm the clinical diagnosis of brucellosis and not to form the basis of the diagnosis. The antigen used in the *Brucella* serum agglutination test (SAT) is from *B. abortus*. Antibodies directed against *B. melitensis* or *B. suis* cross-react with this antigen; however, there is no cross-reactivity with *B. canis*. The specific *B. canis* antigen must be used to diagnose infections with this organism. Antibodies directed against other genera of bacteria (e.g., some strains of *Escherichia*, *Salmonella*, *Vibrio*, *Yersinia*, *Stenotrophomonas*, and *Francisella*) are also reported to cross-react with the *B. abortus* antigen.

Treatment, Prevention, and Control

Tetracyclines, with doxycycline the preferred agent, are generally active against most strains of *Brucella*; however, because this is a bacteriostatic drug, relapse is common after an initially successful response. The World Health Organization currently recommends the combination of **doxycycline with rifampin**. Because the tetracyclines are toxic to young children and fetuses, doxycycline should be replaced with trimethoprim-sulfamethoxazole for pregnant women and for children younger than 8 years. Treatment must be continued for 6 weeks or longer for it to be successful. Fluoroquinolones, macrolides, penicillins, and cephalosporins are either ineffective or have unpredictable activity. Relapse of disease is caused by inadequate therapy and not the development of antibiotic resistance.

Control of human brucellosis is accomplished through control of the disease in livestock, as demonstrated in the United States. This requires systematic identification (by serologic testing) and elimination of infected herds and animal vaccination (currently with the rough strain of *B. abortus* strain RB51). The avoidance of unpasteurized dairy products, the observance of appropriate safety procedures in the clinical laboratory, and the wearing of protective clothing by abattoir workers are further ways to prevent brucellosis. The live attenuated *B. abortus* and *B. melitensis* vaccines have been used successfully to prevent infection in animal herds. Vaccines have not been developed against *B. suis* or *B. canis*, and the existing vaccines cannot be used in humans because they produce symptomatic disease. The lack of an effective human vaccine is of concern because *Brucella* (as well as *Francisella*) could be used as an agent of bioterrorism.

SUMMARY

Francisella tularensis

F. tularensis is very small gram-negative coccobacilli (0.2 × 0.2 to 0.7 μm), strict aerobe, non-fermenter. It requires specialized media and prolonged incubation for growth in culture. As intracellular pathogen, it harbors antiphagocytic capsule and is resistant to killing in serum by phagocytes. Clinical symptoms and prognosis are determined by route of infection from ulceroglandular, oculoglandular, glandular, typhoidal, oropharyngeal, to gastrointestinal and pneumonic infection.

Wild mammals, domestic animals, birds, fish, and blood-sucking arthropods are **F. tularensis**'s common reservoirs. Humans are accidental hosts. However, only rabbits, cats, hard ticks, and biting flies are most commonly associated with human tularemia;

Brucella

The initial nonspecific symptoms of **Brucellosis caused by** brucella species are malaise, chills, sweats, fatigue, myalgias, weight loss, arthralgias, and fever; it can be intermittent; then, Brucella patients can progress to systemic involvement (gastrointestinal tract, bones or joints, respiratory tract, other organs). Infected animal tissues are rich in erythritol (e.g., breast, uterus, placenta, epididymis). Animal reservoirs are goats and sheep (*Brucella melitensis*); cattle and American bison (*Brucella abortus*); swine, reindeer, and caribou (*Brucella suis*); and dogs, foxes, and coyotes (*Brucella canis*).

KEYWORDS

English	Chinese
Zoonotic pathogens	人兽共患病原体
Francisella tularensis	野兔热弗朗西丝菌
Tularemia	野兔热
Brucella	布鲁菌属
Brucella abortus	牛布鲁菌（流产布鲁菌）
Brucella melitensis	羊布鲁菌
Brucella suis	猪布鲁菌
Brucella canis	犬布鲁菌
Undulant fever	波浪热

BIBLIOGRAPHY

1. Barker J, et al: The Francisella tularensis pathogenicity island encodes a secretion system that is required for phagosome escape and virulence, Mol Microbiol 74: 1459-1470, 2009.

2. Boschiroli M, et al: Brucellosis: a worldwide zoonosis, Curr Opin Microbiol 4: 58-64, 2001.

3. Dennis D, et al: Tularemia as a biological weapon: medical and public health management, JAMA 285: 2763-2773, 2001.

4. Farlow J et al: *Francisella tularensis* in the United States, Emerg Infect Dis 12: 1835-1841, 2005.

5. Mann B, Ark N: Rationally designed tularemia vaccines, Expert Rev Vaccines 8: 877-885, 2009.

6. Pappas G, et al: Brucellosis, N Engl J Med 352: 2325-2336, 2005.

7. Staples J, et al: Epidemiologic and molecular analysis of human tularemia, United States, 1964-2004, Emerg Infect Dis 12: 1113-1118, 2006.

8. Starr T, et al: *Brucella* intracellular replication requires trafficking through the late endosomal/lysosomal compartment, Traffic 9: 678-694, 2008.

9. Zhou J, et al: Investigation of animal brucellosis in partial areas in China, the 3rd Symposium on Chinese Veterinary Public Health Association (CAAV), 2012.

Legionella

The family Legionellaceae consists of four genera: *Legionella*, *Fluoribacter*, *Tatlockia*, and *Sarcobium*. *Legionella is* the most important genus with 53 species and 3 subspecies. Approximately half of these species have been implicated in human disease, with the others found in environmental sources. *L. pneumophila* is the cause of 90% of all infections; serotypes 1 and 6 are most commonly isolated. *Fluoribacter* consists of 3 species, *Tatlockia* contains 2 species and *Sarcobium* has 1 species. *Fluoribacter bozemanae* and *Tatlockia micdadei*, formerly members of the genus *Legionella*, cause disease similar to *L. pneumophila* and are commonly referred to in the literature by their historical names. The emphasis of this chapter will be on *L. pneumophila*.

Physiology and Structure

Members of the genus *Legionella* are **slender, pleomorphic, gram-negative rods** measuring 0.3 to 0.9 × 2 μm in size. The organisms characteristically appear as short coccobacilli when observed in tissue but are very pleomorphic (up to 20 μm long) on artificial media (Figure 27-1). Legionellae in clinical specimens do not stain with common reagents but can be seen in tissues stained with Dieterle silver stain. One species, *T. micdadei*, can also be stained with acid-fast stains, but the organism loses this property when grown in vitro.

Legionellae are obligatively aerobic and nutritionally fastidious. They require media supplemented with L-cysteine, and growth is enhanced in by iron. Growth of these bacteria on supplemented media but not on conventional blood agar media has been used as the basis for the preliminary identification

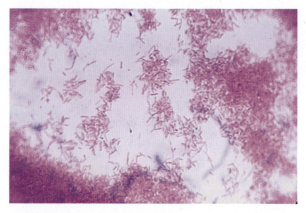

Figure 27-1 Gram stain of *Legionella pneumophila* grown on buffered charcoal yeast extract agar. Note the pleomorphic forms characteristic of *Legionella*. (Courtesy Dr. Janet Stout, Pittsburgh, Penn.)

of clinical isolates. The bacteria have developed multiple methods to acquire iron from their host cells or in vitro media, and loss of this ability is associated with loss of virulence. The organisms derive energy from the metabolism of amino acids but not carbohydrates.

Pathogenesis and Immunity

Respiratory tract disease caused by *Legionella* species develops in susceptible people who inhale infectious aerosols. Legionellae are facultative **intracellular bacteria** that multiply in free-living amoebae in nature, and in alveolar macrophages, monocytes, and alveolar epithelial cells in infected hosts. This ability to infect and replicate in macrophages is critical for pathogenesis. The replicative cycle is initiated by binding complement component C3b to an outer membrane porin protein on the bacterial surface. The bacteria then binds to the CR3 complement receptors on mononuclear phagocytes, after which the organisms penetrate the cell through endocytosis. The bacteria are not killed in the cells by exposure to toxic superoxide, hydrogen peroxide, and hydroxyl radicals because phagolysosome fusion is inhibited. Chemokines and cytokines released by the infected macrophages stimulate a robust inflammatory response that is characteristic of infections with *Legionella*. The organisms proliferate in their intracellular vacuole and produce proteolytic enzymes (phosphatase, lipase, and nuclease) that eventually kill the host cell when the vacuole is lysed. Immunity to disease is primarily cell mediated, with humoral immunity playing a minor role. The bacteria are not killed until sensitized helper T cells (Th$_1$ cells) activate the parasitized macrophages. Production of interferon-γ is critical for elimination of *Legionella* organisms.

Epidemiology

Sporadic and epidemic legionellosis has a **worldwide distribution.** The bacteria are commonly present in natural bodies of water, such as lakes and streams, as well as in air conditioning cooling towers and condensers and in water systems (e.g., showers, hot tubs). Human infections are most commonly associated with **exposure to contaminated aerosols** (e.g., air conditioning cooling towers, whirlpool spas, shower heads, water misters). The organisms can survive in moist environments for a long time, at relatively high temperatures, and in the presence of disinfectants, such as chlorine. One reason for their survival is that the bacteria parasitize amoebae in the water and replicate in this protected environment (similar to their replication in human macrophages). The bacteria also survive in biofilms that develop in the pipes of water systems.

The incidence of infections caused by *Legionella* species is unknown because disease is difficult to document. It is reasonable to conclude that contact with the organism and acquisition of immunity after an asymptomatic infection are common.

Although sporadic outbreaks of the disease occur throughout the year, most epidemics of the infection occur in late summer and autumn because the organism proliferates in water reservoirs during the warm months. More than 80% of the documented infections in the United States are in persons age 40 years or older, presumably because they are more likely to have decreased cellular immunity and compromised pulmonary function. A significant proportion of reported cases are acquired in hospitals because of the predominance of high-risk patients. Person-to-person spread or an animal reservoir has not been demonstrated.

Clinical Diseases

Asymptomatic *Legionella* infections are believed to be relatively common. Symptomatic infections primarily affect the lungs and present in one of two forms (Table 27-1): (1) an influenza-like illness (referred to as **Pontiac fever**) and (2) a severe form of pneumonia (i.e., **Legionnaires' disease**).

Table 27-1 Comparison of Diseases Caused by *Legionella*

	Legionnaires' Disease	Pontiac Fever
Epidemiology		
Presentation	Epidemic, sporadic	Epidemic
Attack rate (%)	<5	>90
Person-to-person spread	No	No
Underlying pulmonary disease	Yes	No
Time of onset	Epidemic disease in late summer or autumn; endemic disease throughout year	Throughout year
Clinical Manifestations		
Incubation period (days)	2-10	1-2
Pneumonia	Yes	No
Course	Requires antibiotic therapy	Self-limited
Mortality (%)	15-20; higher if diagnosis is delayed	<1

Pontiac Fever

L. pneumophila was responsible for causing a self-limited, febrile illness in people working at the Pontiac, Michigan, Public Health Department in 1968. Fever, chills, myalgia, malaise, and headache, but no clinical evidence of pneumonia, are characteristic of the disease. The symptoms developed over 12 hours, persisted for 2 to 5 days, and then resolved spontaneously without antibiotic treatment and with minimal morbidity and no deaths. Other outbreaks of Pontiac fever, with and without *Legionella* pneumonia, have been reported. The precise pathogenesis of this syndrome is unknown, although it is believed that the pathology of this disease is caused by a hypersensitivity reaction to bacterial toxin (e.g., endotoxin).

Legionnaires' Disease

Legionnaires' disease (legionellosis) is characteristically more severe and, if untreated, promptly causes considerable morbidity, often leading to death in 15% of previously healthy individuals and up to 75% in immunocompromised patients. After an incubation period of 2 to 10 days, systemic signs of an acute illness appear abruptly (e.g., fever and chills, a dry, nonproductive cough, headache). Multiorgan disease involving the gastrointestinal tract, central nervous system, liver, and kidneys is common. The primary manifestation is pneumonia, with multilobar consolidation and inflammation and microabscesses in lung tissue observed on histopathologic studies. Pulmonary function steadily deteriorates in susceptible patients with untreated disease. The clinical presentation of pneumonia caused by *Legionella* is not unique, so laboratory tests are required to confirm the diagnosis.

Laboratory Diagnosis

Since *Legionella* was first isolated, the laboratory diagnosis of infections caused by this organism has undergone a significant transition. Initial testing depended on microscopy, culture, and serology. Although culture remains the gold standard for diagnosis, microscopy and serology have been replaced by immunoassays for the detection of *Legionella*-specific antigens in urine and nucleic acid amplification assays.

Legionellae in clinical specimens **stain poorly** with Gram stain and the small, intracellular bacteria are rarely recognized. Immunoassays are used to detect soluble ***Legionella* serogroup 1-specific lipopolysaccharide antigens** excreted in the urine of infected patients. The sensitivity of these assays for *L. pneumophila* serogroup 1 is relatively high (range, 60% to 90%), particularly with concentrated urines, but the assays do not reliably detect other serogroups or *Legionella* species. This is an important distinction because *L. pneumophila* serogroup 1 is responsible for 80% to 90% of community-acquired infections but is responsible for less than 50% of hospital-acquired infections. Antigens persist in the urine of treated patients, with almost 50% of patients remaining positive at 1 month and 25% at 2 months. Persistence is particularly common with immunosuppressed patients, in which antigens can persist for up to 1 year. Nucleic acid amplification (NAA) assays are highly specific and have a sensitivity equivalent to culture for the detection of *Legionella* species in respiratory secretions (i.e., bronchial alveolar lavage fluid). Although these assays are not widely available, it is anticipated that they will be the diagnostic method of choice in the future. The presence of inhibitors in respiratory secretions may cause false-negative reactions, so all specimens should still be cultured. In addition, culture has been demonstrated to be more sensitive than NAA assays for tissue specimens.

Although legionellae were difficult to grow initially, commercially available media now make culture easy (test sensitivity, 80% to >90%). As mentioned above, legionellae require L-cysteine, and recovery is enhanced in the presence of iron salts (supplied in hemoglobin or ferric pyrophosphate). The medium most commonly used for the isolation of legionellae is **buffered charcoal yeast extract (BCYE) agar,** although other supplemented media have been used. Antibiotics can be added to suppress the growth of rapidly growing, contaminating bacteria. Legionellae grow in air or 3% to 5% carbon dioxide at 35°C after 3 to 5 days. The small (1 to 3 mm) colonies have a characteristic ground-glass appearance.

Legionellosis caused by *L. pneumophila* serogroup 1 is commonly diagnosed with the use of enzyme immunoassays or indirect fluorescent antibody tests to measure a serologic response to infection. A fourfold or greater increase in the antibody titer (to a level of 1:128 or greater) is considered diagnostic. However, these tests are relatively insensitive and nonspecific, particularly when polyclonal reagents are used. The response may be delayed. Although a significant increase in the titer can be detected in 25% to 40% of patients in the first week of disease, up to 6 months may be required before seroconversion is demonstrated for the remaining patients. Because high titers can persist for prolonged periods, a single, high-antibody titer cannot be used to define active disease.

Treatment, Prevention, and Control

In vitro susceptibility tests are not performed with legionellae because the organisms grow poorly on the media commonly used for these tests. In addition, some antibiotics that appear active in vitro are ineffective in treating infections. One explanation is that these antibiotics cannot penetrate the macrophages where the legionellae survive and multiply. Accumulated clinical experience indicates that **macrolides** (e.g., azithromycin, clarithromycin) or **fluoroquinolones** (e.g., ciprofloxacin, levofloxacin) should be used to treat *Legionella* infections. β-Lactam antibiotics are ineffective because most isolates produce β-lactamases, and these antibiotics do not penetrate macrophages. Specific therapy for Pontiac fever is generally unnecessary because it is a self-limited hypersensitivity disease.

Prevention of legionellosis requires identification of the environmental source of the organism and reduction of the microbial burden. Hyperchlorination of the water supply and the maintenance of elevated water temperatures have proved moderately successful. However, elimination of *Legionella* organisms from a water supply is often difficult or impossible to achieve. Because the organism has a low potential for causing disease, reducing the number of organisms in the water supply is often an adequate control measure. Hospitals with patients at high risk for disease should monitor their water supply on a regular basis for the presence of *Legionella* and their

hospital population for disease. If hyperchlorination or superheating of the water does not eliminate disease (complete elimination of the organisms in the water supply is probably not possible), continuous copper-silver ionization of the water supply may be necessary.

SUMMARY

Legionella species are slender, pleomorphic, nonfermentative, gram-negative rods, Stains poorly with common reagents and culture is nutritionally fastidious with requirement for L-cysteine and enhanced growth with iron salts. Another specific characteristic of *Legionella* species is capable of replication in alveolar macrophages and amoebae in nature and prevents phagolysosome fusion.

Legionella species are commonly found in natural bodies of water, cooling towers, condensers, and water systems (including hospital systems). *Legionella* species are capable of induce sporadic, epidemic, and nosocomial infections and are primary responsible for Legionnaires' disease and Pontiac fever. Patients at high risk for symptomatic disease include patients with compromised pulmonary function and patients with decreased cellular immunity (particularly transplant patients).

Microscopy is insensitive. Antigen tests are sensitive for *L. pneumophila* serogroup 1 but have poor sensitivity for other serogroups and species. Culture on buffered charcoal yeast extract agar is the diagnostic test of choice. Seroconversion must be demonstrated; this can take as long as 6 months to develop; positive serology may persist for months. Nucleic acid amplification assays are as sensitive and specific as culture.

KEYWORDS

English	Chinese
Intracellular bacteria	胞内寄生菌
Legionella	军团菌属
Legionella pneumophila	嗜肺军团菌
Legionellosis	军团菌病
Pontiac fever	庞蒂亚克热

BIBLIOGRAPHY

1. Edelstein P: Antimicrobial chemotherapy for Legionnaires disease: time for a change, Ann Intern Med 129: 328-330, 1998.

2. Edelstein P: Urine antigen tests positive for Pontiac fever: implications for diagnosis and pathogenesis, Clin Infect Dis 44: 229-231, 2007.

3. Fields BS, Benson RF, Besser RE: Legionella and Legionnaires' disease: 25 years of investigation, Clin Microbiol Rev 15: 506-526, 2002.

4. Greenberg D, et al: Problem pathogens: paediatric legionellosis—implications for improved diagnosis, Lancet 6: 529-535, 2006.

5. Hayden RT, et al: Direct detection of Legionella species from bronchoalveolar lavage and open lung biopsy specimens: comparison of LightCycler PCR, in situ hybridization, direct fluorescence antigen detection, and culture, J Clin Microbiol 39: 2618-2626, 2001.

6. Helbig JH, et al: Clinical utility of urinary antigen detection for diagnosis of community-acquired, travel-associated, and nosocomial Legionnaires' disease, J Clin Microbiol 41: 837-840, 2003.

7. Kim MJ, et al: Characterization of a lipoprotein common to Legionella species as a urinary broad-spectrum antigen for diagnosis of Legionnaires disease, J Clin Microbiol 41: 2974-2979, 2003.

8. Modol J, et al: Hospital-acquired Legionnaires disease in a university hospital: impact of the copper-silver ionization system, Clin Infect Dis 44: 263-265, 2007.

9. Neil K, Berkelman R: Increasing incidence of legionellosis in the United States, 1990-2005: changing epidemiologic trends, Clin Infect Dis 47: 591-599, 2008.

10. Newton H, et al: Molecular pathogenesis of infections caused by Legionella pneumophila, Clin Microbiol Rev 23: 274-298, 2010.

11. Sopena N, et al: Factors related to persistence of Legionella urinary antigen excretion in patients with legionnaires' disease, Eur J Clin Microbiol Infect Dis 21: 845-848, 2002.

12. Stout J, Yu V: Legionellosis, N Engl J Med 337: 681-687, 1997.

Chapter 28

Miscellaneous gram-negative rods

BARTONELLA

As with many groups of bacteria studied in recent years, analysis of the 16S ribosomal ribonucleic acid (rRNA) gene has led to the reorganization of the genus *Bartonella.* Currently, 24 species are included in the genus, with 3 species most commonly associated with human disease: *B. bacilliformis, B. henselae,* and *B. quintana.* Members of the genus are short (0.2 to 0.6 × 0.5 to 1.0 μm), gram-negative, coccobacillary or bacillary rods with fastidious growth requirements. Although the organisms can grow aerobically on enriched blood agar, prolonged incubation (2 to 6 weeks; dividing time, 24 hours) in a humid (37℃) atmosphere supplemented with carbon dioxide is required for their initial recovery.

Members of the genus *Bartonella* are found in a variety of animal reservoirs and are typically present without evidence of disease. The spread of most *Bartonella* species from colonized animals to humans is either by direct contact or by insect vectors (e.g., *B. bacilliformis*—sandflies; *B. quintana*—lice; *B. henselae*—fleas). Most infections with Bartonella are characterized by recurrent fevers and/or angioproliferative lesions (blood filled cysts).

B. bacilliformis, the original member of the genus, is responsible for Carrión disease, an acute, hemolytic bacteremia consisting of fevers and severe anemia (Oroya fever), followed by a chronic vasoproliferative form (verruga peruana, "Peruvian wart"). The disease is restricted to Andes mountain region of Peru, Ecuador, and Colombia, the endemic area of the sandfly vector Phlebotomus. After the bite of an infected sandfly, the bacteria enter the blood, mul-tiply, and penetrate into erythrocytes and endothelial cells. This process increases the fragility of the infected cells and facilitates their clearance by the reticuloendothelial system, leading to acute anemia. Myalgia, arthralgia, and headache are also common. This stage of illness ends with the development of humoral immunity. In the chronic stage of Carrión disease, 1- to 2-cm cutaneous nodules, often engorged with blood ("angioproliferative"), appear over the course of 1 to 2 months and may persist for months to years. The link between verruga peruana skin lesions and Oroya fever was demonstrated by a medical student, Carrión, who infected himself with aspirates from the skin lesions and died of Oroya fever. This act of scientific recklessness immortalized him and illustrates the high mortality associated with this disease if untreated.

Bartonella quintana was originally described as the causative organism of trench fever (also called "5-day" fever), a disease prevalent during World War I. Infection can vary from asymptomatic to a severe, debilitating illness. Typically, patients have severe headache, fever, weakness, and pain in the long bones (particularly the tibia). The fever can recur at 5-day intervals, hence the name of the disease. Although trench fever does not cause death, the illness can be very severe. No animal reservoir for this disease has been identified. Rather, exposure to contaminated feces of the human body louse spreads disease from person-to-person.

B. quintana is also associated with a spectrum of diseases in immunocompromised patients, particular patients infected with the human immunodeficiency virus (HIV): recurrent fevers with bacteremia and bacillary angiomatosis. Bacteremia is characterized by an insidious onset of malaise, body aches, fatigue, weight loss, headaches, and recurrent fevers. This can lead to endocarditis or more commonly vascular proliferative diseases of the skin (bacillary angiomatosis; Figure 28-1), subcutaneous tissues, or bone. The vascular lesions appear as multiple, blood-filled nodules (resembling verruga peruana). As with trench fever, the vector of these diseases appears to be the human body louse, and disease is primarily restricted to the homeless population, in whom personal hygiene is substandard.

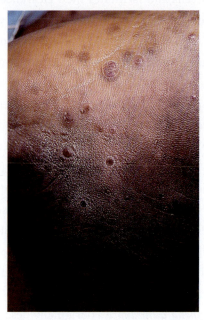

Figure 28-1 Skin lesions of bacillary angiomatosis caused by *Bartonella henselae*. (From Cohen J, Powderly WG: *Infectious diseases*, ed 2, St Louis, 2004, Mosby.)

B. henselae is also responsible for bacillary angiomatosis; however, it primarily involves the skin, lymph nodes, liver (peliosis hepatis), or spleen (splenic peliosis). The reasons for this differential tissue affinity are not known. Also like *B. quantana*, *B. henselae* can cause subacute endocarditis. The reservoirs for *B. henselae* are cats and their fleas. The bacteria are carried asymptomatically in the feline oropharynx and can cause transient bacteremia, particularly in young or feral cats. *B. henselae* is responsible for another disease acquired after exposure to cats (e.g., scratches, bites, contact with the contaminated feces of cat fleas): cat-scratch disease. Typically, cat-scratch

disease is a benign infection in children, characterized by chronic regional adenopathy of the lymph nodes draining the site of contact. Although most infections are self-limited, dissemination can occur to the liver, spleen, eye, or central nervous system. Bacteria may be seen in the lymph node tissues; however, culture is virtually always negative. A definitive diagnosis is based on the characteristic presentation and serologic evidence of a recent infection. Cultures are not useful because relatively few organisms are present in the tissues as a result of the vigorous cellular immune reaction in immunocompetent patients. In contrast, *B. henselae* can be isolated from blood collected from immunocompromised patients with chronic bacteremia, if the cultures are incubated for 4 weeks or more (Figure 28-2).

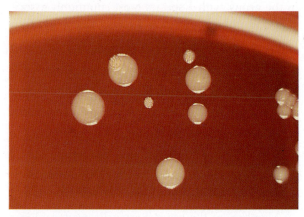

Figure 28-2 *Bartonella henselae* growing on blood agar plates; note the two typical colonial morphologies. (From Cohen J, Powderly WG: *Infectious diseases*, ed 2, St Louis, 2004, Mosby.)

Untreated Oroya fever has a mortality that exceeds 40%, so it is recommended that B. bacilliformis infections should be treated with chloramphenicol combined with a β-lactam antibiotic (e.g., penicillin). Although the value of treating cat-scratch disease is controversial, azithromycin is the drug of choice if treatment is used. Alternative therapy includes treatment with clarithromycin or rifampin. Oral erythromycin, doxycycline or azithromycin is most commonly used for treatment of other *B. quintana* and *B. henselae* infections. Penicillinase-resistant penicillins, first-generation cephalosporins, and clindamycin do not appear active in vitro against Bartonella. The incidence of Bartonella infections in HIV-infected patients has declined in recent years because these patients are treated routinely with azithromycin or clarithromycin for prevention of Mycobacterium avium infections.

CARDIOBACTERIUM

Cardiobacterium hominis is named for the predilection of this bacterium to cause endocarditis in humans. These bacteria are nonmotile, facultatively anaerobic, and characteristically small (1 × 1 to 2 μm) pleomorphic, gram-negative or gram-variable rods. The bacteria are fermentative, oxidase positive, and catalase negative. *C. hominis* is present in the upper respiratory tract of most healthy people.

Endocarditis is the primary human disease caused by *C. hominis* and the related species *Cardiobacterium valvarum*. Many infections are likely to be unreported or undiagnosed because of the low virulence of this organism and its slow growth in vitro. Most patients with Cardiobacterium endocarditis have preexisting heart disease and either a history of oral disease or have undergone a dental procedure before the clinical symptoms developed. The organisms are able to enter the blood from the oropharynx, adhere to the damaged heart tissue, and then slowly multiply. The course of disease is insidious and subacute; patients typically have symptoms (e.g., fatigue, malaise, and low-grade fever) for months before seeking medical care. Complications are rare, and complete recovery after appropriate antibiotic therapy is common.

The isolation of *C. hominis* from blood cultures confirms the diagnosis of endocarditis. The organism grows slowly in culture, requiring 1 week or more for growth to be detected. *C. hominis* appears in broth cultures as discrete clumps that can be easily overlooked. The organism requires enhanced carbon dioxide and humidity levels to grow on agar media, with 1-mm pinpoint colonies seen on blood or chocolate agar plates after 2 days of incubation. The organism does not grow on MacConkey agar or other selective media commonly used for gram-negative rods. *C. hominis* can be readily identified from its growth properties, microscopic morphology, and reactivity in biochemical tests.

C. hominis is susceptible to many antibiotics, and most infections are treated successfully with penicillin or ampicillin for 2 to 6 weeks, although penicillin-resistant strains have been reported. *C. hominis* endocarditis in people with preexisting heart disease is prevented by the maintenance of good oral hygiene and the use of antibiotic prophylaxis at the time of dental procedures. Long-acting penicillin is effective prophylaxis. Erythromycin should not be used because *C. hominis* is commonly resistant to it.

CAPNOCYTOPHAGA AND DYSGONOMONAS

Members of the genus *Capnocytophaga* are filamentous, gram-negative rods capable of aerobic and anaerobic growth in the presence of carbon dioxide. The genus is subdivided into two groups: (1) dysgonic fermenter 1 (DF-1) and (2) dysgonic fermenter 2 (DF-2). DF-1 strains colonize the human oropharynx and are associated with periodontitis, septicemia (particularly in patients who have undergone splenectomy or have compromised hepatic function [cirrhosis]), and rarely endocarditis. DF-2 strains colonize the oral cavities of cats and dogs and are associated with bite wounds. A third group of dysgonic fermenters was transferred from this genus to a new genus, *Dysgonomonas*. These bacteria are associated with gastroenteritis in immunocompromised patients.

Capnocytophaga and Dysgonomonas initially grow slowly in culture, requiring 2 or more days before colonies are observed on blood agar plates. Capnocytophaga appear as long, thin rods with tapered ends ("fusiform" shaped), while Dysgonomonas are small, gram-negative coccobacilli. Dysgonomonas colonies have a characteristic strawberry-like odor. Both genera can be identified at the genus level by biochemical tests. Because some strains of Capnocytophaga and Dysgonomonas produce β-lactamases, treatment with the combination of a β-lactam/β-lactamase inhibitor, such as amoxicillin-clavulanate, is recommended. Resistance of some strains to fluoroquinolones is reported and most strains are resistant to the aminoglycosides.

STREPTOBACILLUS

Streptobacillus moniliformis, the causative agent of rat-bite fever, is a long, thin (0.1 to 0.5 × 1 to 5 μm), gram-negative rod that tends to stain poorly and to be more pleomorphic in older cultures. Granules, bulbous swellings resembling a string of beads, and extremely long filaments may be seen (Figure 28-3).

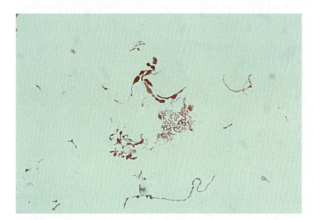

Figure 28-3   Gram stain of *Streptobacillus moniliformis*; note the pleomorphic forms and bulbous swellings.

Streptobacillus is found in the nasopharynx of rats and other small rodents, as well as transiently in animals that feed on rodents (e.g., dogs, cats). Human infections result from rodent bites (rat-bite fever;) or much less commonly from consumption of contaminated food or water (Haverhill fever). Most cases of rat-bite fever in the United States are in children with pet rats, laboratory workers, and pet shop employees. After a 2- to 10-day incubation period, the onset of rat-bite fever is abrupt, characterized by irregular fever, headache, chills, muscle pain, and migratory pain in multiple joints (polyarthralgias). A maculopapular or petechial rash develops a few days later with involvement extending to the hands and feet. This hemorrhagic rash in a patient with a recent history of a rat bite and migratory polyarthralgias is diagnostic. In the absence of effective antibiotics, rat-bite fever is associated with a 10% mortality rate. Despite effective treatment, some patients have persistent polyarthralgias, fatigue, and a slowly resolving rash.

Laboratory confirmation of Streptobacillus infections is difficult. Blood and joint fluid should be collected, and the laboratory should be notified that *S. moniliformis* is suspected because growth of the organism requires use of enriched media supplemented with 15% blood, 20% horse or calf serum, or 5% ascitic fluid. *S. moniliformis* grows slowly, taking at least 3 days to be isolated. When grown in broth, it has the appearance of "puffballs." Small, round colonies are seen when grown on agar, and the colonies of cell wall-defective variants resemble fried eggs (heaped center with spreading edges) on agar media. It is difficult to identify the organisms by biochemical tests because they are relatively inactive, although acid is produced from glucose and other selected carbohydrates. The most reliable method for identifying isolates is to sequence the 16S rRNA gene. *S. moniliformis* is susceptible to many antibiotics, including penicillin (not active against cell wall-defective variants) and tetracycline.

SUMMARY

Bartonella bacilliformis
Bartonella bacilliformis causes a unique clinical syndrome known as Bartonellosis or Carrion's disease in human, including severe anemia (Oroya fever), and chronic cutaneous blood-filled nodules

Bartonella quintana
Clinical manifestations of trench fever caused by *B. quintana* range from asymptomatic infection to severe, life-threatening illness. Few of the common symptoms include severe headache, fever, weakness, and pain in the long bones, constipation, insomnia, dyspnea, and abdominal pain.

Bartonella henselae
Bartonella henselae is responsible for a number of clinical illnesses, such as cat scratch disease or cat scratch fever, bacillary angiomatosis, bacteremia, endocarditis, and peliosis hepatis.

Cardiobacterium hominis
Cardiobacterium hominis is one of the HACEK members (*H. paraphrophilus*, *H. parainfluenzae*, *A. actinomycetemcomitans*, *A. aphrophilus*, *Eikenella corrodens*,

and so on). *C. hominis* causes native valve endocarditis in human.

Capnocytophaga Species

Capnocytophaga species cause a lot of clinical manifestations ranging from periodontitis, bacteremia, and endocarditis (from dysgonic fermenter 1 [DF-1] species) to dog or cat bite wounds (from DF-2 species).

Streptobacillus moniliformis

S. moniliformis causes rat-bite fever (RBF), an infectious disease in North America. The common symptoms of RBF include irregular fever, headache, chills, myalgia, and arthralgia associated with rodent bite; pharyngitis and vomiting are associated with exposure to bacteria in food or water.

KEYWORDS

English	Chinese
Bartonella	巴通体
Bartonella bacilliformis	杆状菌巴通体
Carrión disease	巴尔通体病
Oroya fever	奥罗亚热
Verruga peruana	秘鲁疣
Bartonella quintana	五日热巴通体
Trench fever	战壕热，五日热
Bacillary angiomatosis	杆菌性血管瘤病
Subacute endocarditis	亚急性心内膜炎
Bartonella henselae	汉赛巴通体
Cat-scratch disease	猫抓病
Cardiobacterium hominis	人心杆菌
Capnocytophaga Species	纤维菌
Streptobacillus moniliformis	念珠状链杆菌
Rat-bite fever	鼠咬热

BIBLIOGRAPHY

1. Agan BK, Dolan MJ: Laboratory diagnosis of *Bartonella* infections, Clin Lab Med 22: 937-962, 2002.

2. Anderson B, Neuman M: *Bartonella* spp. as emerging human pathogens, Clin Microbiol Rev 10: 203-219, 1997.

3. Elliott S: Rat bite fever and *Streptobacillus moniliformis*, Clin Microbiol Rev 20: 13-22, 2007.

4. Koehler J, et al: Molecular epidemiology of *Bartonella* infections in patients with bacillary angiomatosis-peliosis, N Engl J Med 337: 1876-1883, 1997.

5. Koehler J, et al: Prevalence of *Bartonella* infection among human immunodeficiency virus-infected patients with fever, Clin Infect Dis 37: 550-666, 2003.

6. La Scola B, Raoult D: Culture of *Bartonella quintana* and *Bartonella henselae* from human samples: a 5-year experience (1993 to 1998), J Clin Microbiol 37: 1899-1905, 1999.

7. Malani A, et al: *Cardiobacterium hominis* endocarditis: two cases and a review of the literature, Eur J Clin Microbiol Infect Dis 25: 587-595, 2006.

8. Maurin M, Raoult D: *Bartonella (Rochalimaea) quintana* infections, Clin Microbiol Rev 9: 273-292, 1996.

9. Metzkor-Cotter E, et al: Long-term serological analysis and clinical follow-up of patients with cat scratch disease, Clin Infect Dis 37: 1149-1154, 2003.

10. Resto-Ruiz S, Burgess A, Anderson B: The role of the host immune response in pathogenesis of *Bartonella henselae*, DNA Cell Biol 22: 431-440, 2003.

11. Spach D, et al: *Bartonella (Rochalimaea)* species as a cause of apparent "culture-negative" endocarditis, Clin Infect Dis 20: 1044-1047, 1995.

12. Zeaiter Z, et al: Phylogenetic classification of *Bartonella* species by comparing groEL sequences, Intl J System Evol Microbiol 52: 165-171, 2002.

Clostridium

Chapter 29

The genus *Clostridium* consists of a large, heterogeneous collection of spore-forming, anaerobic rods. This genus was defined by four properties: (1) presence of endospores, (2) strict anaerobic metabolism, (3) inability to reduce sulfate to sulfite, and (4) gram-positive cell wall structure. The organisms are **ubiquitous** in soil, water, and sewage and are part of the normal microbial flora in the gastrointestinal tracts of animals and humans. Most clostridia are harmless saprophytes, but some are well-recognized human pathogens with a clearly documented history of causing diseases, such as *C. tetani* and *C. botulinum*, the agents responsible for tetanus and botulism, respectively, are well-recognized and have historical significance, and disease caused by *C. difficile* has evolved in recent years as an infectious complication of antibiotic usage both in the hospital and community (Table 29-1).

CLOSTRIDIUM PERFRINGENS

Physiology and Structure

C. perfringens is a large (0.6 to 2.4 × 1.3 to 19.0 μm), rectangular, gram-positive rod (Figure 29-1), with **spores rarely observed** either in vivo or after in vitro cultivation, an important characteristic that differentiates this species from other clostridia. Colonies of *C. perfringens* are also distinctive, with their rapid, spreading growth on laboratory media and β-hemolysis on blood-containing media (Figure 29-2). The produc-

Table 29-1 Pathogenic Clostridia and Their Associated Human Diseases*

Species	Human Disease	Frequency
C. difficile	Antibiotic-associated diarrhea, pseudomembranous colitis	Common
C. perfringens	Soft-tissue infections (e.g., cellulitis, suppurative myositis, myonecrosis, gas gangrene), food poisoning, enteritis necroticans, septicemia	Common
C. septicum	Gas gangrene, septicemia	Uncommon
C. botulinum	Botulism	Uncommon
C. tetani	Tetanus	Uncommon
C. tertium	Opportunistic infections	Uncommon
C. baratii	Botulism	Rare
C. butyricum	Botulism	Rare
C. clostridioforme	Opportunistic infections	Rare
C. histolyticum	Gas gangrene	Rare
C. innocuum	Opportunistic infections	Rare
C. novyi	Gas gangrene	Rare
C. ramosum	Opportunistic infections	Rare
C. sordellii	Gas gangrene, septic shock syndrome	Rare
C. sporogenes	Opportunistic infections	Rare

*Other clostridial species have been associated with human disease but primarily as opportunistic pathogens. In addition, some species (e.g., *C. clostridioforme*, *C. innocuum*, *C. ramosum*) are commonly isolated but are rarely associated with disease.

tion of one or more "major lethal" toxins by *C. perfringens* (alpha, beta, epsilon, and iota toxins) is used to subdivide isolates into five types (A through E).

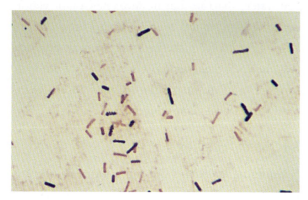

Figure 29-1 Gram stain of *Clostridium perfringens* in a wound specimen. Note the rectangular shape of the rods, the presence of many decolorize rods appearing gram-negative, and the absence of spore and blood cells.

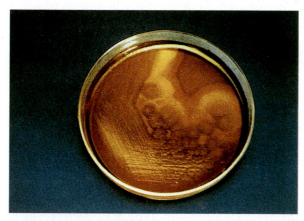

Figure 29-2 Growth of *Clostridium perfringens* on sheep blood agar. Note the flat, spreading colonies and the hemolytic activity of the organism. A presumptive identification of *C. perfringens* can be made by detection of a zone of complete hemolysis (caused by the theta toxin) and a wider zone of partial hemolysis (caused by the alpha toxin), combined with the characteristic microscopic morphology.

Pathogenesis and Immunity

C. perfringens can be associated with asymptomatic colonization or cause a spectrum of diseases, from a self-limited gastroenteritis to an overwhelming destruction of tissue (e.g., clostridial myonecrosis) associated with a very high mortality, even in patients who receive early medical intervention. This pathogenic potential is attributed primarily to at least a dozen toxins and enzymes produced by this organism. **Alpha toxin,** the most important toxin and the one produced by all five types of *C. perfringens,* is a lecithinase (phospholipase C) that lyses erythrocytes, platelets, leukocytes, and endothelial cells. This toxin mediates massive hemolysis, increased vascular permeability and bleeding (augmented by destruction of platelets), tissue destruction (as found in myonecrosis), hepatic toxicity, and myocardial dysfunction (bradycardia, hypotension). The largest quantities of alpha toxin are produced by *C. perfringens* type A. **Beta toxin** is responsible for intestinal stasis, loss of mucosa with formation of the necrotic lesions, and progression to necrotizing enteritis (**enteritis necroticans, pig-bel**). **Epsilon toxin,** a protoxin, is activated by trypsin and increases the vascular permeability of the gastrointestinal wall. **Iota toxin,** the fourth major lethal toxin, is produced by type E *C. perfringens.* This toxin has necrotic activity and increases vascular permeability.

The *C. perfringens* **enterotoxin** is produced primarily by type A strains. The heat-labile toxin is susceptible to pronase. Exposure to trypsin enhances toxin activity threefold. The enterotoxin is produced during the phase transition from vegetative cells to spores and is released with the formed spores when the cells undergo the terminal stages of spore formation (**sporulation**). The alkaline conditions in the small intestine stimulate sporulation. The released enterotoxin binds to receptors on the brush border membrane of the small intestine epithelium in the ileum (primarily) and jejunum but not duodenum. Insertion of the toxin into the cell membrane leads to altered membrane permeability and loss of fluids and ions. The enterotoxin also acts as a superantigen simulating T-lymphocyte activity. Antibodies to enterotoxin, indicating previous exposure, are commonly found in adults but are not protective.

Clinical Diseases

Soft-Tissue Infections

Clostridial species can colonize wounds and skin with no clinical consequences. Indeed, most strains of *C. perfringens* and other clostridial species isolated in wound cultures are insignificant. However, these organisms can also cause a range of soft-tissue infections, including **cellulitis** (Figure 29-3), fasciitis or suppurative **myositis,** and **myonecrosis** or gas gangrene with gas formation in the soft tissue.

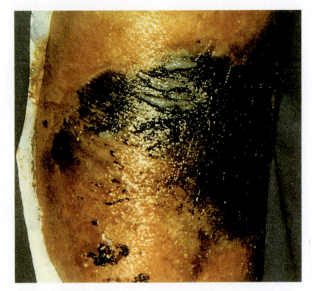

Figure 29-3   Clostridial cellulitis. Clostridia can be introduced into tissue during surgery or by a traumatic injury. This patient suffered a compound fracture of the tibia. Five days after the injury, the skin became discolored, and bullae and necrosis developed. A serosanguineous exudate and subcutaneous gas were present, but there was no evidence of muscle necrosis. The patient had an uneventful recovery. (From Lambert H, Farrar W, editors: *Infectious diseases illustrated,* London, 1982, Gower.)

Cellulitis is localized edema and erythema with gas formation in the soft tissue; generally nonpainful.

Suppurative myositis is accumulation of pus (suppuration) in the muscle planes without muscle necrosis or systemic symptoms.

Clostridial myonecrosis is a life-threatening disease that illustrates the full virulence potential of histotoxic clostridia. The onset of disease, characterized by intense pain, generally develops within a week after clostridia are introduced into tissue by trauma or surgery. The onset is followed rapidly by extensive muscle necrosis, shock, renal failure, and death, often within 2 days of initial onset. Macroscopic examination of muscle reveals devitalized necrotic tissue. Gas was found in the tissue (hence the name gas gangrene).

Gastroenteritis

Food Poisoning

Clostridial food poisoning, a relatively common but underappreciated intoxication, is characterized by (1) a short incubation period (8 to 24 hours); (2) a clinical presentation that includes abdominal cramps and watery diarrhea but no fever, nausea, or vomiting; and (3) a clinical course lasting 24 to 48 hours. Disease results from the ingestion of meat products (e.g., beef, chicken, turkey) contaminated with large numbers (10^8 to 10^9 organisms) of enterotoxin-producing type A *C. perfringens.*

Necrotizing Enteritis

Necrotizing enteritis (also called **enteritis necroticans** or **pig-bel**) is a rare, necrotizing process in the jejunum characterized by acute abdominal pain, vomiting, bloody diarrhea, ulceration of the small intestine, and perforation of the intestinal wall, leading to peritonitis and shock. Mortality in patients with this infection approaches 50%. Beta toxin produced by *C. perfringens* type C is responsible for this disease.

Epidemiology

Type A *C. perfringens* commonly inhabits the intestinal tract of humans and animals and is widely distributed in nature, particularly in **soil and water contaminated with feces.** Spores are formed under adverse environmental conditions and can survive for prolonged periods. **Type A *C. perfringens*** is responsible for most human infections, including soft-tissue infections, food poisoning, and primary septicemia. Type C *C. perfringens* is responsible for one other important infection in humans—**necrotizing enteritis.**

Laboratory Diagnosis

The laboratory performs a confirmatory role in the diagnosis of clostridial soft-tissue diseases because therapy must be initiated immediately. The microscopic detection of gram-positive rods in clinical specimens, usually in the absence of leukocytes, can be a very useful finding because these organisms have a characteristic morphology. It is also relatively simple to culture these anaerobes. The role of *C. perfringens* in food poisoning is documented by recovery of more than 10^5 organisms per gram of food or more than 10^6 bacteria per gram of feces collected within 1 day of the onset of disease. Immunoassays have also been developed for detection of the enterotoxin in fecal specimens; however, clostridial food poisoning is a clinical diagnosis, and culture or immunoassays are not commonly used for this diagnosis.

Treatment, Prevention, and Control

C. perfringens soft-tissue infections, such as suppurative myositis and myonecrosis, must be treated aggressively with **surgical debridement** and **high-dose penicillin therapy.** Hyperbaric oxygen treatment has been used to manage these infections; however, the results are inconclusive. Despite all therapeutic efforts, the prognosis in patients with these diseases is poor, with reported mortality ranging from 40% to almost 100%. Less serious, localized soft-tissue infections can be successfully treated with debridement and penicillin.

Antibiotic therapy for clostridial food poisoning is unnecessary because this is a self-limiting disease.

Exposure to *C. perfringens* is difficult to avoid because the organisms are ubiquitous. Disease requires introduction of the organism into devitalized tissues and maintenance of an anaerobic environment favorable for bacterial growth. Thus proper wound care and the judicious use of prophylactic antibiotics can do much to prevent most infections.

CLOSTRIDIUM TETANI

Physiology and Structure

C. tetani is a large (0.5 to 2 × 2 to 18 µm), motile, spore-forming rod. The organism produces round, terminal spores that give it the appearance of a drumstick. Unlike *C. perfringens*, *C. tetani* is difficult to grow because the organism is extremely sensitive to oxygen toxicity, and when growth is detected on agar media, it typically appears as a film over the surface of the agar rather than discrete colonies. The bacteria are proteolytic but unable to ferment carbohydrates.

Pathogenesis and Immunity

The *C. tetani* produces two toxins, an oxygen-labile hemolysin (**tetanolysin**) and a plasmid-encoded, heat-labile neurotoxin (**tetanospasmin**). However, the clinical significance of tetanolysin is unknown because it is inhibited by oxygen and serum cholesterol.

Tetanospasmin is produced during the stationary phase of growth, released when the cell is lysed, and responsible for the clinical manifestations of tetanus. Tetanospasmin (an **A-B toxin**) is synthesized as a single, 150,000-Da peptide that is cleaved into a light (A-chain) subunit and a heavy (B-chain) subunit by an endogenous protease when the cell releases the neurotoxin. A disulfide bond and noncovalent forces hold the two chains together. The carbohydrate-binding domain of the carboxyl-terminal portion of the heavy (100,000-Da) chain binds to specific sialic acid receptors (e.g., polysialogangliosides) and adjacent glycoproteins on the surface of motor neurons. The intact toxin molecules are internalized in endosomal vesicles and transported in the neuron axon to motor neuron soma located in the spinal cord. In this location, the endosome becomes acidified, resulting in a conformational change in the N-terminus domain of the heavy chain, insertion into the endosome membrane, and passage of the toxin light chain into the cytosol of the cell. The light chain is a **zinc endopeptidase** that cleaves core proteins involved in the trafficking and release of neurotransmitters. Specifically, tetanospasmin **inactivates proteins that regulate release of the inhibitory neurotransmitters** glycine and gamma-aminobutryic acid (GABA). This leads to unregulated excitatory synaptic activity in the motor neurons, resulting in **spastic paralysis.** The toxin binding is irreversible, so recovery depends on whether new axonal terminals form.

Clinical Diseases

The incubation period for tetanus varies from a few days to weeks. The duration of the incubation period is directly related to the distance of the primary wound infection from the central nervous system.

Generalized tetanus is the most common form. Involvement of the masseter muscles (trismus or lockjaw) is the presenting sign in most patients. The characteristic sardonic smile that results from the sustained contraction of the facial muscles is known as *risus sardonicus* (Figure 29-4). Other early signs are drooling, sweating, irritability, and persistent back spasms (*opisthotonos*) (Figure 29-5). The autonomic nervous system is involved in patients with more severe disease; the signs and symptoms include cardiac arrhythmias, fluctuations in blood pressure, profound sweating, and dehydration.

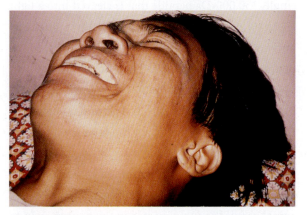

Figure 29-4 Facial spasm and risus sardonicus in a patient with tetanus. (From Cohen J, Powderly WG: *Infectious diseases*, ed 2, St Louis, 2004, Mosby.)

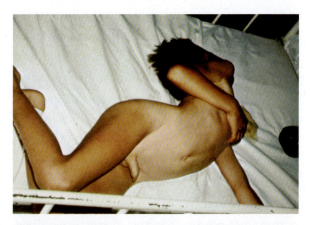

Figure 29-5 A child with tetanus and opisthotonos resulting from persistent spasms of the back muscles. (From Emond RT, Rowland HAK, Welsby P: *Colour atlas of infectious diseases*, ed 3, London, 1995, Wolfe.)

Another form of *C. tetani* disease is **localized tetanus,** in which the disease remains confined to the musculature at the site of primary infection. A variant is **cephalic tetanus,** in which the primary site of infection is the head. In contrast to the prognosis for patients with localized tetanus, the prognosis for patients with cephalic tetanus is very poor.

Neonatal tetanus (tetanus neonatorum) is typi-

cally associated with an initial infection of the umbilical stump that progresses to become generalized. The mortality in infants exceeds 90%, and developmental defects are present in survivors. This is almost exclusively a disease in developing countries.

Epidemiology

C. tetani is **ubiquitous.** It is found in fertile soil and transiently colonizes the gastrointestinal tracts of many animals, including humans. The vegetative forms of *C. tetani* are extremely susceptible to oxygen toxicity, but the organisms sporulate readily and can survive in nature for a long time. Tetanus is still responsible for many deaths in developing countries where vaccination is unavailable or medical practices are lax. It is estimated that more than 1 million cases occur worldwide, with a mortality rate ranging from 30% to 50%. At least half the deaths occur in neonates.

Laboratory Diagnosis

The diagnosis of tetanus, as with that of most other clostridial diseases, is made on the basis of the clinical presentation. The microscopic detection of *C. tetani* or recovery in culture is useful but frequently unsuccessful.

Treatment, Prevention, and Control

Treatment of tetanus requires **debridement** of the primary wound (which may appear innocuous), use of **penicillin** or **metronidazole** to kill the bacteria and reduce toxin production, **passive immunization** with human tetanus immunoglobulin to neutralize unbound toxin, and **vaccination** with tetanus toxoid because infection does not confer immunity. Vaccination with a series of three doses of tetanus toxoid, followed by booster doses every 10 years, is highly effective in preventing tetanus.

CLOSTRIDIUM BOTULINUM

Physiology and Structure

C. botulinum, the etiologic agent of botulism, is a heterogeneous group of large (0.6 to 1.4 × 3.0 to

20.2 μm), fastidious, spore-forming, anaerobic rods. Seven antigenically distinct botulinum toxins (A to G) have been described; human disease is associated with types A, B, E, and F.

Pathogenesis and Immunity

Similar to tetanus toxin, *C. botulinum* toxin is a 150,000-Da progenitor protein (A-B toxin) consisting of a small subunit (light, or A chain) with **zinc-endopeptidase** activity and a large, nontoxic subunit (B, or heavy chain). In contrast with the tetanus neurotoxin, the *C. botulinum* toxin is complexed with nontoxic proteins that protect the neurotoxin during passage through the digestive tract (this is unnecessary for tetanus neurotoxin). The carboxyl-terminal portion of the botulinum heavy chain binds specific sialic acid receptors and glycoproteins (different from those targeted by tetanospasmin) on the surface of motor neurons and stimulates endocytosis of the toxin molecule. Also, in contrast with tetanospasmin, the botulinum neurotoxin remains at the neuromuscular junction. Acidification of the endosome stimulates N-terminal, heavy-chain-mediated release of the light chain. The botulinum endopeptidase then **inactivates the proteins that regulate release of acetylcholine,** blocking neurotransmission at peripheral cholinergic synapses. Because acetylcholine is required for excitation of muscle, the resulting clinical presentation of botulism is a **flaccid paralysis.** As with tetanus, recovery of function after botulism requires regeneration of the nerve endings.

Clinical Diseases

Foodborne Botulism

Patients with foodborne botulism typically become weak and dizzy 1 to 3 days after consuming the contaminated food. The initial signs include blurred vision with fixed, dilated pupils, dry mouth (indicative of the anticholinergic effects of the toxin), constipation, and abdominal pain. Fever is absent. Bilateral descending weakness of the peripheral muscles develops in patients, with progressive disease (flaccid paralysis), and death is most commonly attributed to respiratory paralysis. Patients maintain a clear sensorium throughout the disease. Despite aggressive management of the patient's condition, the disease may continue to progress because the neurotoxin is irreversibly bound and inhibits the release of excitatory neurotransmitters for a prolonged period. Complete recovery in patients often requires many months to years, or until the affected nerve endings regrow. Mortality in patients with foodborne botulism, which once approached 70%, has been reduced to 5 to 10% through the use of better supportive care, particularly in the management of respiratory complications.

Infant Botulism

In contrast with foodborne botulism, this disease is caused by neurotoxin produced in vivo by *C. botulinum* colonizing the gastrointestinal tracts of infants. In the absence of competitive bowel microbes, the organism can become established in the gastrointestinal tracts of infants. The disease typically affects infants younger than 1 year (most between 1 and 6 months), and the symptoms are initially nonspecific (e.g., constipation, weak cry, or "failure to thrive"). Progressive disease with flaccid paralysis and respiratory arrest can develop; however, mortality in documented cases of infant botulism is very low (1% to 2%).

Wound Botulism

Wound botulism develops from toxin production by *C. botulinum* in contaminated wounds. Although the symptoms of disease are identical to those of foodborne disease, the incubation period is generally longer (4 days or more), and the gastrointestinal tract symptoms are less prominent.

Epidemiology

C. botulinum is commonly isolated in soil and water samples throughout the world. Four forms of botulism have been identified: (1) classic or foodborne botulism, (2) infant botulism, (3) wound botulism, and (4) inhalation botulism. **Infant botulism** is more common than foodborne botulism and has been associated with the consumption of foods (e.g., honey, infant milk powder) contaminated with botulinum spores and ingestion of spore-contaminated soil and dust (now the most common source of infant exposure). The incidence of **wound botulism** is unknown, but the disease is very rare. **Inhalation botulism** is a major concern in this era of bioterrorism. Botulinum toxin has been concentrated for purposes of aerosolization as a biologic weapon.

Laboratory Diagnosis

The clinical diagnosis of foodborne botulism is confirmed if toxin activity is demonstrated in the implicated food or in the patient's serum, feces, or gastric fluid. Infant botulism is confirmed if toxin is detected in the infant's feces or serum, or the organism cultured from feces. Wound botulism is confirmed if toxin is detected in the patient's serum or wound, or if the organism is cultured from the wound. Toxin activity is most likely to be found early in the disease.

Isolation of *C. botulinum* from specimens contaminated with other organisms can be improved by heating the specimen for 10 minutes at 80℃ to kill all nonclostridial cells. Culture of the heated specimen on nutritionally enriched anaerobic media allows the heat-resistant *C. botulinum* spores to germinate. Demonstration of toxin production (typically performed at public health laboratories) must be done with a mouse bioassay. Samples of the implicated food, stool specimen, and patient's serum should also be tested for toxin activity.

Treatment, Prevention, and Control

Patients with botulism require the following treatment measures: (1) adequate **ventilatory support;** (2) elimination of the organism from the gastrointestinal tract, through the judicious use of gastric lavage and **metronidazole or penicillin** therapy; and (3) the use of **trivalent botulinum antitoxin** versus toxins A, B, and E to inactivate unbound toxin circulating in the bloodstream. Ventilatory support is extremely important in reducing mortality.

Disease is prevented by destroying the spores in food (virtually impossible for practical reasons), preventing spore germination (by maintaining the food in an acid pH or storage at 4℃ or colder), or destroying the preformed toxin (all botulinum toxins are inactivated by heating at 60℃ to 100℃ for 10 minutes). Infant botulism has been associated with the consumption of honey contaminated with *C. botulinum* spores, so children younger than 1 year should not eat honey.

CLOSTRIDIUM DIFFICILE

Systematic studies now clearly show, however, that toxin-producing *C. difficile* is responsible for antibiotic-associated gastrointestinal diseases, ranging from a relatively benign, self-limited diarrhea to severe, life-threatening pseudomembranous colitis (Figure 29-6 and Figure 29-7).

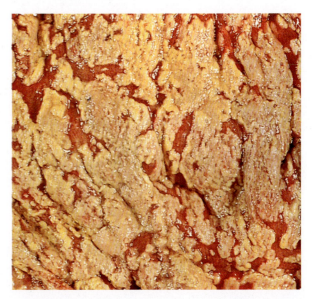

Figure 29-6 Antibiotic-associated colitis: gross section of the lumen of the colon. Note the white plaques of fibrin, mucus, and inflammatory cells overlying the normal red intestinal mucosa.

C. difficile produces two toxins: an **enterotoxin (toxin A)** and a **cytotoxin (toxin B).** The enterotoxin is chemotactic for neutrophils, stimulating the infiltration of polymorphonuclear neutrophils into the ileum with release of cytokines. Toxin A also produces a cytopathic effect, resulting in disruption of the tight cell-to-cell junction, increased permeability of the intestinal wall, and subsequent diarrhea. A

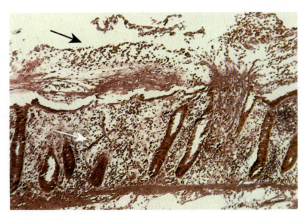

Figure 29-7 Antibiotic-associated colitis caused by *Clostridium difficile*. A histologic section of colon shows an intense inflammatory response, with the characteristic "plaque" *(black arrow)* overlying the intact intestinal mucosa *(white arrow)* (hematoxylin and eosin stain). (From Lambert HP, Farrar WE, editors: *Infectious diseases illustrated*, London, 1982, Gower.)

C. difficile is part of the normal intestinal flora in a small number of healthy people and hospitalized patients. The disease develops in people taking antibiotics because the drugs alter the normal enteric flora, either permitting the overgrowth of these relatively resistant organisms or making the patient more susceptible to the exogenous acquisition of *C. difficile*. The disease occurs if the organisms proliferate in the colon and produce their toxins.

The diagnosis of *C. difficile* disease was confirmed, historically, by demonstration of the enterotoxin or cytotoxin in a stool specimen from a patient with compatible clinical symptoms. Toxin activity can be detected by an in vivo cytotoxicity assay using tissue culture cells and specific neutralizing antibodies for the cytotoxin; however, this assay is technically cumbersome and requires 1 to 2 days before results are available. Both the enterotoxin and cytotoxin can be detected with a number of commercial immunoassays, but these tests are insensitive and not recommended. The current recommended test for defining disease is detection of the *C. difficile* toxin genes directly in clinical specimens by nucleic acid amplification techniques. Commercial assays with high sensitivity and specificity are now available that provide results within a few hours of sample collection.

Discontinuation of the implicated antibiotic (e.g., ampicillin, clindamycin, fluoroquinolones) is gen-erally sufficient to alleviate mild disease. However, specific therapy with **metronidazole** or **vancomycin** is necessary for the management of severe diarrhea or colitis. Relapses may occur in as many as 20% to 30% of patients after the completion of therapy because only the vegetative forms of *C. difficile* are killed by the antibiotics; the spores are resistant. A second course of treatment with the same antibiotic is frequently successful, although multiple relapses are well-documented in some patients. It is difficult to prevent the disease because the organism commonly exists in hospitals, particularly in areas adjacent to infected patients (e.g., beds, bathrooms). The spores of *C. difficile* are difficult to eliminate unless thorough housekeeping measures are used. Thus the organism can contaminate an environment for many months and can be a major source of nosocomial outbreaks of *C. difficile* disease.

SUMMARY

Clostridium perfringens

The *Clostridium perfringens* multiply rapidly in culture and in patients, producing many toxins and enzymes that lyse blood cells and destroy tissues. The bacteria produce a heat-sensitive enterotoxin that binds to receptors on the epithelium of the small intestine, leading to loss of fluids and ions.

The *Clostridium perfringens* can cause a range of soft-tissue infections, including **cellulitis**, fasciitis or suppurative **myositis**, and **myonecrosis** or gas gangrene with gas formation in the soft tissue. The *Clostridium perfringens* can also cause food poisoning and necrotizing enteritis.

The bacteria present in soil, water, and intestinal tract of humans and animals. Type A strains are responsible for most human infections.

Reliably being seen in Gram-stained tissue specimens (large, gram-positive rods) has diagnostic value.

Rapid treatment is essential for serious infections.

Clostridium tetani

The primary virulence factor is tetanospasmin, a heat-labile neurotoxin that blocks release of neurotransmitters (i.e., gamma-aminobutyric acid, glycine) for inhibitory synapses.

The Bacteria can induce generalized tetanus, localized tetanus and neonatal tetanus.

Spores are found in most soils and can colonize gastrointestinal tract of humans and animals. Exposure to spores is common, but disease is uncommon. Risk is greatest for people with inadequate vaccine-induced immunity. Disease does not induce immunity.

Diagnosis is based on clinical presentation and not laboratory tests.

Treatment requires debridement, antibiotic therapy (penicillin, metronidazole), passive immunization with antitoxin globulin, and vaccination with tetanus toxoid.

Prevention through use of vaccination consists of three doses of tetanus toxoid.

Clostridium botulinum

Botulinum toxin prevents release of the neurotransmitter acetylcholine, thus blocking neurotransmission at peripheral cholinergic synapses, leading to a flaccid paralysis.

C. botulinum can cause foodborne botulism, infant botulism, wound botulism and inhalation botulism.

Diagnosis of foodborne botulism is confirmed if toxin activity is demonstrated in the implicated food or in the patient's serum, feces, or gastric fluid. Infant botulism is confirmed if toxin is detected in the infant's feces or serum, or the organism cultured from feces. Wound botulism is confirmed if toxin is detected in the patient's serum or wound, or the organism cultured from the wound.

Treatment involves administration of metronidazole or penicillin, trivalent botulinum antitoxin, and ventilatory support.

Clostridium difficile

Most strains produce two toxins: an enterotoxin that attracts neutrophils and stimulates their release of cytokines, and a cytotoxin that increases permeability of the intestinal wall and subsequent diarrhea. Spore formation allows the organism to persist in the hospital environment and resist decontamination efforts. Resistance to antibiotics such as clindamycin, cepha-

losporins, and fluoroquinolones allows *C. difficile* to overgrow the normal intestinal bacteria in patients exposed to these antibiotics and produce disease.

The *C. difficile* can cause antibiotic-associated diarrhea and even pseudomembranous colitis.

The organism colonizes the intestines of a small proportion of healthy individuals (<5%).

Exposure to antibiotics is associated with overgrowth of *C. difficile* and subsequent disease (endogenous infection). Spores can be detected in hospital rooms of infected patients (particularly around beds and in the bathrooms); these can be an exogenous source of infection.

C. difficile disease is confirmed by detecting cytotoxin or enterotoxin or the toxin genes in the patient's feces.

Treatment with metronidazole or vancomycin should be used in severe disease.

Relapse is common.

KEYWORDS

English	Chinese
Clostridium	梭菌属
Clostridium botulinum	肉毒梭菌
Clostridium difficile	艰难梭菌
Clostridium perfringens	产气荚膜梭菌
Clostridium tetani	破伤风梭菌
Flaccid paralysis	弛缓性麻痹
Gas gangrene	气性坏疽
Infant botulism	婴儿肉毒病
Spastic paralysis	痉挛性麻痹
Tetanospasmin	破伤风痉挛毒素
Tetanus	破伤风

BIBLIOGRAPHY

1. Patrick R. Murray. Medical Microbiology. 7th Edition. ELSEVIER SAUNDERS

2. Martin JS, et al: Clostridium difficile infection: epidemiology, diagnosis and understanding transmission, Nat Rev Gastroenterol Hepatol. 2016 Mar 9.

3. Bakken JS, et al: Treating Clostridiumdifficile infection with fecal microbiota transplantation, Clin Gastroenterol Hepatol. 2011 Dec; 9(12): 1044-9.

4. Bauer M, Kuijper E, van Dissel J: European Society of

Clinical Microbiology and Infectious Diseases (ESCMID): treatment guidance document for *Clostridium difficile* infection, Clin Microbiol Infect 15: 1067-1079, 2009.

5. Boone J, Carman R: *Clostridium perfringens*: food poisoning and antibiotic-associated diarrhea, Clin Microbiol Newslett 19: 65-67, 1997.

6. Bryant A, et al: Clostridial gas gangrene. I. Cellular and molecular mechanisms of microvascular dysfunction induced by exotoxins of *Clostridium perfringens*, J Infect Dis 182: 799-807, 2000.

7. Curry S: *Clostridium difficile*, Clin Lab Med 30: 329-342, 2010.

8. Lalli G, et al: The journey of tetanus and botulinum neurotoxins in neurons, Trends Microbiol 11: 431-437, 2003.

9. Lindstrom M, Korkeala H: Laboratory diagnostics of botulism, Clin Microbiol Rev 19: 298-314, 2006.

10. Midura T: Update: infant botulism, Clin Microbiol Rev 9: 119-125, 1996.

11. Nocak-Weekley S, et al: *Clostridium difficile* testing in the clinical laboratory by use of multiple testing algorithms, J Clin Microbiol 48: 889-893, 2010.

12. Schwan C, et al: *Clostridium difficile* toxin CDT induces formation of microtubule-based protrusions and increases adherence of bacteria, PLoS Pathogens 5: e1000626, 2009.

13. Stevens DL, Bryant AE: The role of clostridial toxins in the pathogenesis of gas gangrene, Clin Infect Dis 35(Suppl 1): S93-S100, 2002.

14. Voth DE, Ballard JD: *Clostridium difficile* toxins: mechanism of action and role in disease, Clin Microbiol Rev 18: 247-263, 2005.

Anaerobic, Non-Spore-Forming, Gram-Positive Bacteria

Chapter

30

ANAEROBIC GRAM-POSITIVE COCCI

At one time, all clinically significant anaerobic cocci were included in the genus *Peptostreptococcus*. Unfortunately, it was recognized that these organisms were organized in a single genus based primarily on their Gram-stain morphology and inability to grow aerobically. More sophisticated methods have since been used to reclassify many of these species into six genera. Although some anaerobic cocci are more virulent than others, and some are associated with specific diseases, specific identification of the different genera is generally unnecessary, and knowledge that anaerobic cocci are associated with an infection is typically sufficient.

The anaerobic gram-positive cocci normally colonize the oral cavity, gastrointestinal tract, genitourinary tract, and skin. They produce infections when they spread from these sites to normally sterile sites. For example, bacteria colonizing the upper airways can cause sinusitis and pleuropulmonary infections; bacteria in the intestines can cause intraabdominal infections; bacteria in the genitourinary tract can cause endometritis, pelvic abscesses, and salpingitis; bacteria on the skin can cause cellulitis and soft-tissue infections; and bacteria that invade the blood can produce infections in bones and solid organs.

Laboratory confirmation of infections with anaerobic cocci is complicated by the following three factors: (1) care must be taken to prevent contamination of the clinical specimen with the anaerobic cocci that normally colonize the skin and mucosal surfaces; (2) the collected specimen must be transported in an oxygen-free container to prevent loss of the organ-

isms; and (3) specimens should be cultured on nutritionally enriched media for a prolonged period (i.e., 5 to 7 days). In addition, some species of staphylococci and streptococci grow initially in an anaerobic atmosphere only and may be mistaken for anaerobic cocci. However, these organisms eventually grow well in air supplemented with 10% carbon dioxide (CO_2), so they cannot be classified as anaerobes.

Anaerobic cocci are usually susceptible to **penicillins** and **carbapenems** (e.g., imipenem, meropenem); have intermediate susceptibility to broad-spectrum cephalosporins, clindamycin, erythromycin, and the tetracyclines; and are resistant to the aminoglycosides (as are all anaerobes). Specific therapy is generally indicated in monomicrobic infections; however, because most infections with these organisms are polymicrobic, broad-spectrum therapy against aerobic and anaerobic bacteria is usually selected.

ANAEROBIC, NON-SPORE-FORMING, GRAM-POSITIVE RODS

The non-spore-forming, gram-positive rods are a diverse collection of facultatively anaerobic or strictly anaerobic bacteria that colonize the skin and mucosal surfaces. *Actinomyces (see Chapter 1)*, *Mobiluncus*, *Lactobacillus*, and *Propionibacterium* are well-recognized opportunistic pathogens, whereas other genera, such as *Bifidobacterium* and *Eubacterium*, can be isolated in clinical specimens but rarely cause human disease.

PROPIONIBACTERIUM

Propionibacteria are small gram-positive rods often

arranged in short chains or clumps (Figure 30-1). They are commonly found on the skin (in contrast with the *Actinomyces*), conjunctiva, external ear, and in the oropharynx and female genital tract. The organisms are anaerobic or aerotolerant, nonmotile, catalase positive, and capable of fermenting carbohydrates, producing propionic acid as their major byproduct (hence the name). The two most commonly isolated species are ***Propionibacterium acnes*** and ***Propionibacterium propionicum.***

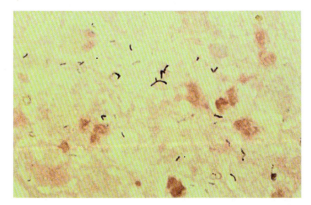

Figure 30-1   Gram stain of *Propionibacterium* in a blood culture.

P. acnes is responsible for two types of infections: (1) **acne vulgaris** (as the name implies) in teenagers and young adults and (2) **opportunistic infections** in patients with prosthetic devices (e.g., artificial heart valves or joints) or intravascular lines (e.g., catheters, cerebrospinal fluid shunts). Propionibacteria are also commonly isolated in blood cultures, but this finding usually represents contamination with bacteria on the skin at the phlebotomy site.

The central role of *P. acnes* in acne is to stimulate an inflammatory response. Production of a low-molecular-weight peptide by the bacteria residing in sebaceous follicles attracts leukocytes. The bacteria are phagocytized and, after release of bacterial hydrolytic enzymes (lipases, proteases, neuraminidase, and hyaluronidase), stimulate a localized inflammatory response. *P. propionicum* is associated with endodontic abscesses and lacrimal canaliculitis (inflammation of the tear duct).

Propionibacteria can grow on most common media, although it may take 2 to 5 days for growth to appear.

Care must be taken to avoid contamination of the specimen with the organisms normally found on the skin. The significance of the recovery of an isolate must also be interpreted in light of the clinical presentation (e.g., a catheter or other foreign body can serve as a focus for these opportunistic pathogens).

Acne is unrelated to the effectiveness of skin cleansing because the lesion develops within the sebaceous follicles. For this reason, acne is managed primarily through the topical application of benzoyl peroxide and antibiotics. Antibiotics such as erythromycin and clindamycin have proved effective for treatment.

MOBILUNCUS

Members of the genus *Mobiluncus* are obligate anaerobic, gram-variable or gram-negative, curved rods with tapered ends. Despite their appearance in Gram-stained specimens (Figure 30-2), they are classified as gram-positive rods because they (1) have a gram-positive cell wall, (2) lack endotoxin, and (3) are susceptible to vancomycin, clindamycin, erythromycin, and ampicillin but resistant to colistin. The organisms are fastidious, growing slowly even on enriched media supplemented with rabbit or horse serum.

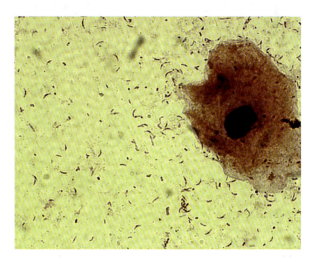

Figure 30-2   Gram stain of *Mobiluncus*. The bacterial cells are curved and have pointed ends.

Of the two species of *Mobiluncus*, **M. curtisii** is rarely found in the vaginas of healthy women but is abundant in women with **bacterial vaginosis** (vaginitis). Their microscopic appearance is a useful marker for this disease, but the precise role of these organisms in the pathogenesis of bacterial vaginosis is unclear.

LACTOBACILLUS

Lactobacillus species are facultatively anaerobic or strictly anaerobic rods. They are found as part of the normal flora of the mouth, stomach, intestines, and genitourinary tract. The organisms are most commonly isolated in urine specimens and blood cultures. Because lactobacilli are the most common organism in the urethra, their recovery in urine cultures usually is a result of contamination of the specimen, even when large numbers of the organisms are present. The reason lactobacilli rarely cause infections of the urinary tract is their inability to grow in urine. Invasion into blood occurs in one of the following three settings: (1) **transient bacteremia** from a genitourinary source (e.g., after childbirth or a gynecologic procedure), (2) **endocarditis** and (3) **opportunistic septicemia** in an immunocompromised patient. Strains of lactobacilli are used as probiotics and have occasionally been associated with human infections, most commonly in immunocompromised patients.

Treatment of endocarditis and opportunistic infections is difficult because lactobacilli are resistant to vancomycin (an antibiotic commonly active against gram-positive bacteria) and are inhibited but not killed by other antibiotics. A combination of **penicillin with an aminoglycoside** is required for bactericidal activity.

BIFIDOBACTERIUM AND EUBACTERIUM

Bifidobacterium and *Eubacterium* species are commonly found in the oropharynx, large intestine, and vagina. These bacteria can be isolated in clinical specimens but have a very low virulence potential and usually represent clinically insignificant contaminants. Confirmation of their etiologic role in an infection requires their repeated isolation in large numbers from multiple specimens and the absence of other pathogenic organisms.

SUMMARY

Anaerobic, Non-Spore-Forming, Gram-Positive Bacteria

Peptostreptococcus spp.	*intraabdominal infections; endometritis, pelvic abscesses, and salpingitis;*
Actinomyces spp.	*Localized oral infections, actinomycosis (cervicofacial, thoracic, abdominal, pelvic, central nervous system)*
Propionibacterium spp.	*Acne, lacrimal canaliculitis, opportunistic infections*
Mobiluncus spp.	*Bacterial vaginosis, opportunistic infections*
Lactobacillus spp.	*Endocarditis, opportunistic infections*
Eubacterium spp.	*Opportunistic infections*
Bifidobacterium spp.	*Opportunistic infections*

KEYWORDS

English	Chinese
Peptostreptococcus	消化链球菌属
Actinomyces	放线菌属
Mobiluncus	动弯杆菌属
Lactobacillus	乳杆菌属
Propionibacterium	痤疮丙酸杆菌属
Bifidobacterium	双歧杆菌属
Eubacterium	真杆菌属
Actinomycosis	放线菌病
Acne vulgaris	寻常性痤疮
Bacterial vaginosis	细菌性阴道病

BIBLIOGRAPHY

1. Brook I, Frazier EH: Infections caused by *Propionibacterium* species, Rev Infect Dis 3: 819-822, 1991.
2. Cannon JP, et al: Pathogenic relevance of *Lactobacillus*: a retrospective review of over 200 cases, Eur J Clin Microbiol Infect Dis 24: 31-40, 2005.
3. Murdoch D: Gram-positive anaerobic cocci, Clin Microbiol Rev 11: 81-120, 1998.
4. Pulverer G, Schütt-Gerowitt H, Schaal KP: Human cervicofacial actinomycoses: microbiological data for 1997 cases, Clin Infect Dis 37: 490-497, 2003.

5. Reichenbach J, et al: *Actinomyces* in chronic granulomatous disease: an emerging and unanticipated pathogen, Clin Infect Dis 49: 1703-1710, 2009.

6. Tiveljung A, Forsum U, Monstein H-J: Classification of the genus *Mobiluncus* based on comparative partial 16S rRNA gene analysis, Int J Syst Bacteriol 46: 332-336, 1996.

Anaerobic Gram-Negative Bacteria

The most important gram-negative anaerobes that colonize the human upper respiratory, gastrointestinal, and genitourinary tracts are the rods in the genera *Bacteroides*, *Fusobacterium*, *Parabacteroides*, *Porphyromonas*, and *Prevotella* and the cocci in the genus *Veillonella*. Anaerobes are the predominant bacteria at each of these sites, outnumbering aerobic bacteria 10- to 1000-fold. The diversity of species is also great, with as many as 500 different species of bacteria estimated to colonize the periodontal pocket, many of which are anaerobes. Despite the abundance and diversity of these bacteria, most infections are caused by relatively few species

PHYSIOLOGY AND STRUCTURE

The genus *Bacteroides* is composed of more than 90 species and subspecies, with *Bacteroides fragilis* the most important member of this genus. A characteristic common to the most species in the genus *Bacteroides* is that their growth is stimulated by 20% bile. *Bacteroides* species are pleomorphic in size and shape and resemble a mixed population of organisms in a casually examined Gram stain (Figure 31-1). Other anaerobic gram-negative rods can be very small (e.g., *Porphyromonas*, *Prevotella*) or elongated (e.g., *Fusobacterium*; Figure 31-2). Most gram-negative anaerobes respond weakly to Gram stain, so stained specimens must be carefully examined. Although *Bacteroides* species grow rapidly in culture, the other anaerobic gram-negative rods are fastidious, and cultures may have to be incubated for 3 days or longer before the bacteria can be detected.

Bacteroides have a typical gram-negative cell wall structure, which can be surrounded by a **polysaccharide capsule**. A major component of the cell wall is a surface lipopolysaccharide (LPS). In contrast to the LPS molecules in *Fusobacterium* and the aerobic gram-negative rods, the *Bacteroides* LPS has little

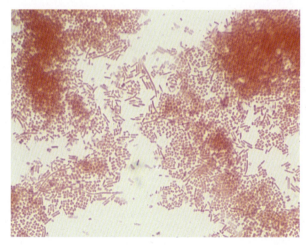

Figure 31-1 *Bacteroides fragilis.* Organisms appear as faintly staining, pleomorphic, gram-negative rods.

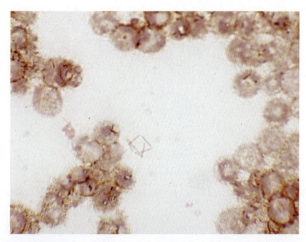

Figure 31-2 *Fusobacterium nucleatum.* Organisms are thin, faintly staining, and elongated with tapered ends (e.g., fusiform).

or no endotoxin activity. This is because the lipid A component of LPS lacks phosphate groups on the glucosamine residues, and the number of fatty acids linked to the amino sugars is reduced; both factors are correlated with the loss of pyrogenic activity.

The anaerobic gram-negative cocci are rarely isolated in clinical specimens except when present as contaminants. Members of the genus *Veillonella* are the predominant anaerobes in the oropharynx, but they represent less than 1% of all anaerobes isolated in clinical specimens. The other anaerobic cocci are rarely isolated.

PATHOGENESIS AND IMMUNITY

Despite the variety of anaerobic species that colonize the human body, relatively few are responsible for causing disease. For example, *Parabacteroides distasonis* and *Bacteroides thetaiotaomicron* are the predominant anaerobic gram-negative rods found in the gastrointestinal tract; however, the majority of intraabdominal infections are associated with *B. fragilis*, an organism that is a minor member of the gastrointestinal flora. The enhanced virulence of this and other pathogenic anaerobes is attributed to a variety of virulence factors that facilitate adherence of the organisms to host tissues, protection from the host immune response, and tissue destruction.

B. fragilis and *Prevotella melaninogenica* strains can adhere to peritoneal surfaces more effectively than other anaerobes because their surface is covered with a polysaccharide capsule. *B. fragilis*, other *Bacteroides* species, and *Porphyromonas gingivalis* can adhere to epithelial cells and extracellular molecules (e.g., fibrinogen, fibronectin, lactoferrin) by means of fimbriae. The fimbriae of *P. gingivalis* are also important for inducing expression of proinflammatory cytokines, such as tumor necrosis factor-α and interleukin-1β (IL-1β).

The polysaccharide capsule of these organisms is antiphagocytic, similar to other bacterial capsules. In addition, the short-chain fatty acids (e.g., succinic acid) produced during anaerobic metabolism inhibit phagocytosis and intracellular killing. Finally, proteases are produced by some *Porphyromonas* and *Prevotella* species that degrade immunoglobulins.

In general, anaerobes capable of causing disease can tolerate exposure to oxygen. Catalase and superoxide dismutase, which inactivate hydrogen peroxide and the superoxide free radicals (O_2^-), respectively, are present in many pathogenic strains.

A variety of cytotoxic enzymes have been associated with gram-negative anaerobes. Many of these enzymes are found in both virulent and avirulent isolates, so the role they play in disease is unclear.

Strains of enterotoxigenic *B. fragilis* that cause diarrheal disease produce a **heat-labile zinc metalloprotease toxin (*B. fragilis* toxin)**. This toxin causes morphologic changes of the intestinal epithelium via F-actin rearrangement, with the resultant stimulation of chloride secretion and fluid loss. The enterotoxin also induces IL-8 secretion by intestinal epithelial cells, thus contributing to inflammatory damage to the epithelium.

EPIDEMIOLOGY

As already stated, anaerobic gram-negative cocci and rods colonize the human body in large numbers. Their numerous important functions at these sites include stabilizing the resident bacterial flora, preventing colonization by pathogenic organisms from exogenous sources, and aiding in the digestion of food. These normal protective organisms produce disease when they move from their endogenous homes to normally sterile sites (i.e., the same as described for gram-positive, non-spore-forming anaerobes in Chapter 30). Thus the organisms in the resident flora are able to spread by trauma or disease from the normally colonized mucosal surfaces to sterile tissues or fluids.

As expected, these endogenous infections are characterized by the presence of a polymicrobial mixture of organisms. It is important to realize, however, that the mixture of organisms appear on healthy mucosal surfaces differs from the mixture in diseased tissues. Studies of the microbial population, or **microbiome,** of healthy mucosal surfaces show a complex mixture of many species of bacteria. In the disease state, the mixture changes to less diversity (i.e., fewer species are represented) and predominance of the most clinically significant organisms. For example, *B. fragilis* is commonly associated with pleuropulmonary, intraabdominal, and genital infections. However, the organism constitutes less than 1% of the colonic flora and is rarely isolated from the oropharynx or genital tract of healthy people unless highly selective techniques are used.

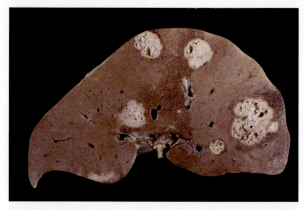

Figure 31-3   Liver abscesses caused by *Bacteroides fragilis*.

CLINICAL DISEASES

Respiratory Tract Infections

Nearly half of the chronic infections of the sinuses and ears, and virtually all periodontal infections, involve mixtures of gram-negative anaerobes, with *Prevotella*, *Porphyromonas*, *Fusobacterium*, and non-fragilis *Bacteroides* the most commonly isolated. Anaerobes are less commonly associated with infections of the lower respiratory tract unless there is a history of aspiration of oral secretions.

Brain Abscess

Anaerobic infections of the brain are typically associated with a history of chronic sinusitis or otitis. Such history is confirmed by radiologic evidence of direct extension into the brain. A less common cause of such infections is bacteremic spread from a pulmonary source. In this case, multiple abscesses are present. The most common anaerobes in these polymicrobial infections are species of *Prevotella*, *Porphyromonas*, and *Fusobacterium* (as well as *Peptostreptococcus* and other anaerobic and aerobic cocci).

Intraabdominal Infections

Despite the diverse population of bacteria that colonize the gastrointestinal tract, relatively few species are associated with intraabdominal infections. Anaerobes are recovered in virtually all of these infections, with *B. fragilis* the most common organism (Figure 31-3). Other important anaerobes are *B. thetaiotaomicron* and *P. melaninogenica*, as well as the anaerobic and aerobic gram-positive cocci.

Gynecologic Infections

Mixtures of anaerobes are often responsible for causing infections of the female genital tract (e.g., pelvic inflammatory disease, abscesses, endometritis, surgical wound infections). Although a variety of anaerobes can be isolated in patients with these infections, *Prevotella bivia* and *Prevotella disiens* are the most important; *B. fragilis* is commonly responsible for abscess formation.

Skin and Soft-Tissue Infections

Although anaerobic gram-negative bacteria are not part of the normal flora of the skin (in contrast to *Peptostreptococcus* and *Propionibacterium* organisms), they can be introduced by a bite or through contamination of a traumatized surface. In some cases, the organisms may simply colonize a wound without producing disease; in other cases, colonization may quickly progress to life-threatening disease, such as myonecrosis (Figure 31-4). *B. fragilis* is the organism most commonly associated with significant disease.

Bacteremia

Anaerobes were at one time responsible for more than 20% of all clinically significant cases of bacteremia; however, these organisms now cause 3% to 5% of such infections. The reduced incidence of disease is not completely understood but probably can be attributed to the widespread use of broad-spectrum antibiotics. *B. fragilis* is the anaerobe most commonly isolated in blood cultures.

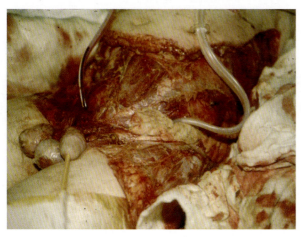

Figure 31-4   Synergistic polymicrobial infection involving *Bacteroides fragilis* and other anaerobes. The infection started at the scrotum and rapidly spread up the trunk and down the thighs, with extensive myonecrosis.

Gastroenteritis

Strains of enterotoxin-producing *B. fragilis* can produce a self-limited watery diarrhea. The majority of infections have been observed in children younger than 5 years of age, although disease has also been reported in adults.

LABORATORY DIAGNOSIS

Microscopic examination of specimens from patients with suspected anaerobic infections can be useful. Although the bacteria may stain faintly and irregularly, the finding of pleomorphic, gram-negative rods can serve as useful preliminary information.

Specimens should be collected and transported to the laboratory in an oxygen-free system, and incubated in an anaerobic environment.

Most *Bacteroides* grow rapidly and should be detected within 2 days; however, recovery of other gram-negative anaerobes may require longer incubation. In addition, it is sometimes difficult to recover all clinically significant bacteria because of the different organisms present in polymicrobial infections. The use of selective media, such as media supplemented with bile, has facilitated the recovery of most important anaerobes (Figure 31-5). In addition, lysed-blood-enriched media stimulates pigment production in organisms such as *Porphyromonas* and *Prevotella* (Figure 31-6).

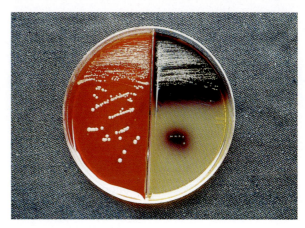

Figure 31-5   Growth of *Bacteroides fragilis* on *Bacteroides* bile-esculin agar. Most aerobic and anaerobic bacteria are inhibited by bile and gentamicin in this medium, whereas the *B. fragilis* group of organisms is stimulated by bile, resistant to gentamicin, and able to hydrolyze esculin, producing a black precipitate.

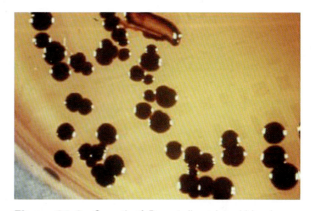

Figure 31-6   Growth of *Prevotella* on lysed blood agar. Note the black pigmentation of the colonies.

Biochemical tests can identify most normal gram-negative anaerobes. Newly-recognized species can be analysis of species-specific genes (e.g., 16S ribosomal RNA gene).

Treatment, Prevention, and Control

Antibiotic therapy combined with surgical intervention is the main approach for managing serious anaerobic infections. Virtually all members of the *B. fragilis* group, many *Prevotella* and *Porphyromonas* species, and some *Fusobacterium* isolates produce β-lactamases. This enzyme renders the bacteria resistant to penicillin and many cephalosporins. Antibiotics with the best activity against gram-negative anaerobic rods are **metronidazole**, **carbapenems** (e.g., imipenem, meropenem), and **β-lactam-β-**

lactamase inhibitors (e.g., piperacillin-tazobactam). Clindamycin resistance in *Bacteroides*, which is plasmid mediated, has become more prevalent; an average of 20% to 25% of the isolates in the United States are now resistant.

Because *Bacteroides* species constitute an important part of the normal microbial flora, and because infections result from the endogenous spread of the organisms, disease is virtually impossible to control. It is important to recognize, however, that disruption of the natural barriers around the mucosal surfaces by diagnostic or surgical procedures can introduce these organisms into normally sterile sites. If the barriers are invaded, prophylactic treatment with antibiotics may be indicated.

SUMMARY

Predominant Anaerobic Gram-Negative Bacteria Responsible for Human Disease

Head and neck infections	*Bacteroides ureolyticus; Fusobacterium nucleatum; Fusobacterium necrophorum; Porphyromonas asaccharolytica; Porphyromonas gingivalis; Prevotella intermedia; Prevotella melaninogenica Veillonella parvula*
Intraabdominal infections	*Bacteroides fragilis; Bacteroides thetaiotaomicron; P. melaninogenica*
Gynecologic infections	*B. fragilis; Prevotella bivia; Prevotella disiens*
Skin and soft tissue infections	*B. fragilis*
Bacteremia	*B. fragilis; B. thetaiotaomicron; Fusobacterium spp.*

KEYWORDS

English	Chinese
Bacteroides	拟杆菌属
Fusobacterium	梭杆菌属
Parabacteroides	副拟杆菌属
Porphyromonas	紫单胞菌属
Prevotella	普雷沃菌属
Veillonella	韦荣菌属

BIBLIOGRAPHY

1. Aldridge KE, et al: Bacteremia due to *Bacteroides fragilis* group: distribution of species, β-lactamase production, and antimicrobial susceptibility patterns, Antimicrob Agents Chemother 47: 148-156, 2003.

2. Aldridge KE, O'Brien M: In vitro susceptibilities of the *Bacteroides fragilis* group species: change in isolation rates significantly affects overall susceptibility data, J Clin Microbiol 40: 4349-4352, 2002.

3. Duerden B: Virulence factors in anaerobes, Clin Infect Dis 18(Suppl 4): S253-S259, 1994.

4. Jousimies-Somer H, Summanen P: Recent taxonomic changes and terminology update of clinically significant anaerobic gram-negative bacteria (excluding spirochetes), Clin Infect Dis 35(Suppl 1): S17-S21, 2002.

5. Sears C: Enterotoxigenic *Bacteroides fragilis*: a rogue among symbiotes, Clin Microbiol Rev 22: 349-369, 2009.

6. Wexler H: *Bacteroides*: the good, the bad, and the nitty-gritty, Clin Microbiol Rev 20: 593-621, 2007.

Chapter 32

Treponema, Borrelia, and *Leptospira*

The bacteria in the order Spirochaetales have been grouped together on the basis of their common morphologic properties. These spirochetes are thin, helical (0.1 to 0.5 × 5 to 20 μm), gram-negative bacteria. The order Spirochaetales is subdivided into 4 families and 14 genera, of which 3 genera (*Treponema* and *Borrelia* in the family Spirochaetaceae, and *Leptospira* in the family Leptospiraceae) are responsible for human disease (Tables 32-1).

TREPONEMA

The two treponemal species that cause human disease are *Treponema pallidum* (with three subspecies) and *Treponema carateum*. All are morphologically identical, produce the same serologic response in humans, and are susceptible to penicillin. The organisms are distinguished by their epidemiologic characteristics, clinical presentation, and host range in experimental animals. *T. pallidum* subspecies *pallidum* (referred to as *T. pallidum* in this chapter) is the etiologic agent of the venereal disease **syphilis;** *T. pallidum* subspecies *endemicum* causes endemic syphilis (**bejel**); *T. pallidum* subspecies *pertenue* causes **yaws;** and *T. carateum* causes **pinta.** Bejel, yaws, and pinta are nonvenereal diseases. Syphilis is discussed initially; the other treponemal diseases are discussed at the end of the section.

Physiology and Structure

T. pallidum and related pathogenic treponemes are thin, tightly coiled spirochetes (0.1 to 0.2 × 6 to 20 μm) with pointed, straight ends. Three periplasmic flagellae are inserted at each end. These spirochetes do not grow in cell-free cultures. Limited growth of the organisms has been achieved in cultured rabbit epithelial cells, but replication is slow (doubling time is 30 hours) and can be maintained for only a few generations. The reason for this failure to grow *T. pallidum* in vitro is because the tricarboxylic acid cycle is missing in the bacteria, and they are dependent on host cells for all purines, pyrimidines, and most

Table 32-1 Medically Important Genera in the Order Spirochaetales

Spirochaetales	Human Disease	Etiologic Agent
Family Spirochaetaceae		
Genus *Borrelia*	Epidemic relapsing fever	*B. recurrentis*
	Endemic relapsing fever	Many *Borrelia* species
	Lyme borreliosis	*B. burgdorferi, B. garinii, B. afzelii*
Genus *Treponema*	Venereal syphilis	*T. pallidum* subsp. *pallidum*
	Endemic syphilis (bejel)	*T. pallidum* subsp. *endemicum*
	Yaws	*T. pallidum* subsp. *pertenue*
	Pinta	*T. carateum*
Family Leptospiraceae		
Genus *Leptospira*	Leptospirosis	*Leptospira* spp.

amino acids. In addition, the spirochetes are micro-aerophilic or anaerobic and are extremely sensitive to oxygen toxicity. The complete genome sequence has revealed there are no genes for catalase or superoxide dismutase.

The spirochetes are too thin to be seen with light microscopy in specimens stained with Gram or Giemsa stain. However, motile forms can be visualized by darkfield illumination or by staining with specific anti-treponemal antibodies labeled with fluorescent dyes.

Pathogenesis and Immunity

The inability to grow *T. pallidum* to high concentrations in vitro has limited detection of specific virulence factors in this organism. However, analysis of the entire genome sequence and the unique structural properties of this spirochete have revealed some insights. Although a number of lipoproteins are anchored in the bacterial cytoplasmic membrane, most or all are not exposed on the surface of the outer membrane. Thus the lack of species-specific antigens on the cell surface allows the spirochete to evade the immune system. Although the bacteria are able to resist phagocytosis, they can adhere to host fibronectin, allowing direct interaction with the host tissues. Analysis of the genome sequence demonstrates the presence of at least five hemolysins, but it is unclear if they mediate tissue damage. Likewise, it has been proposed that production of hyaluronidase facilitates perivascular infiltration, but this remains to be demonstrated. Most investigators believe that the tissue destruction and lesions observed in syphilis are primarily the consequence of the patient's immune response to infection.

The clinical course of syphilis evolves through three phases. The initial or **primary phase** is characterized by one or more skin lesions (**chancres**) at the site where the spirochete penetrated (Figure 32-1). Although spirochetes are disseminated in the blood soon after infection, the chancre represents the primary site of initial replication. Histologic examination of the lesion reveals endarteritis and periarteritis (characteristic of syphilitic lesions at all stages) and infiltration of the ulcer with polymorphonuclear

leukocytes and macrophages. Phagocytic cells ingest spirochetes, but the organisms often survive. In the **secondary phase,** the clinical signs of disseminated disease appear, with prominent skin lesions dispersed over the entire body surface (Figure 32-2). Spontaneous remission may occur after the primary or sec-

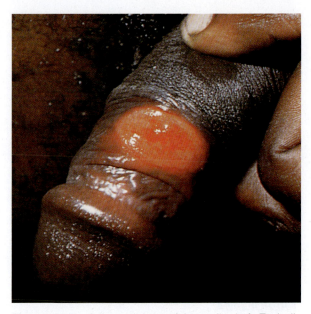

Figure 32-1   Primary chancre of the penile shaft. Typically the lesion is painless unless secondary bacterial infection is present. Large numbers of spirochetes are present in the lesion. (From Morse S, et al: *Atlas of sexually transmitted diseases and AIDS*, St Louis, 2003, Mosby.)

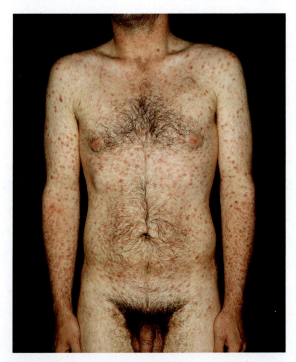

Figure 32-2   Disseminated rash in secondary syphilis. (From Habif TP: *Clinical dermatology: a color guide to diagnosis and therapy*, St Louis, 1996, Mosby.)

ondary stages, or the disease may progress to the **late phase** of disease, in which virtually all tissues may be involved. Each stage represents localized multiplication of the spirochete and tissue destruction. Although replication is slow, numerous organisms are present in the initial chancre, as well as in the secondary lesions, making the patient highly infectious at these stages.

Epidemiology

Syphilis is found worldwide and is the third most common sexually transmitted bacterial disease in the United States (after *Chlamydia trachomatis* and *Neisseria gonorrhoeae* infections). Overall, the incidence of disease has decreased since the advent of penicillin therapy in the early 1940s, although periodic increases have been observed that correspond to changes in sexual practices (e.g., use of birth control pills in the 1960s, gay bath houses in the 1970s, increased prostitution related to crack cocaine use in the 1990s). A troubling trend is evolving now. Between 2000 and 2010, the incidence of newly acquired disease (i.e., primary and secondary syphilis) has more than doubled, with almost 14,000 cases reported in 2010, primarily in homosexual males. This likely reflects the mistaken perception that sexually acquired diseases, including human immunodeficiency virus (HIV) infections, can be controlled effectively with antibiotics, so unprotected sex is a low-risk activity. Unfortunately, patients infected with syphilis are at increased risk for transmitting and acquiring HIV when genital lesions are present. Thus, despite a concerted public health effort to eliminate syphilis, this disease remains a serious problem in sexually active populations.

Natural syphilis is exclusive to humans and has no other known natural hosts. *T. pallidum* is extremely labile, unable to survive exposure to drying or disinfectants. Thus syphilis cannot be spread through contact with inanimate objects, such as toilet seats. The most common route of spread is by direct sexual contact. The disease can also be acquired congenitally or by transfusion with contaminated blood. Syphilis is not highly contagious; the risk of contracting the disease after a single sexual contact is estimated to be 30%. However, contagiousness is influenced by the stage of disease in the infectious person. As mentioned previously, the spirochetes cannot survive on dry skin surfaces. Thus *T. pallidum* is transferred primarily during the early stages of disease, when many organisms are present in moist, cutaneous or mucosal lesions. During the early stages of disease, the patient becomes bacteremic and, if the disease is untreated, bacteremia can persist for as long as 8 years. Congenital transmission from mother to fetus can occur at any time during this period. After 8 years, the disease can remain active, but bacteremia is not believed to occur.

Clinical Diseases

Primary Syphilis

As already noted, the initial syphilitic chancre develops at the site where the spirochete is inoculated. The lesion develops 10 to 90 days after the initial infection and starts as a papule but then erodes to become a **painless ulcer** with raised borders (see Figure 32-1). In most patients, a painless regional lymphadenopathy develops 1 to 2 weeks after the appearance of the chancre, which represents a local focus for the proliferation of spirochetes. Abundant spirochetes are present in the chancre and can be disseminated throughout the patient via the lymphatic system and blood. The fact that this ulcer heals spontaneously within 2 months gives the patient a false sense of relief.

Secondary Syphilis

The clinical evidence of disseminated disease marks the second stage of syphilis. In this stage, patients typically experience a flulike syndrome with sore throat, headache, fever, myalgias (muscle aches), anorexia, lymphadenopathy (swollen lymph nodes), and a generalized mucocutaneous rash (see Figure 32-2). The flulike syndrome and lymphadenopathy generally appear first and then are followed a few days later by the disseminated skin rash. The rash can be variable (macular, papular, pustular), cover the entire skin surface (including the palms and soles), and may resolve slowly over a period of weeks to months.

Raised lesions, called **condylomata lata,** may occur in moist skin folds, and erosions may develop in the mouth and on other mucosal surfaces. As with the primary chancre, these lesions are highly infectious. The rash and symptoms resolve spontaneously within a few weeks, and the patient enters the latent or clinically inactive stage of disease.

Tertiary (Late) Syphilis

Approximately one third of untreated patients progress to the tertiary stage of syphilis. Clinical symptoms of the diffuse, chronic inflammation characteristic of late syphilis develop after an asymptomatic period of a few years to decades and can cause devastating destruction of virtually any organ or tissue (e.g., arteritis, dementia, blindness). Granulomatous lesions (**gummas**) may be found in bone, skin, and other tissues. The nomenclature of late syphilis reflects the organs of primary involvement (e.g., neurosyphilis, cardiovascular syphilis). An increased incidence of neurosyphilis despite adequate therapy for early syphilis has been documented in patients with acquired immunodeficiency syndrome (AIDS). In addition, spirochetes are introduced into the central nervous system during the early stages of disease, and neurologic symptoms, such as meningitis, can develop within the first few months of disease. Thus neurosyphilis is not exclusively a late manifestation.

Congenital Syphilis

In utero infections can lead to serious fetal disease, resulting in latent infections, multiorgan malformations, or death of the fetus. Most infected infants are born without clinical evidence of the disease, but rhinitis then develops and is followed by a widespread desquamating maculopapular rash. Teeth and bone malformation, blindness, deafness, and cardiovascular syphilis are common in untreated infants who survive the initial phase of disease.

Laboratory Diagnosis

Microscopy

Because *T. pallidum* is too thin to be seen by light microscopy, **darkfield microscopy** or **special fluorescent stains** must be used. The diagnosis of primary, secondary, or congenital syphilis can be made rapidly by darkfield examination of the exudate from skin lesions; however, the test is reliable only when an experienced microscopist immediately examines the clinical material with actively motile spirochetes. The spirochetes do not survive transport to the laboratory, and tissue debris can be mistaken for nonviable spirochetes. Material collected from oral and rectal lesions should not be examined because nonpathogenic spirochetes can contaminate the specimen. Because of the limitations of darkfield microscopy, a more useful test for detecting *T. pallidum* is the **direct fluorescent antibody test.** Fluorescein-labeled antitreponemal antibodies are used to stain the bacteria (Figure 32-3). A monoclonal antibody reagent is available that is specific for pathogenic treponemes, so oral and rectal specimens can be examined. Nonviable spirochetes will also stain; therefore specimens do not need to be examined immediately after collection.

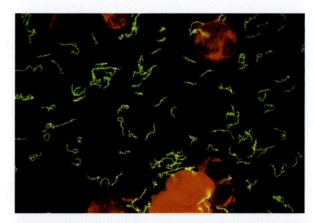

Figure 32-3 *Treponema pallidum* in the direct fluorescent antibody test for *T. pallidum*. (From Morse S, et al: *Atlas of sexually transmitted diseases and AIDS*, St Louis, 2003, Mosby.)

Culture

Efforts to culture *T. pallidum* in vitro should not be attempted because the organism does not grow in artificial cultures.

Nucleic Acid-Based Tests

Nucleic acid amplification tests (i.e., polymerase chain reaction [PCR]) have been developed for detecting *T. pallidum* in genital lesions, infant blood, and cerebrospinal fluid (CSF) but are only available in research or reference laboratories.

Antibody Detection

Syphilis is diagnosed in most patients on the basis of serologic tests. The two general types of tests used are biologically nonspecific (nontreponemal) tests and specific treponemal tests. The nontreponemal tests are used as screening tests because they are rapid to perform and inexpensive. Positive reactivity with one of these tests is confirmed with a treponemal test.

Nontreponemal tests measure immunoglobulin G (IgG) and IgM antibodies (also called **reaginic antibodies**) developed against lipids released from damaged cells during the early stage of disease and that appear on the cell surface of treponemes. The antigen used for the nontreponemal tests is **cardiolipin,** which is derived from beef heart. The two tests used most commonly are the **Venereal Disease Research Laboratory (VDRL) test** and the **rapid plasma reagin (RPR) test.** Both tests measure the flocculation of cardiolipin antigen by the patient's serum. Both tests can be performed rapidly, although complement in serum must be inactivated for 30 minutes before the VDRL test can be performed. Only the VDRL test should be used to test CSF from patients with suspected neurosyphilis. Other nontreponemal tests in use include the unheated serum reagin (USR) test and the toluidine red unheated serum test (TRUST). All nontreponemal tests have essentially the same sensitivity (70% to 85% for primary disease, 100% for secondary disease, 70% to 75% for late syphilis) and specificity (98% to 99%).

Treponemal tests use *T. pallidum* as the antigen and detect specific anti-*T. pallidum* antibodies. The treponemal test results can be positive before the nontreponemal test results become positive in early syphilis, and they can remain positive when the nonspecific test results revert to negative in some patients who have late syphilis. Historically, the most commonly used treponemal test was the **fluorescent treponemal antibody-absorption (FTA-ABS) test.** The FTA-ABS test is an indirect fluores-

cent antibody test. *T. pallidum* immobilized on glass slides is used as the antigen. The slide is overlayed with the patient's serum, which has been mixed with an extract of nonpathogenic treponemes. The fluorescein-labeled antihuman antibodies are then added to detect the presence of specific antibodies in the patient's serum. Because these tests are technically difficult to interpret, most laboratories now use either the ***Treponema pallidum* particle agglutination (TP-PA) test** or one of a number of specific **enzyme immunoassays (EIAs).** The TP-PA test is a microtiter agglutination test. Gelatin particles sensitized with *T. pallidum* antigens are mixed with dilutions of the patient's serum. If antibodies are present, the particles agglutinate. A variety of specific EIAs have been developed and appear to have sensitivities (80% to 95% for primary disease, 100% for secondary and late syphilis) and specificities (96% to 99%) similar to the FTA-ABS and TP-PA tests.

Because positive reactions with the nontreponemal tests develop late during the first phase of disease, the serologic findings are negative in many patients who initially have chancres. However, serologic results are positive within 3 months in all patients and remain positive in untreated patients with secondary syphilis. The antibody titers decrease slowly in patients with untreated syphilis, and serologic results are negative in approximately 25% to 30% of patients with late syphilis. Thus the limitation of the nontreponemal tests is reduced sensitivity in early primary disease and late syphilis. Although the results of treponemal tests generally remain positive for the life of the person who has syphilis, a negative test is unreliable in patients with AIDS.

Successful treatment of primary or secondary syphilis and, to a lesser extent, late syphilis, leads to reduced titers measured in the VDRL and RPR tests. Thus these tests can be used to monitor the effectiveness of therapy, although seroreversion is slowed in patients in an advanced stage of disease, those with high initial titers, and those who have previously had syphilis. The treponemal tests are influenced less by therapy than are the VDRL and RPR tests, with seroreversion observed in less than 25% of patients successfully treated during the primary stage of the disease.

Transient false-positive reactions with the nontreponemal tests are seen in patients with acute febrile diseases, after immunizations, and in pregnant women. Long-term false-positive reactions occur most often in patients with chronic autoimmune diseases or infections that involve the liver or that cause extensive tissue destruction. Most false-positive reactions with the treponemal tests are observed in patients with elevated immunoglobin levels and autoimmune diseases (Box 39-2). Many of the false-positive reactions can be resolved using the Western blot assay.

Diagnosis of neurosyphilis and congenital syphilis can be problematic. The diagnosis of neurosyphilis is based on clinical symptoms and laboratory findings. A VDRL test on CSF is highly specific but not sensitive. Thus a positive VDRL confirms the diagnosis, but a negative test does not rule out neurosyphilis. In contrast, the FTA-ABS CSF test has high sensitivity but low specificity because of passive transfer of antitreponemal antibodies from blood to CSF. In this case, a positive FTA-ABS CSF test is consistent with neurosyphilis but is not diagnostic, and a negative test would essentially rule out the diagnosis. Positive serologic test results in infants of infected mothers can represent a passive transfer of antibodies or a specific immunologic response to a congenital infection. These two possibilities are distinguished by measuring the antibody titers in the sera of the infant during a 6-month period. The antibody titers in noninfected infants decrease to undetectable levels within 3 months of birth but remain elevated in infants who have congenital syphilis.

Treatment, Prevention, and Control

Penicillin is the drug of choice for treating *T. pallidum* infections. Long-acting benzathine **penicillin** is used for the early stages of syphilis, and penicillin G is recommended for congenital and late syphilis. **Doxycycline** or **azithromycin** can be used as alternative antibiotics for patients allergic to penicillin. Only penicillin can be used for the treatment of neurosyphilis; thus, penicillin-allergic patients must

undergo desensitization. This is also true for pregnant women, who should not be treated with the tetracyclines. Treatment failures with the macrolides have been observed, so patients treated with azithromycin should be closely monitored.

Because protective vaccines are not available, syphilis can be controlled only through the practice of safe-sex techniques and adequate contact and treatment of the sex partners of patients who have been documented with infection. The control of syphilis and other venereal diseases has been complicated by an increase in prostitution among drug abusers and high-risk sexual practices in homosexual males.

OTHER TREPONEMES

Three other nonvenereal treponemal diseases are important: **endemic syphilis (bejel), yaws,** and **pinta.** *T. pallidum* subspecies *endemicum* is responsible for endemic syphilis. Disease is spread person to person by the direct contact of early lesions or use of contaminated eating utensils. The initial oral lesions are rarely observed, but secondary lesions include oral papules and mucosal patches. Gummas of the skin, bones, and nasopharynx are late manifestations. The disease is present in desert and temperate regions of North Africa and the Middle East and is primarily a disease of children.

T. pertenue is the etiologic agent of **yaws,** a granulomatous disease in which patients have skin lesions early in the disease (Figure 32-4) and then late destructive lesions of the skin, lymph nodes, and bones. The disease is present in tropical and desert areas of South America, Central Africa, and Indonesia and is spread among children by direct contact with infected skin lesions.

T. carateum is responsible for causing **pinta,** a disease that primarily affects the skin. Small pruritic papules develop on the skin surface after a 1- to 3-week incubation period. These lesions enlarge and persist for months to years before resolving. Disseminated, recurrent, hypopigmented lesions can develop over years, resulting in scarring and disfigurement. Pinta is present in tropical areas of Central

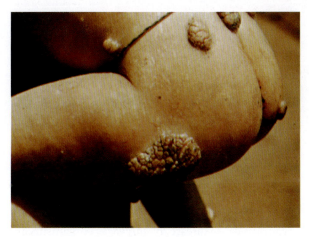

Figure 32-4   The elevated papillomatous nodules characteristic of early yaws are widely distributed and painless. They contain numerous spirochetes that are easily seen on darkfield microscopy studies. (From Peters W, Gilles HM: *A color atlas of tropical medicine and parasitology,* ed 4, London, 1995, Wolfe.)

and South America, is spread by direct contact with infected lesions, and is a disease of young adults (15 to 30 years of age).

Bejel, yaws, and pinta are diagnosed by their typical clinical manifestation in an endemic area. The diagnoses of yaws and pinta are confirmed by the detection of spirochetes in skin lesions by darkfield microscopy, but this test cannot be used to detect spirochetes in patients with the oral lesions of bejel. The results of serologic tests for syphilis are also positive.

Penicillin, tetracycline, and chloramphenicol have been used to treat these diseases. The diseases are controlled through the treatment of infected people and the elimination of person-to-person spread.

BORRELIA

Members of the genus *Borrelia* cause two important human diseases: **Lyme disease** and **relapsing fever.** The history of Lyme disease began in 1977, when an unusual cluster of children with arthritis was noted in Lyme, Connecticut. Five years later, W. Burgdorfer discovered the spirochete responsible for this disease. Lyme disease is a tick-borne disease with protean manifestations, including dermatologic, rheumatologic, neurologic, and cardiac abnormalities. Ini-

tially, it was believed that all cases of Lyme disease (or Lyme borreliosis) were caused by one organism, *B. burgdorferi*. However, subsequent studies have determined that a complex of at least 10 *Borrelia* species is responsible for Lyme disease in animals and humans. Three species (i.e., *B. burgdorferi, Borrelia garinii,* and *Borrelia afzelii*) cause human disease, with *B. burgdorferi* found in the United States and Europe and *B. garinii* and *B. afzelii* found in Europe and central to eastern Asia. This chapter focuses on *B. burgdorferi* infections. Relapsing fever is a febrile illness characterized by recurrent episodes of fever and septicemia separated by afebrile periods. Two forms of the disease are recognized. *Borrelia recurrentis* is the etiologic agent of **epidemic** or **louse-borne relapsing fever** and is spread person-to-person by the human body **louse** (*Pediculus humanus*). **Endemic relapsing fever** is caused by as many as 15 species of borreliae and is spread by infected **soft ticks** of the genus *Ornithodoros*.

Physiology and Structure

Members of the genus *Borrelia* stain poorly with the Gram stain reagents and are considered neither gram-positive nor gram-negative, even though they have an outer membrane similar to gram-negative bacteria. They tend to be larger than other spirochetes (0.2 to 0.5 × 8 to 30 μm), stain well with aniline dyes (e.g., Giemsa or Wright stain), and can be easily seen by light microscopy when present in smears of peripheral blood from patients with relapsing fever (Figure 32-5) but not those with Lyme disease. From 7 to 20 periplasmic flagella (depending on the species) are present between the periplasmic cylinder and the outer envelope and are responsible for the organism's twisting motility (Figure 32-6). Borreliae are microaerophilic and have complex nutritional needs (i.e., requiring N-acetylglucosamine, long-chain saturated and unsaturated fatty acids, glucose, and amino acids). The species that have been successfully cultured have generation times of 18 hours or longer. Because culture is generally unsuccessful, diagnosis of diseases caused by borreliae is by microscopy (relapsing fever) or serology (Lyme disease).

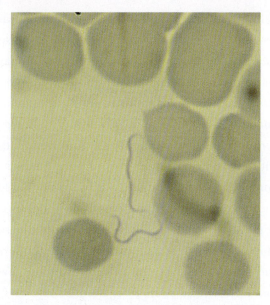

Figure 32-5 *Borrelia* organisms are present in the blood of this patient with endemic relapsing fever (Giemsa stain).

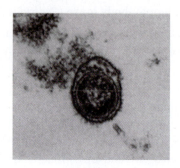

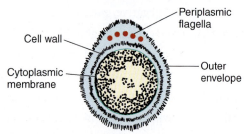

Figure 32-6 Electron micrograph and drawing of a cross-section through *Borrelia burgdorferi*, the agent that causes Lyme borreliosis. The protoplasmic core of the bacterium is enclosed in a cytoplasmic membrane and conventional cell wall. This in turn, is surrounded by an outer envelope, or sheath. Between the protoplasmic core and outer sheath are periplasmic flagella (also called *axial fibrils*), which are anchored at either end of the bacterium and wrap around the protoplasmic core. (From Steere AC, et al: The spirochetal etiology of Lyme disease, *N Engl J Med* 308: 733-740, 1983.)

Pathogenesis and Immunity

The growth of borreliae in both arthropod vectors and mammalian hosts is regulated by differential gene expression with up-regulation or down-regulation of outer surface proteins. For example, outer surface protein A (OspA) is expressed on the surface of *B. burgdorferi* residing in the midgut of unfed ticks. This protein binds specifically to gut proteins. Upon feeding, expression of this protein is repressed, allowing the spirochete to migrate to the salivary glands, and outer surface protein C (OspC) expression, which appears critical for transmission from ticks to mammals, is up-regulated. Unfortunately, knowledge of the complete genome sequence of *B. burgdorferi* has not led to a clear understanding of how these organisms cause disease. *B. burgdorferi* organisms are present in low numbers in the skin when erythema migrans develops. This has been shown by culture of the organism from skin lesions or detection of bacterial nucleic acids by PCR amplification; however, culture and PCR tests are relatively insensitive in the early phase of disease and are not widely available in clinical laboratories. In addition, spirochetes are infrequently isolated from clinical material late in the disease. It is not known whether the viable organisms cause these late manifestations of disease or whether they represent immunologic cross-reactivity to *Borrelia* antigens. Although the immune response to the organism is depressed at the time that skin lesions initially develop, antibodies develop over months to years and are responsible for producing the complement-mediated clearance of the borreliae.

Our understanding of mechanisms by which borreliae cause relapsing fever is also incomplete. Members of the genus do not produce recognized toxins and are removed rapidly when a specific antibody response is mounted. The periodic febrile and afebrile cycles of relapsing fever result from the ability of the borreliae to undergo antigenic variation. These spirochetes carry a large number of genes homologous to the OspC gene, but only one gene is expressed at a time. When specific antibodies are formed, agglutination with complement-mediated lysis occurs, and the borreliae are cleared rapidly from the blood. However, switching of the expression of the gene family occurs at a frequency of 10^{-3} to 10^{-4} per generation. Thus a new population of spirochetes with a new lipoprotein coat will appear in the blood heralding a new febrile episode.

Epidemiology

Despite the relatively recent recognition of Lyme disease in the United States, retrospective studies have shown that the disease was present for many years in this and other countries. Lyme disease has been described on 6 continents, in at least 20 countries, and in 49 states of the United States. The incidence of disease has risen dramatically between 1982 (497 cases were reported) and 2010 (more than 30,000 cases were reported). **Lyme disease is the leading vector-borne disease in the United States.** The three principal foci of infection in the United States are the Northeast and mid-Atlantic states (Massachusetts to Maryland), the upper Midwest (Minnesota and Wisconsin), and the Pacific West (northern California and Oregon). **Hard ticks are the major vectors** of Lyme disease: *Ixodes scapularis* in the Northeast, mid-Atlantic, and Midwest and *Ixodes pacificus* on the West Coast. *Ixodes ricinus* is the major tick vector in Europe, and *Ixodes persulcatus* is the major tick vector in Eastern Europe and Asia. The major reservoir hosts in the United States are the white-footed mouse and the white-tailed deer. The **white-footed mouse** is the primary host of larval and nymph forms of *Ixodes* species, and the adult *Ixodes* species infest the **white-tailed deer.** Because the nymph stage causes more than 90% of the cases of documented disease, the mouse host is more relevant for human disease.

Ixodes larvae become infected when they feed on the mouse reservoir. The larva molts to a nymph in late spring and takes a second blood meal; in this case, humans can be accidental hosts. Although the borreliae are transmitted in the tick's saliva during a prolonged period of feeding (48 hours or more), most patients do not remember having had a specific tick bite because the nymph is the size of a poppy seed. The nymphs mature into adults in the late summer and take a third feeding. Although the white-tailed deer is the natural host, humans can also be infected at this stage. Most infected patients are identified in May to August, although disease can be encountered throughout the year.

As previously mentioned, the etiologic agent of louse-borne epidemic relapsing fever is *B. recurrentis*, the vector is the human body louse, and humans are the only reservoir (Figure 32-7). Lice become infected after feeding on an infected person. The organisms are ingested, pass through the wall of the gut, and multiply in hemolymph. Disseminated disease is not believed to occur in lice; thus human infection occurs when the lice are crushed during feeding. Because infected lice do not survive for more than a few months, maintenance of the disease requires crowded, unsanitary conditions (e.g., wars, natural disasters) that permit frequent human contact with infected lice. Although epidemics of louse-borne relapsing fever swept from Eastern to Western Europe in the past century, the disease now appears to be restricted to Ethiopia, Rwanda, and the Andean foothills.

Infection	Reservoir	Vector
Relapsing fever epidemic (louse-borne)	Humans	Body louse 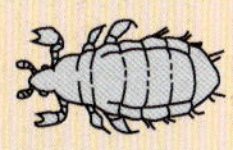
Relapsing fever endemic (tick-borne)	Rodents, soft ticks	Soft tick 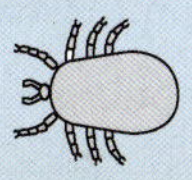
Lyme disease	Rodents, deer, domestic pets, hard ticks	Hard tick 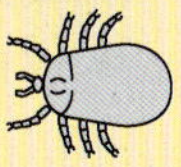

Figure 32-7   Epidemiology of *Borrelia* infections.

Several features distinguish **endemic relapsing fever** from epidemic disease. Tick-borne endemic relapsing fever is a **zoonotic disease,** with rodents, small mammals, and soft ticks (*Ornithodoros* species) the main reservoirs and **many species of *Borrelia*** responsible for the disease. Unlike the louse-borne infections, the borreliae that cause endemic disease produce a disseminated infection in ticks. In addition, the arthropods can survive and maintain an endemic reservoir of infection by transovarian transmission. Furthermore, ticks can survive for months between feedings. A history of a tick bite may also not be elicited because soft ticks are primarily nocturnal feeders and remain attached for only a few minutes. The ticks contaminate the bite wound with borreliae present in saliva or feces. Tick-borne disease is found worldwide, corresponding to the distribution of the *Ornithodoros* tick. In the United States, disease is primarily found in the western states.

Clinical Diseases

Lyme Disease

Clinical diagnosis of Lyme disease is complicated by the varied manifestations of disease caused by *B. burgdorferi* and other *Borrelia* species, as well as the lack of reliable diagnostic tests. The following paragraph is a description of Lyme disease in the United States. The frequency of the skin lesions and late manifestations differ in disease observed in other countries.

Lyme disease begins as an early localized infection, progresses to an early disseminated stage, and, if untreated, can progress to a late manifestation stage. After an incubation period of 3 to 30 days, one or more skin lesions typically develop at the site of the tick bite. The lesion (**erythema migrans**) begins as a small macule or papule and then enlarges over the next few weeks, ultimately covering an area ranging from 5 cm to more than 50 cm in diameter (Figure 32-8). The lesion typically has a flat, red border and central clearing as it develops; however, erythema, vesicle formation, and central necrosis can also be seen. The lesion fades and disappears within weeks, although new transient lesions may subsequently appear. Although the skin lesion is characteristic of Lyme disease, it is not pathognomonic. A similar skin lesion associated with disease of unknown etiology (STARI, or southern tick-associated rash illness) occurs after the bite of the *Amblyomma americanum* tick (lone star tick). These ticks, found in the southeast and south central regions of the United States, are not infected with *B. burgdorferi*. Other early signs and symptoms of Lyme disease include malaise, severe fatigue, headache, fever, chills, musculoskeletal pains, myalgias, and lymphadenopathy. These symptoms last for an average of 4 weeks.

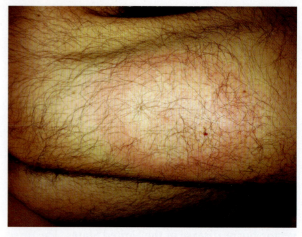

Figure 32-8 Erythema migrans rash on the thigh of the author's son (PRM). An engorged nymph stage of an *Ixodes* tick was found 3 days after exposure. Twelve days later, the rash appeared with accompanying localized pain and progressed to 5 cm in diameter with central clearing. The rash faded over the next week with doxycycline treatment, and the infection, confirmed by culture of the biopsy, resolved with no secondary complications.

Hematogenous dissemination will occur in untreated patients within days to weeks of the primary infection. This stage is characterized by systemic signs of disease (e.g., severe fatigue, headache, fever, malaise), arthritis and arthralgia, myalgia, erythematous skins lesions, cardiac dysfunction, and neurologic signs. Approximately 60% of patients with untreated Lyme disease will develop **arthritis,** typically involving the knee; approximately 10% to 20% will develop **neurologic manifestations** (most commonly facial nerve palsy); and 5% will have **cardiac complications** (usually varying degrees of atrioventricular block).

Late-stage manifestations of Lyme disease in untreated patients can develop months to years after the initial infection. Arthritis can involve one or more joints intermittently. Chronic skin involvement with discoloration and swelling (**acrodermatitis chronica atrophicans**; Figure 32-9) is more common in Lyme disease seen in Europe. The existence of chronic, symptomatic Lyme disease in appropriately treated patients has not been demonstrated definitively.

Relapsing Fever

The clinical presentations of epidemic louse-borne and endemic tick-borne relapsing fever are essentially the same, although a small, pruritic eschar may

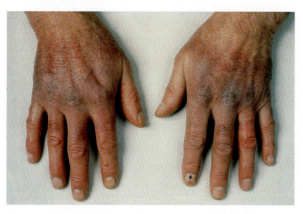

Figure 32-9 Acrodermatitis chronica atrophicans. Bluish-red skin lesions characteristic of late, disseminated manifestations of Lyme borreliosis. (From Cohen J, Powderly W: *Infectious diseases*, ed 2, St Louis, 2004, Mosby.)

develop at the site of the tick bite. After a 1-week incubation period, the disease is heralded by the abrupt onset of shaking chills, fever, muscle aches, and headache. Splenomegaly and hepatomegaly are common. These symptoms correspond to the bacteremic phase of the disease and resolve after 3 to 7 days, when the borreliae are cleared from the blood. Bacteremia and fever return after a 1-week afebrile period. The clinical symptoms are generally milder and last a shorter time during this and subsequent **febrile episodes.** A single relapse is characteristic of epidemic louse-borne disease, and as many as 10 relapses occur in endemic tick-borne disease. The clinical course and outcome of epidemic relapsing fever tend to be more severe than they are in those with endemic disease, but this may be related to the patients' underlying poor state of health. Mortality with endemic disease is less than 5% but can be as high as 40% in louse-borne epidemic disease. Deaths are caused by cardiac failure, hepatic necrosis, or cerebral hemorrhage.

Laboratory Diagnosis

Microscopy

Borreliae that cause relapsing fever can be seen during the febrile period on Giemsa- or Wright-stained preparation of blood. This is the most sensitive method for diagnosing relapsing fever, with smears positive for organisms in more than 70% of patients. Micro-

scopic examination of blood or tissues from patients with Lyme disease is not recommended because *B. burgdorferi* is rarely seen in clinical specimens.

Culture

Some borreliae, including *B. recurrentis* and *Borrelia hermsii* (a common cause of endemic relapsing fever in the United States), can be cultured in vitro on specialized media. The cultures are rarely performed in most clinical laboratories, however, because the media are not readily available and the organisms grow slowly on them. There has been limited success with the culture of *B. burgdorferi*, although isolation of the organism has been improved through the use of specialized media. However, the sensitivity of culture is low for all specimens except the initial skin lesion.

Nucleic Acid-Based Tests

Nucleic acid amplification techniques have a sensitivity of approximately 65% to 75% with skin biopsies, 50% to 85% with synovial fluid, and 25% with CSF specimens from patients with documented Lyme disease. These tests are generally restricted to research and reference laboratories, and the test results should be confirmed by culture or serology.

Antibody Detection

Serologic tests are not useful in the diagnosis of relapsing fever because the borreliae that cause this condition undergo antigenic phase variation. In contrast, serologic testing is the diagnostic test of choice for patients with suspected Lyme disease. The tests most commonly used are the immunofluorescence assay (IFA) and EIA. The U.S. Food and Drug Administration has cleared more than 70 serologic assays for the diagnosis of Lyme disease. Unfortunately, all serologic tests are relatively insensitive during the early acute stage of disease. IgM antibodies appear 2 to 4 weeks after the onset of erythema migrans in untreated patients; the levels peak after 6 to 8 weeks of illness and then decline to a normal range after 4 to 6 months. The IgM level may remain elevated in some patients with a persistent infection.

The IgG antibodies appear later. Their levels peak after 4 to 6 months of illness and persist during the late manifestations of the disease. Thus most patients with late complications of Lyme disease have detectable antibodies to *B. burgdorferi*, although the antibody level may be ablated in patients treated with antibiotics. Detection of antibodies in CSF is strong evidence for neuroborreliosis.

Although cross-reactions are uncommon, positive serologic results must be interpreted carefully, particularly if the titers are low. Most false-positive reactions occur in patients with syphilis. These false results can be excluded by performing a nontreponemal test for syphilis; the result is negative in patients with Lyme disease. Western blot analysis has been used to confirm the specificity of a positive EIA or IFA reaction. A specimen with a negative EIA or IFA reaction does not require further testing. Guidelines for interpretation of Western immunoblots are available on the CDC website (www.cdc.gov). Antigenic heterogeneity in *B. burgdorferi* and other *Borrelia* species that cause Lyme disease affects the test sensitivity. The magnitude of this problem in the United States is unknown, but it should be significant in Europe and Asia, where multiple *Borrelia* species are found to cause Lyme disease. At present, serologic tests should be considered confirmatory and should not be performed in the absence of an appropriate history and clinical symptoms of Lyme disease.

Treatment, Prevention, and Control

Relapsing fever has been treated most effectively with tetracyclines or penicillins. Tetracyclines are the drugs of choice but are contraindicated for pregnant women and young children. A Jarisch-Herxheimer reaction (shocklike profile with rigors, leukopenia, an increase in temperature, and a decrease in blood pressure) can occur in patients within a few hours after therapy is started and must be carefully managed. This reaction corresponds to the rapid killing of borreliae and the possible release of toxic products.

The early manifestations of Lyme disease are managed effectively with orally administered amoxicillin, doxycycline, or cefuroxime. Antibiotic treatment lessens the likelihood and the severity of late complications. Despite this intervention, Lyme arthritis and acrodermatitis chronica atrophicans occur in a small number of patients. Oral cefuroxime, doxycycline, or amoxicillin has been used for the treatment of these manifestations. Patients with recurrent arthritis or central or peripheral nervous system disease typically require parenteral treatment with intravenous ceftriaxone, cefotaxime, or penicillin G. Previously treated patients with chronic symptoms ("post-Lyme disease syndrome") should be treated symptomatically because there is no evidence that multiple courses of oral or parenteral antibiotics relieve the symptoms.

Prevention of tick-borne *Borrelia* diseases includes avoiding ticks and their natural habitats; wearing protective clothing, such as long pants tucked into socks; and applying insect repellents. Rodent control is also important in the prevention of endemic relapsing fever. Epidemic louse-borne disease is controlled through the use of delousing sprays and improvements in hygienic conditions.

Vaccines are not available for relapsing fever. A recombinant vaccine directed against the OspA antigen of *B. burgdorferi* was removed from the market in 2002.

LEPTOSPIRA

The taxonomy of the genus *Leptospira* is a source of great confusion. Traditionally, the genus has been grouped by phenotypic properties, serologic relationships, and pathogenicity. Pathogenic strains were placed in the species *Leptospira interrogans*, and nonpathogenic strains were placed in the species *Leptospira biflexa*. Each of the two species contained many serovars (i.e., serologically distinct groups). Although to this classification scheme exists in the literature, it is not consistent with nucleic acid analysis that supports subdividing the genus into three genera with 17 species in the genus *Leptospira*. To avoid confusion, leptospires will be referred to as pathogenic (for humans) or nonpathogenic without reference to either specific species or serovars.

Physiology and Structure

Leptospires are thin, coiled spirochetes (0.1 × 6.0 to 20.0 μm) with a hook at one or both pointed ends (Figure 32-10). Motility is by means of two periplasmic flagella extending the length of the bacteria and anchored at opposite ends. Leptospires are obligate aerobes with optimum growth at 28℃ to 30℃ in media supplemented with vitamins (i.e., B_2, B_{12}), long-chain fatty acids, and ammonium salts. The practical significance of this is that these organisms can be cultured in a specialized medium from clinical specimens collected from infected patients.

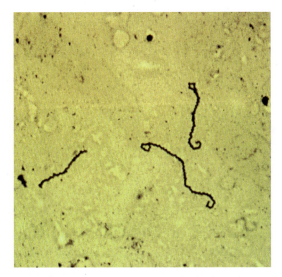

Figure 32-10   Silver staining of leptospires grown in culture. Notice the tightly coiled body with hooked ends. (From Emond R, Rowland H: *Color atlas of infectious diseases*, ed 3, London, 1995, Wolfe.)

Pathogenesis and Immunity

Pathogenic leptospires can cause subclinical infection, a mild influenza-like febrile illness, or severe systemic disease (Weil disease), with renal and hepatic failure, extensive vasculitis, myocarditis, and death. The number of infecting organisms, the host's immunologic defenses, and the virulence of the infecting strain influence the severity of the disease.

Because leptospires are thin and highly motile, they can penetrate intact mucous membranes or skin through small cuts or abrasions. They can then spread in the blood to all tissues, including the central nervous system. *L. interrogans* multiply rapidly and damage the endothelium of small blood vessels, resulting in

the major clinical manifestations of disease (e.g., meningitis, hepatic and renal dysfunction, hemorrhage). Organisms can be found in blood and CSF early in the disease and in urine during the later stages. Clearance of leptospires occurs when humoral immunity develops. However, some clinical manifestations may stem from immunologic reactions with the organisms. For example, meningitis develops after the organisms have been removed from the CSF and immune complexes have been detected in renal lesions.

Epidemiology

Leptospirosis has a worldwide distribution. Between 100 and 200 human infections occur in the United States each year, with more than half the cases reported in Hawaii. However, the incidence of disease is significantly underestimated because most infections are mild and misdiagnosed as a "viral syndrome" or viral aseptic meningitis. Because many states failed to report this disease to the public health service, mandatory reporting was discontinued in 1995. Thus the true prevalence of this disease cannot be determined.

Leptospires infect two types of hosts: reservoir hosts and incidental hosts. Endemic, chronic infections are established in reservoir hosts, which serve as a permanent reservoir for maintaining the bacteria. Different species and serovars of leptospires are associated with specific reservoir hosts (important for epidemiologic investigations). The most common reservoirs are rodents and other small mammals. Leptospires usually cause asymptomatic infections in their reservoir host, in which the spirochetes colonize the renal tubules and are shed in urine in large numbers. Streams, rivers, standing water, and moist soil can be contaminated with urine from infected animals, with organisms surviving for as long as 6 weeks in such sites. Contaminated water or direct exposure to infected animals can serve as a source for infection in incidental hosts (e.g., dogs, farm animals, humans). Most human infections result from recreational exposure to contaminated water (e.g., lakes) or occupational exposure to infected animals (farmers, slaughterhouse workers, veterinarians). Most human infections occur during the warm months, when recreational exposure is greatest. Person-to-person spread has not been documented. By definition, chronic carriage is not established in incidental hosts.

Clinical Diseases

Most human infections with leptospires are clinically inapparent and detected only through the demonstration of specific antibodies. Infection is introduced through skin abrasions or the conjunctiva. Symptomatic infections develop after a 1- to 2-week incubation period and in two phases. The initial phase is similar to an influenza-like illness with fever and myalgia (muscle pain). During this phase, the patient is bacteremic with the leptospires, and the organisms can frequently be isolated in CSF, even though no meningeal symptoms are present. The fever and myalgia may remit after 1 week, or the patient may progress to the second phase, which is characterized by sudden onset of headache, myalgia, chills, abdominal pain, and conjunctival suffusion (i.e., reddening of the eye). Severe disease can progress to vascular collapse, thrombocytopenia, hemorrhage, and hepatic and renal dysfunction.

Leptospirosis confined to the central nervous system can be mistaken for viral aseptic meningitis because the course of the disease is generally uncomplicated and has a very low mortality rate. Culture of CSF is usually negative at this stage. In contrast, the icteric form of generalized disease (approximately 10% of all symptomatic infections) is more severe and is associated with a mortality approaching 10% to 15%. Although hepatic involvement with jaundice (icteric disease, or Weil disease) is striking in patients with severe leptospirosis, hepatic necrosis is not seen, and surviving patients do not suffer permanent hepatic damage. Similarly, most patients recover full renal function. Congenital leptospirosis can also occur. This disease is characterized by the sudden onset of headache, fever, myalgias, and a diffuse rash.

Laboratory Diagnosis

Microscopy

Because leptospires are thin, they are at the limit of the resolving power of a light microscope and thus cannot be seen by conventional light microscopy. Neither Gram stain nor silver stain is reliable in the detection of leptospires. Darkfield microscopy is also relatively insensitive, capable of yielding nonspecific findings. Although leptospires can be seen in blood specimens early in the disease, protein filaments from erythrocytes can be easily mistaken for organisms. Fluorescein-labeled antibody preparations have been used to stain leptospires but are not available in most clinical laboratories.

Culture

Leptospires can be cultured on specially formulated media (e.g., Fletcher, EMJH [Ellinghausen-McCullough-Johnson-Harris], Tween 80-albumin). They grow slowly (generation time, 6 to 16 hours), requiring incubation at 28℃ to 30℃ for as long as 4 months; however, most cultures are positive within 2 weeks. Consistent with the two phases of illness, leptospires are present in blood or CSF during the first 10 days of infection and in urine after the first week and for as long as 3 months. Because the concentration of organisms in blood, CSF, and urine may be low, several specimens should be collected if leptospirosis is suspected. In addition, inhibitors present in blood and urine may delay or prevent recovery of leptospires. Likewise, urine must be treated to neutralize the pH and concentrated by centrifugation. A few drops of the sediment are then inoculated into the culture medium. Growth of the bacteria in culture is detected by darkfield microscopy.

Nucleic Acid-Based Tests

Preliminary work with the detection of leptospires using nucleic acid probes has had limited success. Techniques using nucleic acid amplification (e.g., PCR) are more sensitive than culture. Unfortunately, this technique is not widely available at this time.

Antibody Detection

Because of the need for specialized media and prolonged incubation, most laboratories do not attempt to culture leptospires and thus rely on serologic techniques. The reference method for all serologic tests is the microscopic agglutination test (MAT). This test measures the ability of the patient's serum to agglutinate live leptospires. Because the test is directed against specific serotypes, it is necessary to use pools of leptospiral antigens. In this test, serial dilutions of the patient's serum are mixed with the test antigens and then examined microscopically for agglutination. Agglutinins appear in the blood of untreated patients after 5 to 7 days of illness, although this response may be delayed for as long as several months. Infected patients have a titer of at least 1:200 (i.e., agglutinins are detected in a 1:200 dilution of the patient's serum), and it may be 1: 25,000 or higher. Patients treated with antibiotics may have a diminished antibody response or nondiagnostic titers. Agglutinating antibodies are detectable for many years after the acute illness; thus their presence may represent either a blunted antibody response in a treated patient with acute disease or residual antibodies in a person with a distant, unrecognized infection with leptospires. Because the microscopic agglutination test uses live organisms, it is performed only in reference laboratories. Alternative tests, such as indirect hemagglutination, slide agglutination, and enzyme-linked immunosorbent assay (ELISA), are less sensitive and specific. These tests can be used to screen a patient, but positive reactions must be confirmed with the MAT or preferably culture. Serologic cross-reactions occur with other spirochetal infections (i.e., syphilis, relapsing fever, Lyme disease) and legionellosis.

Treatment, Prevention, and Control

Leptospirosis is usually not fatal, particularly in the absence of icteric disease. Patients should be treated with either intravenously administered penicillin or doxycycline. Doxycycline, but not penicillin, can be used to prevent disease in persons exposed to infected animals or water contaminated with urine. It is difficult to eradicate leptospirosis because the disease is widespread in wild and domestic animals. However, vaccination of livestock and pets has proved successful in reducing the incidence of dis-

ease in these populations and therefore subsequent human exposure. Rodent control is also effective in eliminating leptospirosis in communities.

SUMMARY

Treponema pallidum
Outer membrane proteins promote adherence to host cells; Hyaluronidase facilitates perivascular infiltration; Coating of fibronectin protects *Treponema pallidum* against phagocytosis; Tissue destruction primarily results from host's immune response to infection.

Human is the only natural host; Venereal syphilis is transmitted by sexual contact or congenitally; Syphilis occurs worldwide with no seasonal incidence.

Borrelia
Borrelia species responsible for relapsing fever are able to undergo antigenic shift and escape immune clearance; periodic febrile and afebrile periods result from antigenic variation; immune reactivity against the Lyme disease agents may be responsible for the clinical disease. *Lyme disease* caused by *Borrelia burgdorferi*, *Borrelia garinii* and *Borrelia afzelii*; Transmitted by hard ticks from mice to humans; Epidemic relapsing fever is caused by *Borrelia recurrentis*, and transmitted by person-to-person; The vector is human body louse; Many Borrelia species are responsible for endemic relapsing fever, which is transmitted from rodents to humans.

For relapsing fever, treatment is tetracycline or erythromycin; For early localized or *disseminated Lyme* disease, treatment is amoxicillin, tetracycline, cefuroxime; late manifestations are treated with intravenous penicillin or ceftriaxone; Exposure to the insect vector can be decreased by using insecticides and applying insect repellents to clothing and by wearing protective clothing that reduces exposure of skin to insects.

Leptospira
The *Leptospira* can directly invade and replicate in tissues, inducing an inflammatory response; Immune complex produces renal disease (glomerulonephri-

tis); Most cases present mild, virus-like syndrome. Systemic leptospirosis presents most commonly as aseptic meningitis; Overwhelming disease (Weil disease) is characterized by vascular collapse, thrombocytopenia, hemorrhage, and hepatic and renal dysfunction. Reservoirs are rodents (particularly rats), dogs, farm animals, and wild animals; Human is accidental end-stage host. Organism can penetrate the skin through minor breaks in the epidermis.

KEYWORDS

English	Chinese
Treponema pallidum	苍白密螺旋体
Syphilis	梅毒
Borrelia burgdorferi	伯氏疏螺旋体
Lyme Disease	莱姆病
Borrelia recurrentis	回归热疏螺旋体
Relapsing Fever	回归热
Leptospira	钩端螺旋体
Leptospirosis	钩端螺旋体病

BIBLIOGRAPHY

1. Aguero-Rosenfeld ME, et al: Diagnosis of Lyme borreliosis, Clin Microbiol Rev 18: 484-509, 2005.

2. Antal GM, Lukehart SA, Meheus AZ: The endemic treponematoses, Microbes Infect 4: 83-94, 2002.

3. Butler T, et al: Infection with *Borrelia recurrentis*: pathogenesis of fever and petechiae, J Infect Dis 140: 665-672, 1979.

4. Centers for Disease Control and Prevention: Sexually transmitted disease surveillance 2003, Atlanta, 2004, U.S. Department of Health and Human Services.

5. Cutler S, et al: *Borrelia recurrentis* characterization and comparison with relapsing fever, Lyme-associated, and other *Borrelia* spp., Int J Syst Bacteriol 47: 958-968, 1997.

6. Feder H, et al: Review article: a critical appraisal of "chronic Lyme disease", N Engl J Med 357: 1422-1430, 2007.

7. LaFond RE, Lukehart SA: Biological basis for syphilis, Clin Microbiol Rev 19: 29-49, 2006.

8. Levitt PN: Leptospirosis, Clin Microbiol Rev 14: 296-326, 2001.

9. Rothschild BM: History of syphilis, Clin Inf Dis 40: 1454-1463, 2005.

10. Spach D, et al: Tick-borne diseases in the United States, N Engl J Med 329: 936-947, 1993.

11. Steere A: Lyme disease, N Engl J Med 345: 115-125, 2001.

12. Steere A, et al: Prospective study of serologic tests for Lyme disease, Clin Infect Dis 47: 188-195, 2008.

13. Toner B: Current controversies in the management of adult syphilis, Clin Infect Dis 44: S130-S146, 2007.

14. Wormser GP: Early Lyme disease, N Engl J Med 354: 2794-2801, 2006.

15. Wormser GP, et al: The clinical assessment, treatment, and prevention of Lyme disease, human granulocytic anaplasmosis, and babesiosis: clinical practice guidelines by the Infectious Diseases Society of America, Clin Infect Dis 43: 1089-1134, 2006.

Chapter 33

Mycoplasma and *Ureaplasma*

The order Mycoplasmatales is subdivided into four genera: *Eperythrozoon*, *Haemobartonella*, *Mycoplasma*, and *Ureaplasma*. The most clinically significant genera are *Mycoplasma* and *Ureaplasma*, and the most important species is *Mycoplasma pneumoniae*. *M. pneumoniae* causes respiratory tract diseases, such as tracheobronchitis and pneumonia. Other commonly isolated pathogens include *Mycoplasma genitalium*, *Mycoplasma hominis*, and *Ureaplasma urealyticum* (Table 33-1).

PHYSIOLOGY AND STRUCTURE

Mycoplasma and *Ureaplasma* are the smallest free-living bacteria. They are unique among bacteria because they do not have a cell wall and their cell membrane contains sterols. In contrast, other cell wall-deficient bacteria (called L forms) do not have sterols in their cell membrane and can form cell walls under the appropriate growth conditions. The absence of the cell wall renders the mycoplasmas resistant to penicillins, cephalosporins, vancomycin, and other antibiotics that interfere with synthesis of the cell wall.

The mycoplasmas form pleomorphic shapes varying from 0.2 to 0.3 µm coccoid forms to rods 0.1 to 0.2 µm in width and 1 to 2 µm long. Mycoplasmas are facultatively anaerobic (except *M. pneumoniae*, which is a strict aerobe), and require exogenous sterols supplied by animal serum added to the growth medium. The mycoplasmas grow slowly, with a generation time of 1 to 16 hours, and most form small colonies that are difficult to detect without extended incubation.

PATHOGENESIS AND IMMUNITY

M. pneumoniae is an extracellular pathogen that adheres to the respiratory epithelium by means of a specialized attachment structure that forms at one end of the cell. The structure consists of a complex of adhesions proteins, with the P1 adhesin the most important. The adhesions interact specifically with sialated glycoprotein receptors at the base of cilia on the epithelial cell surface (and on the surface of erythrocytes). Ciliostasis then occurs, after which first the cilia, then the ciliated epithelial cells, are destroyed. *M. pneumoniae* functions as a superanti-

Table 33-1 Clinically Important Mycoplasmataceae

Organism	Site	Human Disease
Mycoplasma pneumoniae	Respiratory tract	Tracheobronchitis, pharyngitis, pneumonia, secondary complications (neurologic, pericarditis, hemolytic anemia, arthritis, mucocutaneous lesions)
Mycoplasma genitalium	Genitourinary tract	Nongonococcal urethritis, pelvic inflammatory disease
Mycoplasma hominis	Respiratory tract, genitourinary tract	Pyelonephritis, postpartum fever, systemic infections in immunocompromised patients
Ureaplasma urealyticum	Respiratory tract, genitourinary tract	Nongonococcal urethritis, pyelonephritis, spontaneous abortion, premature birth

gen, stimulating inflammatory cells to migrate to the site of infection and release cytokines, initially tumor necrosis factor-α and interleukin-1 (IL-1) and later, IL-6. This process contributes to both the clearance of the bacteria and the observed disease.

A number of *Mycoplasma* species are able to rapidly change expression of surface lipoproteins, which is believed to be important for evading the host immune response and establishing persistent or chronic infections.

EPIDEMIOLOGY

M. pneumoniae is a strict human pathogen. Respiratory disease (e.g., tracheobronchitis, pneumonia) caused by *M. pneumoniae* occurs worldwide throughout the year, but proportionally common during the summer and fall. Disease is most common in school-age children and young adults (ages 5 to 15 years), although all age groups are susceptible.

M. pneumoniae colonizes the nose, throat, trachea, and lower airways of infected individuals and is spread via large respiratory droplets during coughing episodes. The attack rate is higher in children than in adults (overall average, approximately 60%), presumably because most adults are partially immune from previous exposure. Infants, particularly females, are colonized with *M. hominis*, *M. genitalium*, and *Ureaplasma* species, with *Ureaplasma* organisms being isolated most often. Although carriage of these mycoplasmas usually does not persist, a small proportion of prepubertal children remains colonized. The incidence of genital mycoplasmas rises after puberty, corresponding to sexual activity. Approximately 15% of sexually active men and women are colonized with *M. hominis*, and 45% to 75% are colonized with *Ureaplasma*. *M. pneumoniae* is not part of the normal mucosa flora of humans; however, prolonged carriage can occur following symptomatic disease.

CLINICAL DISEASES

Exposure to *M. pneumoniae* typically results in asymptomatic carriage. The most common clinical presenta-tion of *M. pneumoniae* infection is tracheobronchitis. Low-grade fever, malaise, headache, and a dry, non-productive cough develop 2 to 3 weeks after exposure. Acute pharyngitis may also be present. Symptoms gradually worsen over the next few days and can persist for 2 weeks or longer. Pneumonia (referred to as primary atypical pneumonia) can also develop. Myalgias and gastrointestinal tract symptoms are uncommon. Secondary complications include neurologic abnormalities (e.g., meningoencephalitis, paralysis, myelitis), pericarditis, hemolytic anemia, arthritis, and mucocutaneous lesions.

Because the genitourinary tract is colonized with other *Mycoplasma* species and *Ureaplasma*, it is difficult to determine the role of these organisms in disease in individual patients. However, it is generally accepted that *M. genitalium* can cause nongonococcal urethritis (NGU) and pelvic inflammatory disease; *U. urealyticum* can cause NGU, pyelonephritis, and spontaneous abortion or premature birth; and *M. hominis* can cause pyelonephritis, postpartum fevers, and systemic infections in immunocompromised patients.

LABORATORY DIAGNOSIS

The diagnostic tests for *M. pneumoniae* infections are summarized in Table 33-2.

Microscopy

Microscopy is of no diagnostic value. Mycoplasmas stain poorly because they have no cell wall.

Antigen Detection

Although antigen tests have been developed for the rapid diagnosis of *M. pneumoniae*, the tests have poor sensitivity and specificity and are not recommended.

Nucleic Acid-Based Tests

Polymerase chain reaction (PCR) amplification tests of species-specific targets have been developed for all pathogenic *Mycoplasma* and *Ureaplasma* species. The tests have excellent sensitivity, but the specificity is

Table 33-2 Diagnostic Tests for *Mycoplasma pneumoniae* Infections

Test	Assessment
Microscopy	Test is not useful because organisms do not have a cell wall and do not stain with conventional reagents
Culture	Test is slow (2-6 wk before positive diagnosis) and insensitive; it is not available in most laboratories
Molecular diagnosis	Polymerase chain reaction-based amplification assays with excellent sensitivity; specificity is not well defined; expected to be the diagnostic test of choice when assays become more widely available
Serology	
Complement fixation	Antibody titers versus glycolipid antigens peak in 4 weeks and persist for 6-12 mo; poor sensitivity and specificity
Enzyme immunoassays	Multiple assays available with varying sensitivity and specificity; assays directed versus P1 adhesin protein may be most specific
Cold agglutinin	Sensitivity and specificity poor with cross-reactions with other respiratory pathogens (e.g., Epstein-Barr virus, cytomegalovirus, adenovirus); test commonly used but not recommended

not well defined; that is, these assays may cross-react with avirulent species that colonize humans.

Culture

Unlike other mycoplasmas, *M. pneumoniae* is a strict aerobe. These mycoplasmas can be isolated from throat washings, bronchial washings, or expectorated sputum. Washings are more reliable than sputum specimens because most infected patients have a dry, nonproductive cough and do not produce sputum. A positive culture result is definitive evidence of disease, but it is relatively insensitive.

Colonies of *M. pneumoniae* are small and have a homogeneous granular appearance ("mulberry shaped"), unlike the fried-egg morphology of other mycoplasmas. Identification of isolates can be confirmed by inhibition of their growth with specific antisera, however, most laboratories do not perform cultures.

M. hominis is a facultative anaerobe that grows within 1 to 4 days and metabolizes arginine but not glucose. The colonies have a typical, large fried-egg appearance. Inhibition of their growth with specific antisera is used to differentiate them from other genital mycoplasmas. *Ureaplasma* requires urea for growth but is inhibited by the higher alkalinity resulting from the metabolism of urea. Thus the growth medium must be supplemented with urea and be highly buffered.

Antibody Detection

Antibody-specific tests are available only for *M. pneumoniae*. Detection of antibodies directed against *M. pneumoniae* by complement fixation is the traditional serologic reference standard. However, the test has poor sensitivity, and antibodies directed against the target glycolipid antigen are also elicited by other *Mycoplasma* species and by host tissues. A number of enzyme immunoassays for the detection of immunoglobulin M (IgM) and IgG antibodies are available. In general, the tests are more sensitive than complement fixation tests and culture.

Historically, it was also possible to measure nonspecific reactions to the outer membrane glycolipids of *M. pneumoniae*. The most useful of these reactions is the production of cold agglutinins (e.g., IgM antibodies that bind the I antigen on the surface of human erythrocytes at 4°C). This test is insensitive and nonspecific, so it should not performed.

TREATMENT, PREVENTION, AND CONTROL

Erythromycin, tetracyclines (particularly doxycycline), and fluoroquinolones are equally effective in treating *M. pneumoniae* infections. Tetracyclines have the advantage of also being active against most other mycoplasmas and chlamydia, a common cause of NGU. Erythromycin is used to treat *Ureaplasma* infections because these organisms are resistant to tetracycline. Unlike the other mycoplasmas, *M. hominis* is resistant to erythromycin and occasionally to the tetracyclines. Clindamycin has been used to treat infections caused by these resistant strains.

The prevention of *Mycoplasma* disease is problematic. *M. pneumoniae* infections are spread by close contact; thus the isolation of infected people could theoretically reduce the risk of infection. Infections with *M. hominis*, *M. genitalium*, and *Ureaplasma* are transmitted by sexual contact. Therefore these diseases can be prevented by avoidance of unprotected sexual activity.

SUMMARY

Mycoplasma and *Ureaplasma* are the smallest free-living bacteria. Absence of cell wall and existence of sterols in cell membrane are unique among bacteria. The mycoplasmas grow slowly in culture, with a generation time of 1 to 16 hours.

P1 adhesin of *M. pneumoniae* is the most important adhesion proteins, which can bind to base of cilia on epithelial cells, leading to eventual loss of ciliated epithelial cells. *M. pneumoniae* can function as a superantigen, stimulating migration of inflammatory cells and release of cytokines. *M. pneumoniae* causes tracheobronchitis, pharyngitis and pneumonia; *M. genitalium* can cause NGU and pelvic inflammatory disease; *U. urealyticum* can cause NGU, pyelonephritis, and spontaneous abortion or premature birth; and *M. hominis* can cause pyelonephritis, postpartum fevers, and systemic infections in immunocompromised patients.

Erythromycin, doxycycline, or newer fluoroquinolones can be used for treatment. Immunity to reinfection is not lifelong, and vaccines have proved ineffective.

KEYWORDS

English	Chinese
Mycoplasma	支原体
Ureaplasma	脲原体
Mycoplasma pneumoniae	肺炎支原体
Mycoplasma genitalium	生殖支原体
Mycoplasma hominis	人型支原体
Ureaplasma urealyticum	解脲脲原体
P1 adhesin	P1 黏附素
Tracheobronchitis	气管支气管炎
Pharyngitis	咽炎
Atypical pneumonia	非典型性肺炎
Nongonococcal urethritis	非淋菌性尿道炎

Rickettsia and *Orientia*

*R*ickettsia, *Ehrlichia*, and *Coxiella* were historically classified in a single family, Rickettsiaceae, based on the observation that they were obligate intracellular, aerobic, gram-negative rods. It was observed that *Rickettsia* should be subdivided into two genera (*Rickettsia* and *Orientia*) and *Ehrlichia* into two genera (*Ehrlichia* and *Anaplasma*). *Rickettsia* and *Orientia* are discussed in this chapter and the other two genera are discussed in Chapter 35.

The organisms of the family Rickettsiaceae are small (0.3 × 1 to 2 μm), structurally similar to gram-negative rods, although they stain poorly with the Gram stain and grow only in the cytoplasm of eukaryotic cells. The pathogenic species of *Rickettsia* and *Orientia* are maintained in animal and arthropod reservoirs and are transmitted by arthropod vectors (e.g., ticks, mites, lice, fleas). Humans are accidental hosts. *Rickettsia* species are subdivided into the **spotted fever group** and the **typhus group**. At least 12 species of *Rickettsia* in the spotted fever group have been associated with human disease, with **Rickettsia rickettsia** and **Rickettsia akari** discussed in this chapter. Two species of *Rickettsia* are members of the typhus group—**R. prowazekii** and **R. typhi**. A single species is in the genus *Orientia*, **Orientia tsutsugamushi**.

Rickettsiae are maintained in reservoir hosts (primarily rodents) and their arthropod vectors (Figure 34-1). Because **transovarian transmission** occurs in arthropods, they can serve as both vector and host. The exception to this is *Rickettsia prowazekii*, for which humans are the primary host and the arthropod vector is the human body louse. The distribution of rickettsial diseases is determined by the distribution of the arthropod host/vector. Most infections with tick vectors have a restricted geographic distribution, whereas rickettsial infections with other vectors, such as lice (*R. prowazekii*), fleas (*R. typhi*), and mites (*R. akari*, *O. tsutsugamushi*), have worldwide distribution (Table 34-1).

PHYSIOLOGY AND STRUCTURE

The cell wall structures of *Rickettsia* are typical of gram-negative rods, with a peptidoglycan layer and lipopolysaccharide (LPS). However, the peptidoglycan layer is minimal, and the LPS has only weak

Table 34-1 Distribution of *Rickettsia* and *Orientia* Species

Organism	Human Disease	Distribution
R. rickettsii	Rocky Mountain spotted fever	Western Hemisphere (United States, Canada, Mexico, Panama, Costa Rica, Brazil, Colombia, Argentina)
R. akari	Rickettsialpox	United States, Ukraine, Croatia, Korea
R. prowazekii	Epidemic typhus	Worldwide
	Recrudescent typhus	Worldwide
	Sporadic typhus	United States
R. typhi	Endemic (murine) typhus	Worldwide
O. tsutsugamushi	Scrub typhus	Japan, eastern Asia, northern Australia, western and southwestern Pacific

Disease	Organism	Vector	Reservoir
Rocky Mountain spotted fever	*R. rickettsii*	Tick-borne 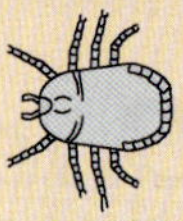	Ticks, wild rodents
Rickettsialpox	*R. akari*	Mite-borne 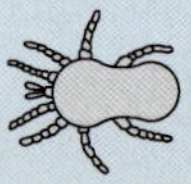	Mites, wild rodents
Scrub typhus	*O. tsutsugamushi*		Mites (chiggers), wild rodents
Epidemic typhus	*R. prowazekii*	Louse-borne 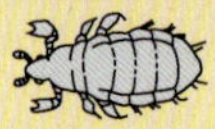	Humans, squirrel fleas, flying squirrels
Murine endemic typhus	*R. typhi*	Flea-borne 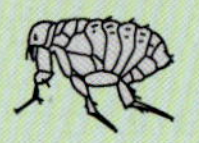	Wild rodents

Figure 34-1 Epidemiology of common *Rickettsia* and *Orientia* infections.

endotoxin activity. *Orientia* lacks both the peptidoglycan layer and LPS. The organisms are seen best with Giemsa or Gimenez stains (Figure 34-2). The bacteria do not have flagella, and *Rickettsia* is surrounded by a loosely adherent slime layer. *Rickettsia* and *Orientia* are strict intracellular parasites found free in the cytoplasm of infected cells.

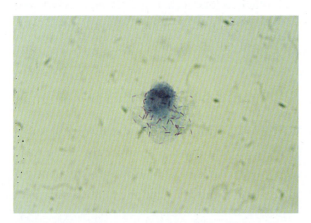

Figure 34-2 Gimenez stain of tissue culture cells infected with spotted fever group *Rickettsia*. (From Cohen J, Powderly WG: *Infectious diseases*, ed 2, St Louis, 2004, Mosby.)

The bacteria enter eukaryotic cells by attaching to host cell surface receptors and stimulating phagocytosis. After engulfment, *Rickettsia* and *Orientia* degrade the phagosome membrane by producing a phospholipase and must be released into the cytoplasm, or the organism will not survive. Multiplication in the host cell by binary fission is slow (genera-

tion time, 9 to 12 hours). *Orientia* and the spotted fever group of *Rickettsia* grow in the cytoplasm and nucleus of infected cells and are continually released from cells through long, cytoplasmic projections. In contrast, the typhus group accumulates in the cell cytoplasm until the cell membranes lyse, signaling cell death and bacterial release. Once these bacteria are released from the host cell, they are unstable and die quickly.

RICKETTSIA RICKETTSII

Pathogenesis and Immunity

R. rickettsii is the agent of **Rocky Mountain spotted fever.** There is no evidence that *R. rickettsii* produces toxins or that the host's immune response is responsible for the pathologic manifestations of Rocky Mountain spotted fever. The **outer membrane protein A (OmpA)** expressed on the surface of *R. rickettsii* is responsible for the ability of the bacteria to adhere to endothelial cells. After the bacteria penetrate into the cell, they are released from the phagosome, freely multiply in both the cytoplasm and nucleus, and move from cell to adjacent cell. The primary clinical manifestations appear to result from the replication of bacteria in endothelial cells, with subsequent damage to the cells and leakage of the blood vessels. Hypovolemia and hypoproteinemia caused by the loss of plasma into tissues can lead to reduced perfusion of various organs and organ failure. The host immune response to infection is based on cytokine-mediated intracellular killing and clearance by cytotoxic CD8 lymphocytes. Antibody response to rickettsial outer membrane proteins may also be important.

Epidemiology

R. rickettsii is transmitted by the bite of an infected tick with most infections occurring from April through September. The distribution of disease mimics the distribution of the principal reservoir and vector for *R. rickettsii*, **hard ticks** in the family Ixodidae. A person must be exposed to the tick for a lengthy period (e.g., 6 hours or more) before transmission occurs. The dormant avirulent rickettsiae are activated by the warm blood meal and then released from the tick salivary glands into the blood of the human host.

Clinical Diseases

Symptomatic disease develops 7 days (range, 2 to 14 days) after the tick bite (Table 34-2), although the patient may not recall the painless tick bite. The onset of disease is heralded by a high fever and headache that may be associated with malaise, myalgias, nausea, vomiting, abdominal pain, and diarrhea. A macular rash develops in 90% of patients after 3 days, initially on the wrists, arms, and ankles and then spreads to the trunk. The palms and soles can also be involved. The rash can evolve to the "spotted" or petechial form, which is a harbinger of more severe disease. Complications of Rocky Mountain spotted fever include neurologic manifestations, pulmonary and renal failure, and cardiac abnormalities. A delay in diagnosis, either because the clinical presentation is not characteristic or the physician does not recognize the disease, is associated with a worse prognosis. The fatality rate in untreated disease is 10% to 25%.

Laboratory Diagnosis

Microscopy

Rickettsiae can be stained with Giemsa or Gimenez stains. Specific fluorescein-labeled antibodies can also be used to stain the intracellular bacteria in biopsy tissue specimens. This direct detection of rickettsial antigens is a rapid, specific method for confirming the clinical diagnosis of Rocky Mountain spotted fever but is primarily available only through reference laboratories.

Nucleic Acid-Based Tests

Specific nucleic acid amplification tests are now used in many reference laboratories for the diagnosis of rickettsial diseases. A variety of gene targets are used, including gene sequences for outer membrane proteins (OmpA, OmpB), the 17-kDa lipoprotein, and citrate synthase. Unfortunately, these polymerase chain reaction assays are relatively insensitive when blood samples are used.

Culture

Although isolation of rickettsiae in tissue culture systems or embryonated eggs is relatively easy, only reference laboratories with extensive experience with rickettsiae routinely perform these cultures. If culture is attempted, buffy coat preparations of blood or skin biopsy specimens should be processed.

Antibody Detection

Although the **Weil-Felix test** (which involves the differential agglutination of cross-reacting *Proteus* antigens) has been used historically for the diagnosis of rickettsial infections, it is no longer recommended

Table 34-2 Clinical Course of Human Diseases Caused by *Rickettsia* and *Orientia* Species

Disease	Average Incubation Period (days)	Clinical Presentation	Rash	Eschar	Mortality without Treatment (%)
Rocky Mountain spotted fever	7	Abrupt onset; fever, headache, malaise, myalgias, nausea, vomiting, abdominal pain	>90%; macular; centripetal spread	No	10-25
Rickettsialpox	9-14	Abrupt onset; fever, headache, chills, myalgias, photophobia	100%; papulovesicular; generalized	Yes	Low
Epidemic typhus	8	Abrupt onset; fever, headache, chills, myalgias, arthralgia	20%-80%; macular; centrifugal spread	No	20
Endemic typhus	7-14	Gradual onset; fever, headache, myalgias, cough	50%; maculopapular rash on trunk	No	Low
Scrub typhus	10-12	Abrupt onset; fever, headache, myalgias	<50%; maculopapular rash; centrifugal	No	1-15

because it is insensitive and nonspecific. The serology test that is considered the reference method is the microimmunofluorescence (MIF) test. The test detects antibodies directed against outer membrane proteins (species-specific) and the LPS antigen. The sensitivity and specificity of MIF is high, with diagnostic levels of antibodies generally detected in the second week of illness.

Treatment, Prevention, and Control

The drug of choice for treating all rickettsial infections is **doxycycline.** Although the tetracyclines are generally contraindicated for pregnant women and young children, this antibiotic is recommended for all patients with suspected rickettsial disease because it is the most effective antibiotic and inadequately treated disease is associated with a high morbidity and mortality. Fluoroquinolones (e.g., ciprofloxacin) have good in vitro activity but clinical experience is inadequate to recommend this for primary therapy. Chloramphenicol also has activity in vitro against rickettsiae, but its use for treatment of infections is associated with a higher incidence of relapse. It is recommended that empiric therapy with doxycycline be started as soon as the diagnosis is considered.

There is no vaccine for Rocky Mountain spotted fever. Thus avoidance of tick-infected areas, the use of protective clothing and insect repellents, and the prompt removal of attached ticks are the best preventive measures. It is virtually impossible to eliminate the tick reservoir because the ticks can survive for as long as 4 years without feeding.

RICKETTSIA AKARI

R. akari, the agent responsible for causing **rickettsialpox,** is one of the few rickettsiae in the spotted fever group that has a **cosmopolitan** distribution and is transmitted by infected **mites.** Infections with *R. akari* are maintained in the rodent population through the bite of mouse ectoparasites (e.g., mites) and in mites by transovarian transmission. Humans become accidental hosts when bitten by infected mites.

Clinical infection with *R. akari* is biphasic. First,

a papule develops at the site where the mite bites the host. The papule appears approximately 1 week after the bite and quickly progresses to ulceration and then **eschar formation.** During this period, the rickettsiae spread systemically. After an incubation period of 7 to 24 days (average, 9 to 14 days), the second phase of the disease develops abruptly, with high **fever,** severe headache, chills, sweats, myalgias, and photophobia. A generalized **papulovesicular rash** forms within 2 to 3 days. A poxlike progression of the rash is then seen, in which vesicles form and then crust over. Despite the appearance of the disseminated rash, rickettsialpox is usually mild and uncomplicated, and complete healing is seen within 2 to 3 weeks without treatment. Specific therapy with doxycycline speeds the process.

RICKETTSIA PROWAZEKII

Epidemiology

R. prowazekii, one of two members of the typhus group of rickettsiae, is the etiologic agent of **epidemic** or **louse-borne typhus. Humans** are the principal reservoir of this disease, and the vector is the **human body louse,** *Pediculus humanus.* Epidemic typhus occurs among people living in crowded, unsanitary conditions that favor the spread of body lice—conditions such as those that arise during wars, famines, and natural disasters. Lice die from their infection within 2 to 3 weeks, preventing the transovarian transmission of *R. prowazekii.*

Clinical Diseases

Clinical disease was found to develop an average of 8 days after exposure (range, 2 to 30 days). Most of the patients initially had nonspecific symptoms; then within 1 to 3 days, high **fever,** severe **headache,** and **myalgias.** Other symptoms can include pneumonia, arthralgia, and neurologic involvement (stupor, confusion, coma). A petechial or macular rash develops in many patients, but this may be obscured in darkly pigmented individuals. The mortality rate in the absence of treatment is 20% to 30% but may be much higher in populations with poor general health and nutrition and lacking proper supportive medical care. In patients with uncomplicated disease, the body temperature returns to normal within 2 weeks, but complete convalescence may take 3 months or longer. The rickettsiae may remain dormant for years and then reactivate to cause recrudescent epidemic typhus or Brill-Zinsser disease.

Laboratory Diagnosis

The MIF test is the diagnostic method of choice for documenting disease with *R. prowazekii*.

Treatment, Prevention, and Control

The tetracyclines are highly effective in the treatment of epidemic typhus; however, antibiotic treatment must be combined with effective louse-control measures for the management of an epidemic. An inactivated typhus vaccine is available and is used in high-risk populations.

RICKETTSIA TYPHI

Epidemiology

Endemic or murine typhus is caused by *R. typhi.* Disease is distributed worldwide primarily in warm, humid areas. Endemic disease continues to be reported in people living in the temperate and subtropical coastal areas of Africa, Asia, Australia, Europe, and South America. **Rodents** are the primary reservoir, and the **rat flea** (*Xenopsylla cheopis*) is the principal vector. Most cases occur during the warm months.

Clinical Disease

The incubation period for *R. typhi* disease is 7 to 14 days. The symptoms appear abruptly, with fever, severe headache, chills, myalgias, and nausea most common. A rash develops in approximately half of infected patients, most commonly late in the illness. It is typically restricted to the chest and abdomen. The course of disease is generally uncomplicated, lasting less than 3 weeks even in untreated patients.

Laboratory Diagnosis

A *R. typhi*-specific indirect fluorescent assay test is used to confirm the diagnosis of murine typhus. Significant titers are usually detectable within 1 to 2 weeks of the onset of disease.

Treatment, Prevention, and Control

The **tetracyclines** are effective in the treatment of murine typhus, and patients respond promptly to these agents. It is difficult to control or prevent endemic typhus because the reservoir and vector are widely distributed. Any such efforts should be directed at controlling the rodent reservoir. An effective vaccine is not available.

ORIENTIA TSUTSUGAMUSHI

O. tsutsugamushi is the etiologic agent for **scrub typhus,** a disease transmitted to humans by **mites** (chiggers, red mites). The reservoir is the mite population, in which the bacteria are transmitted by transovarian means. Infection is also present in the **rodent** population, which can serve as a reservoir for mite infections. Scrub typhus is present in people living in eastern Asia, Australia, and Japan and other western Pacific islands.

O. *tsutsugamushi* disease develops suddenly after a 6- to 18-day incubation period (average, 10 to 12 days), with severe **headache, fever,** and **myalgias.** A macular to papular rash develops on the trunk in less than half of patients and spreads centrifugally to the extremities. Generalized lymphadenopathy, splenomegaly, central nervous system complications, and heart failure can occur. Fever in untreated patients disappears after 2 to 3 weeks, whereas fever in patients who receive appropriate treatment with **doxycycline** responds promptly. No vaccine is available, so the disease is prevented by avoidance of exposure to mites.

SUMMARY

Rickettsia rickettsii

R. Rickettsii is a kind of small, intracellular bacteria and is stained poorly with Gram stain but best with Giemsa or Gimenez. Hard ticks are the primary reservoirs and vectors. Transmission requires prolonged contact. Rocky Mountain spotted fever is characterized by high fever, severe headache, myalgias, and rash; complications are common in untreated patients or where diagnosis is delayed.

Serology (e.g., MIF test) is used most commonly for diagnosis. Doxycycline is the drug of choice. No vaccine is currently available, so people should avoid tick-infected areas, wear protective clothing, use effective insecticides, and remove attached ticks immediately.

Rickettsia akari

R. akari is the agent responsible for causing **rickettsial pox** which transmitted by infected **mites.** Two forms of clinical infection with R. akari exist: papule and eschar formation. Rickettsialpox is usually mild and uncomplicated. Doxycycline is the drug of choice.

Rickettsia prowazekii

The biological characteristics of **R. prowazekii** are similar to that of **R. Rickettsii.** R. prowazekii causes epidemic typhus. Humans are the primary reservoir, with person-to-person transmission by louse vector. Epidemic typhus is characterized by high fever, severe headache, and myalgias. Recrudescent typhus (Brill-Zinsser disease) is a milder form of the disease. Disease is worldwide.

Doxycycline is the drug of choice. Diseases can effectively controlled through improvements in living conditions and reduction of the lice population. Inactivated vaccine is available for high-risk populations.

Rickettsia typhi and Orientia tsutsugamushi

R. typhi causes endemic or murine typhus. Rodents are the primary reservoir, and the rat flea is the principal vector. Tetracyclines is the drug of choice. Efforts to prevent endemic typhus should be directed at controlling the rodent reservoir. Effective vaccine is not available.

O. tsutsugamushi causes scrub typhus, a disease transmitted to humans by mites. O. tsutsugamushi disease is characterized by severe headache, fever, and myalgias. Doxycycline is the drug of choice. No vaccine is available.

KEYWORDS

English	Chinese
Rickettsia rickettsii	立氏立克次体
Rickettsia akari	小蛛立克次体
Rickettsia prowazekii	普氏立克次体
Rickettsia typhi	斑疹伤寒立克次体
Orientia tsutsugamushi	恙虫病东方体
Weil-Felix test	外斐反应
Rocky Mountain spotted fever	落基山斑疹热
Louse-borne typhus	虱传斑疹伤寒
Murine typhus	鼠型斑疹伤寒
Epidemic typhus	流行性斑疹伤寒
Scrub typhus	恙虫病

BIBLIOGRAPHY

1. Luce-Fedrow A, et al: Strategies for detecting rickettsiae and diagnosing rickettsial diseases, Future Microbiol 4: 537-64,2015.

2. Walker DH, et al: The role of CD8 T lymphocytes in rickettsial infections, Semin Immunopathol 3: 289-289,2015.

3. Mahajan SK. Rickettsial diseases, J Assoc Physicians India 60: 37-44,2012.

4. Archibald L, Sexton D: Long-term sequelae of Rocky Mountain spotted fever, Clin Infect Dis 20: 1122-1125, 1995.

5. Dumler JS, Walker D: Rocky Mountain spotted fever—changing ecology and persisting virulence, N Engl J Med 353: 551-553, 2005.

6. Paddock C, et al: Isolation of Rickettsia akari from eschars of patients with rickettsialpox, Am J Trop Med Hyg 75: 732-738, 2006.

7. Raoult D, Dumler JS: Rickettsia and Orientia. In Borriello SP, Murray P, Funke G, editors: Topley and Wilson's microbiology and microbial infections, ed 10, London, 2005, Holder-Arnold, pp 2026-2047.

8. Richards A: Rickettsial vaccines: the old and the new, Expert Rev Vaccines 3: 541-555, 2004.

9. Rolain J, et al: In vitro susceptibilities of 27 rickettsiae to 13 antimicrobials, Antimicrob Agents Chemother 42: 1537-1541, 1998.

Chapter 35

Ehrlichia, Anaplasma, and Coxiella

All tick-borne bacteria in the family Anaplasmataceae are grouped in two genera: *Ehrlichia* and *Anaplasma*. They are **obligate intracellular** bacteria, able to **survive in cytoplasmic vacuoles** of mammalian **hematopoietic cells.** *Coxiella* is an intracellular pathogen that was once thought to be closely related to *Rickettsia* and *Ehrlichia*. Although it is now recognized that *Coxiella* is not a member of the families Rickettsiaceae or Anaplasmataceae, it will also be discussed in this chapter.

EHRLICHIA AND ANAPLASMA

Physiology and Structure

The genera *Ehrlichia* and *Anaplasma* consist of intracellular bacteria that parasitize granulocytes, monocytes, erythrocytes, and platelets. In contrast with *Rickettsia* and *Orientia*, *Ehrlichia* and *Anaplasma* remain in the phagocytic vacuole after entry into the host cell. Fusion with lysosomes is prevented because expression of appropriate receptors on the phagocytic vacuole surface is interrupted. Two morphologic forms of the bacteria exist: small (0.2 to 0.4 μm) elementary bodies and larger (0.8 to 1.5 μm) reticulate bodies. A few days after the cell is infected, the elementary bodies assemble into membrane-enclosed masses called morulae (Figure 35-1). Progressive infection leads to lysis of the infected cell, release of bacteria, and subsequent infection of new cells. Detection of morulae when the cells are stained with Giemsa or Wright stains is a rapid, specific diagnostic test; however, relatively few infected cells may be seen, so a negative test is not helpful.

The cell wall structure of *Ehrlichia* and *Anaplasma*

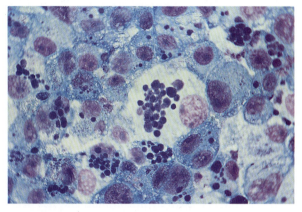

Figure 35-1 Multiple morulae of *Ehrlichia canis* in DH82 tissue culture cells. (From Cohen J, Powderly WG: *Infectious diseases*, ed 2, St Louis, 2004, Mosby.)

is similar to that of gram-negative bacteria; however, the bacteria lack genes for synthesis of peptidoglycan or lipopolysaccharide (LPS). In addition, many of the genes of the glycolytic pathway are also absent. A number of protein antigens are shared among species in these genera, as well as with species of other genera. For this reason, cross-reactive antibodies are commonly observed in serologic assays.

Pathogenesis and Immunity

The intracellular location of the organisms protects them from the host's antibody response. However, bacterial stimulation of proinflammatory cytokine production is believed to play an important role in activating macrophages that act either directly on infected cells or on antibody-opsonized bacteria during their extracellular phase.

Epidemiology (Table 35-1)

Ehrlichia chaffeensis is the etiologic agent of human monocytic ehrlichiosis. *Amblyomma americanum*

Table 35-1 Epidemiology of *Ehrlichia* and *Anaplasma*

	E. chaffeensis	*E. ewingii*	*A. phagocytophilum*
Disease	Human monocytic ehrlichiosis	Human ewingii ehrlichiosis	Human granulocytic anaplasmosis
Geographic distribution	North and South America, Asia	North America	North and South America, Europe, Asia
Reservoir host	Deer, dogs, other candis	Dogs, deer	Small rodents, deer, sheep
Vector (ticks)	*Amblyomma americanum*	*Amblyomma americanum*	*Ixodes* species
Host with clinical symptoms	Humans, dogs	Dogs, humans	Ruminants, horses, dogs, humans
Infected host cell	Monocytes, macrophages	Neutrophils	Neutrophils, eosinophils, basophils

(Lone Star tick) is the primary vector responsible for transmitting the organism, and of white-tailed deer, an important reservoir for *E. chaffeensis*. Other animals that can serve as hosts include domestic dogs, foxes, coyotes, and wolves.

Granulocytic ehrlichiosis is caused by two bacteria—Ehrlichia ewingii and *Anaplasma phagocytophilum. E. ewingii* is relatively uncommon and has been primarily reported in Missouri. Disease caused by *A. phagocytophilum* is found primarily in the upper midwestern states (Minnesota, Wisconsin) and northeast Atlantic states (Massachusetts, Connecticut, New York, New Jersey). The reservoirs are small mammals (e.g., white-footed mouse, chipmunks, voles), and the vectors are Ixodes ticks.

Transovarian transmission of *Ehrlichia* and *Anaplasma* in ticks does not occur, so these bacteria must be maintained in reservoir vertebrate hosts. Ticks become infected when an immature stage (e.g., larva, nymph) ingests blood from a naturally infected host and then transmits the bacteria to another mammalian host (e.g., human) during the next blood meal. Humans are accidental hosts and thus transmission terminates at this stage.

Clinical Diseases

Human Monocytic Ehrlichiosis

Human monocytic ehrlichiosis is caused by *E. chaffeensis* after infection of blood monocytes and mononuclear phagocytes in tissues and organs. Approximately 1 to 2 weeks after a tick bite, patients develop

a flulike illness with high fever, headache, malaise, and myalgias. A late-onset rash develops in 30% to 40% of patients (more common in children than in adults). Leukopenia, thrombocytopenia, and elevated serum transaminases develop in the majority of patients and can range from mild to severe. Although mortality is low (2% to 3%), more than half the infected patients require hospitalization and experience a prolonged recovery period. A fulminant septic syndrome can develop, particularly in immunocompromised patients. It is believed that *E. chaffeensis* disturbs mononuclear phagocytic function and the regulation of the inflammatory response. Thus the immune response both eliminates the pathogen and produces much of the tissue damage.

Canine Granulocytic Ehrlichiosis

E. ewingii primarily causes disease in canines, with humans the accidental hosts. Because there is serologic cross-reactivity between *E. ewingii* and *E. chaffeensis*, the incidence of infections with this organism is likely to be underestimated. The clinical presentation is similar to that of *E. chaffeensis*, with fever, headaches, and myalgias. Leukopenia, thrombocytopenia, and elevated serum transaminases are also seen.

Human Anaplasmosis

Human anaplasmosis, formerly called human granulocytic ehrlichiosis, is caused by *A. phagocytophilum*. Granulocytes are primarily infected. The disease presents 5 to 10 days after exposure as a flulike illness, with a high fever, headache, malaise, and myalgias; a skin rash is observed in less than 10% of the patients. As with human monocytic ehrlichiosis, leukopenia, thrombocytopenia, and serum transaminase elevation are observed in most patients. More than half the infected patients require hospitalization, and severe complications, particularly peripheral neuropathies (e.g., demyelinating polyneuropathy, facial palsy) can occur. Despite the potential severity of this disease, mortality is less than 1%. As with *E. chaffeensis* infections, the pathology of this disease appears related to macrophage activation.

Laboratory Diagnosis

The clinical presentation of *Ehrlichia* and *Anaplasma* infections is not distinctive, laboratory testing is required for a definitive diagnosis. Microscopy has limited value because the bacteria stain poorly with the Gram stain and detection of intracytoplasmic inclusions in Giemsa-stained preparations of peripheral blood is only useful during the first week of illness. Morulae are detected in less than 10% of patients with monocytic ehrlichiosis and in 25% to 75% of patients with granulocytic anaplasmosis. Likewise, although *Ehrlichia* organisms have been cultured in vitro in established cell lines, this procedure is not performed in most clinical laboratories. The most common methods for the laboratory diagnosis of ehrlichiosis are nucleic acid amplification (NAA) tests and serology. Species-specific DNA amplification tests can provide a sensitive, specific diagnostic test for acute disease. An increase in the antibody titer is typically observed 3 to 6 weeks after the initial presentation, so these serologic tests are primarily confirmatory. *E. chaffeensis* and *E. ewingii* are closely related and cannot be differentiated by serology.

Treatment, Prevention, and Control

Patients with suspected ehrlichiosis should be treated with doxycycline. Rifampin has been used to treat patients who are unable to tolerate doxycycline. Fluoroquinolones, penicillins, cephalosporins, chloramphenicol, aminoglycosides, and macrolides are ineffective. Infection is prevented by avoidance of tick-infested areas, wearing of protective clothing, and use of insect repellents. Embedded ticks should be removed promptly. Vaccines are not available.

COXIELLA BURNETII

Coxiella burnetii was originally classified with *Rickettsia* because the gram-negative bacteria stain weakly with the Gram stain, grow intracellularly in eukaryotic cells, and are associated with arthropods (e.g., ticks). However, it is now recognized that these bacteria are not related to *Rickettsia* but rather to *Legionella*. The disease caused by *C. burnetii* is Q (query) fever, so named because the initial investigation of an outbreak in Australian abattoir workers did not identify the causal organism.

Physiology and Structure

Two structural forms of *C. burnetii* are recognized: small cell variants that are resistant to environmental stress (e.g., heat, desiccation, chemical agents) and large cell variants that are the metabolically active form. Additionally, *C. burnetii* undergoes a phase transition similar to what is observed in some other gram-negative bacteria. In the phase observed in nature (phase I), *C. burnetii* has an intact LPS; however, mutations can occur in the LPS genes, resulting in a molecule with lipid A and core sugars but missing the outermost O-antigen sugars (phase II). This phase variation is important for understanding the progression of disease and for diagnostic purposes.

Small cell variants attach to macrophages and monocytes and are internalized in a phagocytic vacuole. The normal progression after phagocytosis of most organisms is fusion of the phagosome with a series of endosomes, resulting in a drop in intracellular pH, followed by fusion with lysosomes containing hydrolytic enzymes and resultant bacterial death. This occurs with *C. burnetii* if phase II organisms are ingested; however, phase I *Coxiella* is able to arrest this process before lysosomal fusion. In addition, the organisms require acid pH for their metabolic activities, which, in turn, protects them from the killing activities of most antibiotics.

Pathogenesis and Immunity

Coxiella is able to regulate the cell signaling pathways in its phagocytic home so that cell death is delayed. The ability of *C. burnetii* to cause either acute or chronic disease is determined in part by the organism's ability to survive intracellularly. In the presence of interferon-γ, phagosome-lysosome fusion occurs, leading to bacterial death; however, in chronic infections interleukin-10 is overproduced by the host cell, which interferes with fusion and allows intracellular survival of *C. burnetii.*

Epidemiology

C. burnetii is extremely stable in harsh environmentalconditions and can survive in soil and milk for months to years. The range of hosts for *C. burnetii* is wide, with infections being found in mammals, birds, and numerous species of ticks. Farm animals, such as sheep, cattle, and goats, and recently infected cats, dogs, and rabbits, are the primary reservoirs for human disease. The bacteria can reach high concentrations in the placenta of infected livestock. Human infections occur after the inhalation of airborne particles from a contaminated environmental source or, less commonly, after ingestion of contaminated unpasteurized milk or other dairy products. Ticks do not transmit disease to humans.

Q fever has a worldwide distribution. Human exposure particularly for ranchers, veterinarians, and food handlers is frequent, and experimental studies have shown that the infectious dose of *C. burnetii* is small (10 or fewer bacteria). Thus most human infections are asymptomatic or mild, a finding confirmed by serologic studies, which have shown that most persons with detectable antibodies do not have a history of disease. Infections also go undetected because diagnostic tests for *C. burnetii* are often not considered.

Clinical Diseases

The majority of individuals exposed to *C. burnetii* have an **asymptomatic infection,** and most symptomatic infections are mild, presenting with non-specific **flulike symptoms** with an abrupt onset, high-grade fever, fatigue, headache, and myalgias. Less than 5% of infected persons develop symptoms severe enough to require hospitalization, with the most common presentations being **hepatitis, pneumonia,** or isolated **fevers.** Chronic Q fever (symptoms lasting more than 6 months) can develop months to years after the initial exposure and occurs almost exclusively in patients with predisposing conditions, such as underlying valvular heart disease or immunosuppression. **Subacute endocarditis** is the most common presentation and can be difficult to diagnose because of the lack of specific signs and symptoms. However, chronic Q fever is a serious illness with significant mortality and morbidity, even in patients with rapid diagnosis and appropriate treatment.

Laboratory Diagnosis

Q fever can be diagnosed by culture, serology, or the polymerase chain reaction (PCR). Culture can be performed in tissue culture cells and recently in a cell-free medium; however, culture is rarely performed except in research laboratories licensed to work with these highly contagious organisms. **Serology** is the most commonly used diagnostic test. A variety of methods are used to measure antibody production: the microagglutination tests, indirect immunofluorescence antibody (IFA) test, and enzyme-linked immunosorbent assay (ELISA). IFA is the test of choice, although ELISA is used in many laboratories and appears to be as sensitive. In acute Q fever, immunoglobulin M (IgM) and IgG antibodies are developed primarily against **phase II antigens.** A diagnosis of chronic Q fever is confirmed by the demonstration of antibodies against both **phase I and II antigens,** with the titers to the phase I antigen typically higher. NAA techniques, such as PCR, are generally not available for routine diagnosis. In addition, although the tests are sensitive when tissue samples are examined, the sensitivity is poor with serum. PCR-based tests are not required for the diagnosis of chronic *C. burnetii* infections because these patients characteristically have high levels of antibodies present.

Treatment, Prevention, and Control

Treatment of acute and chronic *C. burnetii* infections is guided by clinical experience, not in vitro susceptibility tests. Currently, it is recommended that acute infections be treated for 14 days with **doxycycline.** Chronic disease should be treated for a prolonged period with a bactericidal combination of drugs, **doxycycline and the alkalinizing agent hydroxychloroquine.** Fluoroquinolones (e.g., ofloxacin, pefloxacin) have been used as an alternative to doxycycline but are contraindicated in children and pregnant women.

Inactivated whole-cell vaccines and partially purified antigen vaccines for Q fever have been developed, and the vaccines prepared from phase I organisms have been shown to provide the best protection. Vaccination of previously infected individuals is contraindicated because immune stimulation can lead to an increase in adverse reactions. For this reason, a single-dose vaccine with no booster immunizations is recommended.

SUMMARY

Ehrlichia and Anaplasma

Ehrlichia and *Anaplasma* are small, intracellular bacteria, able to prevent fusion of phagosome with lysosome of monocytes or granulocytes. The bacteria can initiate inflammatory response that contributes to pathology. Diseases are human monocytic ehrlichiosis and human anaplasmosis. Depending on the species of *Ehrlichia*, important reservoirs are white-tailed deer, white-footed mouse, chipmunks, voles, and canines. Ticks are important vectors, but transovarian transmission in inefficient. Serology and DNA probe tests are methods of choice. Doxycycline is the drug of choice. Prevention involves avoidance of tick-infested areas, use of protective clothing and insect repellents, and prompt removal of embedded ticks. Vaccines are not available.

Coxiella

Coxiella is a kind of small, intracellular bacteria that stains poorly with Gram stain. *Coxiella* exists in two forms: small cell variant and large cell variant. Most infections are asymptomatic; Endocarditis is the most common form of chronic disease. There are many reservoirs including mammals, birds, and ticks. Most diseases are acquired through inhalation; possible disease from consumption of contaminated milk. Q fever has a worldwide distribution, and no seasonal incidence.

Detection of antibody response to phase I and phase II antigens is test of choice. Doxycycline is the drug of choice for acute infections; hydroxychloroquine combined with doxycycline is used to treat chronic infections. Phase I antigen vaccines are protective and safe if administered in a single dose before the animal or human has been exposed to *Coxiella.*

KEYWORDS

English	Chinese
Ehrlichia	埃立克体属
Anaplasma	无形体属
Coxiella	柯克斯体属
Ehrlichia canis	犬埃立克体
Ehrlichia chaffeensis	查菲埃立克体
Ehrlichia ewingii	伊文埃立克体
Anaplasma phagocytophilum	嗜吞噬细胞无形体
Coxiella burnetii	贝纳柯克斯体
Canine Granulocytic Ehrlichiosis	犬粒细胞埃立克体病
Human monocytic ehrlichiosis	人单核细胞埃立克体病
Anaplasmosis	无形体病
Ehrlichiosis	埃立克体病

BIBLIOGRAPHY

1. Lina TT, et al. Hacker within! *Ehrlichia chaffeensis* Effector Driven Phagocyte Reprogramming Strategy. Front Cell Infect Microbiol, 6: 58, 2016.

2. Beare PA. Genetic manipulation of Coxiella burnetii, Adv Exp Med Biol 984: 249-271, 2012.

3. Angelakis E, Raoult D: Review: Q fever, Vet Microbiol 140: 297-309, 2010.

4. Bakken J, Dumler S: Human granulocytic anaplasmosis, Infect Dis Clin N Am 22: 433-448, 2008.

5. Dumler JS, et al: Ehrlichioses in humans: epidemiology, clinical presentation, diagnosis, and treatment, Clin Infect Dis 45: S45-S51, 2007.

6. Ghigo E, et al: Intracellular life of *Coxiella burnetii* in macrophages: an update, Ann NY Acad Sci 1166: 55-66, 2009.

7. Ismail N, Bloch K, McBride J: Human ehrlichiosis and anaplasmosis, Clin Lab Med 30: 261-292, 2010.

8. Marrie T: Q fever pneumonia, Infect Dis Clin N Am 24: 27-41, 2010.

9. Rikihisa Y: *Anaplasma phagocytophilum* and *Ehrlichia chaffeensis*: subversive manipulators of host cells, Nat Rev

Microbiol 8: 328-339, 2010.

10. Shannon J, Heinzen R: Adaptive immunity to the obligate intracellular pathogen *Coxiella burnetii*, Immunol Res 43: 138-148, 2009.

11. Thomas R, Dumler JS, Carlyon J: Current management of human granulocytic anaplasmosis, human monocytic ehrlichiosis and *Ehrlichia ewingii* ehrlichiosis, Expert Rev Anti Infect Ther 7: 709-772, 2009.

Chapter 36

Chlamydia and *Chlamydophila*

The family Chlamydiaceae consists of two clinically important genera, *Chlamydia* and *Chlamydophila*, with three species responsible for human disease: ***Chlamydia trachomatis***, ***Chlamydophila psittaci***, and ***Chlamydophila pneumoniae***. Properties that differentiate the three important human pathogens in this family are summarized in Table 36-1.

Chlamydiaceae are **obligate intracellular parasites**. The organisms have the following properties: (1) possess inner and outer membranes similar to those of gram-negative bacteria; (2) contain both deoxyribonucleic acid (DNA) and ribonucleic acid (RNA); (3) possess prokaryotic ribosomes; (4) synthesize their own proteins, nucleic acids, and lipids; and (5) are susceptible to numerous antibacterial antibiotics.

Physiology and Structure

Chlamydiaceae exist in two morphologically distinct forms: a small, metabolically inactive infectious forms termed the elementary bodies (EBs) about 300 to 400 nm, and metabolically active, noninfectious forms termed the reticulate bodies (RBs) about 800 to 1000 nm. EBs are resistant to many harsh environmental factors. The cell wall contains a lipopolysaccharide (LPS) that is common to all members of the family. The LPS has only weak endotoxin activity. The major outer membrane protein (MOMP) in the cell wall is an important structural component of the outer membrane and is unique for each species. Variable regions in the gene encoding this protein are found in *C. trachomatis* and are responsible for

Table 36-1 Differentiation of Chlamydiaceae That Cause Human Disease

Property	*Chlamydia trachomatis*	*Chlamydophila pneumoniae*	*Chlamydophila psittaci*
Host range	Primarily human pathogen	Primarily human pathogen	Primarily animal pathogen; occasionally infects humans
Biovars	LGV and trachoma	TWAR	Many
Diseases	LGV; ocular trachoma, oculogenital disease, infant pneumonia	Bronchitis, pneumonia, sinusitis, pharyngitis, coronary artery disease (?)	Pneumonia (psittacosis)
Elementary body morphology	Round, narrow periplasmic space	Pear-shaped, large periplasmic space	Round, narrow periplasmic space
Inclusion body morphology	Single, round inclusion per cell	Multiple, uniform inclusions per cell	Multiple, variably sized inclusions per cell
Plasmid DNA	Yes	No	Yes
Iodine-staining glycogen in inclusions	Yes	No	No
Susceptibility to sulfonamides	Yes	No	No

DNA, Deoxyribonucleic acid; *LGV*, lymphogranuloma venereum.

18 serologic variants (called serovars). Similar variable regions are found in *C. psittaci* MOMP; in contrast, the *C. pneumoniae* MOMP is homogenous and only a single serovar has been described. A second, highly conserved outer membrane protein, OMP 2, is shared by all members of the family Chlamydiaceae. This cysteine-rich protein is responsible for the extensive disulfide cross-links that provide the stability in the EBs.

The Chlamydiaceae multiply by means of a unique growth cycle that occurs within susceptible host cells (Figure 36-1). The cycle is initiated when the small, infectious EBs become attached to the microvilli of susceptible cells, followed by active penetration into the host cell. After they are internalized, the bacteria remain within cytoplasmic phagosomes, where the replicative cycle proceeds. If the outer membrane of the EB is intact, fusion of cellular lysosomes with the EB-containing phagosome is inhibited, thus preventing intracellular killing. Within 6 to 8 hours after entering the cell, the EBs reorganize into the larger, metabolically active RBs. The RBs replicate by binary fission, and histologic stains can readily detect the phagosome with accumulated RBs, called an inclusion. Approximately 18 to 24 hours after infection, the RBs begin reorganizing into the smaller EBs, and between 48 and 72 hours, the cell ruptures and then releases the infectious bacteria.

CHLAMYDIA TRACHOMATIS

C. trachomatis has a limited host range, with infections restricted to humans. The species responsible for human disease are subdivided into two biovars: trachoma and lymphogranuloma venereum (LGV). The biovars have been further divided into serovars based on antigenic differences in the MOMP. Specific serovars are associated with specific diseases (Table 36-2).

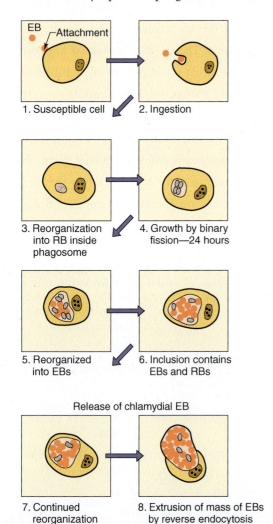

1. Susceptible cell
2. Ingestion
3. Reorganization into RB inside phagosome
4. Growth by binary fission—24 hours
5. Reorganized into EBs
6. Inclusion contains EBs and RBs

Release of chlamydial EB

7. Continued reorganization
8. Extrusion of mass of EBs by reverse endocytosis

Figure 36-1 The growth cycle of *Chlamydia trachomatis*. *EB*, Elementary body; *RB*, reticulate body. (Modified from Batteiger B, Jones R: Chlamydial infections, *Infect Dis Clin North Am* 1: 55-81, 1987.)

Table 36-2 Clinical Spectrum of *Chlamydia trachomatis* Infections

Serovars	Disease
A, B, Ba, C	Trachoma
D-K	Urogenital tract disease
L1, L2, L2a, L2b, L3	Lymphogranuloma venereum

Pathogenesis and Immunity

The range of cells that *C. trachomatis* can infect is limited. Receptors for EBs are primarily restricted to nonciliated columnar, cuboidal, and transitional epithelial cells, which are found on the mucous membranes of the urethra, endocervix, endometrium, fallopian tubes, anorectum, respiratory tract, and conjunctivae. The LGV serovars are more invasive than the other serovars because they replicate in mononuclear phagocytes. The clinical manifestations of chlamydial infections are caused by (1) the direct destruction of cells during replication and (2) the proinflammatory cytokine response they stimulate.

Chlamydiae gain access through minute abrasions

or lacerations. In LGV, the lesions form in the lymph nodes, draining the site of primary infection (Figure 36-2). Granuloma formation is characteristic. The lesions may become necrotic, attract polymorphonuclear leukocytes, and cause the inflammatory process to spread to surrounding tissues. Subsequent rupture of the lymph node leads to formation of abscesses or sinus tracts. Infection with non-LGV serovars of *C. trachomatis* stimulates a severe inflammatory response consisting of neutrophils, lymphocytes, and plasma cells.

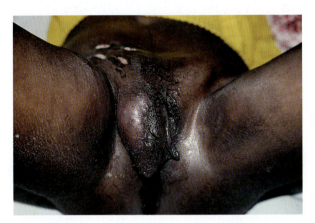

Figure 36-2   Patient with lymphogranuloma venereum causing unilateral vulvar lymphedema and inguinal buboes. (From Cohen J, Powderly W: *Infectious diseases*, ed 2, St Louis, 2004, Mosby.)

Infection does not confer long-lasting immunity; rather, reinfection characteristically induces a vigorous inflammatory response with subsequent tissue damage. This response produces the vision loss in patients with chronic ocular infections, and scarring with sterility and sexual dysfunction in patients with genital infections.

Epidemiology

C. trachomatis is found worldwide and causes trachoma, oculogenital disease, pneumonia, and LGV. The World Health Organization estimates six million people are blind due to trachoma, and more than 150 million people are in need of treatment. Trachoma is the leading cause of preventable blindness. Infections occur predominantly in children, who are the chief reservoir of *C. trachomatis* in endemic areas. Trachoma is transmitted eye-to-eye by droplet, hands, contaminated clothing, and flies that transmit ocular discharges from the eyes of infected children to the eyes of uninfected children. Because a high percentage of children in endemic areas harbor *C. trachomatis* in their respiratory and gastrointestinal tracts, the pathogen may also be transmitted by respiratory droplet or through fecal contamination. Trachoma generally is endemic in communities where the living conditions are crowded, sanitation is poor, and the personal hygiene of the people is poor—all risk factors that promote the transmission of infections.

Most cases of *C. trachomatis* adult inclusion conjunctivitis occur in people who are 18 to 30 years of age, and genital infection probably precedes eye involvement. Autoinoculation and oral-genital contact are believed to be the routes of transmission. A third form of *C. trachomatis* eye infections is newborn inclusion conjunctivitis, an infection acquired during passage of the infant through an infected birth canal. *C. trachomatis* conjunctivitis develops in approximately 25% of infants whose mothers have active genital infections.

Pulmonary infection with *C. trachomatis* also occurs in newborns. A diffuse interstitial pneumonia develops in 10% to 20% of infants exposed to the pathogen at birth.

C. trachomatis infections are the most common bacterial sexually transmitted disease in the world. It is estimated that about 50 million new infections occur annually worldwide. Most genital tract infections are caused by serotypes D to K.

LGV is a chronic sexually transmitted disease caused by *C. trachomatis* serotypes L1, L2, L2a, L2b, and L3. It occurs sporadically in the United States and other industrialized countries but is highly prevalent in Africa, Asia, and South America. Acute LGV is seen more frequently in men, primarily because symptomatic infection is less common in women.

Clinical Diseases

Trachoma

Trachoma is a chronic disease caused by serovars A, B, Ba, and C. Initially, patients have a follicular conjunctivitis with diffuse inflammation that involves the entire conjunctiva. The conjunctivae become scarred as the disease progresses, causing the patient's eyelids to turn inward. The turned-in eyelashes abrade the cornea, eventually resulting in corneal ulceration, scarring, pannus formation (invasion of vessels into the cornea), and loss of vision.

Adult Inclusion Conjunctivitis

An acute follicular conjunctivitis caused by the *C. trachomatis* strains associated with genital infections (serovars A, B, Ba, D to K) has been documented in sexually active adults. The infection is characterized by mucopurulent discharge, keratitis, corneal infiltrates, and, occasionally, some corneal vascularization. Corneal scarring has been observed in patients with chronic infection.

Neonatal Conjunctivitis

Eye infections can also develop in infants exposed to *C. trachomatis* at birth. After an incubation of 5 to 12 days, the infant's eyelids swell, hyperemia occurs, and copious purulent discharge appears. Untreated infections may run a course as long as 12 months, during which time conjunctival scarring and corneal vascularization occur.

Infant Pneumonia

The incubation period for infant pneumonia is variable, but the onset generally occurs 2 to 3 weeks after birth. Rhinitis is initially observed in such infants, after which a distinctive staccato cough develops. The child remains afebrile throughout the clinical illness, which can last for several weeks. Radiographic signs of infection can persist for months.

Lymphogranuloma Venereum

The LGV serotypes of *C. trachomatis* have been implicated in Parinaud oculoglandular conjunctivitis, a conjunctival inflammation associated with preauricular, submandibular, and cervical lymphadenopathy.

Urogenital Infections

Most genital tract infections in women are asymptomatic (as many as 80%). The clinical manifestations include bartholinitis, cervicitis, endometritis, perihepatitis, salpingitis, and urethritis. Asymptomatic patients with chlamydial infection are an important reservoir for the spread of *C. trachomatis*. A mucopurulent discharge (Figure 36-3) is seen in patients with symptomatic infection whose specimens generally yield more organisms on cultures than specimens from patients with asymptomatic infections. Urethritis caused by *C. trachomatis* may occur with or without a concurrent cervical infection.

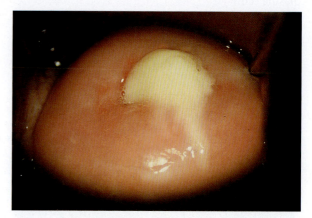

Figure 36-3 Mucopurulent cervicitis caused by *Chlamydia trachomatis*. (From Cohen J, Powderly W: *Infectious diseases*, ed 2, St Louis, 2004, Mosby. Photo by J. Paavonen.)

Although most *C. trachomatis* genital infections in men are symptomatic, as many as 25% of the infections will be inapparent. Approximately 35% to 50% of cases of nongonococcal urethritis are caused by *C. trachomatis*; dual infections with both *C. trachomatis* and *Neisseria gonorrhoeae* are not uncommon.

It is believed that Reiter syndrome (urethritis, conjunctivitis, polyarthritis, and mucocutaneous lesions) is initiated by genital infection with *C. trachomatis*. Approximately 50% to 65% of patients with Reiter syndrome have a chlamydial genital infection at the onset of arthritis, and serologic studies indicate that more than 80% of men with Reiter syndrome have evidence of a preceding or concurrent infection with *C. trachomatis*.

Lymphogranuloma Venereum

After an incubation of 1 to 4 weeks, a primary lesion appears at the site of infection (e.g., penis, urethra, glans, scrotum, vaginal wall, cervix, vulva) in patients with LGV. The lesion (either a papule or an ulcer) is often overlooked because it is small, painless, and heals rapidly. The patient may experience fever, headache, and myalgia when the lesion is present.

The second stage of infection is marked by inflammation and swelling of the lymph nodes draining the site of initial infection. The inguinal nodes are most commonly involved, becoming painful, fluctuant buboes that gradually enlarge and can rupture, forming draining fistulas. Systemic manifestations include fever, chills, anorexia, headache, meningismus, myalgias, and arthralgia.

Proctitis is common in women with LGV, resulting from lymphatic spread from the cervix or the vagina. Proctitis develops in men after anal intercourse or as the result of lymphatic spread from the urethra. Untreated LGV may resolve at this stage or may progress to a chronic ulcerative phase, in which genital ulcers, fistulas, strictures, or genital elephantiasis develop.

Laboratory Diagnosis

C. trachomatis infection can be diagnosed (1) on the basis of cytologic, serologic, or culture findings, (2) through the direct detection of antigen in clinical specimens, and (3) through the use of nucleic acid–based tests. The sensitivity of each method depends on the patient population examined, the site where the specimen is obtained, and the nature of the disease.

Cytology

Examination of Giemsa-stained cell scrapings for the presence of inclusions was the first method used for the diagnosis of *C. trachomatis* infection; however, this method is insensitive and is not recommended. Likewise, Papanicolaou staining of cervical material has been found to be an insensitive and nonspecific method.

Antigen Detection

Two general approaches have been used to detect chlamydial antigens in clinical specimens: direct immunofluorescence staining with fluorescein-conjugated monoclonal antibodies (Figure 36-4) and enzyme-

linked immunosorbent assays. In both assays, antibodies are used that have been prepared against either the chlamydial MOMP or the cell wall LPS. The sensitivity of each assay method has been reported to vary enormously, but neither is considered as sensitive as culture or nucleic acid-based tests, particularly if male urethral specimens or specimens from asymptomatic patients are used.

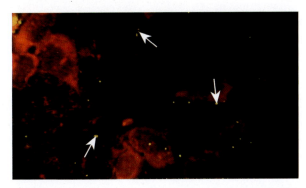

Figure 36-4 Fluorescent-stained elementary bodies *(arrows)* in a clinical sample. (From Hart T, Shears P: *Color atlas of medical microbiology*, London, 2000, Mosby-Wolfe.)

Nucleic Acid-Based Tests

Nucleic acid probe tests most commonly measure the presence of a species-specific sequence of 16S ribosomal RNA. These tests are relatively insensitive for the detection of small numbers of chlamydiae. Nucleic acid amplification tests (NAATs) are more sensitive (generally reported to be 90% to 98% sensitive) and, if properly monitored, are very specific. NAATs are currently considered the tests of choice for the laboratory diagnosis of genital *C. trachomatis* infection.

Culture

The isolation of *C. trachomatis* in cell culture remains the most specific method of diagnosing *C. trachomatis* infections but is relatively insensitive compared with nucleic acid amplification techniques (Figure 36-5). The sensitivity of culture is compromised if inadequate specimens are used and if chlamydial viability has been lost during transport of the specimen. It has been estimated that the sensitivity of the findings yielded by a single endocervical specimen may be only 70% to 85%.

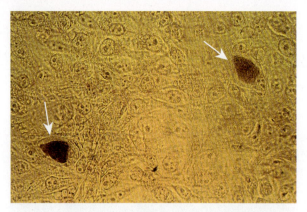

Figure 36-5 *Chlamydia trachomatis* is grown in cell cultures and detected by staining inclusion bodies *(arrows)* with either iodine- or specific fluorescein-labeled antibodies.

Antibody Detection

Serologic testing is of limited value in the diagnosis of *C. trachomatis* urogenital infections in adults because the test cannot differentiate between current and past infections. Testing for immunoglobulin M (IgM) antibodies is also usually not helpful because these antibodies may not be detected in adolescents and adults. An exception is the detection of IgM antibodies in infants with chlamydial pneumonitis.

Antibody tests for the diagnosis of LGV can be helpful. Infected patients produce a vigorous antibody response that can be detected by complement fixation (CF), microimmunofluorescence (MIF), or enzyme immunoassay (EIA). The CF test is directed against the genus-specific LPS antigen. Thus a positive result (i.e., fourfold increase in titer or a single titer≥1:256) is highly suggestive of LGV. Confirmation is determined by the MIF test, which is directed against species- and serovar-specific antigens (the chlamydial MOMPs). Similar to the CF test, EIAs are genus specific. The advantage of these tests is that they are less technically cumbersome; however, the results must be confirmed by MIF.

Treatment, Prevention, and Control

It is recommended that patients with LGV be treated with doxycycline for 21 days. Treatment with erythromycin is recommended for children younger than 9 years, pregnant women, and patients unable to tolerate doxycycline. Ocular and genital infections in adults should be treated with one dose of azithromycin or doxycycline for 7 days. Newborn conjunctivitis and pneumonia should be treated with erythromycin for 10 to 14 days.

The blindness associated with advanced stages of trachoma can be prevented only by prompt treatment of early disease and the prevention of reexposure. *Chlamydia* conjunctivitis and genital infections are prevented through the use of safe sex practices and the prompt treatment of symptomatic patients and their sexual partners.

CHLAMYDOPHILA PNEUMONIAE

C. pneumoniae was first isolated from the conjunctiva of a child in Taiwan. It was subsequently shown that the Taiwan isolate (TW-183) was related serologically to a pharyngeal isolate, designated AR-3. This new organism was initially called TWAR, then classified as *Chlamydia pneumoniae*, and, finally, placed in the new genus *Chlamydophila*. Only a single serotype (TWAR) has been identified.

C. pneumoniae is a human pathogen that causes sinusitis, pharyngitis, bronchitis, and pneumonia. Infections are believed to be transmitted person to person by respiratory secretions. Most *C. pneumoniae* infections are asymptomatic or mild, causing a persistent cough and malaise; most patients do not require hospitalization. More severe respiratory tract infections typically involve a single lobe of the lungs.

The role of *C. pneumoniae* in the pathogenesis of atherosclerosis remains to be defined. The organism has been demonstrated in biopsy specimens of atherosclerotic lesions, thus the association of *C. pneumoniae* with atherosclerotic lesions is clear. What is not clear is the role of the organism in the development of atherosclerosis.

Diagnosis of *C. pneumoniae* infections is difficult. Although *C. pneumoniae* will grow in the HEp-2 cell line, this cell line is not used in most clinical laboratories. Detection of *C. pneumoniae* by NAATs has been successful. The MIF test is the only acceptable test for serodiagnosis. The criteria for the diagnosis of acute *C. pneumoniae* infection is a single IgM titer of greater than 1:16 or a fourfold increase in IgG titer.

Macrolides (erythromycin, azithromycin, clarithromycin), doxycycline, or levofloxacin are recommended for treatment of *C. pneumoniae* infections, although evidence supporting their use is limited. Control of exposure to *C. pneumoniae* is likely to be difficult because the bacterium is ubiquitous.

CHLAMYDOPHILA PSITTACI

C. psittaci is the cause of psittacosis, which can be transmitted to humans. The disease was first observed in parrots, thus the name psittacosis. In reality, however, the natural reservoir of *C. psittaci* is virtually any species of bird, and the disease has been referred to more appropriately as ornithosis. Other animals, such as sheep, cows, and goats, as well as humans, can become infected. The organism is present in the blood, tissues, feces, and feathers of infected birds that may appear either ill or healthy.

Infection occurs by means of the respiratory tract, after which the bacteria spread to the reticuloendothelial cells of the liver and spleen. The organisms multiply in these sites, producing focal necrosis. The lung and other organs are then seeded as the result of hematogenous spread, which causes a predominantly lymphocytic inflammatory response in the alveolar and interstitial spaces.

The bacterium is usually transmitted to humans through the inhalation of dried excrement, urine, or respiratory secretions from psittacine birds. Person-to-person transmission is rare. Veterinarians, zookeepers, pet shop workers, and employees of poultry-processing plants are at increased risk for this infection.

The illness develops after an incubation of 5 to 14 days and usually manifests as headache, high fever, chills, malaise, and myalgias. Pulmonary signs include a nonproductive cough, rales, and consolidation. Central nervous system involvement is common, usually consisting of headache, but encephalitis, convulsions, coma, and death may occur in severe, untreated cases. Patients may suffer gastrointestinal tract symptoms, such as nausea, vomiting, and diarrhea. Other systemic symptoms include carditis,

hepatomegaly, splenomegaly, and follicular keratoconjunctivitis.

Psittacosis is usually diagnosed on the basis of serologic findings. A fourfold increase in titer, shown by the CF testing of paired acute and convalescent phase sera, is suggestive of *C. psittaci* infection, but the species-specific MIF test must be performed to confirm the diagnosis. *C. psittaci* can be isolated in cell culture after 5 to 10 days of incubation, although this procedure is rarely performed in clinical laboratories.

Infections can be treated successfully with doxycycline or macrolides. Psittacosis can be prevented only through the control of infections in domestic and imported pet birds. Such control can be achieved by treating birds with chlortetracycline hydrochloride for 45 days. No vaccine currently exists for this disease.

SUMMARY

Chlamydia trachomatis

C. trachomatis is a kind of small, gram-negative organism with no peptidoglycan layer in cell wall, which is a strict intracellular parasite of humans, and exists in two distinct forms: infectious EBs and noninfectious RBs. Two biovars are associated with human disease: trachoma and LGV. *C. trachomatis* can cause many diseases including trachoma, adult inclusion conjunctivitis, neonatal conjunctivitis, infant pneumonia, urogenital infections and LGV.

Culture is highly specific but is relatively insensitive, and antigen tests (DFA, ELISA) are also relatively insensitive, while molecular amplification tests are the most sensitive and specific tests currently available. Doxycycline or erythromycin are recommended for treatment of LGV infections, ocular or genital infections should be treated with azithromycin or doxycycline, newborn conjunctivitis or pneumonia should be treat with erythromycin. Safe sex practices and prompt treatment of patient and sexual partners help control infections.

Chlamydophila pneumoniae

C. pneumoniae is a human pathogen that causes respiratory infections. Respiratory infections can range from asymptomatic or mild disease to severe, atypical pneumonia requiring hospitalization. *C. pneumoniae* has been associated with inflammatory plaques in blood vessels; the etiologic role in this disease is controversial.

Chlamydophila psittaci

*C. psittaci*can is transmitted to humans and causes respiratory infections, ranging from asymptomatic colonization to severe bronchopneumonia with localized infiltration of inflammatory cells, necrosis, and hemorrhage.

KEYWORDS

English	Chinese
Chlamydia trachomatis	沙眼衣原体
Chlamydophila psittaci	鹦鹉热衣原体
Chlamydophila pneumoniae	肺炎衣原体
Elementary body	原体
Reticulate body	网状体
Major outer membrane protein	主要外膜蛋白
Trachoma	沙眼
Lymphogranuloma venereum	性病淋巴肉芽肿
Adult inclusion conjunctivitis	成人包涵体结膜炎
Psittacosis	鹦鹉热
Ornithosis	鸟疫

BIBLIOGRAPHY

1. Kreuter A, et al: Azithromycin versus Doxycycline for Chlamydia, N Engl J Med 18: 1786-1787, 2016.
2. Elwell C, et al: Chlamydia cell biology and pathogenesis Nat Rev Microbiol 6: 385-400, 2016.
3. Bebear C, de Barbeyrac B: Genital *Chlamydia trachomatis* infections, Clin Microbiol Infect 15: 4-10, 2009.
4. Beeckman D, Vanrompay D: Zoonotic *Chlamydophila psittaci* infections from a clinical perspective, Clin Microbiol Infect 15: 11-17, 2009.
5. Boman J, Hammerschlag MR: *Chlamydia pneumoniae* and atherosclerosis: critical assessment of diagnostic methods and relevance to treatment studies, Clin Microbiol Rev 15: 1-20, 2002.
6. Byrne G: *Chlamydia trachomatis* strains and virulence: rethinking links to infection prevalence and disease severity, J Infect Dis 201: S126-S133, 2010.
7. Gambhir M, et al: Trachoma: transmission, infection, and control, Lancet Infect Dis 7: 420-427, 2007.
8. Kern J, Maass V, Maass M: Molecular pathogenesis of chronic *Chlamydia pneumoniae* infections: a brief overview, Clin Microbiol Infect 15: 36-41, 2009.
9. Kumar S, Hammerschlag M: Acute respiratory infection due to *Chlamydia pneumoniae*: current status of diagnostic methods, Clin Infect Dis 44: 568-576, 2007.
10. Morre S, et al: Urogenital *Chlamydia trachomatis* serovars in men and women with a symptomatic or asymptomatic infection: an association with clinical manifestations? J Clin Microbiol 38: 2292-2296, 2000.
11. Van der Bij A, et al: Diagnostic and clinical implications of anorectal lymphogranuloma venereum in men who have sex with men: a retrospective case-control study, Clin Infect Dis 42: 186-194, 2006.
12. Knittler MR, et al: *Chlamydia psittaci*: update on an underestimated zoonotic agent, Pathog Dis 1: 1-15, 2015.

SECTION 2

Virology

Viral Classification, Structure, and Replication

Viruses **are obligate intracellular parasites** that depend on the biochemical machinery of the host cell for replication. In addition, reproduction of viruses occurs by assembly of the individual components rather than by binary fission (Boxes 37-1 and 37-2).

The simplest viruses consist of a genome of deoxyribonucleic acid (DNA) or ribonucleic acid (RNA) packaged in a protective shell of protein and, for some viruses, a membrane (Figure 37-1). To use the cell's biosynthetic machinery, the virus must be adapted to the biochemical rules of the cell.

The physical structure and genetics of viruses have been optimized by mutation and selection to infect humans and other hosts. To do this, the virus must be capable of transmission through potentially harsh environmental conditions, must traverse the skin or other protective barriers of the host, must be adapted to the biochemical machinery of the host cell for replication, and must escape elimination by the host immune response.

Knowledge of the structural (**size and morphology**) and genetic (**type and structure of nucleic acid**) features of a virus provides insight into how the virus replicates, spreads, and causes disease.

CLASSIFICATION

Viruses range from the structurally simple and small parvoviruses and picornaviruses to the large and complex poxviruses and herpesviruses. Their names may describe viral characteristics, the diseases they are associated with, or even the tissue or geographic locale where they were first identified. Names such as **picornavirus** (*pico*, "small"; *rna*, "ribonucleic acid") or **togavirus** (*toga*, Greek for "mantle," referring to a membrane envelope surrounding the virus) describe the structure of the virus. The name **retrovirus** (*retro*, "reverse") refers to the virus-directed synthesis of DNA from an RNA template, whereas the *poxviruses* are named for the disease smallpox, caused by one of its members. The **adenoviruses** (*adenoids*) and the **reoviruses** (*r*espiratory, *e*nteric, *o*rphan) are named for the body site from which they were first isolated.

Box 37-1

Definition and Properties of a Virus

Viruses are filterable agents.
Viruses are obligate intracellular parasites.
Viruses cannot make energy or proteins independently of a host cell.
Viral genomes may be RNA or DNA but not both.
Viruses have a naked capsid or an envelope morphology.
Viral components are assembled and do not replicate by "division."

Box 37-2

Consequences of Viral Properties

Viruses are not living.
Viruses must be infectious to endure in nature.
Viruses must be able to use host cell processes to produce their components (viral messenger RNA, protein, and identical copies of the genome).
Viruses must encode any required processes not provided by the cell.
Viral components must self-assemble.

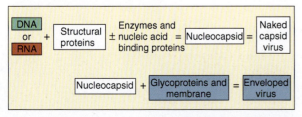

Figure 37-1 Components of the basic virion.

Reovirus was discovered before it was associated with a specific disease, and thus it was designated an "orphan" virus. Norwalk virus is named for Norwalk, Ohio; coxsackievirus is named for Coxsackie, New York; and many of the togaviruses, arenaviruses, and bunyaviruses are named after African places where they were first isolated.

Viruses can be grouped by characteristics such as disease (e.g., hepatitis), target tissue, means of transmission (e.g., enteric, respiratory), or vector (e.g., arboviruses; arthropod-borne virus) (Box 37-3). *The most consistent and current means of classification is by physical and biochemical characteristics, such as size, morphology (e.g., presence or absence of a membrane envelope), type of genome, and means of replication* (Figures 37-2 and 37-3). DNA viruses associated with

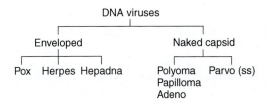

Figure 37-2   The DNA viruses and their morphology. The viral families are determined by the structure of the genome and the morphology of the virion.

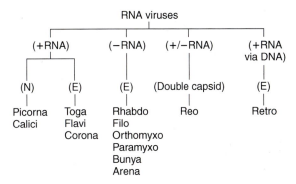

Figure 37-3   The RNA viruses, their genome structure, and their morphology. The viral families are determined by the structure of the genome and the morphology of the virion. *E*, Enveloped; *N*, naked capsid.

human disease are divided into seven families (Tables 37-1 and 37-2). The RNA viruses may be divided into at least 13 families (Tables 37-3 and 37-4).

VIRION STRUCTURE

The units for measurement of virion size are nanometers (nm). The clinically important viruses range from 18 nm (parvoviruses) to 300 nm (poxviruses) (Figure 37-4).

The virion (the virus particle) consists of a nucleic acid genome packaged into a protein coat (capsid) or a membrane (envelope) (Figure 37-5). The virion may also contain certain essential or accessory enzymes or other proteins to facilitate initial replication in the cell. Capsid or nucleic acid-binding proteins may associate with the genome to form a nucleocapsid, which may be the same as the virion or surrounded by an envelope.

The genome of the virus consists either of DNA or RNA. The DNA can be single or double stranded, linear or circular. The RNA can be either positive sense (+) (like messenger RNA [mRNA]) or negative

---

Box 37-3

Means of Classification and Naming of Viruses

Structure: size, morphology, and nucleic acid (e.g., picornavirus [small RNA], togavirus)

Biochemical characteristics: structure and mode of replication*

Disease: encephalitis and hepatitis viruses, for example

Means of transmission: arbovirus spread by insects, for example

Host cell (host range): animal (human, mouse, bird), plant, bacteria

Tissue or organ (tropism): adenovirus and enterovirus, for example.

*This is the current means of taxonomic classification of viruses.

Table 37-1   Families of DNA Viruses and Some Important Members

Family	Members*
POXVIRIDAE†	*Smallpox virus*, vaccinia virus, monkeypox, canarypox, molluscum contagiosum
Herpesviridae	*Herpes simplex virus types 1 and 2*, varicella-zoster virus, Epstein-Barr virus, cytomegalovirus, human herpesviruses 6, 7, and 8
Adenoviridae	*Adenovirus*
Hepadnaviridae	*Hepatitis B virus*
Papillomaviridae	*Papilloma virus*
Polyomaviridae	*JC virus*, BK virus, SV40
Parvoviridae	*Parvovirus B19*, adeno-associated virus

*The italicized virus is the prototype virus for the family.
†The size of type is indicative of the relative size of the virus.

Table 37-2   Properties of Virions of Human DNA Viruses

| Family | Genome* | | Virion | | |
	Molecular Mass × 10^6 Daltons	Nature	Shape	Size (nm)	DNA Poly-merase[†]
Poxviridae	85-140	ds, linear	Brick-shaped, enveloped	300 × 240 × 100	+[‡]
Herpesviridae	100-150	ds, linear	Icosadeltahedral, enveloped	Capsid, 100-110 Envelope, 120-200	+
Adenoviridae	20-25	ds, linear	Icosadeltahedral	70-90	+
Hepadnaviridae	1.8	ds, circular[§]	Spherical, enveloped	42	+[‡¶]
Polyoma and papilloma viridae	3-5	ds, circular	Icosadeltahedral	45-55	−
Parvoviridae	1.5-2.0	ss, linear	Icosahedral	18-26	−

ds, Double-stranded; *ss*, single-stranded.
*Genome invariably a single molecule.
[†]Polymerase encoded by virus.
[‡]Polymerase carried in the virion.
[§]Circular molecule is double stranded for most of its length but contains a single-stranded region.
[¶]Reverse transcriptase.

Table 37-3   Families of RNA Viruses and Some Important Members

Family*	Members[†]
PARAMYXOVIRIDAE	Parainfluenza virus, Sendai virus, *measles virus*, mumps virus, respiratory syncytial virus, metapneumovirus
ORTHOMYXOVIRIDAE	*Influenza virus* types A, B, and C
CORONAVIRIDAE	*Coronavirus*, severe acute respiratory syndrome
Arenaviridae	*Lassa fever virus*, Tacaribe virus complex (Junin and Machupo viruses), lymphocytic chorio-meningitis virus
Rhabdoviridae	*Rabies virus*, vesicular stomatitis virus
Filoviridae	*Ebola virus*, Marburg virus
Bunyaviridae	*California encephalitis virus*, La Crosse virus, sandfly fever virus, hemorrhagic fever virus, Hanta virus
Retroviridae	Human T-cell leukemia virus types I and II, *human immunodeficiency virus*, animal oncoviruses
Reoviridae	*Rotavirus*, Colorado tick fever virus
Togaviridae	*Rubella virus*; western, eastern, and Venezuelan equine encephalitis virus; Ross River virus; Sindbis virus; Semliki Forest virus
Flaviviridae	*Yellow fever virus*, dengue virus, St. Louis encephalitis virus, West Nile virus, hepatitis C virus
Caliciviridae	*Norwalk virus*, calicivirus
Picornaviridae	Rhinoviruses, *poliovirus*, echoviruses, coxsackievirus, hepatitis A virus
Delta	Delta agent

*The size of the type is indicative of the relative size of the virus.
[†]The italicized virus is the prototype virus for the family.

sense (−) (analogous to a photographic negative), double stranded (+/−) or ambisense (containing + and − regions of RNA attached end to end). The RNA genome may also be segmented into pieces, with each piece encoding one or more genes. The outer layer of the virion is the capsid or envelope. These structures are the package, protection, and delivery vehicle during transmission of the virus from one host to another and for spread within the host to the target cell. The surface structures of the capsid and envelope mediate the interaction of the virus with the target cell through a viral attachment protein (VAP) or structure. The capsid is a rigid structure able to withstand harsh environmental conditions. Viruses

Reovirus was discovered before it was associated with a specific disease, and thus it was designated an "orphan" virus. Norwalk virus is named for Norwalk, Ohio; coxsackievirus is named for Coxsackie, New York; and many of the togaviruses, arenaviruses, and bunyaviruses are named after African places where they were first isolated.

Viruses can be grouped by characteristics such as disease (e.g., hepatitis), target tissue, means of transmission (e.g., enteric, respiratory), or vector (e.g., arboviruses; arthropod-borne virus) (Box 37-3). *The most consistent and current means of classification is by physical and biochemical characteristics, such as size, morphology (e.g., presence or absence of a membrane envelope), type of genome, and means of replication* (Figures 37-2 and 37-3). DNA viruses associated with

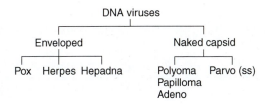

Figure 37-2   The DNA viruses and their morphology. The viral families are determined by the structure of the genome and the morphology of the virion.

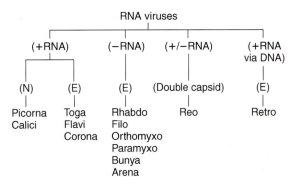

Figure 37-3   The RNA viruses, their genome structure, and their morphology. The viral families are determined by the structure of the genome and the morphology of the virion. *E*, Enveloped; *N*, naked capsid.

human disease are divided into seven families (Tables 37-1 and 37-2). The RNA viruses may be divided into at least 13 families (Tables 37-3 and 37-4).

VIRION STRUCTURE

The units for measurement of virion size are nanometers (nm). The clinically important viruses range from 18 nm (parvoviruses) to 300 nm (poxviruses) (Figure 37-4).

The virion (the virus particle) consists of a nucleic acid genome packaged into a protein coat (capsid) or a membrane (envelope) (Figure 37-5). The virion may also contain certain essential or accessory enzymes or other proteins to facilitate initial replication in the cell. Capsid or nucleic acid-binding proteins may associate with the genome to form a nucleocapsid, which may be the same as the virion or surrounded by an envelope.

The genome of the virus consists either of DNA or RNA. The DNA can be single or double stranded, linear or circular. The RNA can be either positive sense (+) (like messenger RNA [mRNA]) or negative

Box 37-3

Means of Classification and Naming of Viruses

Structure: size, morphology, and nucleic acid (e.g., picornavirus [small RNA], togavirus)
Biochemical characteristics: structure and mode of replication[*]
Disease: encephalitis and hepatitis viruses, for example
Means of transmission: arbovirus spread by insects, for example
Host cell (host range): animal (human, mouse, bird), plant, bacteria
Tissue or organ (tropism): adenovirus and enterovirus, for example.

[*]This is the current means of taxonomic classification of viruses.

Table 37-1   Families of DNA Viruses and Some Important Members

Family	Members[*]
POXVIRIDAE[†]	*Smallpox virus*, vaccinia virus, monkeypox, canarypox, molluscum contagiosum
Herpesviridae	*Herpes simplex virus types 1 and 2*, varicella-zoster virus, Epstein-Barr virus, cytomegalovirus, human herpesviruses 6, 7, and 8
Adenoviridae	*Adenovirus*
Hepadnaviridae	*Hepatitis B virus*
Papillomaviridae	*Papilloma virus*
Polyomaviridae	*JC virus*, BK virus, SV40
Parvoviridae	*Parvovirus B19*, adeno-associated virus

[*]The italicized virus is the prototype virus for the family.
[†]The size of type is indicative of the relative size of the virus.

Table 37-2 Properties of Virions of Human DNA Viruses

Family	Genome*		Virion		
	Molecular Mass × 10⁶ Daltons	Nature	Shape	Size (nm)	DNA Polymerase[†]
Poxviridae	85-140	ds, linear	Brick-shaped, enveloped	300 × 240 × 100	+[‡]
Herpesviridae	100-150	ds, linear	Icosadeltahedral, enveloped	Capsid, 100-110 Envelope, 120-200	+
Adenoviridae	20-25	ds, linear	Icosadeltahedral	70-90	+
Hepadnaviridae	1.8	ds, circular[§]	Spherical, enveloped	42	+[†¶]
Polyoma and papilloma viridae	3-5	ds, circular	Icosadeltahedral	45-55	−
Parvoviridae	1.5-2.0	ss, linear	Icosahedral	18-26	−

ds, Double-stranded; *ss*, single-stranded.
*Genome invariably a single molecule.
[†]Polymerase encoded by virus.
[‡]Polymerase carried in the virion.
[§]Circular molecule is double stranded for most of its length but contains a single-stranded region.
[¶]Reverse transcriptase.

Table 37-3 Families of RNA Viruses and Some Important Members

Family*	Members[†]
PARAMYXOVIRIDAE	Parainfluenza virus, Sendai virus, *measles virus*, mumps virus, respiratory syncytial virus, metapneumovirus
ORTHOMYXOVIRIDAE	*Influenza virus* types A, B, and C
CORONAVIRIDAE	*Coronavirus*, severe acute respiratory syndrome
Arenaviridae	*Lassa fever virus*, Tacaribe virus complex (Junin and Machupo viruses), lymphocytic choriomeningitis virus
Rhabdoviridae	*Rabies virus*, vesicular stomatitis virus
Filoviridae	*Ebola virus*, Marburg virus
Bunyaviridae	*California encephalitis virus*, La Crosse virus, sandfly fever virus, hemorrhagic fever virus, Hanta virus
Retroviridae	Human T-cell leukemia virus types I and II, *human immunodeficiency virus*, animal oncoviruses
Reoviridae	*Rotavirus*, Colorado tick fever virus
Togaviridae	*Rubella virus*; western, eastern, and Venezuelan equine encephalitis virus; Ross River virus; Sindbis virus; Semliki Forest virus
Flaviviridae	*Yellow fever virus*, dengue virus, St. Louis encephalitis virus, West Nile virus, hepatitis C virus
Caliciviridae	*Norwalk virus*, calicivirus
Picornaviridae	Rhinoviruses, *poliovirus*, echoviruses, coxsackievirus, hepatitis A virus
Delta	Delta agent

*The size of the type is indicative of the relative size of the virus.
[†]The italicized virus is the prototype virus for the family.

sense (−) (analogous to a photographic negative), double stranded (+/−) or ambisense (containing + and − regions of RNA attached end to end). The RNA genome may also be segmented into pieces, with each piece encoding one or more genes. The outer layer of the virion is the capsid or envelope. These structures are the package, protection, and delivery vehicle during transmission of the virus from one host to another and for spread within the host to the target cell. The surface structures of the capsid and envelope mediate the interaction of the virus with the target cell through a viral attachment protein (VAP) or structure. The capsid is a rigid structure able to withstand harsh environmental conditions. Viruses

Table 37-4 Properties of Virions of Human RNA Viruses

Family	Genome* Molecular Mass × 10^6 Daltons	Genome* Nature	Virion Shape*	Virion Size (nm)	Virion Polymerase in Virion	Virion Envelope
Paramyxoviridae	5-7	ss, −	Spherical	150-300	+	+
Orthomyxoviridae	5-7	ss, −, seg	Spherical	80-120	+	+
Coronaviridae	6-7	ss, +	Spherical	80-130	−	+[†]
Arenaviridae	3-5	ss, −, seg	Spherical	50-300	+	+[†]
Rhabdoviridae	4-7	ss, −	Bullet-shaped	180 × 75	+	+
Filoviridae	4-7	ss, −	Filamentous	800 × 80	+	+
Bunyaviridae	4-7	ss, −	Spherical	90-100	+	+[†]
Retroviridae	2 × (2-3)[‡]	ss, +	Spherical	80-110	+[§]	+
Reoviridae	11-15	ds, seg	Icosahedral	60-80	+	−
Picornaviridae	2.5	ss, +	Icosahedral	25-30	−	−
Togaviridae	4-5	ss, +	Icosahedral	60-70	−	+
Flaviviridae	4-7	ss, +	Spherical	40-50	−	+
Caliciviridae	2.6	ss, +	Icosahedral	35-40	−	−

ds, Double-stranded; *seg*, segmented; *ss*, single-stranded; *+ or −*, polarity of single-stranded nucleic acid.
*Some enveloped viruses are very pleomorphic (sometimes filamentous).
[†]No matrix protein.
[‡]Genome has two identical single-stranded RNA molecules.
[§]Reverse transcriptase.

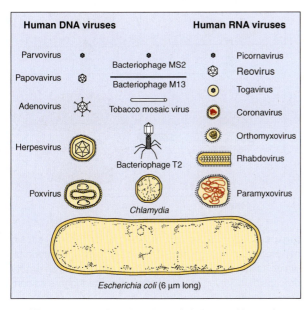

Figure 37-4 Relative sizes of viruses and bacteria.

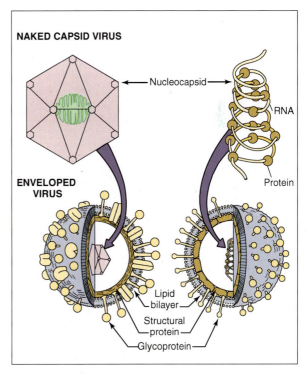

Figure 37-5 The structures of a naked capsid virus (*top left*) and enveloped viruses (*bottom*) with an icosahedral (*left*) nucleocapsid or a helical (*right*) ribonucleocapsid. The helical ribonucleocapsid is formed by viral proteins associated with an RNA genome.

with naked capsids are generally resistant to drying, acid, and detergents, including the acid and bile of the enteric tract. Many of these viruses are transmitted by the fecal-oral route and can endure transmission even in sewage.

The envelope is a membrane composed of lipids, proteins, and glycoproteins. The membranous structure of the envelope can be maintained only in aqueous solutions. It is readily disrupted by drying, acidic conditions, detergents, and solvents such as ether, which results in inactivation of the virus. As a result, enveloped viruses must remain wet and are generally transmitted in fluids, respiratory droplets, blood, and tissue. Most cannot survive the harsh conditions of the gastrointestinal tract. The influence of virion structure on viral properties is summarized in Boxes 37-4 and 37-5.

Capsid Viruses

The viral capsid is assembled from individual proteins associated into progressively larger units. All of the components of the capsid have chemical features that allow them to fit together and to assemble into a larger unit. Individual structural proteins associate into subunits, which associate into protomers, capsomeres (distinguishable in electron micrographs), and finally, a recognizable procapsid or capsid (Figure 37-6). A procapsid requires further processing to the final, transmissible capsid.

Box 37-4

Virion Structure: Naked Capsid

Component
Protein

Properties*
Is environmentally stable to the following:
  Temperature
  Acid
  Proteases
  Detergents
  Drying
Is released from cell by lysis

Consequences*
Can be spread easily (on fomites, from hand to hand, by dust, by small droplets)
Can dry out and retain infectivity
Can survive the adverse conditions of the gut
Can be resistant to detergents and poor sewage treatment
Antibody may be sufficient for immunoprotection

*Exceptions exist.

Box 37-5

Virion Structure: Envelope

Components
Membrane
Lipids
Proteins
Glycoproteins

Properties*
Is environmentally labile—disrupted by the following:
  Acid
  Detergents
  Drying
  Heat
Modifies cell membrane during replication
Is released by budding and cell lysis

Consequences*
Must stay wet
Cannot survive the gastrointestinal tract
Spreads in large droplets, secretions, organ transplants, and blood transfusions
Does not need to kill the cell to spread
May need antibody and cell-mediated immune response for protection and control
Elicits hypersensitivity and inflammation to cause immunopathogenesis

*Exceptions exist.

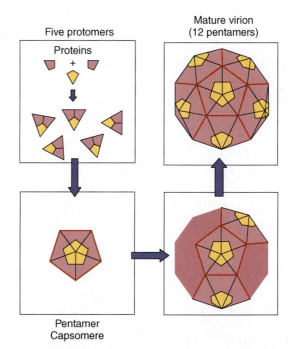

Figure 37-6 Capsid assembly of the icosahedral capsid of a picornavirus. Individual proteins associate into subunits, which associate into protomers, capsomeres, and an empty procapsid. Inclusion of the (+) RNA genome triggers its conversion to the final capsid form.

The simplest viral structures that can be built stepwise are symmetric and include helical and icosahedral structures. Helical structures appear as rods, whereas the icosahedron is an approximation of a sphere assembled from symmetric subunits (Figure 37-7). Nonsymmetric capsids are complex forms and are associated with certain bacterial viruses (phages).

The classic example of a virus with helical sym-

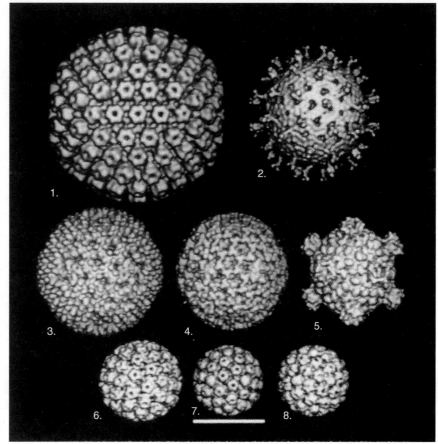

Figure 37-7   Cryoelectron microscopy and computer-generated three-dimensional image reconstructions of several icosahedral capsids. These images show the symmetry of capsids and the individual capsomeres. During assembly, the genome may fill the capsid through the holes in the herpesvirus and papovavirus capsomeres. *1,* Equine herpesvirus nucleocapsid; *2,* simian rotavirus; *3,* reovirus type 1 (Lang) virion; *4,* intermediate subviral particle (reovirus); *5,* core (inner capsid) particle (reovirus); *6,* human papillomavirus type 19; *7,* mouse polyomavirus; *8,* cauliflower mosaic virus. Bar = 50 nm. (Courtesy Dr. Tim Baker, Purdue University, West Lafayette, Ind.)

metry is the tobacco mosaic plant virus. Its capsomeres self-assemble on the RNA genome into rods that extend the length of the genome. Helical nucleocapsids are observed within the envelope of most negative-strand RNA viruses.

Simple icosahedrons are used by small viruses such as the picornaviruses and parvoviruses. The icosahedron is made of 12 capsomeres, each with fivefold symmetry (pentamer or penton). For the picornaviruses, every pentamer is made up of five protomers, each of which is composed of three subunits of four separate proteins (see Figure 37-6). The picornavirus capsid t have manycanyon-like clefts, each of which is a "docking site" to bind to the receptor on the surface of the target cell.

Larger capsid virions are constructed by inserting structurally distinct capsomeres between the pentons at the vertices. These capsomeres have six nearest neighbors (hexons). This extends the icosahedron and is called an icosadeltahedron, and its size is determined by the number of hexons inserted along the edges and within the surfaces between the pentons. For example, the herpesvirus nucleocapsid has 12 pentons and 150 hexons. The adenovirus capsid is composed of 252 capsomeres, with 12 pentons and 240 hexons. A long fiber is attached to each penton of adenovirus to serve as the VAP to bind to target cells, and it also contains the type-specific antigen. The reoviruses have an icosahedral double capsid with fiber-like proteins partially extended from each vertex. The outer capsid protects the virus and promotes its uptake across the gastrointestinal tract and into target cells, whereas the inner capsid contains enzymes for the synthesis of RNA (see Figures 37-7).

Enveloped Viruses

The virion envelope is composed of lipids, proteins, and glycoproteins (see Figure 37-5 and Box 37-5). It has a membrane structure similar to cellular membranes. Cellular proteins are rarely found in the viral envelope, even though the envelope is obtained from cellular membranes. Most enveloped viruses are round or pleomorphic (see Figures 37-2 and 37-3 for the complete listing of enveloped viruses).

Most viral glycoproteins have asparagine-linked (*N*-linked) carbohydrate and extend through the envelope and away from the surface of the virion. For many viruses, these can be observed as spikes (Figure 37-8). Some glycoproteins act as VAPs, capable of binding to structures on target cells. VAPs that also bind to erythrocytes are termed hemagglutinins (HAs). Some glycoproteins have other functions, such as the neuraminidase (NA) of orthomyxoviruses (influenza) and the Fc receptor and the C3b receptor associated with herpes simplex virus (HSV) glycoproteins, or the fusion glycoproteins of paramyxoviruses. Glycoproteins, especially the VAP, are also major antigens that elicit protective immunity.

The envelope of the togaviruses surrounds an icosahedral nucleocapsid containing a positive-strand RNA genome. The envelope contains spikes consisting of two or three glycoprotein subunits anchored to the virion's icosahedral capsid. This causes the envelope to adhere tightly and conform (shrink-wrap) to

an icosahedral structure discernible by cryoelectron microscopy.

All of the negative-strand RNA viruses are enveloped. Components of the viral RNA-dependent RNA polymerase associate with the (−) RNA genome of the orthomyxoviruses, paramyxoviruses, and rhabdoviruses to form helical nucleocapsids (see Figure 37-5). These enzymes are required to initiate virus replication, and their association with the genome ensures their delivery into the cell. Matrix proteins lining the inside of the envelope facilitate the assembly of the ribonucleocapsid into the virion. Influenza A (orthomyxovirus) is an example of a (−) RNA virus with a segmented genome. Its envelope is lined with matrix proteins and has two glycoproteins: the HA, which is the VAP, and an NA. Bunyaviruses do not have matrix proteins.

The herpesvirus envelope is a baglike structure that encloses the icosadeltahedral nucleocapsid. Depending on the specific herpesvirus, the envelope may contain as many as 11 glycoproteins. The interstitial space between the nucleocapsid and the envelope is called the tegument, and it contains enzymes, other proteins, and even RNA that facilitate the viral infection.

The poxviruses are enveloped viruses with large, complex, bricklike shapes. The envelope encloses a dumbbell-shaped, DNA-containing nucleoid structure; lateral bodies; fibrils; and many enzymes and proteins, including the enzymes and transcriptional factors required for mRNA synthesis.

VIRAL REPLICATION

The major steps in viral replication are the same for all viruses (Figure 37-9 and Box 37-6). The cell acts as a factory, providing the substrates, energy, and machinery necessary for the synthesis of viral proteins and replication of the genome. Processes not provided by the cell must be encoded in the genome of the virus. The manner in which each virus accomplishes these steps and overcomes the cell's biochemical limitations is different for different structures of the genome and of the virion (whether it is enveloped or has a naked capsid). This is illustrated in the

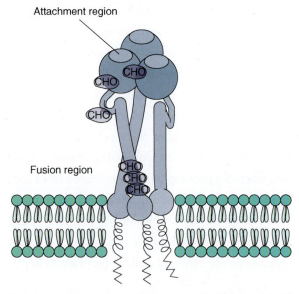

Figure 37-8 Diagram of the hemagglutinin glycoprotein trimer of influenza A virus, a representative spike protein. The region for attachment to the cellular receptor is exposed on the spike protein's surface. Under mild acidic conditions, the hemagglutinin folds over to bring the virion envelope and cellular membrane together and exposes a hydrophobic sequence to promote fusion. *CHO,* *N*-linked carbohydrate attachment sites. (Modified from Schlesinger MJ, Schlesinger S: Domains of virus glycoproteins, *Adv Virus Res* 33: 1-37, 1987.)

examples in Figures 37-12 to 37-14 (see later).

A single round of the viral replication cycle can be separated into several phases. During the early phase of infection, the virus must recognize an appropriate target cell, attach to the cell, penetrate the plasma membrane and be taken up by the cell, release (uncoat) its genome into the cytoplasm, and if necessary, deliver the genome to the nucleus. The late phase begins with the start of genome replication and viral macromolecular synthesis and proceeds through viral assembly and release. Uncoating of the

genome from the capsid or envelope during the early phase abolishes its infectivity and identifiable structure, thus initiating the eclipse period. The eclipse period, like a solar eclipse, ends with the appearance of new virions after virus assembly. The latent period, during which extracellular infectious virus is not detected, includes the eclipse period and ends with the release of new viruses (Figure 37-10). Each infected cell may produce as many as 100,000 particles; however, only 1% to 10% of these particles may be infectious. The noninfectious particles (defective particles) result from mutations and errors in the manufacture and assembly of the virion. The yield of

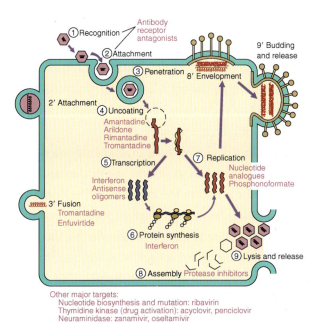

Figure 37-9 A general scheme of viral replication. Enveloped viruses have alternative means of entry *(steps 2' and 3')*, assembly, and exit from the cell (*8'* and *9'*). The antiviral drugs for susceptible steps in viral replication are listed in magenta.

Box 37-6

Steps in Viral Replication

Recognition of the target cell
Attachment
Penetration
Uncoating
Macromolecular synthesis
 Early messenger RNA (mRNA) and nonstructural protein
  synthesis: genes for enzymes and nucleic acid-binding
  proteins
 Replication of genome
 Late mRNA and structural protein synthesis
 Posttranslational modification of protein
Assembly of virus
Budding of enveloped viruses
Release of virus

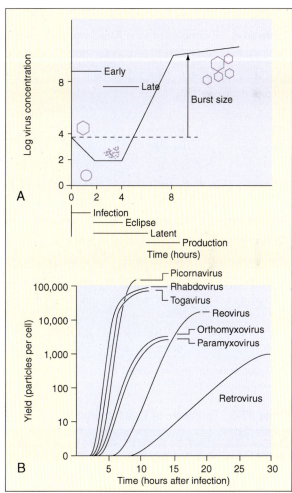

Figure 37-10 A, Single-cycle growth curve of a virus that is released on cell lysis. The different stages are defined by the absence of visible viral components (eclipse period), infectious virus in the media (latent period), or presence of macromolecular synthesis (early/late phases). **B,** Growth curve and burst size of representative viruses. (**A,** Modified from Davis BD, et al: *Microbiology*, ed 4, Philadelphia, 1990, Lippincott; **B,** modified from White DO, Fenner F: *Medical virology*, ed 3, New York, 1986, Academic.)

infectious virus per cell, or burst size, and the time required for a single cycle of virus reproduction are determined by the properties of the virus and the target cell.

Recognition of and Attachment to the Target Cell

The binding of the VAPs or structures on the surface of the virion capsid (Table 37-5) to receptors on the cell (Table 37-6) initially determines which cells can be infected by a virus. *The receptors for the virus on the cell may be proteins or carbohydrates on glycoproteins or glycolipids.* Viruses that bind to receptors expressed on specific cell types may be restricted to certain species (host range) (e.g., human, mouse) or

specific cell types. The susceptible target cell defines the tissue tropism (e.g., neurotropic, lymphotropic).

Penetration

Interactions between multiple VAPs and cellular receptors initiate the internalization of the virus into the cell. The mechanism of internalization depends on the virion structure and cell type. Most nonenveloped viruses enter the cell by receptor-mediated endocytosis or by viropexis. Endocytosis is a normal process used by the cell for the uptake of receptor-bound molecules such as hormones, low-density lipoproteins, and transferrin. Picornaviruses and papovaviruses may enter by viropexis. Hydrophobic structures of capsid proteins may be exposed after viral binding to the cells, and these structures help the virus or the viral genome slip through (direct penetration) the membrane.

Enveloped viruses fuse their membranes with cellular membranes to deliver the nucleocapsid or genome directly into the cytoplasm. The optimum pH for fusion determines whether penetration occurs at the cell surface at neutral pH or whether the virus must be internalized by endocytosis, and fusion occurs in an endosome at acidic pH. The fusion activity may be provided by the VAP or another protein. The HA of influenza A (see Figure 37-8) binds to sialic acid receptors on the target cell. Under the mild acidic conditions of the endosome, the HA undergoes a dramatic conformational change to expose hydrophobic portions capable of promoting membrane fusion.

Table 37-5 Examples of Viral Attachment Proteins

Virus Family	Virus	Viral Attachment Protein
Picornaviridae	Rhinovirus	VP1-VP2-VP3 complex
Adenoviridae	Adenovirus	Fiber protein
Reoviridae	Reovirus	σ-1
	Rotavirus	VP7
Togaviridae	Semliki Forest virus	E1-E2-E3 complex gp
Rhabdoviridae	Rabies virus	G protein gp
Orthomyxoviridae	Influenza A virus	HA gp
Paramyxoviridae	Measles virus	HA gp
Herpesviridae	Epstein-Barr virus	gp350 and gp220
Retroviridae	Murine leukemia virus	gp70
	Human immunodeficiency virus	gp120

gp, Glycoprotein; *HA*, hemagglutinin.

Table 37-6 Examples of Viral Receptors

Virus	Target Cell	Receptor[*]
Epstein-Barr virus	B cell	C3d complement receptor CR2 (CD21)
Human immunodeficiency virus	Helper T cell	CD4 molecule and chemokine coreceptor
Rhinovirus	Epithelial cells	ICAM-1 (immunoglobulin superfamily protein)
Poliovirus	Epithelial cells	Immunoglobulin superfamily protein
Herpes simplex virus	Many cells	Herpesvirus entry mediator (HVEM), nectin-1
Rabies virus	Neuron	Acetylcholine receptor, NCAM
Influenza A virus	Epithelial cells	Sialic acid
B19 parvovirus	Erythroid precursors	Erythrocyte P antigen (globoside)

CD, Cluster of differentiation; *ICAM-1*, intercellular adhesion molecule; *NCAM*, neural cell adhesion molecule.
[*]Other receptors for these viruses may also exist.

Uncoating

Once internalized, the nucleocapsid must be delivered to the site of replication within the cell and the capsid or envelope removed. The genome of DNA viruses, except for poxviruses, must be delivered to the nucleus, whereas most RNA viruses remain in the cytoplasm. The uncoating process may be initiated by attachment to the receptor or promoted by the acidic environment or proteases found in an endosome or lysosome. Picornavirus capsids are weakened by the release of the VP4 capsid protein to allow uncoating. VP4 is released by insertion of the receptor into the keyhole-like canyon attachment site of the capsid. Enveloped viruses are uncoated on fusion with cell membranes. Fusion of the herpesvirus envelope with the plasma membrane releases its nucleocapsid, which then "docks" with the nuclear membrane to deliver its DNA genome directly to the site of replication. The release of the influenza nucleocapsid from its matrix and envelope is facilitated by the passage of protons from inside the endosome through the ion pore formed by the influenza M2 membrane protein to acidify the virion.

Macromolecular Synthesis

Once inside the cell, the genome must direct the synthesis of viral mRNA and protein and generate identical copies of itself. The genome is useless unless it can be transcribed into functional mRNAs capable of binding to ribosomes and being translated into proteins. The means by which each virus accomplishes these steps depends on the structure of the genome (Figure 37-11) and the site of replication.

The cell's machinery for transcription and mRNA processing is found in the nucleus. Most DNA viruses use the cell's DNA-dependent RNA polymerase II and other enzymes to make mRNA. Exceptionally, poxviruses replicate in the cytoplasm and therefore must encode enzymes for all these functions. Most RNA viruses replicate and produce mRNA in the cytoplasm, except for orthomyxoviruses and retroviruses. RNA viruses must encode the necessary enzymes for transcription and replication, because the cell has no means of replicating RNA. The mRNAs for RNA viruses may or may not acquire a 5' cap or polyA tail.

The naked genome of DNA viruses (except poxviruses) and the positive-sense RNA viruses (except retroviruses) are sometimes referred to as infectious nucleic acids because they are sufficient for initiating replication on injection into a cell. These genomes can interact directly with host machinery to promote mRNA or protein synthesis.

In general, mRNA for nonstructural proteins is transcribed first (Figure 37-12). Early gene products (nonstructural proteins) are often DNA-binding proteins and enzymes, including virus-encoded polymerases. These proteins are catalytic, and only a few are required. Replication of the genome usually initiates the transition to transcription of late gene products. Late viral genes encode structural and other proteins. Many copies of these proteins are required to package the virus, but are generally not required before the genome is replicated. Newly replicated genomes also provide new templates for more late gene mRNA synthesis. Different DNA and RNA viruses control the time and amount of viral gene and protein synthesis in different ways.

DNA Viruses

Replication of the DNA genome requires a DNA-dependent DNA polymerase, other enzymes, and deoxyribonucleotide triphosphates, especially thymidine (Box 37-7). Transcription of the DNA virus genome (except for poxviruses) occurs in the nucleus, using host cell polymerases and other enzymes for viral mRNA synthesis. Transcription of the viral genes is regulated by the interaction of specific DNA-binding proteins with promoter and enhancer elements in the viral genome. The viral promoter and enhancer elements are similar in sequence to those of the host cell to allow binding of the cell's transcriptional activation factors and DNA-dependent RNA polymerase. Cells from some tissues do not express the DNA-binding proteins necessary for activating the transcription of viral genes, and replication of the virus in that cell is thus prevented or limited.

Different DNA viruses control the duration, tim-

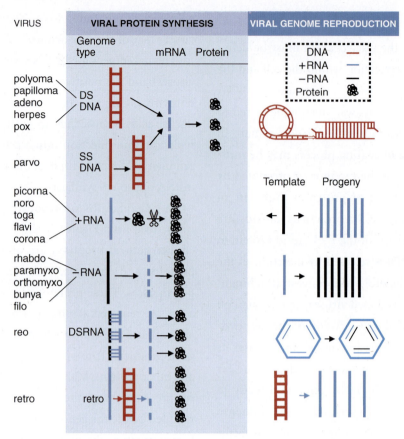

Figure 37-11 Viral macromolecular synthesis steps: the mechanism of viral mRNA and protein synthesis and genome replication are determined by the structure of the genome. *1,* Double-stranded DNA *(DS DNA)* uses host machinery in the nucleus (except poxviruses) to make mRNA, which is translated by host cell ribosomes into proteins. Replication of viral DNA occurs by semiconservative means, by rolling circle, linear, and in other ways. *2,* Single-stranded DNA *(SS DNA)* is converted into DS DNA and replicates like DS DNA. *3,* (+) RNA resembles an mRNA that binds to ribosomes to make a polyprotein that is cleaved into individual proteins. One of the viral proteins is an RNA polymerase that makes a (−) RNA template and then more (+) RNA genome progeny and mRNAs. *4,* (−) RNA is transcribed into mRNAs and a full-length (+) RNA template by the RNA polymerase carried in the virion. The (+) RNA template is used to make (−) RNA genome progeny. *5,* DS RNA acts like (−) RNA. The (−) strands are transcribed into mRNAs by an RNA polymerase in the capsid. New (+) RNAs get encapsidated and (−) RNAs are made in the capsid. *6,* Retroviruses have (+) RNA that is converted to complementary DNA (cDNA) by reverse transcriptase carried in the virion. cDNA integrates into the host chromosome, and the host makes mRNAs, proteins, and full-length RNA genome copies.

ing, and quantity of viral gene and protein synthesis in different ways. The more complex viruses encode their own transcriptional activators, which enhance or regulate the expression of viral genes. Genes may be transcribed from either DNA strand of the genome and in opposite directions. For example, the early and late genes of the SV40 papovavirus are on opposite, nonoverlapping DNA strands. Viral genes may have introns requiring posttranscriptional processing of the mRNA by the cell's nuclear machinery (splicing). The late genes of papovaviruses and adenoviruses are initially transcribed as a large RNA from a single promoter and then processed to pro-

duce several different mRNAs after removal of different intervening sequences (introns).

Replication of viral DNA follows the same biochemical rules as for cellular DNA. Replication is initiated at a unique DNA sequence of the genome called the origin (ori). This is a site recognized by cellular or viral nuclear factors and the DNA-dependent DNA polymerase. Viral DNA synthesis is semiconservative, and viral and cellular *DNA polymerases require a primer* to initiate synthesis of the DNA chain. The parvoviruses have DNA sequences that are inverted and repeated to allow the DNA to fold back and hybridize with itself to provide a primer.

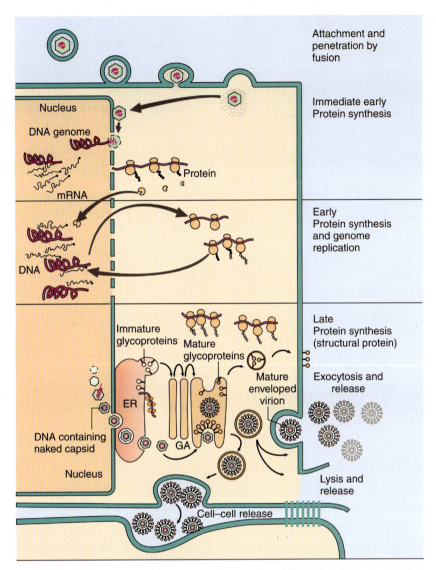

Figure 37-12   Replication of herpes simplex virus, a complex enveloped DNA virus. The virus binds to specific receptors and fuses with the plasma membrane. The nucleocapsid then delivers the DNA genome to the nucleus. Transcription and translation occur in three phases: immediate early, early, and late. Immediate early proteins promote the takeover of the cell; early proteins consist of enzymes, including the DNA-dependent DNA polymerase; and the late proteins are structural and other proteins, including the viral capsid and glycoproteins. The genome is replicated before transcription of the late genes. Capsid proteins migrate into the nucleus, assemble into icosadeltahedral capsids, and are filled with the DNA genome. The capsids filled with genomes bud through the nuclear and endoplasmic reticulum *(ER)* membranes into the cytoplasm, acquire tegument proteins, and then acquire their envelope as they bud through the viral glycoprotein-modified membranes of the trans-Golgi network. The virus is released by exocytosis or cell lysis. *GA,* Golgi apparatus.

Replication of the adenovirus genome is primed by deoxycytidine monophosphate attached to a terminal protein. A cellular enzyme (primase) synthesizes an RNA primer to start the replication of the papovavirus genome, whereas the herpesviruses encode a primase.

Replication of the genome of the simple DNA viruses (e.g., parvoviruses, papovaviruses) uses the host DNA-dependent DNA polymerases, whereas the larger, more complex viruses (e.g., adenoviruses,

herpesviruses, poxviruses) encode their own polymerases. Viral polymerases are usually faster but less precise than host cell polymerases, causing a higher mutation rate in viruses and providing a target for nucleotide analogues as antiviral drugs.

Hepadnavirus replication is unique in that a larger than genome positive-strand RNA copy is first synthesized by the cell's DNA-dependent RNA polymerase and circularizes. Viral proteins surround the RNA, a viral encoded RNA-dependent DNA

Properties of DNA Viruses

DNA is not transient or labile.

Many DNA viruses establish persistent infections (e.g., latent, immortalizing).

DNA genomes reside in the nucleus (except for poxviruses).

Viral DNA resembles host DNA for transcription and replication.

Viral genes must interact with host transcriptional machinery (except for poxviruses).

Viral gene transcription is temporally regulated.

Early genes encode DNA-binding proteins and enzymes.

Late genes encode structural and other proteins.

DNA polymerases require a primer to replicate the viral genome.

The larger DNA viruses encode means to promote efficient replication of their genome.

Parvovirus: requires cells undergoing DNA synthesis to replicate.

Papovavirus: stimulates cell growth and DNA synthesis.

Hepadnavirus: stimulates cell growth, cell makes RNA intermediate, encodes a reverse transcriptase.

Adenovirus: stimulates cellular DNA synthesis and encodes its own polymerase.

Herpesvirus: stimulates cell growth, encodes its own polymerase and enzymes to provide deoxyribonucleotides for DNA synthesis, establishes latent infection in host.

Poxvirus: encodes its own polymerases and enzymes to provide deoxyribonucleotides for DNA synthesis, replication machinery, and transcription machinery in the cytoplasm.

polymerase (reverse transcriptase) in this virion core makes a negative-strand DNA, and then the RNA is degraded. Positive-strand DNA synthesis is initiated but stops when the genome and core are enveloped, yielding a partially double-stranded, circular DNA genome.

Major limitations for replication of a DNA virus include availability of the DNA polymerase and deoxyribonucleotide substrates. Most cells in the resting phase of growth are not undergoing DNA synthesis because the necessary enzymes are not present, and deoxythymidine pools are limited. *The smaller the DNA virus, the more dependent the virus is on the host cell* to provide these functions (see Box 37-7).

RNA Viruses

Replication and transcription of RNA viruses are similar processes, because the viral genomes are usually either an mRNA (positive-strand RNA) (Figure 37-13) or a template for mRNA (negative-strand RNA) (Box 37-8 and Figure 37-14). During replication and

transcription, a double-stranded RNA replicative intermediate is formed. Double-stranded RNA is not normally found in uninfected cells and is a strong inducer of innate host protections.

The RNA virus genome must code for RNA-dependent RNA polymerases (replicases and transcriptases) because the cell has no means of replicating RNA. The replicases and transcriptases are generated by addition of subunits or cleavage of a core polymerase. Because RNA is degraded relatively quickly, the RNA-dependent RNA polymerase must be provided or synthesized soon after uncoating to generate more viral RNA, or the infection will be aborted. Most viral RNA polymerases work at a fast pace but are also error prone, causing mutations. Replication of the genome provides new templates for production

Properties of RNA Viruses

RNA is labile and transient.

Most RNA viruses replicate in the cytoplasm.

Cells cannot replicate RNA. RNA viruses must encode an RNA-dependent RNA polymerase.

The genome structure determines the mechanism of transcription and replication.

RNA viruses are prone to mutation.

The genome structure and polarity determine how viral messenger RNA (mRNA) is generated and proteins are processed.

RNA viruses, except (+) RNA genome, must carry polymerases.

All (−) RNA viruses are enveloped.

Picornaviruses, Togaviruses, Flaviviruses, Caliciviruses, and Coronaviruses

(+) RNA genome resembles mRNA and is translated into a polyprotein, which is proteolyzed. A (−) RNA template is used for replication. For togaviruses, coronaviruses, and caliciviruses, early proteins are transcribed from the genome and late proteins from the template.

Orthomyxoviruses, Paramyxoviruses, Rhabdoviruses, Filoviruses, and Bunyaviruses

(−) RNA genome is a template for individual mRNAs, but full-length (+) RNA template is required for replication. Orthomyxoviruses replicate and transcribe in nucleus, and each segment of the genome encodes one mRNA and template.

Reoviruses

(+/−) Segmented RNA genome is a template for mRNA. (+) RNA may also be encapsulated to generate the (+/−) RNA and then more mRNA.

Retroviruses

(+) Retrovirus RNA genome is converted into DNA, which is integrated into the host chromatin and transcribed as a cellular gene

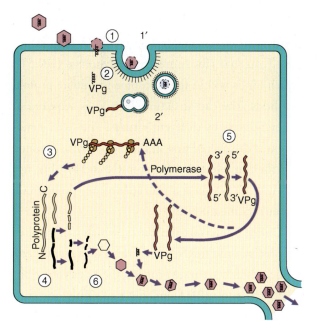

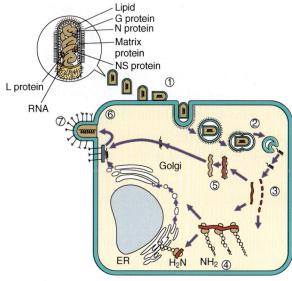

Figure 37-13   Replication of picornaviruses: a simple (+) RNA virus. *1*, Interaction of the picornaviruses with receptors on the cell surface defines the target cell and weakens the capsid. *2*, The genome is injected through the virion and across the cell membrane. *2′*, Alternatively, the virion is endocytosed, and then the genome is released. *3*, The genome is used as mRNA for protein synthesis. One large polyprotein is translated from the virion genome. *4*, Then the polyprotein is proteolytically cleaved into individual proteins, including an RNA-dependent RNA polymerase. *5*, The polymerase makes a (−) strand template from the genome and replicates the genome. A protein *(VPg)* is covalently attached to the 5′ end of the viral genome. *6*, The structural proteins associate into the capsid structure, the genome is inserted, and the virions are released on cell lysis.

Figure 37-14   Replication of rhabdoviruses: a simple enveloped (−) RNA virus. *1*, Rhabdoviruses bind to the cell surface and are *(2)* endocytosed. The envelope fuses with the endosome vesicle membrane to deliver the nucleocapsid to the cytoplasm. The virion must carry a polymerase, which *(3)* produces five individual messenger RNAs (mRNAs) and a full-length (+) RNA template. *4*, Proteins are translated from the mRNAs, including one glycoprotein (G) which is co-translationally glycosylated in the endoplasmic reticulum *(ER)*, processed in the Golgi apparatus, and delivered to the cell membrane. *5*, The genome is replicated from the (+) RNA template, and N, L, and NS proteins associate with the genome to form the nucleocapsid. *6*, The matrix protein associates with the G protein-modified membrane, which is followed by assembly of the nucleocapsid. *7*, The virus buds from the cell in a bullet-shaped virion.

of more mRNA and genomes, which amplifies and accelerates virus replication.

The positive-strand RNA viral genomes of the picornaviruses, caliciviruses, coronaviruses, flaviviruses, and togaviruses act as mRNA, bind to ribosomes, and direct protein synthesis. The naked positive-strand RNA viral genome is sufficient to initiate infection by itself. After the virus-encoded, RNA-dependent RNA polymerase is produced, a negative-strand RNA template (antigenome) is synthesized. The template can then be used to generate more mRNA and to replicate the genome.

The negative-strand RNA virus genomes of the rhabdoviruses, orthomyxoviruses, paramyxoviruses, filoviruses, and bunyaviruses are the templates for production of mRNA. The negative-strand RNA genome is not infectious by itself, and a polymerase

must be carried into the cell with the genome (associated with the genome as part of the nucleocapsid) to make individual mRNA for the different viral proteins. As a result, a full-length positive-strand RNA must also be produced by the viral polymerase to act as a template to generate more copies of the genome. Except for influenza viruses, transcription and replication of negative-strand RNA viruses occur in the cytoplasm. The reoviruses have a segmented, double-stranded RNA genome and undergo a more complex means of replication and transcription. The reovirus RNA polymerase is part of the inner capsid core; mRNA units are transcribed from each of the 10 or more segments of the genome while they are still in the core. The negative strands of the genome segments are used as templates for mRNA in a manner similar to that of the negative-strand RNA viruses.

Reovirus-encoded enzymes contained in the inner capsid core add the 5′ cap to viral mRNA. The mRNA does not have polyA. The mRNAs are released into the cytoplasm, where they direct protein synthesis or are sequestered into new cores. The positive-strand RNA in the new cores acts as a template for negative-strand RNA, and the core polymerase produces the progeny double-stranded RNA.

The arenaviruses have an ambisense genome with (−) sequences adjacent to (+) sequences. The early mRNAs of the virus are transcribed from the negative-sense portion of the genome, a full-length replicative intermediate is produced to generate a new genome, and the late mRNAs of the virus are transcribed from the region complementary to the (+) sequences in the replicative intermediate.

The retroviruses carry two copies of the genome, two transfer RNA (tRNA) molecules, and an RNA-dependent DNA polymerase (reverse transcriptase) in the virion. The tRNA is used as a primer for synthesis of a circular complementary DNA (cDNA) copy of the genome. The cDNA is synthesized in the cytoplasm, travels to the nucleus, and is then integrated into the host chromatin. The viral genome becomes a cellular gene. Promoters at the end of the integrated viral genome enhance the transcription of the viral DNA sequences by the cell. Full-length RNA transcripts are used as new genomes, and individual mRNAs are generated by differential splicing of this RNA.

The most unusual mode of replication is reserved for the deltavirus. The deltavirus resembles a viroid. The genome is a circular, rod-shaped, single-stranded RNA, which is extensively hybridized to itself. As the exception, the deltavirus RNA genome is replicated by the host cell DNA-dependent RNA polymerase II in the nucleus. A portion of the genome forms an RNA structure called a ribozyme, which cleaves the RNA circle to produce an mRNA.

Viral Protein Synthesis

All viruses depend on the host cell ribosomes, tRNA, and mechanisms for posttranslational modification to produce their proteins. The binding of mRNA to the ribosome is mediated by a 5′ cap structure of methylated guanosine or a special RNA loop structure (internal ribosome entry sequence [IRES]), which binds within the ribosome to initiate protein synthesis. The cap structure, if used, is acquired in different ways by different viruses. The IRES structure was discovered first in the picornavirus genome and then in selected cellular mRNAs. Most but not all viral mRNA have a polyadenosine (polyA) tail, like eukaryotic mRNAs.

Unlike bacterial ribosomes, which can bind to a polycistronic mRNA and translate several gene sequences into separate proteins, the eukaryotic ribosome binds to mRNA and can make only one continuous protein, and then it falls off the mRNA. Each virus deals with this limitation differently, depending on the structure of the genome. For example, the entire genome of a positive-strand RNA virus is read by the ribosome and translated into one giant polyprotein. The polyprotein is subsequently cleaved by cellular and viral proteases into functional proteins. DNA viruses, retroviruses, and most negative-strand RNA viruses transcribe separate mRNA for smaller polyproteins or individual proteins. The orthomyxovirus and reovirus genomes are segmented, and most of the segments code for single proteins for this reason.

Viruses use different tactics to promote preferential translation of their viral mRNA instead of cellular mRNA. In many cases, the concentration of viral mRNA in the cell is so large that it occupies most of the ribosomes, preventing translation of cellular mRNA. Adenovirus infection blocks the egress of cellular mRNA from the nucleus. HSV and other viruses inhibit cellular macromolecular synthesis and induce degradation of the cell's DNA and mRNA. To promote selective translation of its mRNA, poliovirus uses a virus-encoded protease to inactivate the 200,000-Da cap-binding protein of the ribosome to prevent binding and translation of the cell's 5′capped cellular mRNA. Togaviruses and many other viruses increase the permeability of the cell's membrane; thus the ribosomal affinity for most cellular mRNA is decreased. All these actions also contribute to the cytopathology of the virus infection. The pathogenic consequences of these actions are discussed further in Chapter 38.

Some viral proteins require posttranslational modifications, such as phosphorylation, glycosylation, acylation, or sulfation. Protein phosphorylation is accomplished by cellular or viral protein kinases and is a means of modulating, activating, or inactivating proteins. Several herpesviruses and other viruses encode their own protein kinase. Viral glycoproteins are synthesized on membrane-bound ribosomes and have the amino acid sequences to allow insertion into the rough endoplasmic reticulum and N-linked glycosylation. The presence of the glycoproteins determines where the virion will assemble within the cell.

Assembly

Virion assembly is analogous to a three-dimensional interlocking puzzle that puts itself together in the box. The virion is built from small, easily manufactured parts that enclose the genome in a functional package. Each part of the virion has recognition structures that allow the virus to form the appropriate protein-protein, protein-nucleic acid, and (for enveloped viruses) protein-membrane interactions needed to assemble into the final structure.

The site and mechanism of virion assembly in the cell depend on where genome replication occurs and whether the final structure is a naked capsid or an enveloped virus. Assembly of the DNA viruses, other than poxviruses, occurs in the nucleus and requires transport of the virion proteins into the nucleus. RNA virus and poxvirus assembly occurs in the cytoplasm.

Capsid viruses may be assembled as empty structures (procapsids) to be filled with the genome (e.g., picornaviruses), or they may be assembled around the genome. Nucleocapsids of the retroviruses, togaviruses, and the negative-strand RNA viruses assemble around the genome and are subsequently enclosed in an envelope. The helical nucleocapsid of negative-strand RNA viruses includes the RNA-dependent RNA polymerase necessary for mRNA synthesis in the target cell.

For enveloped viruses, newly synthesized and processed viral glycoproteins are delivered to cellular membranes by vesicular transport. Acquisition of an envelope occurs after association of the nucleocapsid with the viral glycoprotein-containing regions of host cell membranes in a process called budding. Matrix proteins for negative-strand RNA viruses line and promote the adhesion of nucleocapsids with the glycoprotein-modified membrane. As more interactions occur, the membrane surrounds the nucleocapsid, and the virus buds from the membrane.

Viruses use different tricks to ensure that all the parts of the virus are assembled into complete virions. The RNA polymerase required for infection by negative-strand RNA viruses is carried on the genome as part of a helical nucleocapsid. The human immunodeficiency virus (HIV) and other retrovirus genomes are packaged in a procapsid consisting of a polyprotein containing the protease, polymerase, integrase, and structural proteins. This procapsid binds to viral glycoprotein-modified membranes, and the virion buds from the membrane. The virus-encoded protease is activated within the virion and cleaves the polyprotein to produce the final infectious nucleocapsid and the required proteins within the envelope.

Assembly of viruses with segmented genomes, such as influenza or reovirus, requires accumulation of at least one copy of each gene segment. This can be accomplished if the segments assemble together like capsid subunits or randomly package more segments per virion than necessary. This will statistically generate a small but acceptable percentage of functional viruses.

Release

Viruses can be released from cells after lysis of the cell, by exocytosis, or by budding from the plasma membrane. Naked capsid viruses are generally released after lysis of the cell. Release of most enveloped viruses occurs after budding from the plasma membrane without killing the cell. Survival of the cell allows continual release of virus from the factory. Lysis and plasma membrane budding are efficient means of release. Viruses that bud or acquire their membrane in the cytoplasm (e.g., flaviviruses, poxviruses) remain cell associated and are released by exocytosis or cell lysis. Viruses that bind to sialic acid receptors (e.g., orthomyxoviruses, certain paramyxoviruses) may also have an NA. The NA removes potential sialic acid receptors on the glycoproteins of the virion and the host cell to prevent clumping and facilitate release.

Reinitiation of the Replication

Spread of the infection occurs from virus released to the extracellular medium, but alternatively, the virus, nucleocapsid, or genome can be transmitted *through cell-to-cell bridges, upon cell-to-cell fusion, or vertically to daughter cells*. These alternate routes allow the virus to escape antibody detection. Some herpesviruses, retroviruses, and paramyxoviruses can induce cell-to-cell fusion to merge the cells into multinucleated giant cells (syncytia), which become huge virus factories. The retroviruses and some DNA viruses can transmit their integrated copy of the genome vertically to daughter cells on cell division.

VIRAL GENETICS

Mutations spontaneously and readily occur in viral genomes, creating new virus strains with properties differing from the parental, or wild-type, virus. These variants can be identified by their nucleotide sequences, antigenic differences (serotypes), or differences in functional or structural properties. Most mutations have no effect or are detrimental to the virus. Mutations in essential genes inactivate the virus, but mutations in other genes can produce antiviral drug resistance or alter the antigenicity or pathogenicity of the virus.

Mutations that inactivate essential genes are termed lethal mutations. These mutants are difficult to isolate, because the virus cannot replicate. A deletion mutant results from the loss or selective removal of a portion of the genome and the function that it encodes. Other mutations may produce plaque mutants, which differ from the wild type in the size or appearance of the infected cells; host

range mutants, which differ in the tissue type or species of target cell that can be infected; or attenuated mutants, which are variants that cause less serious disease in animals or humans. Conditional mutants, such as temperature-sensitive (ts) or cold-sensitive mutants, have a mutation in a gene for an essential protein that allows virus production only at certain temperatures. Whereas ts mutants generally grow well or relatively better at 30°C to 35°C, the encoded protein is inactive at elevated temperatures of 38°C to 40°C, preventing virus production. Live virus vaccines are often conditional or host range mutants and attenuated for human disease.

New virus strains can also arise by genetic interactions between viruses or between the virus and the cell (Figure 37-15). Intramolecular genetic exchange between viruses or the virus and the host is termed recombination. Recombination can occur readily between two related DNA viruses. Viruses with segmented genomes (e.g., influenza viruses and reoviruses) form hybrid strains on infection of one cell with more than one virus strain. This process, termed reassortment, is analogous to picking 10 marbles out of a box containing 10 black and 10 white marbles. Very different strains of influenza A virus are created on co-infection with a virus from different species.

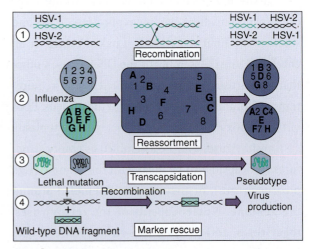

Figure 37-15 Genetic exchange between viral particles can give rise to new viral types, as illustrated. Representative viruses include the following: *1,* intertypic recombination of herpes simplex virus type 1 *(HSV-1)* and type 2 *(HSV-2); 2,* reassortment of two strains of influenza virus; *3,* rescue of a papovavirus defective in assembly by a complementary defective virus (transcapsidation); and *4,* marker rescue of a lethal or conditional mutation.

In some cases, a defective viral strain can be rescued by the replication of another mutant, by the wild-type virus, or by a cell line bearing a replacement viral gene. Replication of the other virus or expression of the gene in the cell provides the missing function required by the mutant (complementation), allowing replication to occur. An experimental disabled infectious single-cycle HSV (DISC-HSV) vaccine lacks an essential gene and is grown in a cell line that expresses that gene product to "complement" the virus. The vaccine virus can infect the normal cells of the individual, but the virions that are produced lack the function necessary for replication in other cells and cannot spread. Rescue of a lethal or conditional-lethal mutant with a defined genetic sequence, such as a restriction endonuclease DNA fragment, is called marker rescue. Marker rescue is used to map the genomes of viruses such as HSV. Virus produced from cells infected with different virus strains may be phenotypically mixed and have the proteins of one strain but the genome of the other (transcapsidation). Pseudotypes are generated when transcapsidation occurs between different types of virus, but this is rare.

Individual virus strains or mutants are selected by their ability to use the host cell machinery and to withstand the conditions of the body and the environment. A small selective advantage in a mutant virus can shortly lead to its becoming the predominant viral strain. The high mutation rate of HIV promotes a switch in target cell tropism to include different types of T cells, the development of antiviral drug-resistant strains, and the generation of antigenic variants during a patient's course of infection.

VIRAL VECTORS FOR THERAPY

Genetically manipulated viruses can be excellent delivery systems for foreign genes. Viruses can provide gene replacement therapy, can be used as vaccines to promote immunity to other agents or tumors, and can act as targeted killers of tumors. The advantages of using viruses are that they can be readily amplified by replication in appropriate cells, and they target specific tissues and deliver the DNA or RNA into the cell. Viruses that are being developed as vectors include retroviruses, adenoviruses, HSV, adeno-associated virus (parvovirus), poxviruses (e.g., vaccinia and canarypox), and even some togaviruses. The viral vectors are usually defective or attenuated viruses, in which the foreign DNA replaces a virulence or unessential gene. The foreign gene may be under the control of a viral promoter or even a tissue-specific promoter. Defective virus vectors are grown in cell lines that express the missing viral functions "complementing" the virus. The progeny can deliver their nucleic acid but not produce infectious virus. Retroviruses and adeno-associated viruses can integrate into cells and permanently deliver a gene into the cell's chromosome. Adenovirus and HSV promote targeted delivery of the foreign gene to receptor-bearing cells. Genetically attenuated HSVs are being developed to specifically kill the growing cells of glioblastomas while sparing the surrounding neurons. Adenovirus and canarypox virus are being used to carry and express HIV genes as vaccines. Vaccinia virus carrying a gene for the rabies glycoprotein is already being used successfully to immunize raccoons, foxes, and skunks in the wild. Some day, virus vectors may be routinely used to treat cystic fibrosis, Duchenne muscular dystrophy, lysosomal storage diseases, and immunologic disorders.

SUMMARY

Viruses are obligate intracellular parasites that depend on the biochemical machinery of the host cell for replication. The virion (the virus particle) consists of a nucleic acid genome packaged into a protein coat (capsid) or a membrane (envelope). The virion may also contain certain essential or accessory enzymes or other proteins to facilitate initial replication in the cell. Capsid or nucleic acid-binding proteins may associate with the genome to form a nucleocapsid, which may be the same as the virion or surrounded by an envelope. The genome of the virus consists either of DNA or RNA. The DNA can be single or double stranded, linear or circular. The RNA can be either positive sense (+) or negative sense (−), double stranded (+/−), or ambisense. The RNA genome may also be segmented into pieces. A single round of the viral replication cycle can be separated into several phases. During the early phase of infection, the virus must recognize an appropriate target cell, attach to the cell, penetrate the plasma membrane and be taken up by the cell, release (uncoat) its genome into the cytoplasm, and if necessary, deliver the genome to the nucleus. The late phase begins with the start of genome replication and viral macromolecular synthesis and proceeds through viral assembly and release.

KEYWORDS

English	Chinese
Virus	病毒
Virion	病毒体
Capsid	衣壳
Envelope	包膜
Nucleocapsid	核衣壳
Replication	复制
Spike	刺突
Helical symmetry	螺旋对称

BIBLIOGRAPHY

1. Cann AJ: Principles of molecular virology, ed 4, San Diego, 2005, Academic.

2. Cohen J, Powderly WG: Infectious diseases, ed 2, St Louis, 2004, Mosby.

3. Flint SJ, et al: Principles of virology: molecular biology, pathogenesis, and control of animal viruses, ed 3, Washington, DC, 2009, American Society for Microbiology Press.

4. Knipe DM, et al: Fields virology, ed 5, Philadelphia, 2006, Lippincott Williams & Wilkins.

5. Richman DD, Whitley RJ, Hayden FG: Clinical virology, ed 3, Washington, DC, 2009, American Society for Microbiology Press.

6. Rosenthal KS: Viruses: microbial spies and saboteurs, Infect Dis Clin Pract 14: 97-106, 2006.

7. Specter S, et al: Clinical virology manual, ed 4, Washington, DC, 2009, American Society for Microbiology Press.

8. Strauss JM, Strauss EG: Viruses and human disease, ed 2, San Diego, 2007, Academic.

Mechanisms of Viral Pathogenesis

Viruses cause disease after they break through the natural protective barriers of the body, evade immune control, and either kill cells of an important tissue (e.g., brain) or trigger a destructive immune and inflammatory response. The outcome of a viral infection is determined by the nature of the virus-host interaction and the host's response to the infection (Box 38-1). The immune response is the best treatment, but it often contributes to the pathogenesis of a viral infection. The tissue targeted by the virus defines the nature of the disease and its symptoms. Viral and host factors govern the severity of the disease; they include the strain of virus, the inoculum size, and the general health of the infected person. The ability of the infected person's immune response to control the infection determines the severity and duration of the disease. A particular disease may be caused by several viruses that have a common tissue **tropism** (preference), such as hepatitis—liver, common cold—upper respiratory tract, encephalitis—central nervous system. On the other hand, a particular virus may cause several different diseases or no observable symptoms. For example, herpes simplex virus type 1 (HSV-1) can cause gingivostomatitis, pharyngitis, herpes labialis (cold sores), genital herpes, encephalitis, or keratoconjunctivitis, depending on the affected tissue, or it can cause no apparent disease at all. Although normally benign, this virus can be life threatening in a newborn or an immunocompromised person.

Viruses encode activities (**virulence factors**) that promote the efficiency of viral replication, viral transmission, the access and binding of the virus to target tissue, or the escape of the virus from host defenses and immune resolution. These activities may not be essential for viral growth in tissue culture but are necessary for the pathogenicity or survival of the virus in the host. Loss of these virulence factors results in **attenuation** of the virus. Many live-virus vaccines are attenuated virus strains.

The discussion in this chapter focuses on viral disease at the cellular level (cytopathogenesis), the host level (mechanisms of disease), and the population level (epidemiology and control).

BASIC STEPS IN VIRAL DISEASE

Viral disease in the body progresses through defined steps, just like viral replication in the cell (Figure 38-1A). These steps are noted in Box 38-2.

Box 38-1

Determinants of Viral Disease

Nature of the Disease
Target tissue
Portal of entry of virus
Access of virus to target tissue
Tissue tropism of virus
Permissiveness of cells for viral replication
Pathogenic activity (strain)

Severity of Disease
Cytopathic ability of virus
Immune status (naive or immunized)
Competence of the immune system
Prior immunity to the virus
Immunopathology
Virus inoculum size
Length of time before resolution of infection
General health of the person
Nutrition
Other diseases influencing immune status
Genetic makeup of the person
Age

The incubation period may proceed without symptoms (**asymptomatic**) or may produce nonspecific early symptoms, such as fever, head or body ache, or chills, termed the **prodrome.** Often, the virus infection is resolved by innate host protections without symptoms. The symptoms of the disease are caused by tissue damage and systemic effects caused by the virus and the immune system. These symptoms may continue through **convalescence** while the body repairs the damage. The individual usually develops a memory immune response for future protection against a similar challenge with this virus.

INFECTION OF THE TARGET TISSUE

The virus gains **entry into the body** through breaks in the skin (cuts, bites, injections) or across the mucoepithelial membranes that line the orifices of the body (eyes, respiratory tract, mouth, genitalia, and gastrointestinal tract). Inhalation is probably the most common route of viral infection.

On entry into the body, the virus replicates in cells that express viral receptors and have the appropriate biosynthetic machinery. Many viruses initiate infection in the oral mucosa or upper respiratory tract. Disease signs may accompany viral replication at the primary site. The virus may replicate and remain at the primary site, may disseminate to other tissues via the bloodstream or within mononuclear phagocytes and lymphocytes, or may disseminate through neurons (Figure 38-1B).

The bloodstream and the lymphatic system are

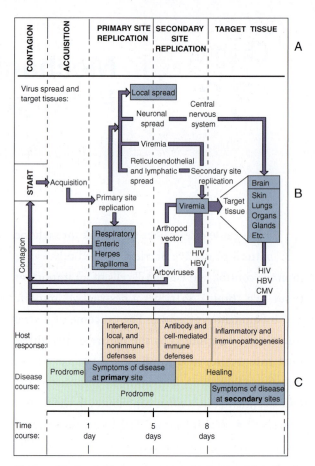

Figure 38-1 **A,** The stages of viral infection. The virus is released from one person, is acquired by another, replicates, and initiates a primary infection at the site of acquisition. Depending on the virus, it may then spread to other body sites and finally to a target tissue characteristic of the disease. **B,** The cycle starts with acquisition, as indicated, and proceeds until the release of new virus. The thickness of the arrow denotes the degree to which the original virus inoculum is amplified on replication. The boxes indicate a site or cause of symptoms. **C,** Time course of viral infection. The time course of symptoms and the immune response correlate with the stage of viral infection and depend on whether the virus causes symptoms at the primary site or only after dissemination to another (secondary) site. *CMV,* Cytomegalovirus; *HBV,* hepatitis B virus; *HIV,* human immunodeficiency virus.

the predominant means of viral transfer in the body. The virus may gain access to them after tissue damage, upon uptake by macrophages, or on transport past the mucoepithelial cells of the oropharynx, gastrointestinal tract, vagina, or anus. Several enteric viruses (picornaviruses and reoviruses) bind to receptors on M cells, which translocate the virus to the underlying Peyer patches of the lymphatic system.

The transport of virus in the blood is termed **viremia.** The virus may either be free in the plasma or be cell associated in lymphocytes or macrophages. Viruses taken up by phagocytic macrophages may be inactivated, may replicate, or may be delivered to other tissues. Replication of a virus in macrophages, the endothelial lining of blood vessels, or the liver can cause the infection to be amplified and initiate the development of a **secondary viremia.** In many cases, a secondary viremia precedes delivery of the virus to the **target tissue** (e.g., liver, brain, skin) and the manifestation of characteristic symptoms.

Viruses can gain access to the central nervous system or brain (1) from the bloodstream (e.g., arbo-encephalitis viruses), (2) from infected meninges or cerebrospinal fluid, (3) by means of the migration of infected macrophages, or (4) the infection of peripheral and sensory (olfactory) neurons. The meninges are accessible to many of the viruses spread by viremia, which may also provide access to neurons. Herpes simplex, varicella-zoster, and rabies viruses initially infect mucoepithelium, skin, or muscle, and then the peripheral innervating neuron, which transports the virus to the central nervous system or brain.

VIRAL PATHOGENESIS

Cytopathogenesis

The four potential outcomes of a viral infection of a cell are as follows (Box 38-3 and Table 38-1):

1. Failed infection (abortive infection)

2. Cell death (lytic infection)

3. Replication without cell death (persistent infection)

4. Presence of virus without virus production but with potential for reactivation (latent-recurrent infection)

Viral mutants, which cause abortive infections, do not multiply and therefore disappear. Persistent infections may be (1) **chronic** (nonlytic, productive), (2) **latent** (limited viral macromolecular but no virus synthesis), (3) **recurrent** (periods of latency then virus production), or (4) **transforming** (immortalizing).

The nature of the infection is determined by the characteristics of the virus and the target cell. A **non-permissive cell** may lack a receptor, important enzyme

pathway, transcriptional activator, or express an antiviral mechanism that will not allow replication of a particular type or strain of virus. A **permissive cell** provides the biosynthetic machinery to support the

---

Box 38-3

Determinants of Viral Pathogenesis

Interaction of Virus with Target Tissue
Access of virus to target tissue
Stability of virus in the body
Temperature
Acid and bile of the gastrointestinal tract
Ability to cross skin or mucous epithelial cells (e.g., cross the gastrointestinal tract into the bloodstream)
Ability to establish viremia
Ability to spread through the reticuloendothelial system
Target tissue
Specificity of viral attachment proteins
Tissue-specific expression of receptors

Cytopathologic Activity of the Virus
Efficiency of viral replication in the cell
Optimum temperature for replication
Permissiveness of cell for replication
Cytotoxic viral proteins
Inhibition of cell's macromolecular synthesis
Accumulation of viral proteins and structures (inclusion bodies)
Altered cell metabolism (e.g., cell immortalization)

Host Protective Responses
Antigen-nonspecific antiviral responses
Interferon
Natural killer cells and macrophages
Antigen-specific immune responses
T-cell responses
Antibody responses
Viral mechanisms of escape of immune responses

Immunopathology
Interferon: flulike systemic symptoms
T-cell responses: cell killing, inflammation
Antibody: complement, antibody-dependent cellular cytotoxicity, immune complexes
Other inflammatory responses

Table 38-1 Types of Viral Infections at the Cellular Level

Type	Virus Production	Fate of Cell
Abortive	–	No effect
Cytolytic	+	Death
Persistent		
Productive	+	Senescence
Latent	–	No effect
Transforming		
DNA viruses	–	Immortalization
RNA viruses	+	Immortalization

complete replicative cycle of the virus. Replication of the virus in a **semipermissive cell** may be very inefficient, or the cell may support some but not all the steps in viral replication.

Replication of the virus can initiate changes in cells that lead to cytolysis or to alterations in the cell's appearance, functional properties, or antigenicity. The effects on the cell may result from viral takeover of macromolecular synthesis, the accumulation of viral proteins or particles, modification or disruption of cellular structures, or manipulation of cellular functions (Table 38-2).

Lytic Infections

Lytic infection results when virus replication kills the target cell. Some viruses damage the cell and prevent repair by inhibiting the synthesis of cellular macromolecules or by producing degradative enzymes and toxic proteins.

Replication of the virus and the accumulation of viral components and progeny within the cell can disrupt the structure and function of the cell or disrupt lysosomes, causing cell death. The expression of viral antigens on the cell surface and disruption of the cytoskeleton can change cell-to-cell interactions and the cell's appearance, making the cell a target for immune cytolysis.

Virus infection or cytolytic immune responses may induce **apoptosis** in the infected cell, and *many viruses (e.g., herpesviruses, adenoviruses, hepatitis C virus) encode methods for inhibiting apoptosis.*

Cell surface expression of the glycoproteins of some paramyxoviruses, herpesviruses, and retroviruses triggers the fusion of neighboring cells into **multinucleated giant cells** called **syncytia.** Syncytia formation allows the virus infection to spread from cell to cell and escape antibody detection. The syncytia that occurs in infection with HIV also causes death of the cells.

Some viral infections cause characteristic changes in the appearance and properties of the target cells. For example, chromosomal aberrations and degradation may occur and can be detected with histologic staining (e.g., marginated chromatin ringing the nuclear membrane in HSV-infected and adenovirus-infected cells). In addition, new stainable structures called **inclusion bodies** may appear within the nucleus or cytoplasm. These structures may result from virus-induced changes in the membrane or chromosomal structure or may represent the sites of viral replication or accumulations of viral capsids. Because the nature and location of these inclusion bodies are characteristic of particular viral infections, the presence of such bodies facilitates laboratory

Table 38-2 Mechanisms of Viral Cytopathogenesis

Mechanism	Examples
Inhibition of cellular protein synthesis	Polioviruses, herpes simplex virus, togaviruses, poxviruses
Inhibition and degradation of cellular DNA	Herpesviruses
Alteration of cell membrane structure	Enveloped viruses
Glycoprotein insertion	All enveloped viruses
Syncytia formation	Herpes simplex virus, varicella-zoster virus, paramyxoviruses, human immunodeficiency virus
Disruption of cytoskeleton	Nonenveloped viruses (accumulation), herpes simplex virus
Permeability	Togaviruses, herpesviruses
Toxicity of virion components	Adenovirus fibers, reovirus NSP4 protein
Inclusion Bodies	Examples
Negri bodies (intracytoplasmic)	Rabies
Intronuclear basophilic (Owl's eye)	Cytomegalovirus (enlarged cells), adenoviruses
Cowdry type A (intranuclear)	Herpes simplex virus, subacute sclerosing panencephalitis (measles) virus
Intracytoplasmic acidophilic	Poxviruses
Perinuclear cytoplasmic acidophilic	Reoviruses

diagnosis (see Table 38-2). Viral infection may also cause vacuolization, rounding of the cells, and other nonspecific histologic changes that are characteristics of sick cells.

Nonlytic Infections

A **persistent infection** occurs in an infected cell that is not killed by the virus. Some viruses cause a persistent productive infection because the virus is released gently from the cell through exocytosis or through budding (many enveloped viruses) from the plasma membrane.

A **latent infection** may result from DNA virus infection of a cell that restricts or lacks the machinery for transcribing all the viral genes. The specific transcription factors required by such a virus may be expressed only in specific tissues, in growing but not resting cells, or after hormone or cytokine induction. For example, HSV establishes a latent infection in neurons that don't express the nuclear factors required to transcribe the immediate early viral genes, but stress and other stimuli can activate the cells to allow viral replication.

Oncogenic Viruses

Some DNA viruses and retroviruses establish persistent infections that can also stimulate uncontrolled cell growth, causing the **transformation** or **immortalization** of the cell (Figure 38-2).

Different **oncogenic** viruses have different mechanisms for immortalizing cells. Viruses immortalize cells by (1) activating or providing growth-stimulating genes, (2) removing the inherent braking mechanisms that limit DNA synthesis and cell growth, or (3) preventing apoptosis. Immortalization by DNA viruses occurs in semipermissive cells, which express only select viral genes but do not produce virus. The synthesis of viral DNA, late mRNA, late proteins, or virus leads to cell death, which precludes immortalization. Several oncogenic DNA viruses integrate into the host cell chromosome. Papillomavirus, SV40 virus, and adenovirus encode proteins that bind and inactivate cell growth-regulatory proteins, such as p53 and the retinoblastoma gene product, thus releasing

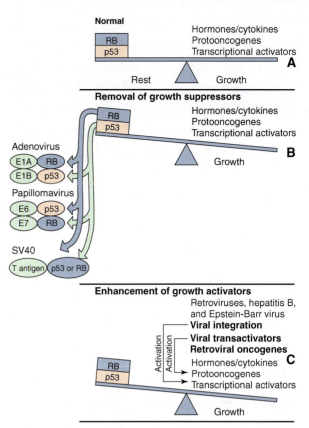

Figure 38-2 Mechanisms of viral transformation and immortalization. Cell growth is controlled **(A)** by the maintenance of a balance in the external and internal growth activators (accelerators) and by growth suppressors, such as p53 and the retinoblastoma *(RB)* gene product (brakes). Oncogenic viruses alter the balance by removing the brakes **(B)** or by enhancing the effects of the accelerators **(C)**.

the brakes on cell growth. Loss of p53 also makes the cell more susceptible to mutation. Epstein-Barr virus immortalizes B cells by stimulating cell growth (as a B-cell mitogen) and by preventing programmed cell death (apoptosis).

Retroviruses (RNA viruses) use two approaches to oncogenesis. Some oncoviruses encode **oncogene** proteins (e.g., SIS, RAS, SRC, MOS, MYC, JUN, FOS), which are almost identical to the cellular proteins involved in cellular growth control (e.g., components of a growth-factor signal cascade [receptors, G proteins, protein kinases], or growth-regulating transcription factors). The overproduction or altered function of these oncogene products stimulates cell growth. These oncogenic viruses *rapidly* cause tumors to form. *However, no human retrovirus of this type has been identified.*

Human T-cell lymphotropic virus 1, the only

human oncogenic retrovirus identified, uses more subtle mechanisms of leukemogenesis. It encodes a protein (**TAX**) that **transactivates** gene expression, including genes for growth-stimulating cytokines (e.g., interleukin-2 [IL-2]). This constitutes the second approach to oncogenesis. The integration of the DNA copy of HTLV-1 near a cellular growth-stimulating gene can also cause the gene to be activated by the strong viral enhancer and promoter sequences encoded at each end of the viral genome (long terminal repeat [LTR] sequences). *HTLV-1-associated leukemias* **develop slowly,** *occurring 20 to 30 years after infection.* Retroviruses continue to produce virus in immortalized or transformed cells.

Some viruses may initiate tumor formation indirectly. Hepatitis B virus (HBV) and hepatitis C virus (HCV) may have mechanisms for direct oncogenesis; however, both viruses establish persistent infections that cause inflammation and require significant tissue repair. Inflammation and continuous stimulation of liver cell growth and repair may promote mutations that lead to tumor formation. Human herpesvirus 8 (HHV-8) promotes the development of Kaposi sarcoma by means of growth-promoting cytokines encoded by the virus; this disease occurs most often in immunosuppressed patients, such as those with acquired immunodeficiency syndrome (AIDS).

Viral transformation is the first step but is generally not sufficient to cause oncogenesis and tumor formation. Instead, over time, immortalized cells are more likely than normal cells to accumulate other mutations or chromosomal rearrangements that promote development of tumor cells. Immortalized cells may also be more susceptible to cofactors and tumor promoters (e.g., phorbol esters, butyrate) that enhance tumor formation. Approximately 15% of human cancers can be related to oncogenic viruses such as HTLV-1, HBV, HCV, papillomaviruses 16 and 18, HHV-8, and Epstein-Barr virus. HSV-2 may be a cofactor for human cervical cancer.

Host Defenses against Viral Infection

The ultimate goals of the host antiviral innate and immune responses are to prevent entry, prevent spread, and to eliminate the virus and the cells harboring or replicating the virus (**resolution).** The immune response is the best and in most cases the only means of controlling a viral infection. Innate, humoral and cellular immune responses are important for antiviral immunity. The longer the virus replicates in the body, the greater the dissemination of the infection, the more rigorous the immune response necessary to control the infection, and the potential for immunopathogenesis.

The skin is the best barrier to infection. The orifices of the body (e.g., mouth, eyes, nose, ears, and anus) are protected by mucous, ciliated epithelium, tears, and the gastric acid and bile of the gastrointestinal tract. After the virus penetrates these natural barriers, it activates the **antigen-nonspecific (innate) host defenses** (e.g., fever, interferon, macrophages, dendritic cells, natural killer [NK] cells), which attempt to limit and control local viral replication and spread. Viral molecules, including double-stranded RNA (which is the replicative intermediate of RNA viruses), certain forms of DNA and single-stranded RNA, and some viral glycoproteins, activate type I interferon production and innate cellular responses through interaction with cytoplasmic receptors or the Toll-like receptors (TLRs) in endosomes and on cell surfaces. *Innate responses prevent most viral infections from causing disease.*

Antigen-specific immune responses take several days to be activated and become effective. The goal of these protective responses is to resolve the infection by eliminating all infectious virus and virus-infected cells from the body. **Antibody** is effective against extracellular virus and may be sufficient to control cytolytic viruses because viral replication will eliminate the virion factory within the infected cell. Antibody is essential to control virus spread to target tissues by viremia. **Cell-mediated immunity** is required for lysis of cells infected with a **noncytolytic virus** (e.g., hepatitis A virus) and infections caused by **enveloped viruses.**

Prior immunity delivers antigen specific immunity much sooner and more effectively than during a primary infection. It may not prevent the initial stages of infection but, in most cases, does prevent disease progression. On rechallenge, cell-mediated responses are more effective at limiting the local spread of virus, and serum antibody can prevent viremic spread of the virus. Memory immune responses can be generated by prior infection or vaccination.

Many viruses, especially the larger viruses, have the means to escape one or more aspects of immune control. These mechanisms include preventing interferon action, changing virus antigens, spreading by cell-to-cell transmission to escape antibody, and suppressing antigen presentation and lymphocyte function.

Immunopathology

The hypersensitivity and inflammatory reactions initiated by antiviral immunity can be the major cause of the pathologic manifestations and symptoms of viral disease (Table 38-3). Early responses to the virus and viral infection, such as interferon and cytokines, can initiate local inflammatory and systemic responses. For example, interferon and cytokines stimulate the flulike systemic symptoms (e.g., fever, malaise, headache) that are usually associated with *respiratory viral infections and viremias* (e.g., arboencephalitis viruses). These symptoms often precede (prodrome) the characteristic symptoms of the viral infection during the viremic stage. Some virus infections induce a large cytokine response, a cytokine storm, and this can dysregulate immune responses and may trigger autoimmune diseases in genetically predisposed individuals. Later, immune complexes and complement activation (classic pathway), CD4

T-cell-induced delayed-type hypersensitivity, and CD8 cytolytic T-cell action may induce tissue damage. These actions often promote neutrophil infiltration and more cell damage.

The inflammatory response initiated by cell-mediated immunity is difficult to control and damages tissue. The presence of large amounts of antigen and antibody in blood during viremias or chronic infections (e.g., HBV infection) can initiate the classic type III immune complex hypersensitivity reactions. These immune complexes can activate the complement system, triggering inflammatory responses and tissue destruction. These immune complexes often accumulate in the kidney and cause glomerulonephritis.

In the case of dengue and measles viruses, partial immunity to a related or inactivated virus can result in a more severe host response and disease on subsequent challenge with a related or virulent virus. This is because antigen-specific T-cell and antibody responses are enhanced and induce significant inflammatory and hypersensitivity damage to infected endothelial cells (dengue hemorrhagic fever) or skin and the lung (atypical measles). In addition, a non-neutralizing antibody can facilitate the uptake of dengue and yellow fever viruses into macrophages through Fc receptors, where they can replicate.

VIRAL DISEASES

The relative susceptibility of a person and the severity of the disease depend on the following factors:

The mechanism of exposure and site of infection

Table 38-3 Viral Immunopathogenesis

Immunopathogenesis	Immune Mediators	Examples
Flulike symptoms	Interferon, cytokines	Respiratory viruses, arboviruses (viremia-inducing viruses)
Delayed-type hypersensitivity and inflammation	T cells, macrophages, and polymorphonuclear leukocytes	Enveloped viruses
Immune complex disease	Antibody, complement	Hepatitis B virus, rubella
Hemorrhagic disease	T cell, antibody, complement	Yellow fever, dengue, Lassa fever, Ebola viruses
Postinfection cytolysis	T cells	Enveloped viruses (e.g., postmeasles encephalitis)
Cytokine storm	–	Dendritic cells, T cells enveloped and other viruses
Immunosuppression	–	Human immunodeficiency virus, cytomegalovirus, measles virus, influenza virus

The immune status, age, and general health of the person

The viral dose

The genetics of the virus and the host

The stages of viral disease are shown in Figure 38-1C. During the incubation period, the virus is replicating but has not reached the target tissue or induced sufficient damage to cause the disease. Nonspecific or flulike symptoms may precede the characteristic symptoms during the prodrome. The incubation periods for many common viral infections are listed in Table 38-4. Specific viral diseases are discussed in subsequent chapters.

Table 38-4 Incubation Periods of Common Viral Infections

Disease	Incubation Period (Days)*
Influenza	1-2
Common cold	1-3
Herpes simplex	2-8
Bronchiolitis, croup	3-5
Acute respiratory disease (adeno-viruses)	5-7
Dengue	5-8
Enteroviruses	6-12
Poliomyelitis	5-20
Measles	9-12
Smallpox	12-14
Chickenpox	13-17
Mumps	16-20
Rubella	17-20
Mononucleosis	30-50
Hepatitis A	15-40
Hepatitis B	50-150
Rabies	30-100+
Papilloma (warts)	50-150
Human immunodeficiency virus	1-15 years
AIDS	1-10 years

*Until first appearance of prodromal symptoms. Diagnostic signs (e.g., rash, paralysis) may not appear until 2 to 4 days later.
Modified from White DO, Fenner F: *Medical Virology*, ed 3, New York, 1986, Academic.

The nature and severity of the symptoms of a viral disease are related to the function of the infected target tissue (e.g., liver—hepatitis, brain—encephalitis) and the extent of the immunopathologic responses

triggered by the infection. Inapparent infections result if (1) the infected tissue is undamaged, (2) the infection is controlled before the virus reaches its target tissue, (3) the target tissue is expendable, (4) the damaged tissue is rapidly repaired, or (5) the extent of damage is below a functional threshold for that particular tissue. Despite the lack of symptoms, virus-specific antibody will be produced. For example, although 97% of adults have antibody (seropositive) to varicella-zoster virus, less than half remember having had chickenpox. *Inapparent or asymptomatic infections are major sources of contagion.*

Viral infections may cause acute or chronic disease (persistent infection). The ability and speed with which a person's immune system controls and resolves a viral infection usually determine whether acute or chronic disease ensues, as well as the severity of the symptoms (Figure 38-3). The acute episode of a persistent infection may be asymptomatic (JC polyomavirus)

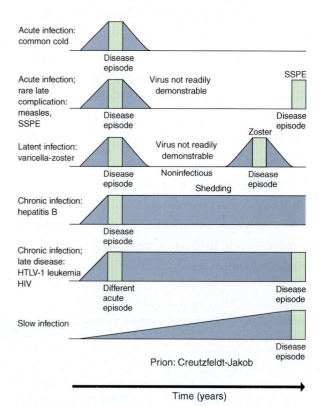

Figure 38-3 Acute infection and various types of persistent infection, as illustrated by the diseases indicated in the column at the left. Blue represents presence of virus; green indicates episode of disease. *HIV*, Human immunodeficiency virus; *HTLV-1*, human T-cell lymphotropic virus 1; *SSPE*, subacute sclerosing panencephalitis. (Modified from White DO, Fenner FJ: *Medical virology*, ed 3, New York, 1986, Academic, 1986.)

or may later in life cause symptoms similar to (vari-cella and zoster) or different from (HIV) those of the acute disease. Slow viruses and prions have long incubation periods, during which sufficient virus or tissue destruction accumulates before a rapid pro-gression of symptoms.

EPIDEMIOLOGY

Epidemiology studies the spread of disease through a population. Infection of a population is similar to infection of a person in that the virus must spread through the population and is controlled by immu-nization of the population (Box 38-4). To endure, viruses must continue to infect new, immunologi-cally naïve, susceptible hosts.

Exposure

People are exposed to viruses throughout their lives. However, some situations, vocations, lifestyles, and living arrangements increase the likelihood that a person will come in contact with certain viruses.

Poor hygiene and crowded living, school, and job conditions promote exposure to respiratory and enteric viruses. Day-care centers are consistent sources of viral infections, especially viruses spread by the respiratory and fecal-oral routes. Travel, sum-mer camp, and vocations that bring people in con-tact with a virus vector (e.g., mosquitoes) put them at particular risk for infection by arboviruses and other zoonoses. Sexual promiscuity also promotes the spread and acquisition of several viruses. Health care workers, such as physicians, dentists, nurses, and technicians, are frequently exposed to respiratory and other viruses but are uniquely at risk for acquir-ing viruses from contaminated blood (HBV, HIV) or vesicle fluid (HSV).

Transmission of Viruses

Viruses are transmitted by direct contact (including sexual contact), injection with contaminated fluids or blood, the transplantation of organs, and the respiratory and fecal-oral routes (Table 38-5). *The route of transmission depends on the source of the virus*

> **Box 38-4**
>
> ### Viral Epidemiology
>
> **Mechanisms of Viral Transmission**
> Aerosols
> Food, water
> Fomites (e.g., tissues, clothes)
> Direct contact with secretions (e.g., saliva, semen)
> Sexual contact, birth
> Blood transfusion or organ transplant
> Zoonoses (animals, insects [arboviruses])
> Genetic (vertical) (e.g. retroviruses)
>
> **Disease and Viral Factors That Promote Transmission**
> Stability of virion in response to the environment (e.g., dry-ing, detergents, temperature)
> Replication and secretion of virus into transmissible aerosols and secretions (e.g., saliva, semen)
> Asymptomatic transmission
> Transience or ineffectiveness of immune response to control reinfection or recurrence
>
> **Risk Factors**
> Age
> Health
> Immune status
> Occupation: contact with agent or vector
> Travel history
> Lifestyle
> Children in day-care centers
> Sexual activity
>
> **Critical Community Size**
> Seronegative, susceptible people
>
> **Geography and Season**
> Presence of cofactors or vectors in the environment
> Habitat and season for arthropod vectors (mosquitoes)
> School session: close proximity and crowding
> Home-heating season
>
> **Modes of Control**
> Quarantine
> Elimination of the vector
> Immunization
> Vaccination
> Treatment
> Education

(the tissue site of viral replication and secretion) and the ability of the virus to endure the hazards and bar-riers of the environment and the body enter route to the target tissue. For example, viruses that replicate in the respiratory tract (e.g., influenza A virus) are released in aerosol droplets, whereas enteric viruses (e.g., picornaviruses and reoviruses) are passed by the fecal-oral route. Cytomegalovirus is transmitted in most bodily secretions because it infects mucoepi-thelial, secretory, and other cells found in the skin, secretory glands, lungs, liver, and other organs.

Table 38-5 Viral Transmission

Mode	Examples
Respiratory transmission	Paramyxoviruses, influenza viruses, picornaviruses, rhinoviruses, varicella-zoster virus, B19 virus
Fecal-oral transmission	Picornaviruses, rotavirus, reovirus, noroviruses, adenovirus
Contact (lesions, fomites)	Herpes simplex virus, rhinoviruses, poxviruses, adenovirus
Zoonoses (animals, insects)	Togaviruses (alpha), flaviviruses, bunyaviruses, orbiviruses, arenaviruses, hantaviruses, rabies virus, influenza A virus, orf (pox)
Transmission via blood	Human immunodeficiency virus, HTLV-1, hepatitis B virus, hepatitis C virus, hepatitis delta virus, cytomegalovirus
Sexual contact	Blood-borne viruses, herpes simplex virus, human papillomavirus, molluscum contagiosum
Maternal-neonatal transmission	Rubella virus, cytomegalovirus, B19 virus, echovirus, herpes simplex virus, varicella-zoster virus, HIV
Genetic	Prions, retroviruses

HTLV-1, Human T-cell lymphotropic virus 1.

Nonenveloped viruses (naked capsid viruses) are generally transmitted by the respiratory and fecal-oral routes and can often be acquired from contaminated objects, termed fomites. For example, hepatitis A virus, a picornavirus, is a nonenveloped virus that is transmitted by the fecal-oral route and acquired from contaminated water, shellfish, and food. Adenoviruses and many other nonenveloped viruses can be spread by contact with fomites, such as handkerchiefs and toys.

Most enveloped viruses must remain wet and are spread (1) in respiratory droplets, blood, mucus, saliva, and semen; (2) by injection; or (3) in organ transplants. Most enveloped viruses are also labile to treatment with acid and detergents, a feature that precludes their being transmitted by the fecal-oral route. Exceptions are HBV and coronaviruses.

Animals can also act as vectors that spread viral disease to other animals and humans and even to other locales. They can also be reservoirs for the virus, which maintain and amplify the virus in the environment. Viral diseases that are shared by animals or insects and humans are called zoonoses. For example, raccoons, foxes, bats, dogs, and cats are reservoirs and vectors for the rabies virus. Arthropods, including mosquitoes, ticks, and sandflies, can act as vectors for togaviruses, flaviviruses, bunyaviruses, or reoviruses. These viruses are often referred to as arboviruses because they are *arthropod borne.*

Other factors that can promote the transmission of viruses are the potential for asymptomatic infection, crowded living conditions, certain occupations, certain lifestyles, day care centers, and travel. Virus transmission during an asymptomatic infection (e.g., HIV, varicella-zoster virus) occurs unknowingly and is difficult to restrict. This is an important characteristic of sexually transmitted diseases.

Maintenance of a Virus in the Population

The persistence of a virus in a community depends on the availability of a critical number of immunologically naïve (seronegative), susceptible people. The efficiency of virus transmission determines the size of the susceptible population necessary for maintenance of the virus in the population. Immunization, produced by natural means or by vaccination, is the best way of reducing the number of such susceptible people.

Age

A person's age is an important factor in determining his or her susceptibility to viral infections. Infants, children, adults, and elderly persons are susceptible to different viruses and have different symptomatic responses to the infection. Differences in lifestyles, habits, school environments, and job settings at different ages also determine when people are exposed to viruses.

Infants and children acquire a series of respiratory and exanthematous viral diseases at first exposure because they are immunologically naïve. Infants are especially prone to more serious presentations of paramyxovirus respiratory infections and viral gastroenteritis because of their small size and physiologic requirements (e.g., nutrients, water, electrolytes). Elderly persons are especially susceptible to new viral infections and the reactivation of latent viruses. Because they are less able to initiate a new immune response, repair damaged tissue, and recover, elderly persons are therefore more susceptible to complications after infection and outbreaks of the new strains of the influenza A and B viruses. Elderly persons are also more prone to zoster (shingles), a recurrence of varicella-zoster virus, as a result of a decline in this specific immune response with age.

Immune Status

The competence of a person's immune response and immune history determine how quickly and efficiently the infection is resolved and can also determine the severity of the symptoms. The rechallenge of a person with prior immunity usually results in asymptomatic or mild disease without transmission. People who are in an immunosuppressed state as a result of AIDS, cancer, or immunosuppressive therapy are at greater risk of suffering more serious disease on primary infection (measles, vaccinia) and are more prone to suffer recurrences of infections with latent viruses (e.g., herpesviruses, papovaviruses).

Other Host Factors

General health plays an important role in determining the competence and nature of the immune response and ability to repair diseased tissue. Poor nutrition can compromise a person's immune system and decrease his or her tissue regenerative capacity. Immunosuppressive diseases and therapies may allow viral replication or recurrence to proceed unchecked. Genetic makeup also plays an important role in determining the response of the immune system to viral infection.

Geographic and Seasonal Considerations

The geographic distribution of a virus is usually determined by whether the requisite cofactors or vectors are present or whether there is an immunologically naïve, susceptible population. For example, many of the arboviruses are limited to the ecologic niche of their arthropod vectors. Extensive global transportation is eliminating many of the geographically determined restrictions to virus distribution.

Seasonal differences in the occurrence of viral disease correspond with behaviors that promote the spread of the virus. For example, respiratory viruses are more prevalent in the winter, because crowding facilitates the spread of such viruses, and the temperature and humid conditions stabilize them. Enteric viruses, on the other hand, are more prevalent during the summer, possibly because hygiene is laxer during this season. The seasonal differences in arboviral diseases reflect the life cycle of the arthropod vector or its reservoir (e.g., birds).

Outbreaks, Epidemics, and Pandemics

Outbreaks of a viral infection often result from the introduction of a virus (e.g., hepatitis A) into a new location. The outbreak originates from a common source (e.g., food preparation) and often can be stopped once the source is identified. Epidemics occur over a larger geographic area and generally result from the introduction of a new strain of virus into an immunologically naïve population. Pandemics are worldwide epidemics, usually resulting from the introduction of a new virus (e.g., HIV). Pandemics of influenza A used to occur approximately every 10 years as the result of the introduction of new strains of the virus.

CONTROL OF VIRAL SPREAD

The spread of a virus can be controlled by quarantine, good hygiene, changes in lifestyle, elimination of the vector, or immunization of the population. Quarantine was once the only means of limiting epidemics of viral infections and is most effective for limiting the spread of viruses that always cause symptomatic disease (e.g., smallpox). It is now used in hospitals to limit the nosocomial spread of viruses, especially to high-risk patients (e.g., immunosuppressed people). The proper sanitation of contaminated items and disinfection of the water supply are means of limiting the spread of enteric viruses. Education and resultant changes in lifestyle have made a difference in the spread of sexually transmitted viruses, such as HIV, HBV, and HSV. Elimination of an arthropod or its ecologic niche (e.g., drainage of the swamps it inhabits) has proved effective for controlling arboviruses.

The best way to limit viral spread, however, is to immunize the population. Immunization, whether produced by natural infection or by vaccination, protects individuals and reduces the size of the immunologically naïve, susceptible population necessary to promote the spread and maintenance of the virus.

SUMMARY

Viruses cause disease after they break through the natural protective barriers of the body, evade immune control, and either kill cells of an important tissue (e.g., brain) or trigger a destructive immune and inflammatory response. Viruses encode activities (virulence factors) that promote the efficiency of viral replication, viral transmission, access and binding of the virus to target tissue, or escape of the virus from host defenses and immune resolution. Viruses are transmitted by direct contact (including sexual contact), injection with contaminated fluids or blood, transplantation of organs, and the respiratory and fecal-oral routes. The outcome of a viral infection is determined by the nature of the virus-host interaction and the host's response to the infection. Viral infections may cause acute or chronic disease (persistent infection). The tissue targeted by the virus defines the nature of the disease and its symptoms. Viral and host factors govern the severity of the disease (viral pathogenesis); they include the strain of virus, the inoculum size, and the general health of the infected person. The ability of the infected person's immune response to control the infection determines the severity and duration of the disease.

KEYWORDS

English	Chinese 1
Viral infections	病毒感染
Persistent infection	持续感染
Abortive infection	顿挫感染
Latent infection	潜伏感染

BIBLIOGRAPHY

1. Cann AJ: Principles of molecular virology, San Diego, 2005, Academic.
2. Carter J, Saunders V: Virology: principles and applications, Chichester, England, 2007, Wiley.
3. Cohen J, Powderly WG: Infectious diseases, ed 3, St Louis, 2004, Mosby.
4. Collier L, Oxford J: Human virology, ed 3, Oxford, England, 2006, Oxford University Press.
5. Emond RT, Welsby PD, Rowland HAK: Color atlas of infectious diseases, ed 4, St Louis, 2003, Mosby.
6. Evans AS, Kaslow RA: Viral infections of humans: epidemiology and control, ed 4, New York, 1997, Plenum.
7. Flint SJ, et al: Principles of virology: molecular biology, pathogenesis and control of animal viruses, ed 3, Washington, DC, 2009, American Society for Microbiology Press.
8. Haller O, Kochs G, Weber F: The interferon response circuit: induction and suppression by pathogenic viruses, Virology 344: 119-130, 2006.
9. Hart CA, Broadhead RL: Color atlas of pediatric infectious diseases, St Louis, 1992, Mosby.
10. Hart CA, Shears P: Color atlas of medical microbiology, London, 2004, Mosby.
11. Gershon AA, Hotez PJ, Katz SL: Krugman's infectious diseases of children, ed 11, St Louis, 2004, Mosby.
12. Knipe DM, et al: Fields virology, ed 5, Philadelphia, 2006, Lippincott Williams & Wilkins.
13. Mandell GL, Bennet JE, Dolin R: Principles and practice of infectious diseases, ed 6, Philadelphia, 2005, Churchill Livingstone.
14. Mims CA, et al: Medical microbiology, ed 4, Edinburgh, 2007, Mosby.
15. Mims CA, White DO: Viral pathogenesis and immunology, Oxford, England, 1984, Blackwell.

16. Richman DD, Whitley RJ, Hayden FG: Clinical virology, ed 3, Washington, DC, 2009, American Society Microbiology Press.

17. Rosenthal KS: Viruses: microbial spies and saboteurs, Infect Dis Clin Pract 14: 97-106, 2006.

18. Sampayrac L: How pathogenic viruses work, Mississauga, Ontario, 2001, Jones and Bartlett.

19. Shulman ST, et al: The biologic and clinical basis of infectious diseases, ed 5, Philadelphia, 1997, WB Saunders.

20. Stark GR, et al: How cells respond to interferons, Ann Rev Biochem 67: 227-264, 1998.

21. Strauss JM, Strauss EG: Viruses and human disease, ed 2, San Diego, 2007, Academic.

22. Voyles BA: The biology of viruses, ed 2, Boston, 2002, McGraw-Hill.

23. White DO, Fenner FJ: Medical virology, ed 4, San Diego, 1994, Academic.

24. Zuckerman AJ, Banatvala JE, Pattison JR: Principles and practice of clinical virology, ed 5, Chichester, England, 2004, Wiley.

Immune Responses to Viruses

The previous chapters have introduced the different mechanism of pathogenesis in viral diseases. This chapter describes the different roles immune response play in host protection from viral infection, their interactions, and the immunopathogenic consequences that may arise as a result of the response. Some infections are controlled by innate responses before adapative immune responses can be initiated, but immune responses are necessary to resolve the more troublesome infections.

Human beings have three basic lines of protection against infection by microbes to block entry, spread in the body, and inappropriate colonization.

Natural barriers, such as skin, ciliated epithelium, gastric acid, and bile, restrict entry of the agent.

Innate, antigen-nonspecific immune defenses such as fever, interferon, complement, neutrophils, macrophages, dendritic cells (DCs), and natural killer (NK) cells provide rapid local responses to act at the infection site in order to restrict the growth and spread of the agent.

Adaptive, antigen-specific immune responses, such as antibody and T cells, reinforce the innate protections and specifically target, attack, and eliminate the invaders that succeed in passing the first two defenses.

Usually, barrier functions and innate responses are sufficient to control most infections before symptoms or disease occurs. Initiation of a new antigen-specific immune response takes time, and infections can grow and spread during this time period. Prior immunity and immune memory elicited by infection or vaccination can activate quickly enough to control most infections.

Host Defenses against Viral Infection

The immune response is the best and, in most cases, the only means of controlling a viral infection (Figure 39-1). Unfortunately, it is also the source of pathogenesis for many viral diseases. The humoral and cellular immune responses are important for antiviral immunity. **The ultimate goal of the immune response in a viral infection is to eliminate both the virus and the host cells harboring or replicating the virus.** Interferons, NK cells, CD4 TH1 responses, and CD8 cytotoxic killer T cells are more important for viral infections than for bacterial infections. Failure to resolve the infection may lead to persistent or chronic infection or death.

Innate Defenses

Body temperature, fever, interferons, other cytokines, the mononuclear phagocyte system, and NK cells provide a local rapid response to viral infection and also activate the specific immune defenses. Often the nonspecific defenses are sufficient to control a viral infection, thus preventing the occurrence of symptoms.

Innate immunity is a first line of host defense against pathogens. It plays a key role in the activation of adaptive immunity and in the maintenance of tissue repair via **pattern-recognition receptors (PRRs)** that recognize **pathogen-associated molecular patterns (PAMP).** PAMP receptorsincludes the cell surface **Toll-like receptors (TLRs)** and the cytoplasmic peptidoglycan receptors—nucleotide-binding oligomerization domain protein (NOD)1, NOD2, and cryopyrin **(Table 39-1).** Binding of these PAMPs to receptors on epithelial cells, macrophages, Langerhans cells,

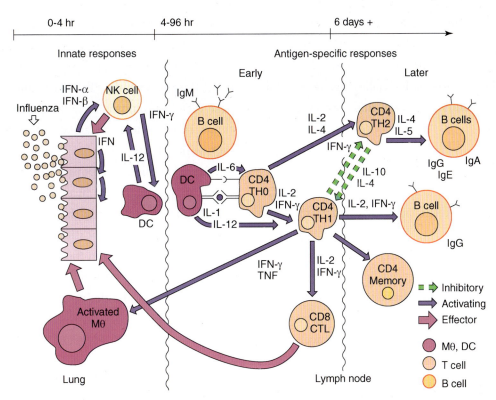

Figure 39-1   Antiviral responses. The response to a virus (e.g., influenza virus) initiates with interferon production and action and natural killer *(NK)* cells. Activation of antigen-specific immunity resembles the antibacterial response, except that CD8 cytotoxic T lymphocytes *(CTLs)* are important antiviral responses. **The time course of events is indicated at the top of the figure.** *IFN*, Interferon, *IL*, interleukin; *Mθ*, macrophage; *TH*, T helper (cell); *TNF*, tumor necrosis factor.

and DCs activate kinase cascades that activate the inflammasome and also promote cytokine production (including the **acute-phase cytokines, interleukin (IL)-1, IL-6, and tumor necrosis factor [TNF]**), protective responses, and maturation of DCs.

Viral infection can induce the release of cytokines (e.g., TNF, IL-1) and interferon from infected cells, iDCs, and macrophages. Viral RNA (especially dsRNA), DNA, and some viral glycoproteins are potent activators of TLRs, and viral nucleic acids can also trigger vesicular and cytoplasmic pathogen pattern receptors to initiate these interferon and cytokine responses. Interferons and other cytokines trigger early local and systemic responses. Induction

Table 39-1   The Functions of Pattern-recognition Receptors

Location	PRRs	PAMPs	Virus
Cell membrane	TLR2	Viral protein	HCMV, MCMV
	TLR4	Viral protein	RSV, MMTV, Leukovirus, Coxsackie virus
Membrane of endosome	TLR3	dsRNA	EMCV, WNV, RSV
	TLR7/8	ssRNA	HIV, VSV, IAV, SeV, CBV, DENV
	TLR9	CpG DNA	MCMV, HSV
Intracytoplasm	RIG-1	5′ ppp-dsRNA	IAV, VSV, NDV, SeV, JEV, HCV, WNV, DENV, RSV
	MDA5	Long dsRNA	EMCV, TMEV, MNV-1, MHV, DENV, WNV
	LGP2	dsRNA	EMCV
	NOD2	5′ ppp-dsRNA	RSV
	NALP3	dsRNA, dsDNA, ssRNA	IAV, SeV, Adenovirus
	cGAS	DNA	DNA viruses
	DAI	AT-rich DNA	HSV
	AIM2	dsDNA	Vaccinia virus, MCMV

of fever and stimulation of the immune system are two of these systemic effects. Body temperature and fever can limit the replication of or destabilize some viruses. Many viruses are less stable (e.g., herpes simplex virus) or cannot replicate (rhinoviruses) at 37°C or higher.

Interferon

Interferon was first described by Isaacs and Lindemann as a very potent factor that "interferes with" the replication of many different viruses. Interferon is the body's first active defense against a viral infection, an "early warning system." In addition to activating a target-cell antiviral defense to block viral replication, interferons activate the immune response and enhance T-cell recognition of the infected cell. Interferon is a very important defense against infection, but it is also a cause of the systemic symptoms associated with many viral infections, such as malaise, myalgia, chills, and fever (nonspecific flulike symptoms), especially during viremia. Type I interferon is also a factor in causing systemic lupus erythematosus.

Interferons comprise a family of proteins that can be subdivided according to several properties, including size, stability, cell of origin, and mode of action (Table 39-2). **IFN-α** and **IFN-β** are type I interferons that share many properties, including structural homology and mode of action. B cells, epithelial cells, monocytes, macrophages, and iDCs make **IFN-α**. Plasmacytoid DCs in blood produce large amounts in response to viremia. Fibroblasts and other cells make **IFN-β** in response to viral infection and other stimuli. **IFN-λ** (interferon lambda) is a type III interferon with activity similar to **IFN-α** and is important for antiinfluenza responses. **IFN-γ** is a type II interferon, a cytokine produced by activated T and NK cells that occurs later in the infection. Although IFN-γ inhibits viral replication, its structure and mode of action differ from those of the other interferons. IFN-γ is also known as macrophage activation factor and is the defining component of the TH1 response.

The best inducer of IFN-α and IFN-β production is **dsRNA**, *produced as the replicative intermediates of RNA viruses* or from the interaction of sense/antisense messenger RNAs (mRNAs) for some DNA viruses. One dsRNA molecule per cell is sufficient to induce the production of interferon. Interaction of some enveloped viruses (e.g., herpes simplex virus and human immunodeficiency virus [HIV]) with iDCs can promote production of IFN-α. Alternatively, inhibition of protein synthesis in a virally infected cell can decrease the production of a repressor protein of the interferon gene, allowing production of interferon. Nonviral interferon inducers include the following:

Table 39-2 Basic Properties of Human Interferons (IFNs)

Property	IFN-α	IFN-β	IFN-γ
Previous designations	Leukocyte IFN type I	Fibroblast IFN type I	Immune IFN type II
Genes	> 20	1	1
Molecular mass (Da)*	16,000-23,000	23,000	20,000-25,000
Cloned†	19,000	19,000	16,000
Glycosylation	No‡	Yes	Yes
pH 2 stability	Stable‡	Stable	Labile
Primary activator	Viruses	Viruses	Immune response
Principal source	Epithelium, leukocytes	Fibroblast	NK or T cell
Introns in gene	No	No	Yes
Homology with human IFN-α	100%	30%-50%	<10%

*Molecular mass of monomeric form.
†Nonglycosylated form, as produced in bacteria by recombinant DNA technology.
‡Most subtypes but not all.
Data from White DO: *Antiviral chemotherapy, interferons and vaccines*, Basel, Switzerland, 1984, Karger; and Samuel CE: Antiviral actions of interferon. Interferon-regulated cellular proteins and their surprisingly selective antiviral activities, *Virology* 183: 1-11, 1991.

Intracellular microorganisms (e.g., mycobacteria, fungi, protozoa)

Activators of certain TLRs or mitogens (e.g., endotoxins, phytohemagglutinin)

Double-stranded polynucleotides (e.g., poly I:C, poly dA:dT)

Synthetic polyanion polymers (e.g., polysulfates, polyphosphates, pyran)

Antibiotics (e.g., kanamycin, cycloheximide)

Low-molecular-weight synthetic compounds (e.g., tilorone, acridine dyes)

IFN-α, IFN-β, and IFN-λ can be induced and released within hours of infection (Figure 39-2). The interferon binds to specific receptors on the neighboring cells and induces the production of antiviral proteins-**the antiviral state**. However, these antiviral proteins are not activated until they bind dsRNA. The major antiviral effects of interferon are produced by two enzymes, **2′,5′-oligoadenylate synthetase** (an unusual polymerase) and **protein kinase R (PKR)** (Figure 39-3), and for influenza, the **mx protein** is also important. Viral infection of the cell and production of dsRNA activate these enzymes and trigger a cascade of biochemical events that leads to (1) the inhibition of protein synthesis by PKR phosphorylation of an important ribosomal initiation factor (elongation initiation factor 2-α [eIF-2α]) and (2) the degradation of mRNA (preferentially, viral mRNA) by ribonuclease L, activated by 2′,5′-oligoadenosine. This process essentially puts the cellular protein synthesis factory "on strike" and prevents

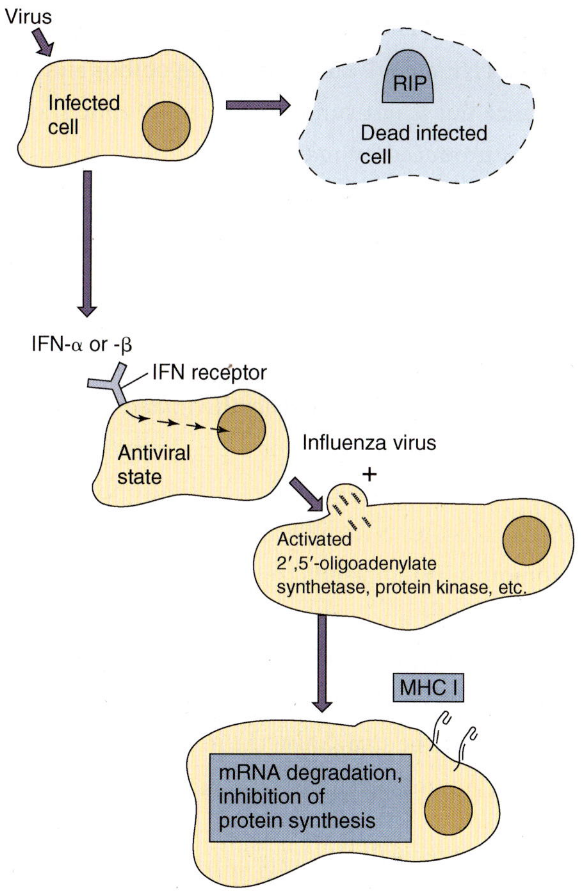

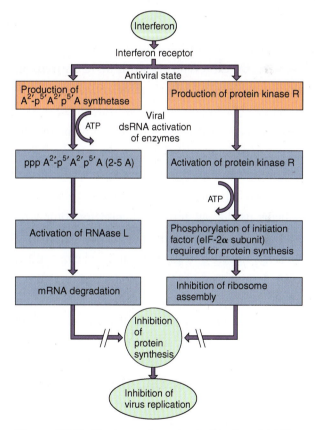

Figure 39-2   Induction of the antiviral state by interferon (*IFN*)-α or IFN-β. Interferon is produced in response to viral infection but does not affect the initially infected cell. The interferon binds to a cell surface receptor on other cells and induces production of antiviral enzymes (antiviral state). The infection and production of double-stranded RNA activates the antiviral activity. *MHC I*, Major histocompatibility antigen type I.

Figure 39-3   The two major routes for interferon inhibition of viral protein synthesis. One mechanism involves the induction of an unusual polymerase (2′,5′-oligoadenylate synthetase [2-5A]) that is activated by double-stranded RNA (*dsRNA*). The activated enzyme synthesizes an unusual adenine chain with a 2′,5′-phosphodiester linkage. The oligomer activates RNAase L that degrades messenger RNA (*mRNA*). The other mechanism involves the induction of protein kinase R (PKR), which prevents assembly of the ribosome by phosphorylation of the elongation initiation factor (eIF-2α) to prevent initiation of protein synthesis from capped mRNAs. *ATP*, Adenosine triphosphate.

viral replication. It must be stressed that interferon does not directly block viral replication. The antiviral state lasts for 2 to 3 days, which may be sufficient for the cell to degrade and eliminate the virus without being killed.

Interferons stimulate cell-mediated immunity by activating effector cells and enhancing recognition of the virally infected target cell. Type I IFNs activate NK cells and assist in activation of CD8 T cells. *IFN and activated NK cells provide an early, local, natural defense against virus infection.* IFN-α and IFN-β increase the expression of class I MHC antigens, enhancing the cell's ability to present antigen and making the cell a better target for cytotoxic T cells (CTLs). Activation of macrophages by IFN-γ promotes production of more IFN-α and IFN-β, secretion of other biologic response modifiers, phagocytosis, recruitment, and inflammatory responses. IFN-γ increases the expression of class II MHC antigens on the macrophage to help promote antigen presentation to T cells. Interferon also has widespread regulatory effects on cell growth, protein synthesis, and the immune response. All three interferon types block cell proliferation at appropriate doses.

Genetically engineered recombinant interferon is being used as an antiviral therapy for some viral infections (e.g., human papilloma and hepatitis C viruses). Effective treatment requires the use of the correct interferon subtype(s) and its prompt delivery at the appropriate concentration. IFN-β is used for treatment of multiple sclerosis. Interferons have also been used in clinical trials for the treatment of certain cancers. However, interferon treatment causes flulike side effects, such as chills, fever, and fatigue.

Cytokines

The proinflammatory cytokines, sometimes referred to as *acute-phase cytokines*, are IL-1, TNF-α, and IL-6. These cytokines are produced by activated macrophages and other cells. IL-1 and TNF-α share properties. Both of these cytokines are endogenous pyrogens capable of stimulating fever; they promote local inflammatory reactions and synthesis of acute-phase proteins.

TNF-α is the ultimate mediator of inflammation and the systemic effects of infection. TNF-α stimulates endothelial cells to express adhesion molecules and chemokines to attract leukocytes to the site of infection, activates neutrophils and macrophages, and promotes apoptosis of certain cell types. Systemically, TNF acts on the hypothalamus to induce fever, can cause systemic metabolic changes, weight loss (cachexia) and loss of appetite, and enhance production of IL-1, IL-6, and chemokines, and it promotes acute-phase protein synthesis by the liver. At high concentrations, TNF-α elicits all of the functions leading to septic shock.

There are two types of IL-1, IL-1α and IL-1β. IL-1 is produced mainly by activated macrophages, also neutrophils, epithelial, and endothelial cells. IL-1β must be cleaved by the inflammasome to become activated. IL-1 shares many of the activities of TNF-α to promote local and systemic inflammatory responses. Unlike TNF-α, IL-1 cannot induce apoptosis and will enhance but is not sufficient to cause septic shock. IL-6 is produced by many cell types, promotes the synthesis of acute-phase proteins in the liver, production of neutrophils in bone marrow, and the activation of T and B lymphocytes. **IL-23 and IL-12** are cytokines that bridge the innate and immune responses. Both cytokines have two subunits, a p40 subunit and a p35 subunit for IL-12 and a p19 subunit for IL-23. IL-23 promotes TH17 responses from memory T cells, which enhance neutrophil action. IL-12 promotes NK-cell function and is required to promote a TH1 immune response, which enhances macrophages and other myeloid cells functions. These cytokines will be discussed further regarding their actions on T cells. IL-18 is produced by macrophages, must be cleaved by the inflammasome to an active form, and promotes NK- and T-cell function.

Innate Immune Cells

Cells of the **dendritic and mononuclear phagocyte system** phagocytose the viral and cell debris from virally infected cells. Macrophages in the liver (Kupffer cells) and spleen rapidly filter many viruses from the blood. Antibody and complement bound to a virus facilitate its uptake and clearance by macrophages (opsonization). DCs and macrophages also present antigen to T cells and release IL-1, IL-12, and IFN-α to expand the innate and initiate the antigen-specific immune responses. Plasmacytoid DCs in the blood produce large amounts of IFN-α in response to a viremia. Activated macrophages can also distinguish and kill infected target cells.

NK cells are activated by (1) IFN-α and IFN-*β* (produced early in response to viral and other infections), (2) TNF-α, (3) IL-12, IL-15, and IL-18 (produced by pre-DCs and activated macrophages), and (4) IL-2 (produced by CD4 TH1 cells). The NK cells express many of the same cell surface markers as T cells (e.g., CD2, CD7, IL-2 receptor [IL-2R], and **FasL [Fas ligand]**) but also the **Fc receptor for IgG (CD16)**, complement receptors for ADCC, and NK-specific inhibitory receptors and activating receptors (including NK immunoglobulin-like receptors [KIR]). Activated NK cells produce IFN-γ, IL-1, and granulocyte-macrophage colony-stimulating factor (GM-CSF). The granules in an NK cell contain **perforin**, a pore-forming protein, and **granzymes** (esterases), which are similar to the contents of the granules of a CD8 cytotoxic T lymphocyte (CTL). These molecules promote the death of the target cell.

The NK cell sees every cell as a potential victim, especially those that appear in distress, unless it receives an inhibitory signal from the target cell. NK cells interact closely with the target cell by binding to carbohydrates and surface proteins on the cell surface. The interaction of a class I MHC molecule on the target cell with a KIR **inhibitory receptor** is like communicating a secret password, indicating that all is normal, and this provides an inhibitory signal to prevent NK killing of the target cell. Virus-infected and tumor cells express "stress-related receptors" and are often deficient in MHC I molecules and become NK-cell targets. Binding of the NK cell to antibody-coated target cells (ADCCs) also initiates killing, but this is not controlled by an inhibitory signal. The **killing mechanisms** are similar to those of CTLs. A synapse (pocket) is formed between the NK and target cell, and **perforin and granzymes** are released to disrupt the target cell and induce apoptosis. In addition,

the interaction of the **FasL** on the NK cell with **Fas** protein on the target cell can also induce apoptosis.

Macrophages mature from blood **monocytes** and, like neutrophils, are decorated with opsonin receptors to promote phagtocytosis of microbes, receptors for PAMPs (see later) to initiate activation and response, cytokine receptors, to promote activation of the macrophages, and express MHC II proteins for antigen presentation to CD4 T cells. Unlike neutrophils, macrophages live longer, must be activated to kill phagocytosed virus. Macrophages can be activated by IFN-γ (classical activation) produced by NK cells and CD4 and CD8 T cells as part of the TH1 response and are then able to kill phagocytosed virus. These are called *M1 macrophages*. **Activated M1 macrophages** produce cytokines, enzymes, and other molecules to promote antimicrobial function. They also reinforce local inflammatory reactions by producing various chemokines to attract neutrophils, iDCs, NK cells, and activated T cells. Activation of the macrophages makes them more efficient killers of phagocytosed microbes, virally infected cells, and tumor cells. **Alternatively activated macrophages (M2 macrophages)** are activated by the TH2-related cytokines, IL-4 and IL-13, and support antiparasitic responses, promote tissue remodeling, and wound repair.

Dendritic cells provide the bridge between the innate and the immune responses. The cytokines they produce determine the nature of the T-cell response. Monocytes and precursor myeloid DCs circulate in the blood and then differentiate into iDCs in tissue and lymphoid organs. **iDCs** are phagocytic, and upon activation by danger signals, they release an early cytokine-mediated warning system and then mature into **DCs. Mature DCs** are the ultimate antigen-presenting cell, the only antigen-presenting cell that can initiate an antigen-specific T-cell response.

Adaptive (Antigen-Specific) Immunity

Humoral immunity and cell-mediated immunity play different roles in resolving viral infections (i.e., eliminating the virus from the body). Humoral immunity (antibody) acts mainly on extracellular virions, whereas cell-mediated immunity (T cells) is directed at the virus-producing cell.

Humoral Immunity

Practically all viral proteins are foreign to the host and are immunogenic (i.e., capable of eliciting an antibody response). However, not all immunogens elicit protective immunity.

Antibody blocks the progression of disease through the **neutralization and opsonization** of cell-free virus. Protective antibody responses are generated toward the viral capsid proteins of naked viruses and the glycoproteins of enveloped viruses that interact with cell surface receptors (viral attachment proteins). These antibodies can neutralize the virus by preventing viral interaction with target cells or by destabilizing the virus, thus initiating its degradation. Binding of antibody to these proteins also opsonizes the virus, promoting its uptake and clearance by macrophages. Antibody recognition of infected cells can also promote antibody-dependent cellular cytotoxicity (ADCC) by NK cells. Antibodies to other viral antigens may be useful for serologic analysis of the viral infection.

The major antiviral role of antibody is to prevent the spread of extracellular virus to other cells. Antibody is especially important in limiting the spread of the virus by **viremia,** preventing the virus from reaching the target tissue for disease production. Antibody is most effective at resolving cytolytic infections. Resolution occurs because the virus kills the cell factory and the antibody eliminates the extracellular virus. Antibody is the primary defense initiated by most vaccines.

T Cell-Immunity

T cell-mediated immunity promotes antibody and inflammatory responses (CD4 helper T cells) and kills infected cells (cytotoxic T cells [primarily CD8 T cells]). The **CD4 TH1** response is generally more important than TH2 responses for controlling a viral infection, especially noncytolytic and enveloped viruses. **CD8** killer T cells promote apoptosis in infected cells after their T-cell receptor binds to a viral peptide presented by a class I MHC protein.

The peptides expressed on class I MHC antigens are obtained from viral proteins synthesized within the infected cell (endogenous route). *The viral protein from which these peptides are derived may not elicit protective antibody* (e.g., intracellular or internal virion proteins, nuclear proteins, improperly folded or processed proteins [cell trash]). For example, the matrix and nucleoproteins of the influenza virus and the infected cell protein 4 (ICP4) (nuclear) of herpes simplex virus are targets for CTLs but do not elicit protective antibody. An **immune synapse** formed by interactions of the TCR and MHC I, the co-receptors, and adhesion molecules creates a space into which **perforin,** a complement-like membrane pore former, and granzymes (degradative enzymes) are released to induce apoptosis in the target cell. Interaction of the Fas ligand protein on CD4 or CD8 T cells with the Fas protein on the target cell can also promote apoptosis. CTLs kill infected cells and, as a result, eliminate the source of new virus.

The CD8 T-cell response probably evolved as a defense against virus infection. Cell-mediated immunity is especially important for resolving infections by syncytia-forming viruses (e.g., measles, herpes simplex virus, varicella-zoster virus, HIV), which can spread from cell to cell without exposure to antibody; and by noncytolytic viruses (e.g., hepatitis A and measles viruses). CD8 T cells also interact with neurons to control, without killing, the recurrence of latent viruses (herpes simplex virus, varicella-zoster virus, and JC papillomaviruses).

Immune Response to Viral Challenge

Primary Viral Challenge

The innate host responses are the earliest responses to viral challenge and are often sufficient to limit viral spread (see Figure 39-3). The **type I interferons** produced in response to most viral infections initiate the protection of adjacent cells, enhances antigen presentation by increasing the expression of MHC antigens, and initiates the clearance of infected cells by activating NK cells and antigen-specific responses. Virus and viral components released from the infected cells are phagocytosed by and activate **iDCs** to produce cytokines and then move to the lymph nodes. Macrophages in the liver and spleen are especially important for clearing virus from the bloodstream (filters). These phagocytic cells degrade and process the viral antigens. DCs present the appropriate peptide fragments bound to class II MHC antigens to CD4 T cells and can also cross-present these antigens on MHC I molecules to CD8 T cells to initiate the response. The APCs also release IL-1, IL-6, and TNF and, with IL-12, promote activation of helper T cells and specific cytokine production (TH1 response). The type I interferons and these cytokines induce the prodromal flulike symptoms of many viral infections. The activated T cells move to the site of infection and B-cell areas of the lymph node, and macrophages and B cells present antigen and become stimulated by the T cells.

Antiviral antigen-specific responses are similar to antibacterial antigen-specific responses, except that the CD8 T cell plays a more important role. **IgM** is produced approximately 3 days after infection. Its production indicates a primary infection. **IgG** and **IgA** are produced 2 to 3 days after IgM. Secretory IgA is made in response to a viral challenge of mucosal surfaces at the natural openings of the body (i.e., eyes, mouth, and respiratory and gastrointestinal systems). Activated **CD4** and **CD8** T cells are present at approximately the same time as serum IgG. During infection, the number of CD8 T cells specific for antigen may increase 50,000 to 100,000 fold. The antigen-specific CD8 T cells move to the site of infection and kill virally infected cells. Recognition and binding to class I MHC viral-peptide complexes promotes apoptotic killing of the target cells, either through the release of perforin and granzymes (to disrupt the cell membrane) or through the binding of the Fas ligand with Fas on the target cell. Resolution of the infection occurs later, when sufficient antibody is available to neutralize all virus progeny or when cellular immunity has been able to reach and eliminate the infected cells. For the resolution of most enveloped and noncytolytic viral infections, TH1-mediated responses are required to kill the viral

factory and resolve infection.

Viral infections of the brain and the eye can cause serious damage because these tissues cannot repair tissue damage and are **immunologically privileged sites** of the body. TH1 responses are suppressed to prevent the serious tissue destruction that accompanies extended inflammation. These sites depend on innate, cytokine, TH17, and antibody control of infection.

Cell-mediated and IgG immune responses do not arise until 6 to 8 days after viral challenge. For many viral infections, this is after innate responses have controlled viral replication. However, for other viral infections, this period allows the virus to expand the infection, spread through the body and infect the target tissue, and cause disease (e.g., brain: encephalitis, liver: hepatitis). The response to the expanded infection may require a larger and more intense immune response, which often includes the immunopathogenesis and tissue damage that cause disease symptoms.

Secondary Viral Challenge

In any war, it is easier to eliminate an enemy if its identity and origin are known and if establishment of its foothold can be prevented. Similarly, in the human body, prior immunity, established by prior infection or vaccination, allows rapid, specific mobilization of defenses to prevent disease symptoms, promote rapid clearance of the virus, and block viremic spread from the primary site of infection to the target tissue to prevent disease. As a result, most secondary viral challenges are asymptomatic. Antibody and memory B and T cells are present in an immune host to generate a more rapid and extensive anamnestic (booster) response to the virus. Secretory IgA is produced quickly to provide an important defense to reinfection through the natural openings of the body, but it is produced only transiently.

Host, viral, and other factors determine the outcome of the immune response to a viral infection. Host factors include genetic background, immune status, age, and the general health of the individual. Viral factors include viral strain, infectious dose, and route of entry. The time required to initiate immune protection, the extent of the response, the level of control of the infection, and the potential for immunopathology (see Chapter 45) resulting from the infection differ after a primary infection and a rechallenge.

Viral Mechanisms for Escaping the Immune Response

A major factor in the virulence of a virus is its ability to escape immune resolution. Viruses may escape immune resolution by evading detection, preventing activation, or blocking the delivery of the immune response. Specific examples are presented in Table 39-3. Some viruses even encode special proteins that suppress the immune response.

Viral Immunopathogenesis

The symptoms of many viral diseases are the conse-

Table 39-3 Examples of Viral Evasion of Immune Responses

Mechanism	Viral Examples	Action
Humoral Response		
Hidden from antibody	Herpesviruses, retroviruses	Latent infection
	Herpes simplex virus, varicella-zoster virus, paramyxoviruses, human immunodeficiency virus	Cell-to-cell infection (syncytia formation)
Antigenic variation	Lentiviruses (human immunodeficiency virus)	Genetic change after infection
	Influenza virus	Annual genetic changes (drift) Pandemic changes (shift)
Secretion of blocking antigen	Hepatitis B virus	Hepatitis B surface antigen
Decay of complement	Herpes simplex virus	Glycoprotein C, which binds and promotes C3 decay
Interferon		
Block production	Hepatitis B virus	Inhibition of IFN transcription
	Epstein-Barr virus	IL-10 analogue (BCRF-1) blocks IFN-γ production
Block action	Adenovirus	Inhibits up-regulation of MHC expression, VA1 blocks double-stranded RNA activation of interferon- induced protein kinase (PKR)
	Herpes simplex virus	Inactivates PKR and activates phosphatase (PP1) to reverse inactivation of initiation factor for protein synthesis
Immune Cell Function		
Impairment of DC function	Measles, hepatitis C	Induction of IFN-β, which limits DC function
Impairment of lymphocyte function	Herpes simplex virus	Prevention of CD8 T-cell killing
	Human immunodeficiency virus	Kills CD4 T cells and alters macrophages
	Measles virus	Suppression of NK, T, and B cells
Immunosuppressive factors	Epstein-Barr virus	BCRF-1 (similar to IL-10) suppression of CD4 TH1 helper T-cell responses
Decreased Antigen Presentation		
Reduced class I MHC expression	Adenovirus 12	Inhibition of class I MHC transcription; 19-kDa protein (E3 gene) binds class I MHC heavy chain, blocking translocation to surface
	Cytomegalovirus	H301 protein blocks surface expression of β_2-microglobulin and class I MHC molecules
	Herpes simplex virus	ICP47 blocks TAP, preventing peptide entry into ER and binding to class I MHC molecules
Inhibition of Inflammation		
	Poxvirus, adenovirus	Blocking of action of IL-1 or tumor necrosis factor

DC, Dendritic cell; *ER*, endoplasmic reticulum; *ICP47*, infected cell protein 47; *IFN*, interferon; *IL*, interleukin; *MHC I*, major histocompatibility complex, antigen type I; *NK*, natural killer; *PMN*, polymorphonuclear neutrophil; *TAP*, transporter associated with antigen production.

quence of cytokine action or overzealous immune responses. The flulike symptoms of influenza and any virus that establishes a viremia (e.g., arboviruses) are a result of the interferon and other cytokine responses induced by the virus. Antibody interactions with large amounts of viral antigen in blood, such as occurs with hepatitis B virus infection, can lead to immune complex diseases. The measles rash, the extensive tissue damage to the brain associated with herpes simplex virus encephalitis (-*itis* means "inflammation"), and the tissue damage and symptoms of hepatitis are a result of cell-mediated immune responses. The more aggressive NK-cell and T-cell responses of adults exacerbate some diseases that are benign in children, such as varicella-zoster virus, Epstein-Barr virus infectious mononucleosis, and hepatitis B infection. Yet, the lack of such a response in children makes them prone to chronic hepatitis B infection because the response is insufficient to kill the infected cells and resolve the infection. Virus infections may also provide the initial activation trigger that allows the immune system to respond to self-antigens and cause autoimmune diseases.

SUMMARY

The host immune system utilizes several defense mechanisms against viruses, including innate and adaptive immunity.

The innate defense encompasses elevated body temperature, interferon and cytokines, as well as innate immune cells. Interferon comprise a family of proteins that can be induced by double-stranded RNA, inhibited cellular protein synthesis and enveloped viruses. Interferon act locally by initiating the antiviral state in cells surrounding the infected cell followed by blockade of local viral replication, and globally activating systemic antiviral responses. NK cells are activated by Interferons and cytokines, thus producing IFN-γ that activates macrophages and meanwhile targeting and killing virus-infected cells (especially enveloped viruses). Upon activation, macrophages produce cytokines, enzymes, chemokines etc to enhance antimicrobial function. They

also inactivate opsonized virus particles and then kill phagocytosed virus. Immature DCs produce IFN-α and other cytokines, which determine the nature of the CD4 and CD8 T-cell response, while mature DCs present antigen to CD4 T cells along with macrophages.

As the mainstay of humoral immunity, antibody neutralizes extracellular virus by blocking viral attachment proteins (e.g., glycoproteins, capsid proteins) or destabilizing the viruses, and then opsonizes virus for phagocytosis, thus blocking viremic spread to target tissue and resolving lytic viral infections. Besides, antibody promotes killing of target cells by the complement cascade and antibody-dependent cellular cytotoxicity. T cells are essential for controlling enveloped and noncytolytic viral infections. CD4 helper T cells are responsible for promoting antibody and inflammatory responses, while CD8 cytotoxic T cells recognize and respond to viral peptides presented by MHC molecules on cell surfaces and promoting apoptosis of infected cells.

KEYWORDS

English	Chinese
Interferon	干扰素
Interleukin	白介素
Perforin	穿孔素
Systemic lupus erythematosus	系统性红斑狼疮
Tumor necrosis factor	肿瘤坏死因子
Viremia	病毒血症

BIBLIOGRAPHY

1. Abbas AK, et al: Cellular and molecular immunology, ed 6, Philadelphia, 2007, WB Saunders.

2. Alcami A, Koszinowski UH: Viral mechanisms of immune evasion, Trends Microbiol 8: 410-418, 2000.

3. DeFranco AL, Locksley RM, Robertson M: Immunity: the immune response in infectious and inflammatory disease, Sunderland, Mass, 2007, Sinauer Associates.

4. Janeway CA, et al: Immunobiology: the immune system in health and disease, ed 6, New York, 2004, Garland Science.

5. Kindt TJ, Goldsby RA, Osborne BA: Kuby immunology, ed 6, New York, 2007, WH Freeman.

6. Kumar V, Abbas AK, Fausto N: Robbins and Cotran pathologic basis of disease, ed 7, Philadelphia, 2005, Elsevier.

7. Male D: Immunology, ed 4, London, 2004, Elsevier.

8. Mims C, et al: Medical microbiology, ed 3, London, 2004, Elsevier.

9. Novak R: Crash course immunology, Philadelphia, 2006, Mosby.

10. Rosenthal KS: Are microbial symptoms "self-inflicted"? The consequences of immunopathology, Infect Dis Clin Pract 13: 306-310, 2005.

11. Rosenthal KS: Vaccines make good immune theater: immunization as described in a three-act play, Infect Dis Clin Pract 14: 35-45, 2006.

12. Rosenthal KS, Wilkinson JG: Flow cytometry and immunospeak, Infect Dis Clin Pract 15: 183-191, 2007.

13. Sompayrac L: How the immune system works, ed 2, Malden, Mass, 2003, Blackwell Scientific.

Laboratory Diagnosis of Viral Diseases

There have been many new developments in laboratory viral diagnosis that provide more rapid and sensitive viral identification from clinical samples. These include better antibody reagents for direct analysis of samples, molecular genetics techniques and genomic sequencing for direct identification of the virus, and assays that can identify multiple viruses (multiplex) and be automated. Often, isolation of the organism is unnecessary and avoided to minimize the risk to laboratory and other personnel. The quicker turnaround allows a more rapid choice of the appropriate antiviral therapy.

Viral laboratory studies are performed to (1) confirm the diagnosis by identifying the viral agent of infection, (2) determine appropriate antiviral therapy, (3) check on the compliance of the patient taking antiviral drugs, (4) define the course of the disease, (5) monitor the disease epidemiologically, and (6) educate physicians and patients.

The laboratory methods accomplish the following results (Box 40-1): (1) description of virus-induced **cytopathologic effects (CPEs)** on cells; (2) detection of viral particles; (3) isolation and growth of the virus; (4) detection and analysis of viral components (e.g., antigens, enzymes, genomes); (5) evaluation of the patient's immune response to the virus (serology).

SPECIMEN COLLECTION

The patient's symptoms and history, including recent travel, the season of the year, and a presumptive diagnosis, help determine the appropriate procedures to be used to identify a viral agent (Table 40-1). The selection of the appropriate specimen for analysis is often complicated because several viruses may cause the same clinical disease.

Specimens should be collected early in the acute phase of infection, before the virus ceases to be shed. Viruses are best transported and stored on ice and in special media that contain antibiotics and proteins, such as serum albumin or gelatin. Significant losses in infectious titers occur when enveloped viruses (e.g., HSV, VZV, influenza virus) are kept at room temperature or frozen at $-20°C$. This is not a risk for nonenveloped viruses (e.g., adenoviruses, enteroviruses).

CYTOLOGY

Many viruses produce a characteristic CPE. Characteristic CPEs in the tissue sample or in cell culture include changes in cell morphology, cell lysis, vacuolation, **syncytia** (Figure 40-1), and inclusion bodies. **Syncytia** are multinucleated giant cells formed by viral fusion of individual cells. Paramyxoviruses, HSV, VZV, and human immunodeficiency virus (HIV) promote syncytia formation. **Inclusion bodies** are either histologic changes in the cells caused

---

Box 40-1

Laboratory Procedures for Diagnosing Viral Infections

Cytologic examination
Electron microscopy
Virus isolation and growth
Detection of viral proteins (antigens and enzymes)
Detection of viral genomes
Serology

Table 40-1 Specimens for Viral Diagnosis

Common Pathogenic Viruses	Specimens for Culture	Procedures and Comments
Respiratory Tract		
Influenza virus; paramyxoviruses; coronavirus; rhinovirus; enterovirus (picornavirus)	Nasal washing, throat swab, nasal swab, sputum	RT-PCR, ELISA, multiplex assays detect several agents; cell culture
Gastrointestinal Tract		
Reovirus; rotavirus; adenovirus; Norwalk virus, other calicivirus	Stool, rectal swab	RT-PCR, ELISA; viruses are not cultured
Maculopapular Rash		
Adenovirus; enterovirus (picornavirus)	Throat swab, rectal swab	PCR, RT-PCR
Rubella virus; measles virus	Urine	RT-PCR, ELISA
Vesicular Rash		
Coxsackievirus; echovirus; HSV; VZV	Vesicle fluid, scraping, or swab, enterovirus in stool	HSV and VZV: vesicle scraping (Tzanck smear), cell culture; HSV typing by PCR, IF
Central Nervous System (Aseptic Meningitis, Encephalitis)		
Enterovirus (picornavirus)	Stool, CSF	RT-PCR
Arboviruses (e.g., togaviruses, bunyavirus)	Blood, CSF; rarely cultured	RT-PCR, serology; multiplex assays detect several agents
Rabies virus	Tissue, saliva, brain biopsy, CSF	IF of biopsy, RT-PCR
HSV; CMV; mumps virus; measles virus	Cerebrospinal fluid	PCR or RT-PCR, virus isolation, and antigen are assayed
Urinary Tract		
Adenovirus; CMV	Urine	PCR; CMV may be shed without apparent disease
Blood		
HIV; human T-cell leukemia virus; hepatitis B, C, and D viruses, EBV, CMV, HHV-6	Blood	ELISA for antigen or antibody, PCR, and RT-PCR; multiplex assays detect several agents

CMV, Cytomegalovirus; *EBV*, Epstein-Barr virus; *ELISA*, enzyme-linked immunosorbent assay; *HIV*, human immunodeficiency virus; *HHV-6*, human herpes virus 6; *HSV*, herpes simplex virus; *IF*, immunofluorescence; *PCR*, polymerase chain reaction; *RT-PCR*, reverse transcriptase polymerase chain reaction; *VZV*, varicella-zoster virus.

by viral components or virus-induced changes in cell structures. For example, intranuclear basophilic (owl's-eye) inclusion bodies found in large cells of tissues with cytomegalovirus (CMV) or in the sediment of urine from patients with the infection are readily identifiable. Rabies may be detected through the finding of cytoplasmic-Negri bodies (rabies virus inclusions) in brain tissue (Figure 40-2).

Often, the cytologic specimens will be examined for the presence of specific viral antigens by immunofluorescence or viral genomes by in situ hybridization or PCR for a rapid, definitive identification. These tests are specific for individual viruses and must be chosen based on the differential diagnosis. These methods are discussed in the following paragraphs.

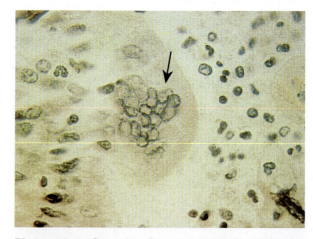

Figure 40-1 Syncytium formation by measles virus. Multinucleated giant cell *(arrow)* visible in a histologic section of lung biopsy tissue from a measles virus-induced giant cell pneumonia in an immunocompromised child. (From Hart C, Broadhead RL: *A color atlas of pediatric infectious diseases,* London, 1992, Wolfe.)

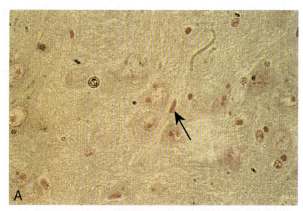

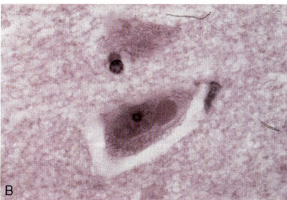

Figure 40-2   Negri bodies caused by rabies. **A,** A section of brain from a patient with rabies shows Negri bodies *(arrow)*. **B,** Higher magnification from another biopsy specimen.(**A,** From Hart C, Broadhead RL: *A color atlas of pediatric infectious diseases*, London, 1992, Wolfe.)

ELECTRON MICROSCOPY

Electron microscopy is not a standard clinical laboratory technique, but it can be used to detect and identify some viruses if sufficient viral particles are present. The addition of virus-specific antibody to a sample can cause viral particles to clump, thereby facilitating the detection and simultaneous identification of the virus (immunoelectron microscopy). Enteric viruses, such as rotavirus, that are produced in abundance and have a characteristic morphology can be detected in stool by these methods. Appropriately processed tissue from a biopsy or clinical specimen can also be examined for the presence of viral structures.

VIRAL ISOLATION AND GROWTH

A virus can be grown in tissue culture, embryonated eggs, and experimental animals (Box 40-2). Although embryonated eggs are still used for the growth of virus for some vaccines (e.g., influenza), they have been replaced by cell cultures for routine virus isolation in clinical laboratories. Experimental animals are rarely used in clinical laboratories for the purpose of isolating viruses.

Box 40-2

Systems for the Propagation of Viruses

People
Animals: cows (e.g., Jenner cowpox vaccine), chickens, mice, rats, suckling mice
Embryonated eggs
Organ culture
Tissue culture
  Primary
  Diploid cell line
  Tumor or immortalized cell line

Cell Culture

Specific types of tissue culture cells are used to grow viruses, such as **primary celllines, Diploid cell lines, tumor cell lines** and **immortalized cell lines.** Many clinically significant viruses, such as influenza viruses, enteroviruses, HSV, VZV, CMV, adenoviruses, can be recovered in at least one of these cell cultures.

Viral Detection

A virus can be detected and initially identified through observation of the virus-induced CPE in the cell monolayer (Box 40-3; Figure 40-3), by immunofluorescence, or genome analysis of the infected cell culture. For example, a single virus infects, spreads, and kills surrounding cells (**plaque**). The type of cell culture, the

---

Box 40-3

Viral Cytopathologic Effects

Cell death
  Cell rounding
  Degeneration
  Aggregation
  Loss of attachments to culture dish
Characteristic histologic changes: inclusion bodies in the nucleus or cytoplasm, margination of chromatin
Syncytia: multinucleated giant cells caused by virusinduced cell-to-cell fusion
Cell surface changes
  Viral antigen expression
  Hemadsorption (hemagglutinin expression)

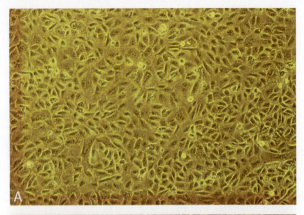

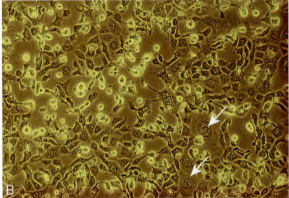

Figure 40-3 Cytopathologic effect of herpes simplex virus (HSV) infection. **A,** Uninfected Vero cells, an African green monkey kidney cell line. **B,** HSV-1-infected Vero cells showing rounded cells, multinucleated cells, and loss of the monolayer. Arrows point to syncytia.

characteristics of the CPE, and the rapidity of viral growth can be used to initially identify many clinically important viruses. This approach to identifying viruses is similar to that used in the identification of bacteria, which is based on the growth and morphology of colonies on selective differential media.

Some viruses grow slowly or not at all or do not readily cause a CPE in cell lines typically used in clinical virology laboratories. Some cause diseases that are hazardous to personnel. These viruses are most frequently diagnosed on the basis of serologic findings or through the detection of viral genomes or proteins.

Characteristic viral properties can also be used to identify viruses that do not have a classic CPE. For example, the rubella virus may not cause a CPE, but it does prevent (interfere with) the replication of picornaviruses in a process known as **heterologous interference,** which can be used to identify the rubella virus. Cells infected with the influenza virus,

parainfluenza virus, mumps virus, and togavirus express a viral glycoprotein (hemagglutinin) that binds erythrocytes of defined animal species to the infected cell surface (**hemadsorption**) (Figure 40-4). When released into the cell culture medium, such viruses can be detected from the agglutination of erythrocytes, a process termed **hemagglutination.** The virus can then be identified from the specific antibody that blocks the hemagglutination, a process called **hemagglutination inhibition (HI).** One can quantitate a virus by determining the greatest dilution that retains the following properties (**titer**):

1. **Tissue culture infectious dose (TCID$_{50}$):** titer of virus that causes cytopathologic effects in half the tissue culture cells

2. **Lethal dose (LD$_{50}$):** titer of virus that kills 50% of a set of test animals

3. **Infectious dose (ID$_{50}$):** titer of virus that initiates a detectable symptom, antibody, or other response in 50% of a set of test animals

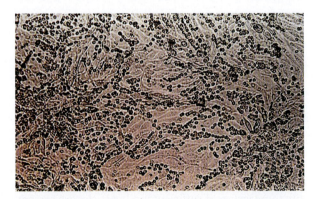

Figure 40-4 Hemadsorption of erythrocytes to cells infected with influenza viruses, mumps virus, parainfluenza viruses, or togaviruses. These viruses express a hemagglutinin on their surfaces, which binds to erythrocytes of selected animal species.

The number of infectious viruses can also be evaluated with a count of the plaques produced by 10-fold dilutions of sample (**plaque-forming units**). The ratio of viral particles (from electron microscopy) to plaque-forming units is always much greater than one because numerous defective viral particles are produced during viral replication.

Interpretation of Culture Results

In general, the detection of any virus in host tissues,

CSF, blood, or vesicular fluid can be considered a highly significant finding. However, viral shedding may occur and be unrelated to the disease symptoms. Similarly, a negative result cannot be conclusive because the sample may have been improperly handled, contain neutralizing antibody, or be acquired before or after viral shedding.

DETECTION OF VIRAL PROTEINS

Enzymes and other proteins are produced during viral replication and can be detected by biochemical, immunologic, and molecular biologic means (Box 40-4). The viral proteins can be separated by electrophoresis and their patterns used to identify and distinguish different viruses. For example, the electrophoretically separated HSV-infected cell proteins and virion proteins exhibit different patterns for different types and strains of HSV-1 and HSV-2.

The detection and assay of characteristic enzymes or activities can identify and quantitate specific viruses. For example, the presence of reverse transcriptase in serum or cell culture indicates the presence of a retrovirus or hepadnavirus. Similarly, hemagglutination or hemadsorption can be used to easily assay the hemagglutinin produced by the influenza virus.

Antibodies can be used as sensitive and specific tools to detect, identify, and quantitate the virus and viral antigen in clinical specimens or cell cultures (immunohistochemistry). Specifically, monoclonal or monospecific antibodies are useful for distinguishing viruses. Viral antigens on the cell surface or within the cell can be detected by **immunofluorescence** and **enzyme immunoassay (EIA)**. Virus or antigen released from infected cells can be detected by **enzyme-linked immunosorbent assay (ELISA)**, **radioimmunoassay (RIA)**, and **latex agglutination (LA)**.

The detection of CMV and other viruses can be enhanced through the use of a combination of cell culture and immunologic means. In this method, the clinical sample is centrifuged onto cells grown on a coverslip on the bottom of a **shell vial** (glass tube). This step increases the efficiency and accelerates the progression of infection of the cells on the coverslip. The cells can then be analyzed with immunofluorescence (**direct fluorescence**) or EIA for early viral antigens, which are detectable within 24 hours, instead of the 7 to 14 days it takes for a CPE to become evident.

DETECTION OF VIRAL GENETIC MATERIAL

The genetic sequence of a virus is a major distinguishing characteristic of the family, type, and strain of virus. The electrophoretic patterns of ribonucleic acid (RNA) (influenza, reovirus) or restriction endonuclease fragment lengths from DNA viral genomes are like genetic fingerprints for these viruses. Different strains of HSV-1 and HSV-2 can be distinguished in this way by restriction fragment length polymorphism. Newer methods for viral genome detection use sequence-specific genetic probes and PCR-like DNA and RNA amplification approaches, which allow more rapid analysis and quantitation with a minimum of risk from infectious virus. Methods for sequencing the genomes of viruses are becoming rapid and inexpensive enough to become a routine viral identification method.

DNA probes, with sequences complementary to specific regions of a viral genome, can be used like antibodies as sensitive and specific tools for detecting a virus. These probes can detect the virus even in the absence of viral replication. DNA probe analysis is especially useful for detecting slowly replicating or

---

Box 40-4

Assays for Viral Proteins and Nucleic Acids

Protein patterns (electrophoresis)
Enzyme activities (e.g., reverse transcriptase)
Hemagglutination and hemadsorption
Antigen detection (e.g., direct and indirect immunofluorescence, enzyme-linked immunosorbent assay, Western blot)

Nucleic Acids

Restriction endonuclease cleavage patterns
Size of RNA for segmented RNA viruses (electrophoresis)
DNA genome hybridization in situ (cytochemistry)
Southern, Northern, and dot blots
PCR (DNA)
Reverse transcriptase polymerase chain reaction (RNA)
Real-time quantitative PCR
Genome sequencing

nonproductive viruses, such as CMV and human papillomavirus, or the viral antigen cannot be detected using immunologic tests. Specific viral genetic sequences in fixed, permeabilized tissue biopsy specimens can be detected by **in situ hybridization** (e.g., **fluorescence in situ hybridization [FISH]**).

Viral genomes can also be detected in clinical samples with the use of **dot blot** or **Southern blot analysis.** For the latter method, the viral genome or electrophoretically separated restriction endonuclease cleavage fragments of the genome are blotted onto nitrocellulose filters and then detected on the filter by their hybridization to DNA probes. For many laboratories, genome amplification techniques, including **PCR** for DNA genomes **and reverse transcriptase PCR (RT-PCR)** for RNA genomes, are the method of choice for detection and identification of viruses. Use of the appropriate primers for PCR can promote a millionfold amplification of a target sequence in a few hours. This technique is especially useful for detecting latent and integrated sequences of viruses, such as retroviruses, herpesviruses, papillomaviruses, and other papovaviruses, as well as evidence of viruses present in low concentrations and viruses that are difficult or too dangerous to isolate in cell culture. RT-PCR uses the retroviral reverse transcriptase to convert viral RNA to DNA and allow PCR amplification of the viral nucleic acid sequences. Quantification of the amount of genomes within a patient (virus load) can be determined by **real-time PCR.** For example, the concentration of viral genome (RNA genomes would be converted to DNA) is proportional to the initial rate of PCR amplification of the genomic DNA. This test is especially important for following the course of HIV infection.

VIRAL SEROLOGY

The humoral immune response provides a history of a patient's infections. Serologic studies are used for the identification of viruses that are difficult to isolate and grow in cell culture, as well as viruses that cause diseases of long duration (see Box 6-2). Serology can be used to identify the virus and its strain or serotype, whether it is an acute or chronic disease, and determine whether it is a primary infection or a reinfection. The detection of **virus-specific immunoglobulin M (IgM) antibody,** which is present during the first 2 or 3 weeks of a primary infection, generally indicates a recent primary infection. **Seroconversion** is indicated by at least **a fourfold increase in the antibody titer** between the serum obtained during the acute phase of disease and that obtained at least 2 to 3 weeks later during the convalescent phase. Reinfection or recurrence later in life causes an anamnestic (secondary or booster) response. Antibody titers may remain high in patients who suffer frequent recurrence of a disease (e.g., herpesviruses).

The course of a chronic infection can also be evaluated by a serologic profile. Specifically, the presence of antibodies to several key viral antigens and their titers can be used to identify the stage of disease caused by certain viruses. This approach is especially useful for the diagnosis of viral diseases with slow courses (e.g., hepatitis B, infectious mononucleosis caused by Epstein-Barr virus).

Serologic Test Methods

Neutralization and **HI tests** assay antibody on the basis of its recognition of and binding to virus. The antibody coating of the virus blocks its binding to indicator cells (Figure 40-5). Antibody neutralization of virus inhibits infection and subsequent cytopathologic effects in tissue culture cells. HI is used for the identification of viruses that can selectively agglutinate erythrocytes of various animal species (e.g., chicken, guinea pig, human). Antibody in serum prevents a standardized amount of virus from binding to and agglutinating erythrocytes.

The indirect fluorescent antibody test and solidphase immunoassays, such as latex agglutination and **ELISA,** are commonly used to detect and quantitate viral antigen and antiviral antibody. The ELISA test is used to screen the blood supply to exclude individuals who are seropositive for hepatitis B and C viruses and HIV. **Western blot** analysis has become very important to confirm seroconversion and hence infection with HIV. The ability of the patient's anti-

Figure 40-5   Neutralization, hemagglutination, and hemagglutination inhibition assays. In the assay shown, 10-fold dilutions of serum were incubated with virus. Aliquots of the mixture were then added to cell cultures or erythrocytes. In the absence of antibody, the virus infected the monolayer (indicated by cytopathologic effect *[CPE]*) or caused hemagglutination (i.e., formed a gel-like suspension of erythrocytes). In the presence of the antibody, infection was blocked, preventing CPE (neutralization), or hemagglutination was inhibited, allowing the erythrocytes to pellet. The titer of antibody of this serum would be 100. *pfu*, Plaque-forming units.

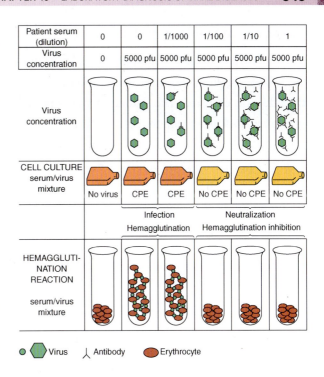

body to recognize specific viral proteins separated by electrophoresis, transferred (blotted) onto a filter paper (e.g., nitrocellulose, nylon), and visualized with an enzyme-conjugated antihuman antibody confirms the ELISA-indicated diagnosis of HIV infection (Figure 40-6).

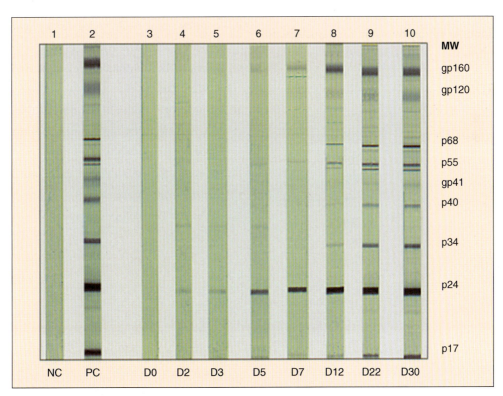

Figure 40-6   Western blot analysis of human immunodeficiency virus (HIV) antigens and antibody. HIV protein antigens are separated by electrophoresis and blotted onto nitrocellulose paper strips. The strip is incubated with patient antibody, washed to remove the unbound antibody, and then reacted with enzyme-conjugated antihuman antibody and chromophoric substrate. Serum from an HIV-infected person binds and identifies the major antigenic proteins of HIV. These data demonstrate the seroconversion of one HIV-infected individual with sera collected on day 0 *(D0)* to day 30 *(D30)* compared to a known positive control *(PC)* and negative control *(NC)*. *MW*, molecular weight. (From Kuritzkes DR: Diagnostic tests for HIV infection and resistance assays. In Cohen J, Powderly WG: *Infectious diseases*, ed 2, St Louis, 2004, Mosby.)

Limitations of Serologic Methods

The presence of an antiviral antibody indicates previous infection but is not sufficient to indicate when the infection occurred. The finding of virus-specific IgM, a fourfold increase in the antibody titer between acute and convalescent sera, or specific antibody profiles is indicative of recent infection. A good understanding of the clinical symptoms and knowledge of the limitations and potential problems with serologic assays aid the diagnosis.

SUMMARY

In the diagnostic laboratory, virus infections are confirmed by several methods that include: observation of virus particles by electron microscopy; growth of the virus in a cell culture from a specimen taken from the patient; detection of virus antigens; detection of virus nucleic acids, or gene sequencing to characterize viral strains; detection of virus-specific antibodies in the blood; hemagglutination assay and hemagglutination inhibition assay for viruses with hemagglutinin.

KEYWORDS

English	Chinese
Cytopathologic effects, CPEs	细胞病变效应
Syncytia	合胞体
Inclusion bodies	包涵体
Intranuclear basophilic	核内嗜碱性包涵体
Negri bodies	内基小体
Plaque	噬斑
Hemagglutinin	血凝素
Hemagglutination inhibition	血凝抑制
Plaque-forming units	空斑形成单位

BIBLIOGRAPHY

1. Carter J, Saunders V: Virology: principles and applications, Chichester, England, 2007, Wiley.
2. Cohen J, Powderly WG: Infectious diseases, ed 2, St Louis, 2004, Mosby.
3. Collier L, Oxford J: Human virology, ed 3, Oxford, England, 2006, Oxford University Press.
4. De Clercq E: A 40-year journey in search of selective antiviral chemotherapy, Ann Rev Pharmacol Toxicol 51: 1-24, 2011.
5. Flint SJ, et al: Principles of virology: molecular biology, pathogenesis and control of animal viruses, ed 3, Washington, DC, 2009, American Society for Microbiology Press.
6. Galasso GJ, Whitley RJ, Merigan TC: Antiviral agents and human viral diseases, ed 4, Philadelphia, 1997, Lippincott.
7. Hodinka RL: What clinicians need to know about antiviral drugs and viral resistance, Infect Dis Clin North Am 11: 945-967, 1997.
8. Knipe DM, et al: Fields virology, ed 5, Philadelphia, 2006, Lippincott Williams & Wilkins.
9. Richman DD: Antiviral drug resistance, Antiviral Res 71: 117-121, 2006.
10. Richman DD, Whitley RJ, Hayden FG: Clinical virology, ed 3, Washington, DC, 2009, American Society for Microbiology Press.
11. Strauss JM, Strauss EG: Viruses and human diseases, ed 2, San Diego, 2007, Academic.
12. Voyles BA: The biology of viruses, ed 2, Boston, 2002, McGraw-Hill.

Antiviral Agents

Unlike bacteria, viruses are obligate intracellular parasites that use the host cell's biosynthetic machinery and enzymes for replication. Hence it is more difficult to inhibit viral replication without also being toxic to the host. Most antiviral drugs (Box 41-1) are targeted toward viral-encoded enzymes or structures of the virus that are important for replication. Most of these compounds are classic biochemical inhibitors of viral-encoded enzymes. Some antiviral drugs are actually stimulators of host innate immune protective responses.

TARGETS FOR ANTIVIRAL DRUGS

The different targets for antiviral drugs (e.g., structures, enzymes, or processes important or essential for virus production) are discussed with respect to the steps of the viral replication cycle they inhibit. These targets and their respective antiviral agents are listed in Table 41-1.

Virion Disruption

Enveloped viruses are susceptible to certain lipid and detergent-like molecules that disperse or disrupt the envelope membrane, thereby preventing acquisition of the virus. Nonoxynol-9, a detergent-like component in birth control jellies, can inactivate herpes simplex virus (HSV) and human immunodeficiency virus (HIV) and prevent sexual acquisition of the viruses. Rhinoviruses are susceptible to acid, and citric acid can be incorporated into facial tissues as a means of blocking virus transmission.

Attachment

The first step in viral replication is mediated by the interaction of a viral attachment protein with its cell surface receptor. This interaction can be blocked by **neutralizing antibodies** of viral attachment protein, the oldest form of antiviral therapy, or by **receptor antagonists**, include peptide or sugar analogues of the cell receptor, **or** compounds that bind to the C-C chemokine receptor 5 (CCR5) molecule to prevent the initial infection of HIV. Acidic polysaccharides, such as heparan and dextran sulfate, interfere with viral binding and have been suggested for the treatment of infection with HIV, HSV, and other viruses.

Penetration and Uncoating

Penetration and uncoating of the virus are required to deliver the viral genome into the cytoplasm of the host cell. **Amantadine, rimantadine,** and other hydrophobic amines (weak organic bases) are antiviral agents that can neutralize the pH of these compartments and inhibit virion uncoating. influenzaA virion uncoating. Penetration and uncoating of HIV are blocked by a 33-amino acid peptide, T20 (**enfuvirtide [Fuzeon]**), which inhibits the action of the viral fusion protein gp41.

Table 41-1 Examples of Targets for Antiviral Drugs

Replication Step or Target	Agent	Targeted Virus[*]
Attachment	Peptide analogues of attachment protein	HIV (CCR5 co-receptor antagonist)
	Neutralizing antibodies	Most viruses
	Heparan and dextran sulfate	HIV, HSV
Penetration and uncoating	Amantadine, rimantadine	Influenza A virus
	Tromantadine	HSV
	Arildone, disoxaril, pleconaril	Picornaviruses
Transcription	Interferon	HCVs, papillomavirus
	Antisense oligonucleotides	—
Protein synthesis	Interferon	HCV, papillomavirus
DNA replication (polymerase)	Nucleoside analogues	Herpesviruses; HIV; hepatitis B virus, poxviruses, etc.
	Phosphonoformate, phosphonoacetic acid	Herpesviruses
Nucleoside biosynthesis	Ribavirin	Respiratory syncytial virus, Lassa fever virus, HCV
Nucleoside scavenging (thymidine kinase)	Nucleoside analogues	HSV, varicella-zoster virus
Glycoprotein processing	—	HIV
Assembly (protease)	Hydrophobic substrate analogues	HIV, HCV
Assembly (neuraminidase)	Oseltamivir, zanamivir	Influenza A, B virus
Virion integrity	Nonoxynol-9	HIV, HSV

CCR5, C-C chemokine receptor 5; *DNA*, deoxyribonucleic acid; *HCV*, hepatitis C virus; *HIV*, human immunodeficiency virus; *HSV*, herpes simplex virus.
[*]Therapies may not have received approval for human use.

RNA Synthesis

Although messenger ribonucleic acid (mRNA) synthesis is essential for the production of virus, it is not a good target for antiviral drugs. It would be difficult to inhibit viral mRNA synthesis without affecting cellular mRNA synthesis. Deoxyribonucleic acid (DNA) viruses use the host cell's transcriptases for mRNA synthesis. The RNA polymerases encoded by RNA viruses may not be sufficiently different from host cell transcriptases to selectively inhibit this activity, and the high rate at which RNA viruses mutate results in the generation of many drug-resistant strains. **Ribavirin** resembles riboguanosine and inhibits nucleoside biosynthesis, mRNA capping, promotes hypermutation, and other processes (cellular and viral) important to the replication of many viruses.

The proper processing (splicing) and translation of viral mRNA can be inhibited by interferon and antisense oligonucleotides. Viral infection of an **interferon**-treated cell triggers a cascade of biochemical events that block viral replication. Specifically, the degradation of viral and cellular mRNA is enhanced, and ribosomal assembly is blocked, preventing protein synthesis and viral replication. Interferon and artificial interferon inducers (**Ampligen, poly rI:rC**) have been approved for clinical use (papilloma, hepatitis B and C) or are in clinical trials.

Genome Replication

Most antiviral drugs are **nucleoside analogues,** which are nucleosides with modifications of the base, sugar, or both (Figure 41-1). The viral **DNA polymerases** of the herpesviruses and the **reverse transcriptases** of HIV and hepatitis B virus (HBV) are the prime targets for most antiviral drugs because they are essential for virus replication and are different from host enzymes. For example, **acyclovir (ACV), azidothymidine (AZT).**

Nucleoside analogues selectively inhibit viral

polymerases because these enzymes are less accurate than host cell enzymes. The viral enzyme binds nucleoside analogues with modifications of the base, sugar, or both several hundred times better than the host cell enzyme. These drugs either **prevent chain elongation,** as a result of the absence of a 3′-hydroxyl on the sugar, or **alter recognition and base pairing,** as a result of a base modification, and induce inactivating mutations (see Figure 41-1). Antiviral drugs that cause termination of the DNA chain by means

of modified nucleoside sugar residues include ACV, ganciclovir (GCV), valacyclovir, famciclovir, adefovir, adenosine arabinoside (vidarabine, ara-A), zidovudine (AZT), lamivudine (3TC). Antiviral drugs that become incorporated into the viral genome and cause errors in replication (mutation) and transcription (inactive mRNA and proteins) because of modified nucleoside bases include **ribavirin, 5-iododeoxyuridine (idoxuridine),** and **trifluorothymidine (trifluridine).**

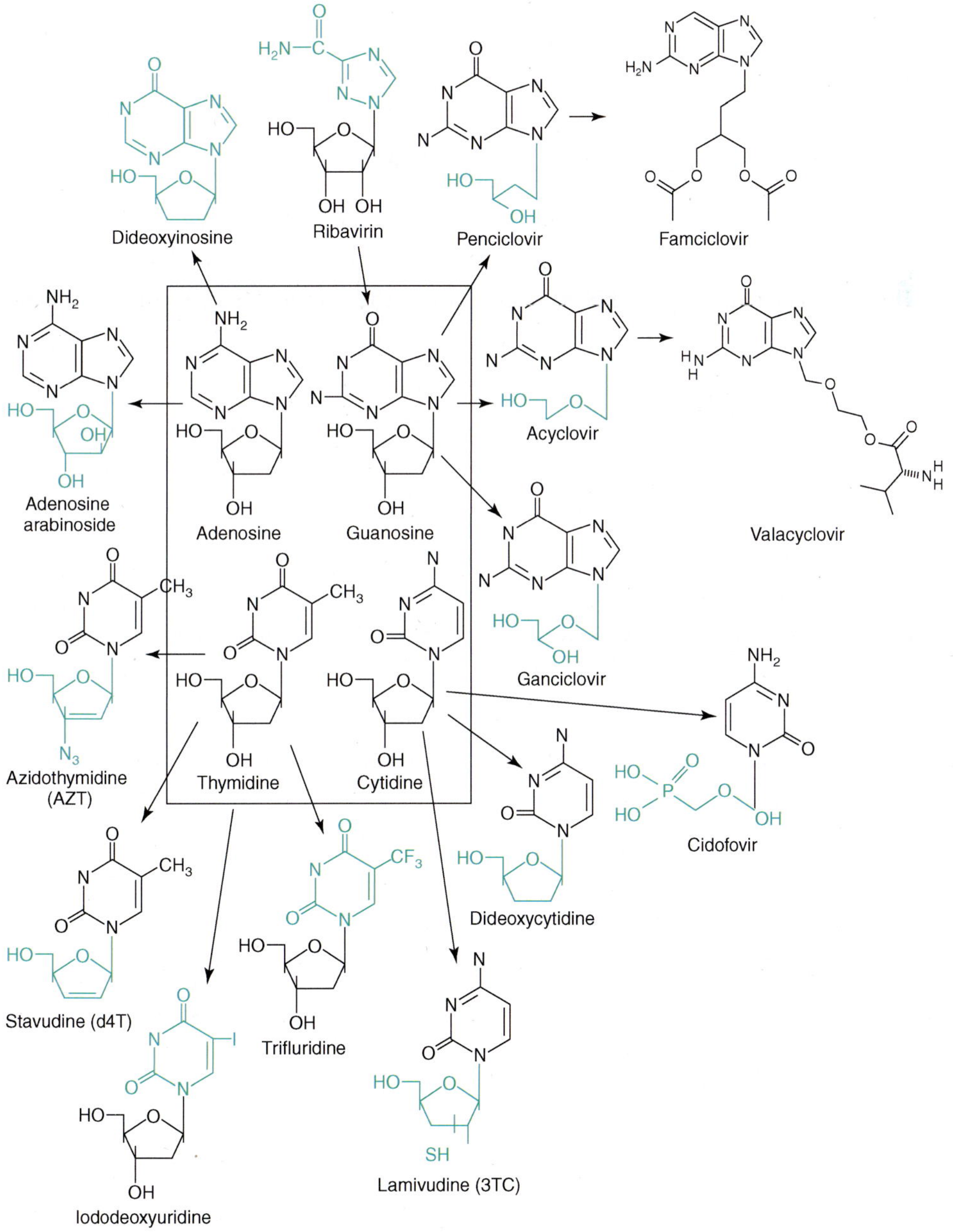

Figure 41-1 Structure of the most common nucleoside analogues that are antiviral drugs. The chemical distinctions between the natural deoxynucleoside and the antiviral drug analogues are highlighted. Arrows indicate related drugs. Valacyclovir is the L-valyl ester of acyclovir. Famciclovir is the diacetyl 6-deoxyanalogue of penciclovir. Both of these drugs are metabolized to the active drug in the liver or intestinal wall.

Deoxyribonucleotide scavenging enzymes (e.g., the thymidine kinase and ribonucleosidereductase of the herpesviruses) are also enzyme targets of antiviral drugs. Inhibition of these enzymes reduces the levels of deoxyribonucleotides necessary for the replication of the DNA virus genome, preventing virus replication.

Integration of the cDNA of HIV into the host chromosome catalyzed by the viral integrase enzyme is essential for virus replication. An inhibitor of the integrase is now approved for anti-HIV therapy.

Protein Synthesis

Although bacterial protein synthesis is the target for several antibacterial compounds, viral protein synthesis is a poor target for antiviral drugs. The virus uses host cell ribosomes and synthetic mechanisms for replication, so selective inhibition is not possible. **Interferon-α (IFN-α)** and **interferon-β (IFN-β)** stop a virus by promoting the inhibition of viral protein synthesis in the infected cell.

Virion Assembly and Release

The **HIV protease** is unique and **essential** to the assembly of virions and the production of infectious virions. **saquinavir, ritonavir,** and **indinavir** (*navir*, "no virus"), are inhibitors of HIV protease. Bocepravir and telaprevir are two new protease inhhibitors for treatment of hepatitis C virus (HCV). Proteases of other viruses are also targets for antiviral drugs.

The **neuraminidase of influenza** has also become a target for antiviral drugs. **Zanamivir (Relenza)** and **oseltamivir (Tamiflu)** act as enzyme inhibitors and, unlike amantadine and rimantadine, can inhibit influenza A and B. Amantadine and rimantadine also inhibit release of influenza A.

Stimulators of Host Innate Immune Protective Responses

The best antiviral agents are those of the host's innate and immune antiviral response. Innate responses of dendritic cells, macrophages, and other cells can be stimulated by **imiquimod, resiquimod, and CpG oligodeoxynucleotides,** which bind to Toll-like receptors

to stimulate release of protective cytokines. **Interferon** and interferon inducers facilitate the treatment of chronic diseases of hepatitis C and papillomaviruses. **Antibodies,** for example, passive immunization is administered after exposure to rabies and hepatitis A virus (HAV) and HBV.

NUCLEOSIDE ANALOGUES

Most of the antiviral drugs in clinical use (Table 41-2) are nucleoside analogues that inhibit viral polymerases. Resistance to the drug is usually caused by a mutation of the polymerase.

Acyclovir, Valacyclovir, Penciclovir, and Famciclovir

ACV (acycloguanosine) and its valyl derivative, valacyclovir, differ in pharmacologic ways. ACV differs from the nucleoside guanosine by having an acyclic (hydroxyethoxymethyl) side chain instead of a ribose or deoxyribose sugar. ACV has selective action against HSV and VZV, the herpesviruses that encode a thymidine kinase (Figure 41-2). The viral thymidine kinase is required to activate the drug by phosphorylation, and host cell enzymes complete the progression to the diphosphate form and finally to the triphosphate form. Because there is no initial phosphorylation in uninfected cells, there is no active drug to inhibit cellular DNA synthesis or to cause toxicity. The ACV triphosphate causes termination of the growing viral DNA chain because there is no 3'-hydroxyl group on the ACV molecule to allow chain elongation. The minimal toxicity of ACV is also a result of a 100-fold or greater use by the viral DNA polymerase than by cellular DNA polymerases. **Resistance to ACV** develops by mutation of either the thymidine kinase, so that activation of ACV cannot occur, or the DNA polymerase, to prevent ACV binding.

ACV is effective against all HSV infections, including encephalitis, disseminated herpes, and other serious herpes diseases. ACV inhibits the replication of HSV but cannot resolve the latent HSV infection.

Valacyclovir, the valyl ester derivative of ACV, is more efficiently absorbed after oral administra-

Table 41-2 Some Antiviral Drug Therapies Approved by the U.S. Food and Drug Administration

Virus	Antiviral Drug	Trade Name
Herpes simplex and varicella-zoster viruses	Acyclovir*	Zovirax
	Valacyclovir*	Valtrex
	Penciclovir	Denavir
	Famciclovir*	Famvir
	Iododeoxyuridine (idoxuridine)†	Stoxil
	Trifluridine	Viroptic
Cytomegalovirus	Ganciclovir	Cytovene
	Valganciclovir	Valcyte
	Cidofovir	Vistide
	Phosphonoformate (foscarnet)	Foscavir
Influenza A virus	Amantadine	Symmetrel
	Rimantadine	Flumadine
Influenza A and B viruses	Zanamivir	Relenza
	Oseltamivir	Tamiflu
Hepatitis B virus	Lamivudine	Epivir
	Adefovirdipivoxil	Hepsera
Hepatitis C virus	Interferon-α, ribavirin boceprevir, telaprevir	Various Victrelis, Incivek
Papillomavirus	Interferon-α	Various
Respiratory syncytial virus and Lassa virus	Ribavirin	Virazole
Picornaviruses	Pleconaril	Picovir
Human immunodeficiency virus		
Nucleoside analogue reverse transcriptase inhibitors	Azidothymidine (zidovudine)	Retrovir
	Dideoxyinosine (didanosine)	Videx
	Dideoxycytidine (zalcitabine)	Hivid
	Stavudine (d4T)	Zerit
	Lamivudine (3TC)	Epivir
Nonnucleoside reverse transcriptase inhibitors	Nevirapine	Viramune
	Delavirdine	Rescriptor
Protease inhibitors	Saquinavir	Invirase
	Ritonavir	Norvir
	Indinavir	Crixivan
	Nelfinavir	Viracept
Integrase inhibitor	Raltegravir	Isentriss
CCR5 co-receptor antagonist	Maraviroc	Selzentry
Fusion inhibitor	Enfuvirtide	Fuzeon

CCR5, C-C chemokine receptor 5.
*Also active against varicella-zoster virus.
†Topical use only.

tion and rapidly converted into ACV, increasing the bioavailability of ACV for the treatment of HSV and serious VZV. VZV is less sensitive to the agent because ACV is phosphorylated less efficiently by the VZV thymidine kinase.

Penciclovir inhibits HSV and VZV in the same way ACV does but is concentrated and persists in the infected cells to a greater extent than ACV. Penciclovir also has some activity against the Epstein-Barr virus and cytomegalovirus (CMV).

Ganciclovir

GCV (dihydroxypropoxymethyl guanine) differs from ACV in having a single hydroxymethyl group in the acyclic side chain (see Figure 41-1). The remarkable result of this addition is that it confers considerable activity against CMV. CMV does not encode a thymidine kinase, but a viral-encoded protein kinase phosphorylates GCV. Once activated by phosphorylation, GCV inhibits all herpesvirus DNA polymerases. The viral DNA polymerases have nearly 30 times greater affinity for the drug than the cellular DNA polymerase.

GCV (**valganciclovir**) is effective in the treatment of CMV retinitis and shows some efficacy in the treatment of CMV esophagitis, colitis, and pneumonia in patients with AIDS.

Cidofovir and Adefovir

Cidofovir and **adefovir** are both nucleotide analogues and contain a phosphate attached to the sugar analogue. This obviates the need for the initial phosphorylation by a viral enzyme. Compounds with this type of sugar analogue are substrates for DNA polymerases or reverse transcriptases and have an expanded spectrum of susceptible viruses. Cidofovir, a cytidine analogue, is approved for CMV infections in AIDS patients but can also inhibit replication of polyomavirus, papillomaviruses, and inhibit the polymerases of herpesviruses, adenoviruses, and poxvirus. Adefovir and adefovirdipivoxil (a diesterprodrug) are analogues of adenosine and are approved for treatment of HBV.

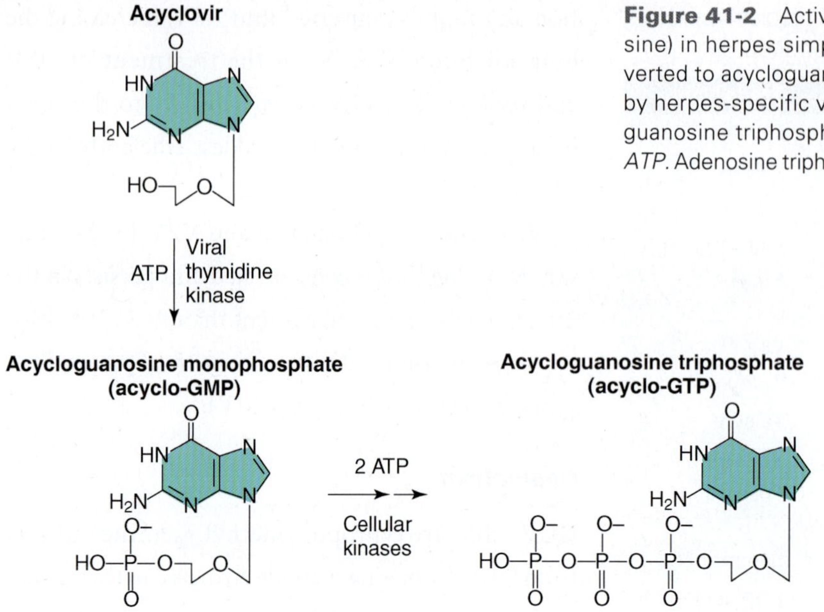

Acyclovir

Figure 41-2 Activation of acyclovir (ACV) (acycloguanosine) in herpes simplex virus-infected cells. ACV is converted to acycloguanosine monophosphate *(acyclo-GMP)* by herpes-specific viral thymidine kinase, then to acycloguanosine triphosphate *(acyclo-GTP)* by cellular kinases. *ATP.* Adenosine triphosphate.

Azidothymidine

AZT was the first useful therapy for HIV infection. AZT (Retrovir), a nucleoside analogue of thymidine, inhibits the reverse transcriptase of HIV (see Figure 41-1). Similar to other nucleosides, AZT must be phosphorylated by host cell enzymes. It lacks the 3′-hydroxyl necessary for DNA chain elongation and prevents complementary DNA synthesis. The selective therapeutic effect of AZT stems from the 100-fold lower sensitivity of the host cell DNA polymerase in comparison with the HIV reverse transcriptase.

Continuous oral AZT treatment is administered to HIV-infected people with depleted CD4 T-cell counts to prevent progression of disease. AZT treatment of pregnant HIV-infected women can reduce the likelihood of or prevent transmission of the virus to the baby. Side effects of AZT range from nausea to life-threatening bone marrow toxicity.

The high error rate of the HIV polymerase creates extensive mutations and promotes the development of antiviral drug-resistant strains. This problem is being addressed by the administration of multidrug therapy as initial therapy (**highly active antiretroviral therapy, HAART**). It is more difficult for the HIV to develop resistance to multiple drugs with multiple target enzymes. Multidrug-resistant HIV strains are likely to be much weaker than the parent strains.

Dideoxyinosine, Dideoxycytidine, Stavudine, and Lamivudine

Several other nucleoside analogues have been approved as anti-HIV agents. **Dideoxyinosine** (didanosine) is a nucleoside analogue that is converted to dideoxyadenosine triphosphate (see Figure 41-1). Similar to AZT, dideoxyinosine, **dideoxycytidine,** and **stavudine** (d4T) lack a 3′-hydroxyl group. The modified sugar attached to **lamivudine** (2′-deoxy-3′-thiacytidine [3TC]) also inhibits the HIV reverse transcriptase by preventing DNA chain elongation and HIV replication. These drugs are available for the treatment of AIDS that is unresponsive to AZT therapy, or they can be given in combination with AZT. Lamivudine is also active on the reverse transcriptase polymerase of HBV. Most of the anti-HIV agents have potential toxic side effects.

Ribavirin

Ribavirin is an analogue of the nucleoside guanosine (see Figure 41-1) but differs from guanosine in that its base ring is incomplete and open. Similar to other nucleoside analogues, ribavirin must be phosphorylated. The drug is active in vitro against a broad range of viruses.

Ribavirin monophosphate resembles guanosine monophosphate and inhibits nucleoside biosynthesis, mRNA capping, and other processes important to the replication of many viruses. Ribavirin depletes the cellular stores of guanine by inhibiting inosine monophosphate dehydrogenase, an enzyme important in the synthetic pathway of guanosine. It also prevents the synthesis of the mRNA 5′ cap by interfering with the guanylation and methylation of the nucleic acid base. In addition, ribavirin triphosphate inhibits RNA polymerases and promotes hypermutation of the viral genome. Its multiple sites of action may explain the lack of ribavirin-resistant mutants.

Ribavirin is administered in an aerosol to children with severe respiratory syncytial virus bronchopneumonia and potentially to adults with severe influenza or measles. The drug may be effective for the treatment of influenza B, as well as Lassa, Rift Valley, Crimean-Congo, Korean, and Argentine hemorrhagic fevers, for which it is administered orally or intravenously. Ribavirin is approved for use against HCV in combination with IFN-α. Treatment can have serious side effects.

Other Nucleoside Analogues

Idoxuridine was the first anti-HSV drug approved for human use but has been replaced by trifluridine and other more effective, less toxic agents. Fluorouracil is an antineoplastic drug that kills rapidly growing cells but has also been used for the topical treatment of warts caused by human papillomaviruses.

NONNUCLEOSIDE POLYMERASE INHIBITORS

Foscarnet (PFA) and the related phosphonoacetic acid (PAA) are simple compounds that resemble pyrophosphate (Figure 41-3). These drugs inhibit viral replication by binding to the pyrophosphate-binding site of the DNA polymerase to block nucleotide binding. PFA and PAA do not inhibit cellular polymerases at pharmacologic concentrations, but they can cause renal and other problems because of their ability to chelate divalent metal ions (e.g., calcium) and become incorporated into bone. PFA inhibits the DNA polymerase of all herpesviruses and the HIV reverse transcriptase without having to

be phosphorylated by nucleoside kinases (e.g., thymidine kinase). PFA has been approved for the treatment of CMV retinitis in patients with AIDS.

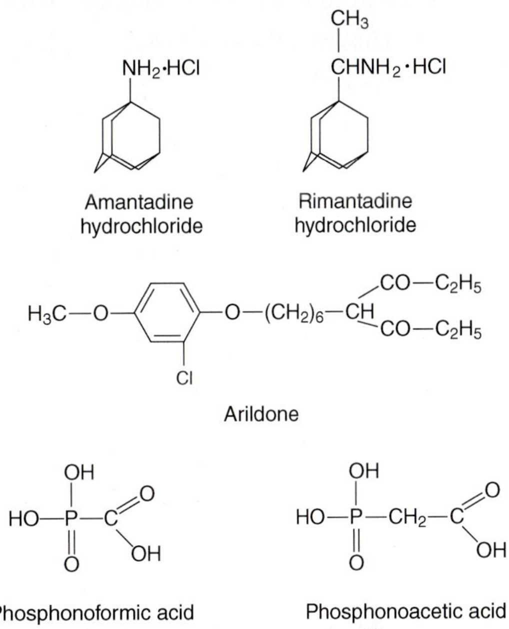

Figure 41-3   Structures of nonnucleoside antiviral drugs.

PROTEASE INHIBITORS

The unique structure of the HIV protease and its essential role in the production of a functional virion have made this enzyme a good target for antiviral drugs. **Saquinavir, indinavir, ritonavir, nelfinavir, amprenavir,** and other agents work by slipping into the hydrophobic active site of the enzyme to inhibit its action. As occurs with the other anti-HIV drugs, drug-resistant strains arise through mutation of the protease. The combination of a protease inhibitor with AZT and a second nucleoside analogue (HAART) can reduce blood levels of HIV to undetectable levels.

ANTIINFLUENZA DRUGS

Amantadine and **rimantadine** are amphipathic amine compounds with clinical efficacy against the influenza A but not the influenza B virus (see Figure 41-3). These drugs have several effects on influenza A replication. Both compounds are acidotrophic and concentrate in and buffer the contents of the endosomal vesicles involved in the uptake of the influenza virus. This effect can inhibit the acid-mediated change in conformation in the hemagglutinin protein that promotes the fusion of the viral envelope with cell membranes. However, the specificity for influenza A is a result of its ability to bind to and block the proton channel formed by the M_2 membrane protein of the influenza A virus. Resistance is the result of an altered M_2 or hemagglutinin protein.

Amantadine and rimantadine may be useful in ameliorating an influenza A infection if either agent is taken within 48 hours of exposure. They are also useful as a prophylactic treatment in lieu of vaccination. In addition, amantadine is an alternative therapy for Parkinson disease. The principal toxic effect is on the central nervous system, with patients experiencing nervousness, irritability, and insomnia.

Zanamivir (Relenza) and **oseltamivir (Tamiflu)** inhibit influenza A and B as enzyme inhibitors of the neuraminidase of influenza. Without the neuraminidase, the hemagglutinin of the virus binds to sialic acid on other glycoproteins, forming clumps and preventing assembly and virus release.

IMMUNOMODULATORS

Genetically engineered forms of IFN-α have been approved for human use. Interferons work by binding to cell surface receptors and initiating a cellular antiviral response. In addition, interferons stimulate the immune response and promote the immune clearance of viral infection.

IFN-α is active against many viral infections, including hepatitis A, B, and C; HSV; papillomavirus; and rhinovirus. It has been approved for the treatment of condylomaacuminatum (genital warts, a presentation of papillomavirus) and hepatitis C (especially with ribavirin). Attachment of polyethylene glycol to IFN-α (pegylated IFN-α) increases its potency. Pegylated IFN-α is used with ribavirin to treat hepatitis C infections. Natural interferon causes the influenza-like symptoms observed during many viremic and respiratory tract infections, and the synthetic agent has similar side effects during treatment. Inter-feron is discussed further in Chapters 10 and 45.

Imiquimod, a Toll-like receptor ligand, stimulates innate responses to attack the virus infection. This therapeutic approach can activate local protective responses against papillomas, which generally escape immune control.

SUMMARY

The majority of antiviral drugs today generally interrupt viral-encoded enzymes or structures of the virus that are important for replication. Some antiviral drugs are actually stimulators of host innate immune protective responses. Currently, treatable virus infections by antiviral drugs are these caused by DNA viruses including herpes simplex virus (HSV) (treatable with nucleoside analogues), varicella-zoster virus (VZV) (treatable with nucleoside analogues), cytomegalovirus (CMV) (treatable with nucleoside analogues), Smallpox virus (treatable with nucleoside analogues), hepatitis B virus (treatable with nucleoside analogues) and RNA viruses including icornaviruses, influenza viruses A and B, respiratory syncytial virus (RSV) (treatable with nucleoside analogues), hepatitis C virus (HCV) (treatable with nucleoside analogues), human immunodeficiency virus (HIV) (treatable with nucleoside analogues). However, resistance to antiviral drugs is becoming more of a problem because of the high rate of mutation for viruses and the long-term treatment of some patients, especially those with the acquired immunodeficiency syndrome (AIDS), or viral hepatitis B and viral hepatitis C.

KEYWORDS

English	Chinese
Acyclovir, ACV	阿昔洛韦
Amantadine	金刚烷胺
Antiviral agents	抗病毒制剂
Azidothymidine, AZT	叠氮胸苷
Ganciclovir, GCV	丙氧鸟苷
Highly active antiretroviral therapy, HAART	高效抗逆转录病毒治疗
Immunomodulator	免疫调节剂

Interferon 干扰素

lamivudine (2'-deoxy-3'-thiacytidine, 拉米夫定
  3TC)

Nucleoside analogues 核苷类似物

Oseltamivir 奥司他韦

Protease Inhibitors 蛋白酶抑制剂

Ribavirin 利巴韦林

Zanamivir 扎那米韦

BIBLIOGRAPHY

1. Carter J, Saunders V: Virology: principles and applications, Chichester, England, 2007, Wiley.

2. Cohen J, Powderly WG: Infectious diseases, ed 2, St Louis, 2004, Mosby.

3. Collier L, Oxford J: Human virology, ed 3, Oxford, England, 2006, Oxford University Press.

4. De Clercq E: A 40-year journey in search of selective antiviral chemotherapy, Ann Rev Pharmacol Toxicol 51: 1-24, 2011.

5. Flint SJ, et al: Principles of virology: molecular biology, pathogenesis and control of animal viruses, ed 3, Washington, DC, 2009, American Society for Microbiology Press.

6. Galasso GJ, Whitley RJ, Merigan TC: Antiviral agents and human viral diseases, ed 4, Philadelphia, 1997, Lippincott.

7. Hodinka RL: What clinicians need to know about antiviral drugs and viral resistance, Infect Dis Clin North Am 11: 945-967, 1997.

8. Knipe DM, et al: Fields virology, ed 5, Philadelphia, 2006, Lippincott Williams & Wilkins.

9. Richman DD: Antiviral drug resistance, Antiviral Res 71: 117-121, 2006.

10. Richman DD, Whitley RJ, Hayden FG: Clinical virology, ed 3, Washington, DC, 2009, American Society for Microbiology Press.

11. Strauss JM, Strauss EG: Viruses and human diseases, ed 2, San Diego, 2007, Academic.

12. Voyles BA: The biology of viruses, ed 2, Boston, 2002, McGraw-Hill.

Antiviral Vaccines

Immunity, whether generated in reaction to immunization or administered as therapy, can prevent or lessen the serious symptoms of disease by **blocking the spread** of a viurs to its target organ or by acting rapidly at the site of infection. The memory immune responses activated upon challenge of an immunized individual are faster and stronger than for an unimmunized individual. The immunization of a population, like personal immunity, stops the spread of the infectious agent by reducing the number of susceptible hosts (**herd immunity**).

In conjunction with immunization programs, measures can be taken to prevent viral disease by limiting the exposure of healthy people to infected people (**quarantine**) and by eliminating the source (e.g., water purification) or means of spread (e.g., mosquito eradication) of the infectious agent. Smallpox is an example of an infection that was controlled by such means. As of 1977, natural smallpox was eliminated through a successful World Health Organization (WHO) program that combined vaccination and quarantine. Polio and measles have also been targeted for elimination.

TYPES OF IMMUNIZATION

The injection of purified antibody or antibody-containing serum to provide rapid, temporary protection or treatment of a person is termed **passive immunization.** Newborns receive natural passive immunity from maternal immunoglobulin that crosses the placenta or is present in the mother's milk.

Active immunization occurs when an immune response is stimulated because of challenge with an immunogen, such as exposure to an infectious agent (**natural immunization**) or through exposure to microbes or their antigens in **vaccines.** On subsequent challenge with the virulent agent, a secondary immune response is activated that is faster and more effective at protecting the individual, or antibody is present to block the spread or function of the agent.

Passive Immunization

Passive immunization may be used as follows:

1. To prevent disease after a known exposure (e.g., needlestick injury with blood that is contaminated with hepatitis B virus [HBV])

2. To ameliorate the symptoms of an ongoing disease

3. To protect immunodeficient individuals

Immune serum globulin preparations derived from seropositive humans or animals (e.g., horses) are available as prophylaxis for several bacterial and viral diseases (Table 42-1). Human serum globulin

Table 42-1 Immune Globulins Available for Postexposure Prophylaxis*

Disease	Source
Hepatitis A	Human
Hepatitis B	Human
Measles	Human
Rabies	Human[†]
Chickenpox, varicella-zoster	Human[†]
Cytomegalovirus	Human
Tetanus	Human,[†] equine
Botulism	Equine
Diphtheria	Equine

*Immune globulins to other agents may also be available.
[†]Specific high-titer antibody is available and is the preferred therapy.

is prepared from pooled plasma and contains the normal repertoire of antibodies for an adult. Special high-titer immune globulin preparations are available for hepatitis B virus (HBIg), varicella-zoster virus (VZIg) and rabies (RIg). Human immunoglobulin is preferable to animal immunoglobulin because there is little risk of a hypersensitivity reaction (serum sickness).

Active Immunization

The term *vaccine* is derived from vaccinia virus, a less virulent member of the poxvirus family that is used to immunize people against smallpox. Classical vaccines can be subdivided into two groups on the basis of whether they elicit an immune response on infection (**live vaccines** such as vaccinia) or not (**inactivated-subunit-killed vaccines**).

Inactivated Vaccines

Inactivated vaccines utilize a large amount of antigen to produce a protective antibody response but without the risk of infection by the agent. Inactivated vaccines can be produced by chemical (e.g., formalin) or heat inactivation of viruses, or by purification or synthesis of the components or subunits of the infectious agents. Inactivated vaccines usually generate antibody (TH2 responses) and limited cell-mediated immune responses.

These vaccines are usually administered with an adjuvant, which boosts their immunogenicity by enhancing uptake by or stimulating dendritic cells (DCs) and macrophages. Many adjuvants stimulate Toll-like receptors to activate these antigen-presenting cells. Most vaccines are precipitated onto alum to promote uptake by DCs and macrophages. MF59 (squalene microfluidized in an oil and water emulsion) and monophosphoryl lipid A (MPL) are adjuvants used in some newer vaccines.

Inactivated, rather than live, vaccines are used to confer protection against most viruses that cannot be attenuated, may cause recurrent infection, or have oncogenic potential. Inactivated vaccines are generally safe, except in people who have allergic reactions to vaccine components. For example, many antiviral vaccines are produced in eggs and therefore cannot be administered to people who are allergic to eggs. The disadvantages of inactivated vaccines are listed below and compared to live vaccines see in Table 8-1.

Immunity is not usually lifelong.

Immunity may be only humoral (TH2) and not cell mediated.

The vaccine does not elicit a local IgA response.

Booster shots are required.

Larger doses must be used.

Inactivated viral vaccines are available for polio, hepatitis A, influenza, and rabies, among other viruses. The Salk polio vaccine (inactivated poliomyelitis vaccine [IPV]) is prepared through the formaldehyde inactivation of virions. A rabies vaccine is prepared through the chemical inactivation of virions grown in human diploid tissue culture cells.

A subunit vaccine consists of the bacterial or viral components that elicit a protective immune response. Surface structures of the viral attachment proteins (capsid or glycoproteins) elicit protective antibodies. T-cell antigens may also be included in a subunit vaccine. The immunogenic component can be isolated from the virus, or virally infected cells by biochemical means, or the vaccine can be prepared through genetic engineering by the expression of cloned viral genes in bacteria or eukaryotic cells. For example, the HBV subunit vaccine was initially prepared from surface antigen obtained from human sera of chronic carriers of the virus. Today HBV vaccine is obtained from yeast bearing the HBsAg gene. The antigen is purified, chemically treated, and absorbed onto alum to be used as a vaccine. The subunit proteins used in the HBV and the human papillomavirus (HPV) vaccines form virus-like particles (VLPs), which are more immunogenic than individual proteins. The HBV and HPV vaccines are also preventing their associated cancers (cervical carcinoma: HPV; primary hepatocellular carcinoma: HBV).

Live Vaccines

Live vaccines are prepared with organisms limited in their ability to cause disease (e.g., avirulent or attenuated organisms). Live vaccines are especially useful for protection against infections caused by enveloped viruses, which require T-cell immune responses for resolution of the infection. Immunization with a live vaccine resembles the natural infection in that the immune response progresses through the natural innate, TH1, and then TH2 immune responses, and humoral, cellular, and memory immune responses are developed. Immunity is generally long lived and, depending on the route of administration, can mimic the normal immune response to the infecting agent. However, the following list includes three problems with live vaccines:

The vaccine virus may still be dangerous for immunosuppressed people or pregnant women, who do not have the immunologic resources to resolve even a weakened virus infection.

The vaccine may revert to a virulent viral form.

The viability of the vaccine must be maintained.

Live virus vaccines consist of less virulent mutants (attenuated) of the wild-type virus, viruses from other species that share antigenic determinants (vaccinia for smallpox, bovine rotavirus), or genetically engineered viruses lacking virulence properties. Wild-type viruses are attenuated by growth in embryonated eggs or tissue culture cells at nonphysiologic temperatures (25°C to 34°C) and away from the selective pressures of the host immune response. These conditions select for or allow the growth of viral strains (mutants) that (1) are less virulent because they grow poorly at 37°C (temperature-sensitive strains [e.g., measles vaccine] and cold-adapted strains [influenza vaccine]), (2) do not replicate well in any human cell (host-range mutants), (3) cannot escape immune control, or (4) can replicate at a benign site but do not disseminate, bind, or replicate in the target tissue characteristically affected by the disease (e.g., polio vaccine replicates in the gastrointestinal tract but does not reach or infect neurons). Table 42-2 lists examples of attenuated live virus vaccines currently in use.

Table 42-2 Viral Vaccines[*]

Virus	Vaccine Components	Who Should Receive Vaccinations
Polio, inactivated	Trivalent (Salk vaccine)	Children
Attenuated polio	Live (oral polio vaccine, Sabin vaccine)	Children
Measles	Attenuated	Children
Mumps	Attenuated	Children
Rubella	Attenuated	Children
Varicella-zoster	Attenuated	Children
Rotavirus	Human-bovine hybrids	Infants
	Attenuated	
Human papilloma-virus	VLP	Girls aged 9-26 yr
Influenza	Inactivated	Children, adults, especially medical personnel, and the elderly
	Attenuated (nasal spray)	2-50 yr
Hepatitis B	Subunit (VLP)	Newborns, health care workers, high-risk groups (e.g., sexually promiscuous, intravenous drug users)
Hepatitis A	Inactivated	Children, child care workers, travelers to endemic areas, Native Americans, and Alaskans
Adenovirus	Attenuated	Military personnel
Yellow fever	Attenuated	Travelers at risk to exposure, military personnel
Rabies	Inactivated	Anyone exposed to virus Preexposure: veterinarians, animal handlers
Smallpox	Live vaccinia virus	Protection from bioterrorism, military
Japanese encephalitis	Inactivated	Travelers at risk to exposure

VLP, Virus-like particle.
[*]Listed in order of frequency of use.

The first vaccine—that for smallpox—was developed by Edward Jenner. The idea for the vaccine came to him when he noted that cowpox (vaccinia), a virulent virus from another species that shares antigenic determinants with smallpox, caused benign infections in humans but conferred protective immunity against smallpox. Albert Sabin developed the first live oral polio vaccine (OPV) in the 1950s. The attenuated virus vaccine was obtained by multiple passages of the three types of poliovirus through monkey kidney tissue culture cells. At least 57 mutations accumulated in the polio type 1 vaccine strain. When this vaccine is administered orally, IgA is secreted in the gut and IgG in the serum, providing protection along the normal route of infection by the wild-type virus. This vaccine is inexpensive, easy to administer, and relatively stable and can spread to contacts of the immunized individual. Effective immunization programs have led to the elimination of wild-type polio in most of the world. The IPV is used in most of the world for routine well-baby immunizations because of the risk of vaccine-virus-induced polio disease by the OPV.

Live vaccines for measles, mumps, and rubella (administered together as the MMR vaccine), varicella-zoster, and now influenza have been developed. Protection against these infections requires a potent cellular immune response. To elicit a mature T-cell response, the vaccine must be administered after 1 year of age, when there will be no interference by maternal antibodies and cell-mediated immunity is sufficiently mature.

Future Directions for Vaccination

Molecular biology techniques are being used to develop new vaccines. New live vaccines can be created by genetic engineering mutations to inactivate or delete a virulence gene instead of through random attenuation of the virus by passage through tissue culture. Genes from infectious agents that cannot be properly attenuated can be inserted into safe viruses (e.g., vaccinia, canarypox, attenuated adenovirus) to form hybrid virus vaccines. This approach holds the promise of allowing the development of a polyvalent vaccine to many agents in a single, safe, inexpensive, and relatively stable vector. On infection, the hybrid virus vaccine need not complete a replication cycle but simply promote the expression of the inserted gene to initiate an immune response to the antigens. The vaccinia, canarypox, and adenovirus virus vector systems have been used in several experimental hybrid vaccines. A canarypox human immunodeficiency virus (HIV) vaccine followed by two booster immunizations with recombinant HIV glycoprotein 120 showed modest but promising results. A vaccinia-based vaccine is used to immunize forest animals against rabies. Other viruses have also been considered as vectors.

Genetically engineered subunit vaccines are being developed through cloning of genes that encode immunogenic proteins into bacterial and eukaryotic vectors. The greatest difficulties in the development of such vaccines are (1) identifying the appropriate subunit or peptide immunogen that can elicit protective antibody and, ideally, T-cell responses and (2) presenting the antigen in the correct conformation. Once identified, the gene can be isolated, cloned, and expressed in bacteria or yeast cells, and then large quantities of these proteins can be produced. The envelope protein gp120 of HIV, the hemagglutinin of influenza, the G antigen of rabies, and the glycoprotein D of herpes simplex virus have been cloned, and their proteins have been generated in bacteria or eukaryotic cells for use (or potential use) as subunit vaccines.

Peptide subunit vaccines contain *specific epitopes* of microbial proteins that elicit neutralizing antibody or desired T-cell responses. To generate such a response, the peptide must contain sequences that bind to MHC I or MHC II (class I or class II major histocompatibility complex) proteins on DCs for presentation and recognition by T cells to initiate an immune response. The immunogenicity of the peptide can be enhanced by its covalent attachment to a carrier protein (e.g., tetanus toxoid or keyhole limpet hemocyanin [KLH]), a ligand for a Toll-like receptor (e.g., flagellin) or an immunologic peptide that can specifically present the epitope to the appropriate immune response. Better vaccines are being developed as the mechanisms of antigen presentation and T-cell receptor-specific antigens are better understood.

Adjuvants in addition to alum are being developed to enhance the immunogenicity and direct the response of vaccines to a TH1- or TH2-type of response. These include activators of Toll-like receptors, such as oligodeoxynucleotides of CpG, derivatives of lipid A from lipopolysaccharide, cytokines, liposomes, nanoparticles, etc. DNA vaccines offer great potential for immunization against infectious agents that require T-cell responses but are not appropriate for use in live vaccines. For these vaccines, the gene for a protein that elicits protective responses is cloned into a plasmid that allows the protein to be expressed in eukaryotic cells. The naked DNA is injected into the muscle or skin of the vaccine recipient, where the DNA is taken up by cells, the gene is expressed, and the protein is produced, presented to, and activates T-cell responses. DNA vaccines usually require a boost with antigenic protein to produce antibody.

IMMUNIZATION PROGRAMS

An effective vaccine program can save millions of dollars in health care costs. Such a program not only protects each vaccinated person against infection and disease but also reduces the number of susceptible people in the population, thereby preventing the spread of the infectious agent within the population. Although immunization may be the best means of protecting people against infection, vaccines cannot be developed for all infectious agents. One reason is that it is very time consuming and costly to develop vaccines.

Natural smallpox was eliminated by means of an effective vaccine program because it was a good candidate for such a program; the virus existed in only one serotype, symptoms were always present in infected people, and the vaccine was relatively benign and stable. However, its elimination came about only as the result of a concerted, cooperative effort on the part of the WHO and local health agencies worldwide. Rhinovirus is an example of a poor candidate for vaccine development, because the viral disease is not serious and there are too many serotypes for vaccination to be successful. From the standpoint of the individual, the ideal vaccine should elicit dependable, lifelong immunity to infection without serious side effects. Factors that influence the success of an immunization program include not only the composition of the vaccine but also the timing, site, and conditions of its administration. Misinformation regarding safety issues with vaccines has deterred some individuals from being vaccinated putting them at risk to disease.

SUMMARY

A vaccine is a biological preparation that provides active immunization to a particular disease. The memory immune responses activated upon challenge of a vaccine-immunized individual are faster and stronger than for an unimmunized individual.

Classical vaccines can be subdivided into two groups on the basis of whether they elicit an immune response on infection (live vaccines) or not (inactivated-subunit-killed vaccines). Live vaccines are prepared with organisms limited in their ability to cause disease. Live vaccines are especially useful for protection against infections caused by enveloped viruses, which require T-cell immune responses for resolution of the infection. Inactivated vaccines utilize a large amount of antigen to produce a protective antibody response but without the risk of infection by the agent. Nowadays, molecular biology techniques are being used to develop new vaccines, which include hybrid virus vaccines, genetically engineered subunit vaccines, Peptide subunit vaccines and DNA vaccines.

KEYWORDS

English	Chinese
Adjuvant	佐剂
Booster immunization	加强免疫
Herd immunity	群体免疫

Inactivated poliomyelitis vaccine, IPV	灭活脊髓灰质炎疫苗
Oral polio vaccine, OPV	口服脊髓灰质炎减毒活疫苗
Live vaccine	活疫苗
Virus-like particles, VLPs	病毒样颗粒

BIBLIOGRAPHY

1. Plotkin SA, Orenstein WA: Vaccines, ed 5, Philadelphia, 2005, WB Saunders.

2. Centers for Disease Control and Prevention, Atkinson W, Wolfe S, Hamborsky J, editors: Epidemiology and prevention of vaccine-preventable diseases (the pink book), ed 12, Washington, DC, 2011, Public Health Foundation.

3. Rosenthal KS: Vaccines make good immune theater: immunization as described in a three-act play, Infect Dis Clin Pract 14: 35-45, 2006.

4. Rosenthal KS, Zimmerman DH: Vaccines: all things considered, Clin Vaccine Immunol 13: 821-829, 2006.

Papillomaviruses and Polyomaviruses

Chapter

43

What used to be called the **papovavirus family** (*Papovaviridae*) has been divided into two families, *Papillomaviridae* and *Polyomaviridae* (Table 43-1). These viruses are capable of causing lytic, chronic, latent, and transforming infections, depending on the host cell. Human papillomaviruses (HPVs) cause **warts**, and several genotypes are associated with human cancer (e.g., **cervical carcinoma**). **BK** and **JC** viruses, members of the *Polyomaviridae*, usually cause asymptomatic infection but are associated with renal disease and **progressive multifocal leukoencephalopathy (PML)**, respectively, in immunosuppressed people. Simian virus 40 (SV40) is the prototype polyomavirus.

The papillomaviruses and polyomaviruses are small, nonenveloped, icosahedral capsid viruses with double-stranded circular deoxyribonucleic acid (DNA) genomes. They encode proteins that promote cell growth. The promotion of cell growth facilitates lytic viral replication in a permissive cell type but **may oncogenically transform a cell that is nonpermissive.** The polyomaviruses, especially SV40, have been studied extensively as model oncogenic viruses.

Table 43-1 Human Papillomaviruses and Polyomaviruses and Their Diseases

Virus	Disease
Papillomavirus	Warts, condylomas, papillomas, cervical cancer*
Polyomavirus	
BK virus	Renal disease†
JC virus	Progressive multifocal leukoencephalopathy†

*High-risk genotypes are present in 99.7% of cervical carcinomas.
†Disease occurs in immunosuppressed patients.

HUMAN PAPILLOMAVIRUSES

Structure and Replication

Classification of the HPVs is based on DNA sequence homology. At least 100 types have been identified and classified into 16 (A through P) groups. HPV can be distinguished further as cutaneous HPV or mucosal HPV on the basis of the susceptible tissue. Within the mucosal HPV, there is a group associated with cervical cancer. Viruses in a group cause similar types of warts. The icosahedral capsid of HPV is 50 to 55 nm in diameter and consists of two structural proteins that form 72 capsomeres (Figure 43-1). The HPV genome is circular and has approximately 8000 base pairs. The HPV DNA encodes seven or eight early genes (E1 to E8), depending on the virus, and two late or structural genes (L1 and L2). An upstream regulatory region contains the control sequences for transcription, the shared N-terminal sequence for the early proteins, and the origin of replication. All the genes are located on one strand (the plus strand) (Figure 43-2).

The L1 protein of HPV is the viral attachment protein and initiates replication by binding to integrins on the cell surface. Replication is also controlled by the host cell's transcriptional machinery, as determined by the differentiation state of the skin or mucosal epithelial cells (Figure 43-3). The virus accesses the basal cell layer through breaks in the skin. The early genes of the virus stimulate cell growth, which facilitates replication of the viral genome by the host cell DNA polymerase when the cells divide. The virus-induced increase in cell number causes the basal and the prickle cell layer (stratum spinosum) to thicken

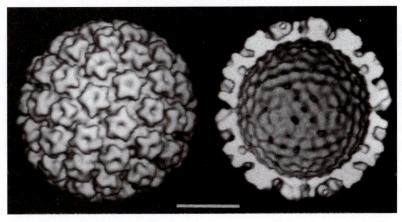

Figure 43-1   Computer reconstruction of cryoelectron micrographs of human papillomavirus (HPV). *Left*, View of the surface of HPV shows 72 capsomeres arranged in an icosadeltahedron. All the capsomeres (pentons and hexons) appear to form a regular five-point star shape. *Right*, Computer cross-section of the capsid shows the interaction of the capsomeres and channels in the capsid. (From Baker TS, et al: Structures of bovine and human papillomaviruses. Analysis by cryoelectron microscopy and three-dimensional image reconstruction, *Biophys J* 60: 1445-1456, 1991.)

(wart, condyloma, or papilloma). As the basal cell differentiates, the specific nuclear factors expressed in the different layers and types of skin and mucosa promote transcription of different viral genes. Expression of the viral genes correlates with the expression of specific keratins. The late genes encoding the structural proteins are expressed only in the terminally differentiated upper layer, and the virus assembles in the nucleus. As the infected skin cell matures and works its way to the surface, the virus matures and is shed with the dead cells of the upper layer.

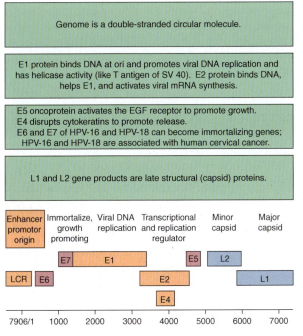

Figure 43-2   Genome of human papillomavirus type 16 (HPV-16). DNA is normally a double-stranded circular molecule, but it is shown here in a linear form. *E5*, Oncogene protein that enhances cell growth by stabilizing and activating the epidermal growth factor receptor; *E6*, oncogene protein that binds p53 and promotes its degradation; *E7*, oncogene protein that binds p105RB (p105 retinoblastoma gene product). *EGF*, epidermal growth factor; *L1*, major capsid protein; *L2*, minor capsid protein; *LCR* (URR), long control region (upstream regulatory region); *ori*, origin of replication. (Courtesy Tom Broker, Baltimore.)

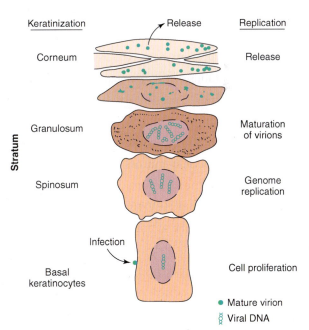

Figure 43-3   Development of papilloma (wart). Human papillomavirus infection promotes the outgrowth of the basal layer, increasing the number of prickle cells of the stratum spinosum (acanthosis). These changes cause the skin to thicken and promote the production of keratin (hyperkeratosis), thereby causing epithelial spikes to form (papillomatosis). Virus is produced in the granular cells close to the final keratin layer.

Pathogenesis

Papillomaviruses infect and replicate in the squamous epithelium of skin (warts) and mucous membranes (genital, oral, and conjunctival papillomas) to induce epithelial proliferation. The HPV types are very tissue specific, causing different disease presentations. The wart develops because of virus stimulation of cell growth and thickening of the basal and prickle layers (stratum spinosum), as well as the stratum granulosum. Koilocytes, characteristic of papillomavirus infection, are enlarged keratinocytes with clear haloes around shrunken nuclei. It usually takes 3 to 4 months for the wart to develop (Figure 43-4). The viral infection remains local and generally regresses spontaneously but can recur.

Innate and cell-mediated immunity are important for control and resolution of HPV infections. HPV can suppress or hide from protective immune responses. In addition to very low levels of antigen expression (except in the "near-dead" terminally differentiated skin cell), the keratinocyte is an immunologically privileged site for replication. Inflammatory responses are required to activate protective cytolytic responses and promote resolution of warts. Immunosuppressed persons have recurrences and more severe presentations of papillomavirus infections.

High-risk HPV types (for example HPV-16 and HPV-18) can initiate the development of cervical carcinoma. Viral DNA is found in benign and malignant tumors, especially mucosal papillomas. Almost all cervical carcinomas contain integrated HPV DNA, with 70% from HPV-16 or HPV-18. Breaking of the circular genome within the *E1* or *E2* genes to promote integration often causes these genes to be inactivated, thereby preventing viral replication without preventing the expression of other HPV genes, including the *E5*, *E6*, and *E7* genes (Figure 43-5). The E5, E6, and E7 proteins of HPV-16 and HPV-18 have been identified as oncogenes. The E5 protein enhances cell growth by stabilizing the epidermal growth factor receptor to make the cell more sensitive to growth signals, while the E6 and E7 proteins bind and inactivate the cellular growth-suppressor (transformation-suppressor) proteins, p53 and the *p105* retinoblastoma gene product (RB). E6 binds the p53 protein and targets it for degradation, and E7 binds and inactivates p105. Cell growth and inactivation of p53 makes the cell more susceptible to mutation, chromosomal aberrations, or the action of a cofactor and thereby develops into cancer.

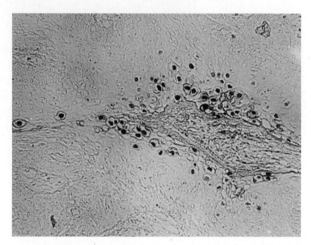

Figure 43-4 DNA probe analysis of an HPV-6-induced anogenital condyloma. A biotin-labeled DNA probe was localized by horseradish peroxidase-conjugated avidin conversion of a substrate to a chromogen precipitate. Dark staining is seen over the nuclei of koilocytotic cells. (From Belshe RB: *Textbook of human virology,* ed 2, St Louis, 1991, Mosby.)

Epidemiology

HPV resists inactivation and can be transmitted on fomites, such as the surfaces of countertops or furniture, bathroom floors, and towels. Asymptomatic shedding may promote transmission. HPV infection is acquired (1) by direct contact through small breaks in the skin or mucosa, (2) during sexual intercourse, or (3) while an infant is passing through an infected birth canal.

Common, plantar, and flat warts are most common in children and young adults. Laryngeal papillomas occur in young children and middle-aged adults.

HPV is possibly the most prevalent sexually transmitted infection in the world, with certain HPV types common among sexually active people. HPV is present in 99.7% of all cervical cancers, with HPV-16 and HPV-18 in 70% of them. Other high-risk strains

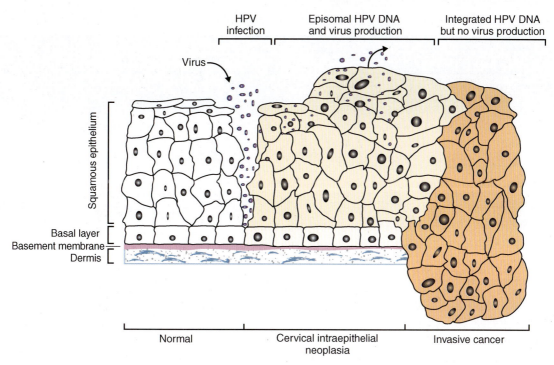

Figure 43-5 Progression of human papilloomavirus *(HPV)*-mediated cervical carcinoma. HPV infects and replicates in the epithelial cells of the cervix, maturing and releasing virus as the epithelial cells progress through terminal differentiation. Growth stimulation of the basal cells produces a wart. In some cells, the circular genome integrates into host chromosomes, inactivating the *E2* gene. Expression of the other genes without virus production stimulates growth of the cells and possible progression to neoplasia. (Adapted from Woodman CBJ, Collins SI, Young LS: The natural history of cervical HPV infection: unresolved issues, *Nat Rev Cancer* 7: 11-22, 2007.)

are listed in Table 43-2. HPV-6 and HPV-11 are low-risk HPV types for cervical carcinoma but cause condyloma acuminatum and oral and laryngeal papillomas. Cervical cancer is the second leading cause of cancer death in women. Approximately 5% of all Pap smears contain HPV-infected cells, and 10% of women infected with the high-risk HPV types will develop cervical dysplasia, a precancerous state. Multiple sexual partners, smoking, a family history of cervical cancer, and immunosuppression are the major risk factors for infection and progression to cancer.

Clinical Syndromes

The clinical syndromes and the HPV types that cause them are summarized in Table 43-2.

Warts

A wart is a benign, self-limited proliferation of skin that regresses with time. Most people with HPV infection have the common types of the virus (HPV-1

through HPV-4), which infect keratinized surfaces, usually on the hands and feet (Figure 43-6).

Benign Head and Neck Tumors

Single oral papillomas are the most benign epithelial tumors of the oral cavity. They are pedunculated with a fibrovascular stalk, and their surface usually has a rough, papillary appearance. They can occur in people of any age group, are usually solitary, and rarely recur after surgical excision. Laryngeal papillomas are commonly associated with HPV-6 and HPV-11 and are the most common benign epithelial tumors of the larynx. Infection of children probably occurs at birth and can be life threatening if the papillomas obstruct the airway. Occasionally, papillomas may be found farther down in the trachea and into the bronchi.

Anogenital Warts

Genital warts (condylomata acuminata) occur almost exclusively on the squamous epithelium of the exter-

Table 43-2 Clinical Syndromes Associated with Papillomaviruses

Syndrome	Human Papillomavirus Types	
	Common	Less Common
Cutaneous Syndromes		
Skin Warts		
Plantar wart	1	2, 4
Common wart	2, 4	1, 7, 26, 29
Flat wart	3, 10	27, 28, 41
Epidermodysplasia verruciformis	5, 8, 17, 20, 36	9, 12, 14, 15, 19, 21-25, 38, 46
Mucosal Syndromes		
Benign Head and Neck Tumors		
Laryngeal papilloma	6, 11	—
Oral papilloma	6, 11	2, 16
Conjunctival papilloma	11	—
Anogenital Warts		
Condyloma acuminatum	6, 11	1, 2, 10, 16, 30, 44, 45
Cervical intraepithelial neoplasia, cancer	16, 18 (high risk)	31, 33, 35, 39, 45, 51, 52, 56, 58, 59, 68, 69, 73, 82

Modified from Balows A, et al, editors: *Laboratory diagnosis of infectious diseases: principles and practice*, vol 2, New York, 1988, Springer-Verlag. Data from Centers for Disease Control and Prevention: *Epidemiology and prevention of vaccine-preventable diseases*, ed 12, Washington, DC, 2001, Public Health Foundation.

nal genitalia and perianal areas. Approximately 90% are caused by HPV-6 and HPV-11. Anogenital lesions infected with these types of HPV can be problematic but rarely become malignant in otherwise healthy people.

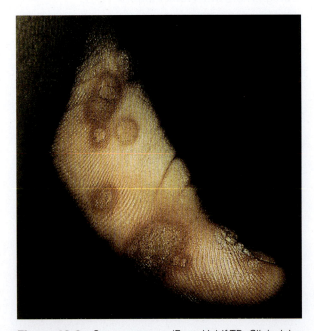

Figure 43-6 Common warts. (From Habif TP: *Clinical dermatology: a color guide to diagnosis and therapy*, St Louis, 1985, Mosby.)

Cervical Dysplasia and Neoplasia

HPV infection of the genital tract is a very common sexually transmitted disease. Infection is usually asymptomatic but may result in slight itching. Genital warts may appear as soft, flesh-colored warts that are flat, raised, and sometimes cauliflower shaped. The warts can appear within weeks or months of sexual contact with an infected person. Cytologic changes indicating HPV infection (koilocytotic cells) are detected in Papanicolaou-stained cervical smears (Pap smears) (Figure 43-7). Infection of the female genital tract by high-risk HPV types is associated with intraepithelial cervical neoplasia and cancer. The first neoplastic changes noted on light microscopy are termed dysplasia. Approximately 40% to 70% of the mild dysplasias spontaneously regress.

Cervical cancer is thought to develop through a continuum of progressive cellular changes, from mild (cervical intraepithelial neoplasia [CIN I]) to moderate neoplasia (CIN II) to severe neoplasia or carcinoma in situ (see Figure 43-5). This sequence of events can occur over 1 to 4 years. Routine and regular Pap smears can prevent or promote early treatment and cure of cervical cancer.

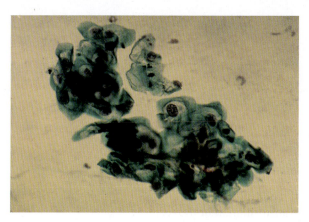

Figure 43-7 Papanicolaou stain of the exfoliated cervico-vaginal squamous epithelial cells, showing the perinuclear cytoplasmic vacuolization termed koilocytosis (vacuolated cytoplasm), which is characteristic of human papillomavirus infection (400× magnification).

Laboratory Diagnosis

A wart can be confirmed microscopically on the basis of its characteristic histologic appearance, which consists of hyperplasia of the prickle cells and an excess production of keratin (hyperkeratosis) (see Figure 43-7). Papillomavirus infection can be detected in Pap smears by the presence of koilocytotic (vacuolated cytoplasm) squamous epithelial cells, which are rounded and occur in clumps (Table 43-3; see Figure 43-4). DNA molecular probe and polymerase chain reaction analysis of cervical swabs and tissue specimens are the methods of choice for establishing the diagnosis and typing of the HPV infection. Papillomaviruses do not grow in cell cultures, and tests for HPV antibodies are rarely used except in research studies.

Table 43-3   Laboratory Diagnosis of Papillomavirus Infections

Test	Detects
Cytology	Koilocytotic cells
In situ DNA probe analysis*	Viral nucleic acid
Polymerase chain reaction*	Viral nucleic acid
Southern blot hybridization	Viral nucleic acid
Culture	Not useful

*Method of choice.

Treatment, Prevention, and Control

Warts spontaneously regress, but the regression may take many months to years. Warts are removed because of pain and discomfort, for cosmetic reasons, and to prevent spread to other parts of the body or to other people. They are removed through the use of surgical cryotherapy, electrocautery, or chemical means (e.g., 10% to 25% solution of podophyllin), although recurrences are common. Surgery may be necessary for the removal of laryngeal papillomas.

Topical or intralesional delivery of cidofovir can treat warts by selectively killing the HPV-infected cells. Cidofovir induces apoptosis by inhibiting the host cell DNA polymerase.

Immunization with either a tetravalent (Gardasil: HPV-6, -11, -16, and -18) or divalent (Cervarix: HPV-16 and -18) HPV vaccine is recommended for girls, starting at age 11 years, before sexual activity to prevent cervical cancer and anogenital warts. The vaccines consist of the L1 major capsid protein assembled into virus-like particles. Vaccination is also recommended for boys to prevent penile and anogenital warts. The HPV vaccine is not a replacement for a Pap smear, and women should continue to be tested.

At present, the best way to prevent transmission of warts is to avoid coming in direct contact with infected tissue. Proper precautions (e.g., the use of condoms) can prevent the sexual transmission of HPV.

POLYOMAVIRIDAE

The human polyomaviruses, BK and JC viruses, are ubiquitous but usually do not cause disease. Less prevalent human polyoma viruses include the KI, WU, and the Merkel cell carcinoma polyomaviruses. SV40, a simian polyomavirus, and murine polyomaviruses, in particular, have been studied extensively as models of tumor-causing viruses, but only recently has a polyomavirus been associated with human cancers.

Structure and Replication

The polyomaviruses are smaller (45 nm in diameter), contain less nucleic acid (5000 base pairs), and are less complex than the papillomaviruses. The genomes of BK virus, JC virus, and SV40 are closely related and are divided into early, late, and noncoding regions

(Figure 43-8). The early region on one-strand codes for nonstructural T (transformation) proteins (including large T, T′, and small t antigens), and the late region, which is on the other strand, codes for three viral capsid proteins (VP1, VP2, and VP3). The noncoding region contains the origin of DNA replication and transcriptional control sequences for both early and late genes.

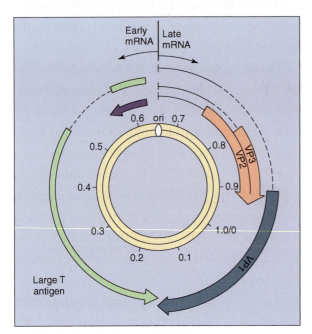

Figure 43-8   Genome of the SV40 virus. The genome is a prototype of other polyomaviruses and contains early, late, and noncoding regions. The noncoding region contains the start sequence for the early and late genes and for DNA replication *(ori)*. The individual early and late mRNAs are processed from the larger nested transcripts. (Modified from Butel JS, Jarvis DL: *Biochim Biophys Acta* 865: 171-195, 1986.)

For JC virus infection of glial cells, the virus binds to sialylated carbohydrates and serotonin receptors and then enters the cell by endocytosis. The DNA genome is uncoated and delivered to the nucleus. The early genes encode the large T and small t antigens, proteins that promote cell growth. Viral replication requires the transcriptional and DNA replication machinery provided by a growing cell. The large T antigens of SV40, BK, and JC viruses have several functions. For example, the T antigen of SV40 binds to DNA and controls early and late gene transcription, as well as viral DNA replication. In addition, the T antigen binds to and inactivates the two major cellular growth-suppressor proteins, p53 and p105RB,

promoting cell growth.

Similar to replication of the HPVs, replication of polyomavirus is highly dependent on host cell factors. Permissive cells allow the transcription of late viral messenger ribonucleic acid (mRNA) and viral replication, which results in cell death. Some nonpermissive cells, however, allow only the early genes, including the T antigen, to be expressed, promoting cell growth and potentially leading to oncogenic transformation of the cell.

Pathogenesis

Each polyomavirus is limited to specific hosts and cell types within that host. For example, JC and BK viruses are human viruses that probably enter the respiratory tract or tonsils, after which they infect lymphocytes and then the kidney with a minimal cytopathologic effect. The BK virus establishes latent infection in the kidney, and the JC virus establishes infection in the kidneys, in B cells, in monocyte-lineage cells, and other cells. Replication is blocked in immunocompetent persons.

In T-cell-deficient patients, such as those with the acquired immunodeficiency syndrome (AIDS), reactivation of the virus in the kidney leads to viral shedding in the urine and potentially severe urinary tract infections (BK virus) or viremia and central nervous system infection (JC virus) (Figure 43-9). JC virus crosses the blood-brain barrier by replicating in the

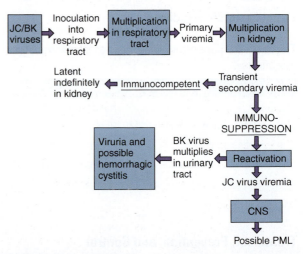

Figure 43-9   Mechanisms of spread of polyomaviruses within the body. *CNS*, Central nervous system; *PML*, progressive multifocal leukoencephalopathy.

endothelial cells of capillaries. An abortive infection of astrocytes results in partial transformation, yielding enlarged cells with abnormal nuclei resembling glioblastomas. Productive lytic infections of oligodendrocytes cause demyelination. Although SV40, BK, and JC viruses can cause tumors in hamsters, these viruses are not associated with any human tumors.

Epidemiology

Polyomavirus infections are ubiquitous, and most people are infected with both the JC and BK viruses by the age of 15 years. Respiratory transmission is the probable mode of spread. Latent infections can be reactivated in people whose immune systems are suppressed because of AIDS, organ transplantation, or pregnancy. Approximately 10% of people with AIDS develop PML, and the disease is fatal in approximately 90% of all cases. The incidence has decreased with the success of the highly active antiretroviral therapy (HAART).

Clinical Syndromes

Primary infection is almost always asymptomatic. The BK and JC viruses are activated in immunocompromised patients, as indicated by the presence of virus in the urine of as many as 40% of these patients. The viruses are also reactivated during pregnancy, but no effects on the fetus have been noted.

The ureteral stenosis observed in renal transplant recipients appears to be associated with BK virus, as is the hemorrhagic cystitis observed in bone marrow transplant recipients. PML caused by the JC virus is a subacute demyelinating disease that occurs in immunocompromised patients, including those with AIDS.

The genome of a new polyomavirus, Merkel cell polyoma virus (MCV or MCPyV), was recently discovered integrated into the chromatin of Merkel cell carcinomas. This is the first example of a polyoma virus associated with a human cancer.

Laboratory Diagnosis

The diagnosis of PML is confirmed by the presence of PCR-amplified viral DNA in cerebrospinal fluid and magnetic resonance imaging or computed tomographic evidence of lesions. In situ immunofluorescence, immunoperoxidase, DNA probe analysis, and PCR analysis of cerebrospinal fluid, urine, or biopsy material for the particular genetic sequences can also be used to detect virus. Urine cytologic tests can reveal the presence of JC or BK virus infection by revealing the existence of enlarged cells with dense, basophilic intranuclear inclusions resembling those induced by cytomegalovirus. It is difficult to isolate BK and JC viruses in tissue cultures.

Treatment, Prevention, and Control

As for papillomaviruses, cidofovir can be used to treat polyomavirus infections. Decreasing the immunosuppression responsible for allowing the polyomavirus to be reactivated is also helpful.

SUMMARY

Human papillomavirus (HPV) causes papillomas, which are nonenveloped viruses with double-stranded circular DNA and an icosahedral nucleocapsid. There are at least 100 types of papillomaviruses, Some HPV types cause benign tumors of squamous cells (e.g., warts on the skin). Some HPV types, especially types 16 and 18, cause carcinoma of the cervix, penis, and anus. Two of the early genes, E6 and E7, are implicated in carcinogenesis. Papillomavirus E6 protein binds to p53, activates telomerase, and suppresses apoptosis, and E7 protein binds to p105RB. Inactivation of the p53 and p105RB is an important step in the process by which a normal cell becomes a cancer cell. Immunization with either a tetravalent (Gardasil: HPV-6, -11, -16, and -18) or bivalent (Cervarix: HPV-16 and -18) HPV vaccine is recommended.

Polyomaviruses, including BK virus and JC virus, are ubiquitous but rarely cause disease in healthy individuals. Less prevalent human polyoma viruses include the KI, WU, and the Merkel cell carcinoma polyomaviruses. In immunocompromised people, JC virus is activated, spreads to the brain, and causes PML, a conventional slow virus disease. BK virus is benign but may cause kidney disease in immunocompromised patients.

KEYWORDS

English	Chinese
Papillomaviruses	乳头瘤病毒
Polyomaviruses	多瘤病毒
Cervical cancer	宫颈癌
Warts	疣
Condylomata acuminata	尖锐湿疣
Progressive multifocal leukoencephalopathy	进行性多灶性白质脑病

BIBLIOGRAPHY

1. Balows A, Hausler WJ, Lennette EH. Laboratory diagnosis of infectious diseases: principles and practice, New York, 1988, Springer-Verlag.

2. Benihoud K, Yeh P, Perricaudet M. Adenovirus vectors for gene delivery, Curr Opin Biotechnol 10: 440-447, 1999.

3. Carter J, Saunders V. Virology: principles and applications, Chichester, England, 1988, Wiley.

4. Cohen J, Powderly WG. Infectious diseases, ed 3, St Louis, 2004, Mosby.

5. Collier L, Oxford J. Human virology, ed 3, Oxford, England, 2006, Oxford University Press.

6. Doerfler W, Böhm P. Adenoviruses: model and vectors in virus-host interactions, *Curr Top Microbiol Immunol*, vols 272-273, New York, 2003, Springer-Verlag.

7. Flint SJ, et al. Principles of virology: molecular biology, pathogenesis, and control of animal viruses, ed 2, Washington, DC, 2003, American Society of Microbiology Press.

8. Ginsberg HS. The adenoviruses, New York, 1984, Plenum.

9. Gorbach SL, Bartlett JG, Blacklow NR. Infectious diseases, ed 3, Philadelphia, 2004, WB Saunders.

10. Knipe DM, et al. Fields virology, ed 5, Philadelphia, 2006, Lippincott Williams & Wilkins.

11. Kolavic-Gray SA, et al. Large epidemic of adenovirus type 4 infection among military trainees: epidemiological, clinical, and laboratory studies, Clin Infect Dis 35: 808-818, 2002.

12. Lenaerts L, De Clercq E, Naesens L. Clinical features and treatment of adenovirus infections, Rev Med Virol 18: 357-374, 2008.

13. Mandell GL, Bennet JE, Dolin R. Principles and practice of infectious diseases, ed 6, Philadelphia, 2005, Churchill Livingstone.

14. Robbins PD, Ghivizzani SC. Viral vectors for gene therapy, Pharmacol Ther 80: 35-47, 1998.

15. Strauss JM, Strauss EG. Viruses and human disease, ed 2, San Diego, 2007, Academic.

16. Voyles BA: The biology of viruses, ed 2, Boston, 2002, McGraw-Hill.

Chapter 44

Adenoviruses

Adenoviruses were first isolated in 1953 in a human adenoid cell culture. Since then, approximately 100 serotypes have been recognized, at least 52 of which infect humans. All human serotypes are included in a single genus within the family *Adenoviridae*. There are 7 subgroups for human adenoviruses (A through G) (Table 44-1).

STRUCTURE AND REPLICATION

Adenoviruses are double-stranded DNA viruses with a genome of approximately 36,000 base pairs, large enough to encode 30 to 40 genes. The adenovirus genome is a **linear, double-stranded DNA** with a 55 kDa of **terminal protein** covalently attached at each 5′ end. The virions are **nonenveloped icosadeltahedrons** with a diameter of 70 to 90 nm (Figure 44-1). The capsid comprises 240 capsomeres, which consist of hexons and pentons. The 12 pentons, which are located at each of the vertices, have a penton base and a fiber. The **fiber** contains the **viral attachment proteins** and can act as a hemagglutinin. The penton base and fiber are toxic to cells. The pentons and fibers also carry type-specific antigens.

The core complex within the capsid includes viral DNA and at least two major proteins. There are at least 11 proteins in the adenovirus virion, 9 of which have an identified structural function.

A map of the adenovirus genome shows the locations of the viral genes (Figure 44-2). The genes are transcribed from both DNA strands and in both directions at different times during the replication cycle. Genes for related functions are clustered together. Most of the RNA transcribed from the adenovirus genome is processed into several individual mRNAs in the nucleus. Early proteins promote

Table 44-1 Illnesses Associated with Adenoviruses

Disease	Types	Patient Population
Respiratory Diseases		
Febrile, undifferentiated upper respiratory tract infection	1, 3, 5, 7, 14, 21, etc.	Infants, young children
Pharyngoconjunctival fever	1, 2, 3, 4, 5, 7	Children, adults
Acute respiratory disease	4, 7, 14, 21	Infants, young children; military recruits
Pertussis-like syndrome	5	Infants, young children
Pneumonia	3, 4, 7, 21	Infants, young children; military recruits; immunocompromised patients
Other Diseases		
Acute hemorrhagic cystitis	11, 21	Children; immunocompromised patients
Epidemic keratoconjunctivitis	8, 9, 11, 19, 35, 37	Any age
Gastroenteritis	40, 41	Infants, young children, immunocompromised patients
Hepatitis	1-5, 7, 31	Immunocompromised patients
Meningoencephalitis	2, 7	Children; immunocompromised patients

Adenovirus

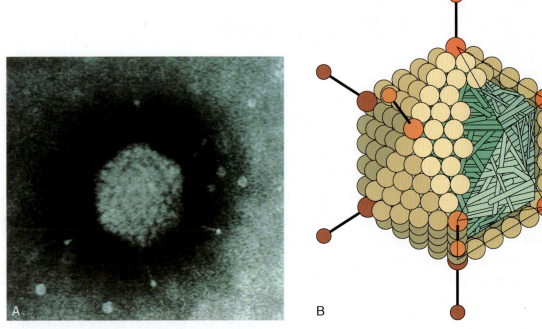

Figure 44-1 A, Electron micrograph of adenovirus virion with fibers. **B,** Model of adenovirus virion with fibers. (**A,** From Valentine RC, Pereira HG: Antigens and structure of the adenovirus, *J Mol Biol* 13: 13-20, 1965. **B,** From Armstrong D, Cohen J: *Infectious diseases*, St Louis, 1999, Mosby.)(original Figure 50-1, 7th)

cell growth and include a **DNA polymerase** that is involved in the replication of the genome. Adenovirus also encodes proteins that suppress apoptosis and host immune and inflammatory responses. Late proteins, which are synthesized after the onset of

viral DNA replication, are primarily components of the capsid. Viral DNA replication occurs in the nucleus and is mediated by the viral-encoded DNA polymerase. Capsid proteins are produced in the cytoplasm and then transported to the nucleus for viral assembly. Empty procapsids first assemble, and then the viral DNA and core proteins enter the capsid through an opening at one of the vertices. The virus remains in the cell and is released when the cell degenerates and lyses.

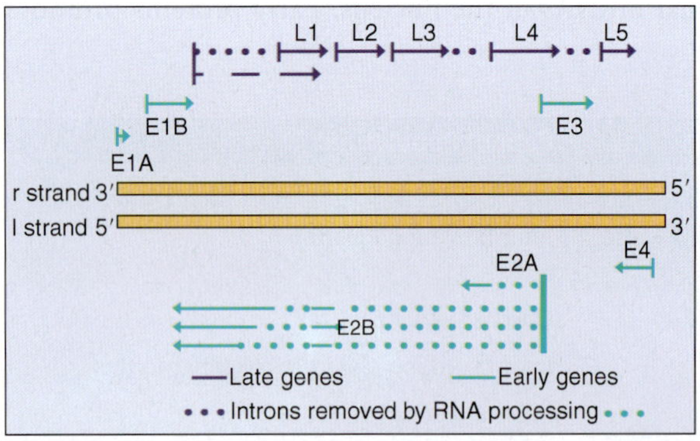

PATHOGENESIS AND IMMUNITY

Adenoviruses are capable of causing lytic (e.g., muco-epithelial cells), latent (e.g., lymphoid and adenoid cells), and transforming (hamster, not human) infections. These viruses infect epithelial cells lining the oropharynx, as well as the respiratory and enteric organs. The viral fiber proteins determine the target cell specificity. The toxic activity of the penton base protein can result in inhibition of cellular mRNA transport and protein synthesis, cell rounding, and tissue damage.

Figure 44-2 Simplified genome map of adenovirus type 2. Genes are transcribed from both strands (*l* and *r*) in opposite directions. The early genes are transcribed from four promoter sequences, and each generates several messenger RNAs by processing the primary RNA transcripts. This produces the full repertoire of viral proteins. The splicing pattern for only the E2 transcript is shown as an example. All of the late genes are transcribed from one promoter sequence. *E*, Early protein; *L*, late protein.(Modified from Jawetz E, et al: *Review of medical microbiology*, ed 17, Norwalk, Conn, 1987, Appleton & Lange.)

The histologic hallmark of adenovirus infection is a dense, central intranuclear inclusion (that consists of viral DNA and protein) within an infected epithelial cell. Mononuclear cell infiltrates and epithelial cell necrosis are seen at the site of infection.

Viremia may occur after local replication of the virus, with subsequent spread to visceral organs (Figure 44-3). This dissemination is more likely to occur in immunocompromised patients than in immunocompetent ones. The virus has a propensity to become latent and persist in lymphoid and other tissue, such as adenoids, tonsils, and Peyer patches, and can be reactivated in immunosuppressed patients. Although certain adenoviruses (groups A and B) are oncogenic in certain rodents, adenovirus transformation of human cells has not been observed.

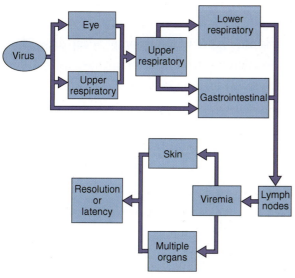

Figure 44-3 Mechanism of adenovirus spread within the body.

Antibody is important for resolving lytic adenovirus infections and protects the person from reinfection with the same serotype but not other serotypes. Cell-mediated immunity is important in limiting virus outgrowth, and immunosuppressed people suffer more serious and recurrent disease.

Epidemiology

Adenovirus virions resist drying, detergents, gastrointestinal tract secretions (acid, protease, and bile), and even mild chlorine treatment. These virions are spread in aerosols and by the fecal-oral route, by fingers, by fomites (including towels and medical instruments), and in poorly chlorinated swimming pools. Crowds and close proximity, as occurs in classrooms and military barracks, promotes spread of the virus. Adenoviruses may be shed intermittently and over long periods from the pharynx and especially in feces. Most infections are asymptomatic, a feature that greatly facilitates their spread in the community.

Adenoviruses 1 through 7 are the most prevalent serotypes. From 5% to 10% of cases of pediatric respiratory tract disease is caused by adenovirus types 1, 2, 5, and 6, and the infected children shed virus for months after infection. Adenovirus causes 15% of the cases of gastroenteritis requiring hospitalization. Serotypes 4 and 7 seem especially able to spread among military recruits because of their close proximity and rigorous lifestyle.

Clinical Syndromes

Adenoviruses primarily infect children and, less commonly, infect adults. Disease from reactivated virus occurs in immunocompromised children and adults. Specific clinical syndromes are associated with specific adenovirus types (see Table 44-1).

Acute Febrile Pharyngitis and Pharyngoconjunctival Fever

Adenovirus causes pharyngitis, which is often accompanied by conjunctivitis and pharyngoconjunctival fever. Pharyngitis alone occurs in young children, particularly those younger than 3 years, and may mimic streptococcal infection. Affected patients have mild, flulike symptoms that may last 3 to 5 days. Pharyngoconjunctival fever occurs more often in outbreaks involving older children.

Acute Respiratory Disease

Acute respiratory disease is a syndrome consisting of fever, runny nose, cough, pharyngitis, and possible conjunctivitis.

Adenoviruses can also cause coldlike symptoms, laryngitis, croup, and bronchiolitis, or a pertussis-like illness in children and adults that consists of a prolonged clinical course and true viral pneumonia.

Conjunctivitis and Epidemic Keratoconjunctivitis

Adenoviruses cause a follicular conjunctivitis in which the mucosa of the palpebral conjunctiva becomes pebbled or nodular, and both conjunctivae (palpebral and bulbar) become inflamed. Such conjunctivitis may occur sporadically or in outbreaks that can be traced to a common source. Swimming pool conjunctivitis is a familiar example of a common-source adenovirus infection. Epidemic keratoconjunctivitis may be an occupational hazard for industrial workers. Irritation of the eye by a foreign body, dust, debris, and so forth is a risk factor for the acquisition of this infection.

Gastroenteritis and Diarrhea

Adenovirus is a major cause of acute viral gastroenteritis especially in infants. The enteric adenoviruses (types 40 to 42) do not replicate in the same tissue culture cells as do other adenoviruses and rarely cause fever or respiratory tract symptoms.

Other Manifestations

Adenovirus has also been associated with intussusception in young children, acute hemorrhagic cystitis with dysuria and hematuria in young boys, musculoskeletal disorders, and genital and skin infections. Adenovirus (type 36) is also associated with obesity.

Systemic Infection in Immunocompromised Patients

Immunocompromised patients are at risk for serious adenovirus infections, although not as much as they are for infections caused by herpesviruses. Adenoviral disease in immunocompromised patients includes pneumonia and hepatitis. Infection can originate from exogenous or endogenous (reactivation) sources.

Laboratory Diagnosis

For the results of virus isolation to be significant, the isolate should be obtained from a site or secretion relevant to the disease symptoms. The isolation of most adenovirus types is best accomplished in cell cultures derived from epithelial cells (e.g., primary human embryonic kidney cells, continuous [transformed] lines, such as HeLa).

Direct analysis of the clinical sample without virus isolation can be used for rapid detection and identification of adenoviruses. Immunoassays, including fluorescent antibody and enzyme-linked immunosorbent assay, and genome assays, including different variations of the polymerase chain reaction (PCR) and DNA probe analysis, can be used to detect, type, and group the virus in clinical samples and tissue cultures.

TREATMENT, PREVENTION, AND CONTROL

Careful handwashing and chlorination of swimming pools can reduce transmission of adenovirus. There is no approved treatment for adenovirus infection. The vaccine that can be used in civilian populations is not available.

THERAPEUTIC ADENOVIRUSES

Adenoviruses have been used and are being considered for gene delivery for correction of human diseases, including immune deficiencies, cystic fibrosis, and lysosomal storage diseases.

SUMMARY

Adenoviruses are double-stranded DNA viruses. Common disorders caused by the adenoviruses include respiratory tract infection, pharyngoconjunctivitis (pinkeye), hemorrhagic cystitis, and gastroenteritis. The predominant route of transmission of adenovirus is aerosols inhalation, but adenovirus is also transmitted by contact and the fecal-oral route. Antibody is sufficient to control the spread of adenoviruses. However, adenovirus can also establish chronic infection, and natural killer and T cells are important in killing and controlling the chronic and latent infection. Several adenoviruses have oncogenic potential in animals, but not humans. Adenovirus is also being used in genetic therapies to deliver DNA. Virus isolation, immunoassays, and genome assays can be used for laboratory diagnosis. There are no approved drugs and vaccine for adenovirus infection.

KEYWORDS

English	Chinese
Adenovirus	腺病毒
Hexon	六邻体
Penton	五邻体
Pharyngoconjunctivitis	咽结膜炎
Epidemic keratoconjunctivitis	流行性角膜结膜炎
Hemorrhagic cystitis	出血性膀胱炎

BIBLIOGRAPHY

1. Balows A, Hausler WJ, Lennette EH. Laboratory diagnosis of infectious diseases: principles and practice, New York, 1988, Springer-Verlag.

2. Benihoud K, Yeh P, Perricaudet M. Adenovirus vectors for gene delivery, Curr Opin Biotechnol 10: 440-447, 1999.

3. Carter J, Saunders V. Virology: principles and applications, Chichester, England, 1988, Wiley.

4. Cohen J, Powderly WG. Infectious diseases, ed 3, St Louis, 2004, Mosby.

5. Collier L, Oxford J. Human virology, ed 3, Oxford, England, 2006, Oxford University Press.

6. Doerfler W, Böhm P. Adenoviruses: model and vectors in virus-host interactions, *Curr Top Microbiol Immunol*, vols 272-273, New York, 2003, Springer-Verlag.

7. Flint SJ, et al. Principles of virology: molecular biology, pathogenesis, and control of animal viruses, ed 2, Washington, DC, 2003, American Society of Microbiology Press.

8. Ginsberg HS. The adenoviruses, New York, 1984, Plenum.

9. Gorbach SL, Bartlett JG, Blacklow NR. Infectious diseases, ed 3, Philadelphia, 2004, WB Saunders.

10. Knipe DM, et al. Fields virology, ed 5, Philadelphia, 2006, Lippincott Williams & Wilkins.

11. Kolavic-Gray SA, et al. Large epidemic of adenovirus type 4 infection among military trainees: epidemiological, clinical, and laboratory studies, Clin Infect Dis 35: 808-818, 2002.

12. Lenaerts L, De Clercq E, Naesens L. Clinical features and treatment of adenovirus infections, Rev Med Virol 18: 357-374, 2008.

13. Mandell GL, Bennet JE, Dolin R. Principles and practice of infectious diseases, ed 6, Philadelphia, 2005, Churchill Livingstone.

14. Robbins PD, Ghivizzani SC. Viral vectors for gene therapy, Pharmacol Ther 80: 35-47, 1998.

15. Strauss JM, Strauss EG. Viruses and human disease, ed 2, San Diego, 2007, Academic.

16. Voyles BA: The biology of viruses, ed 2, Boston, 2002, McGraw-Hill.

Human Herpesviruses

The human herpesviruses are grouped into three subfamilies on the basis of differences in viral characteristics (genome structure, tissue tropism, cytopathologic effect, and site of latent infection), as well as the pathogenesis of the disease and disease manifestation (Table 45-1).

The herpesviruses are an important group of large, deoxyribonucleic acid (DNA)-enveloped viruses with the following features in common: virion morphology, basic mode of replication, and capacity to establish latent and recurrent infections. Cell-mediated immunity is important for causing symptoms and controlling infection with these viruses. Herpesviruses encode proteins and enzymes that facilitate the replication and interaction of the virus with the host.

Epstein-Barr virus (EBV) and human herpesvirus 8 (HHV-8) are associated with human cancers.

STRUCTURE OF HERPESVIRUSES

The herpesviruses are large, enveloped viruses that contain double-stranded DNA. The virion is approximately 150 nm in diameter and has the characteristic morphology shown in Figure 45-1. The DNA core is surrounded by an icosadeltahedral capsid containing 162 capsomeres. This capsid is enclosed by a glycoprotein-containing envelope. Herpesviruses encode several glycoproteins for viral attachment, fusion, and for escaping immune control. Attached to the capsid and in the space between the envelope

Table 45-1 Properties Distinguishing the Herpesviruses

Subfamily	Virus	Primary Target Cell	Site of Latency	Means of Spread
Alphaherpesvirinae				
Human herpesvirus 1	Herpes simplex type 1	Mucoepithelial cells	Neuron	Close contact (sexually transmitted disease)
Human herpesvirus 2	Herpes simplex type 2	Mucoepithelial cells	Neuron	
Human herpesvirus 3	Varicella-zoster virus	Mucoepithelial and T cells	Neuron	Respiratory and close contact
Gammaherpesvirinae				
Human herpesvirus 4	Epstein-Barr virus	B cells and epithelial cells	B cell	Saliva (kissing disease)
Human herpesvirus 8	Kaposi sarcoma-related virus	Lymphocyte and other cells	B cell	Close contact (sexual), saliva?
Betaherpesvirinae				
Human herpesvirus 5	Cytomegalovirus	Monocyte, granulocyte, lymphocyte, and epithelial cells	Monocyte, myeloid stem cell, and ?	Close contact, transfusions, tissue transplant, and congenital
Human herpesvirus 6	Herpes lymphotropic virus	Lymphocytes and ?	T cells and ?	Saliva
Human herpesvirus 7	Human herpesvirus 7	Like human herpesvirus 6	T cells and ?	Saliva

Indicates that other cells may also be the primary target or site of latency.

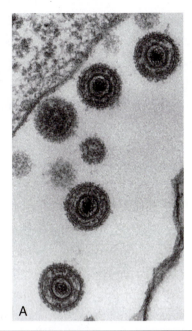

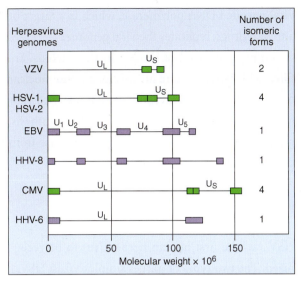

Figure 45-2 Herpesvirus genomes. The genomes of the herpesvirus are doubled-stranded DNA. The length and complexity of the genome differ for each virus. Inverted repeats in herpes simplex virus *(HSV)*, varicella-zoster virus *(VZV)*, and cytomegalovirus *(CMV)* allow the genome to recombine with itself to form isomers. Large genetic repeat sequences are boxed. The genomes of HSV and CMV have two sections, the unique long *(U_L)* and the unique short *(U_S)*, each of which is bracketed by two sets of inverted repeats of DNA. The inverted repeats facilitate the replication of the genome but also allow the U_L and U_S regions to invert independently of each other to yield four different genomic configurations, or isomers. VZV has only one set of inverted repeats and can form two isomers. Epstein-Barr virus *(EBV)* exists in only one configuration, with several unique regions surrounded by direct repeats. Purple bars indicate direct repeat DNA sequences; green bars indicate inverted repeated DNA sequences. *HHV-6*, Human herpesvirus 6; *HHV-8*, human herpesvirus 8.

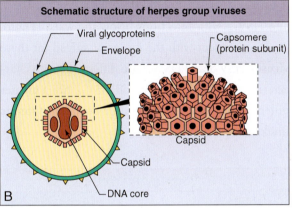

Figure 45-1 Electron micrograph **(A)** and general structure **(B)** of the herpesviruses. The DNA genome of the herpesvirus in the core is surrounded by an icosadeltahedral capsid and an envelope. Glycoproteins are inserted into the envelope. (**A,** From Armstrong D, Cohen J: *Infectious diseases*, St Louis, 1999, Mosby.)

and the capsid (the tegument) are viral proteins and enzymes that help initiate replication. As enveloped viruses, the herpesviruses are sensitive to acid, solvents, detergents, and drying.

Herpesviral genomes differ in size and gene orientation (Figure 45-2). Direct or inverted repeat sequences bracket unique regions of the genome (unique long [U_L], unique short [U_S]), allowing circularization and recombination within the genome. Recombination among inverted repeats of HSV, CMV, and VZV allows large portions of the genome to flip the orientation of their U_L and U_S gene segments with respect to each other to form isomeric genomes.

HERPESVIRUS REPLICATION

Herpesvirus replication is initiated by the interaction of viral glycoproteins with cell surface receptors. The virus can fuse its envelope with the plasma membrane, releasing the nucleocapsid into the cytoplasm. Enzymes and transcription factors are carried into the cell in the tegument of the virion. The nucleocapsid docks with the nuclear membrane and delivers the genome into the nucleus, where the genome is transcribed and replicated.

Transcription of the viral genome and viral protein synthesis proceeds in a coordinated and regulated manner in three phases including immediate early proteins, early proteins, and late proteins. The viral-encoded DNA polymerase, which is a target of antiviral drugs, replicates the viral genome.

Empty procapsids assemble in the nucleus, are filled with DNA, acquire an envelope at the nuclear or Golgi membrane, and exit the cell by exocytosis or by lysis of the cell. Transcription, protein synthesis, glycoprotein processing, and exocytotic release from the cell are performed by cellular machinery.

HERPES SIMPLEX VIRUS

HSV was the first human herpesvirus to be recognized. The two types of herpes simplex virus, HSV-1 and HSV-2, share many characteristics, including DNA homology, antigenic determinants, tissue tropism, and disease signs. However, they can still be distinguished by subtle but significant differences in these properties.

Proteins and Replication

The HSV genome is large enough to encode approximately 80 proteins. Only half the proteins are required for viral replication; the others facilitate HSV's interaction with different host cells and the immune response. The HSV genome encodes enzymes, including a DNA-dependent DNA polymerase and scavenging enzymes, such as deoxyribonuclease, thymidine kinase, ribonucleotide reductase, and protease. Ribonucleotide reductase converts ribonucleotides to deoxyribonucleotides, and thymidine kinase phosphorylates the deoxyribonucleosides to provide substrates for replication of the viral genome. The substrate specificities of these enzymes and the DNA polymerase differ significantly from those of their cellular analogues and thus represent potentially good targets for antiviral chemotherapy.

HSV encodes at least 11 glycoproteins that serve as viral attachment proteins (gB, gC, gD, gE/gI), fusion proteins (gB, gH/gL), structural proteins, immune escape proteins (gC, gE, gI), type-specific proteins (gG1 and gG2 for HSV-1 and HSV-2, respectively), and other functions. For example, the C3 component of the complement system binds to gC and is depleted from serum. The Fc portion of

immunoglobulin G (IgG) binds to a gE/gI complex, thereby camouflaging the virus and virus-infected cells. These actions reduce the antiviral effectiveness of antibody.

HSV can infect most types of human cells and even cells of other species. The virus generally causes lytic infections of fibroblasts and epithelial cells and latent infections of neurons.

Pathogenesis and Immunity

The mechanisms involved in the pathogenesis of HSV-1 and HSV-2 are very similar. Both viruses initially infect, replicate in mucoepithelial cells, cause disease at the site of infection, and then establish latent infection of the innervating neurons. HSV-1 is usually associated with infections above the waist, and HSV-2 with infections below the waist (Figure 45-3), consistent with the means of spread for these viruses. HSV-1 and HSV-2 also differ in growth characteristics and antigenicity, and HSV-2 has a greater potential to cause viremia with associated systemic flulike symptoms.

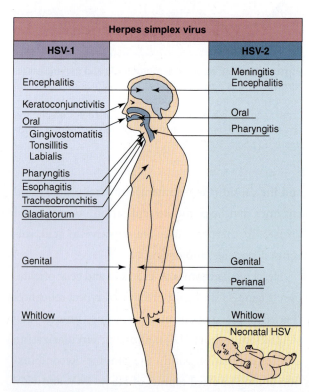

Figure 45-3 Disease syndromes of herpes simplex virus *(HSV)*. HSV-1 and HSV-2 can infect the same tissues and cause similar diseases but have a predilection for the sites and diseases indicated.

HSV can cause lytic infections of most cells and latent infection of neurons. Cytolysis generally results from the virus-induced inhibition of cellular macromolecular synthesis, the degradation of host cell DNA, membrane permeation, cytoskeletal disruption, and senescence of the cell. Visible changes in the nuclear structure and margination of the chromatin occur, and acidophilic intranuclear inclusion bodies are produced. Many strains of HSV also initiate syncytia formation. In tissue culture, HSV rapidly kills cells, causing them to appear rounded.

HSV initiates infection through mucosal membranes or breaks in the skin. The virus replicates in the cells at the base of the lesion and infects the innervating neuron, traveling by retrograde transport to the ganglion (the trigeminal ganglia for oral HSV and the sacral ganglia for genital HSV) (see Figure 45-5 later). CD8 T cells and interferon-γ are important to maintaining HSV in latency. Upon reactivation, the virus then returns to the initial site of infection, and the infection may be inapparent or may produce vesicular lesions. The vesicle fluid contains infectious virions. Tissue damage is caused by a combination of viral pathology and immunopathology. The lesion generally heals without producing a scar.

Innate protections, including interferon and natural killer cells, may be sufficient to limit the initial progression of the infection. T-helper 1 (Th1)-associated and CD8 cytotoxic killer T-cell responses are required to kill infected cells and resolve the current disease. The immunopathologic effects of the cell-mediated and inflammatory responses are also a major cause of the disease signs. Antibody directed against the glycoproteins of the virus neutralizes extracellular virus, limiting its spread, but is not sufficient to resolve the infection. In the absence of functional cell-mediated immunity, HSV infection is likely to recur, be more severe, and may disseminate to the vital organs and the brain.

Latent infection occurs in neurons and results in no detectable damage. A recurrence can be activated by various stimuli (e.g., stress, trauma, fever, sunlight [ultraviolet B]). These events trigger virus replication in an individual nerve cell within the bundle and allow the virus to travel back down the nerve to cause lesions to develop at the same dermatome and location each time. The stress triggers reactivation by promoting replication of the virus in the nerve, by transiently depressing cell-mediated immunity, or by inducing both processes. The virus can be reactivated despite the presence of antibody. However, recurrent infections are generally less severe, more localized, and of shorter duration than the primary episodes because of the nature of the spread and the existence of memory immune responses.

Epidemiology

Because HSV can establish latency with the potential for asymptomatic recurrence, the infected person is a lifelong source of contagion. As an enveloped virus, HSV is transmitted in secretions and by close contact. The virus is very labile and is readily inactivated by drying, detergents, and the conditions of the gastrointestinal tract. Although HSV can infect animal cells, HSV infection is exclusively a human disease.

HSV is transmitted in vesicle fluid, saliva, and vaginal secretions (the "mixing and matching of mucous membranes"). The site of infection, and hence the disease, is determined primarily by which mucous membranes are mixed. Both types of HSV can cause oral and genital lesions.

HSV-1 infection is common. It is usually spread by oral contact (kissing) or through the sharing of drinking glasses, toothbrushes, or other saliva-contaminated items. HSV-1 can infect the fingers or body through a cut or abraded skin. Autoinoculation may also cause infection of the eyes or fingers.

HSV-2 is spread mainly by sexual contact or autoinoculation or from an infected mother to her infant at birth. Depending on a person's sexual practices and hygiene, HSV-2 may infect the genitalia, anorectal tissues, or oropharynx. The incidence of HSV-1 genital infection is approaching that of HSV-2. HSV may cause symptomatic or asymptomatic primary genital infection or recurrences. Neonatal infection usually results from the excretion of HSV-2 from the cervix during vaginal delivery but can occur from an ascending in utero infection during a primary infection of the mother. Neonatal infection results in disseminated and neurologic disease with severe consequences.

Clinical Syndromes

HSV-1 and HSV-2 are common human pathogens that can cause painful but benign manifestations and recurrent disease. In the classic manifestation, the lesion is a clear vesicle on an erythematous base ("dewdrop on a rose petal") and then progresses to pustular lesions, ulcers, and crusted lesions (Figure 45-4). Both viruses can cause significant morbidity and mortality on infection of the eye or brain and on disseminated infection of an immunosuppressed person or a neonate.

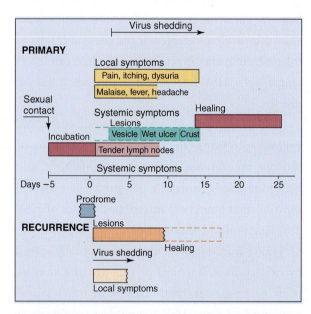

Figure 45-4 Clinical course of genital herpes infection. The time course and symptoms of primary and recurrent genital infection with herpes simplex virus type 2 are compared. *Top,* Primary infection; *bottom,* recurrent disease. (Data from Corey L, et al: Genital herpes simplex virus infection: clinical manifestations, course and complications, *Ann Intern Med* 98: 958-973, 1983.)

Oral Herpes

Primary Oral Herpes

Oral herpes can be caused by HSV-1 or HSV-2. The lesions of herpes labialis or gingivostomatitis begin

as clear vesicles that rapidly ulcerate. The vesicles may be widely distributed around or throughout the mouth, involving the palate, pharynx, gingivae, buccal mucosa, and tongue (Figure 45-5). Many other conditions (e.g., Coxsackie virus lesions, canker sores, acne) may resemble HSV lesions.

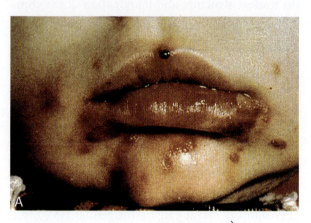

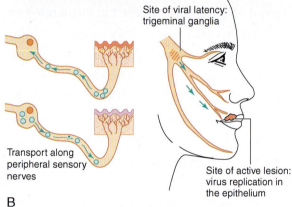

Figure 45-5 **A,** Primary herpes gingivostomatitis. **B,** Herpes simplex virus establishes latent infection and can recur from the trigeminal ganglia. (**A,** From Hart CA, Broadhead RL: *A color atlas of pediatric infectious diseases,* London, 1992, Wolfe. **B,** Modified from Straus SE: Herpes simplex virus and its relatives. In Schaechter M, Eisenstein BI, Medoff G, editors: *Mechanisms of microbial disease,* ed 2, Baltimore, 1993, Williams & Wilkins.)

Recurrent Oral Herpes

Infected people may experience recurrent mucocutaneous HSV infection (cold sores, fever blisters) (Figure 45-6), even though they never had a clinically apparent primary infection. The lesions usually occur at the corners of the mouth or next to the lips. Recurrent facial herpes infections are generally activated from the trigeminal ganglia. As noted earlier, the symptoms of a recurrent episode are less severe, more localized, and of shorter duration than those of a primary episode.

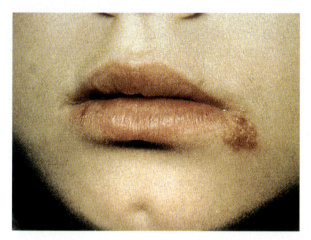

Figure 45-6 Cold sore of recurrent herpes labialis. It is less severe than that of primary disease. (From Hart CA, Broadhead RL: *A color atlas of pediatric infectious diseases*, London, 1992, Wolfe.) (original Figure 51-6, 7th)

Genital Herpes

There also are primary and recurrent genital herpes.

Genital herpes can be caused by HSV-1 or HSV-2. In male patients, the lesions typically develop on the glans or shaft of the penis and occasionally in the urethra. In female patients, the lesions may be seen on the vulva, vagina, cervix, perianal area, or inner thigh and are frequently accompanied by itching and a mucoid vaginal discharge. Anal sex can lead to HSV proctitis, a condition in which the lesions are found in the lower rectum and anus. The lesions are usually painful. In patients of both sexes, a primary infection may be accompanied by fever, malaise, and myalgia, which are symptoms related to a transient viremia. The symptoms and time course of primary and recurrent genital herpes are compared in Figure 45-4.

Recurrent genital HSV disease is shorter in duration and less severe than the primary episode. In approximately 50% of patients, recurrences are preceded by a characteristic prodrome of burning or tingling in the area in which the lesions eventually erupt. Episodes of recurrence may be as frequent as every 2 to 3 weeks or may be infrequent. Unfortunately, any infected person may shed virus asymptomatically. Such individuals may be important vectors for spread of this virus.

Others

Herpetic keratitis is almost always limited to one eye. It can cause recurrent disease, leading to permanent scarring, corneal damage, and blindness.

Herpetic whitlow is an infection of the finger, and herpes gladiatorum is an infection of the body. The virus establishes infection through cuts or abrasions in the skin. Herpetic whitlow often occurs in nurses or physicians who attend patients with HSV infections, in thumb-sucking children, and in people who have genital HSV infections. Herpes gladiatorum is often acquired during wrestling or rugby.

Eczema herpeticum is acquired by children with active eczema. The underlying disease promotes the spread of the infection along the skin and potentially to the adrenal glands, liver, and other organs.

Herpes encephalitis is usually caused by HSV-1. The lesions are generally limited to one of the temporal lobes. The viral pathology and immunopathology cause the destruction of the temporal lobe and give rise to erythrocytes in the cerebrospinal fluid, seizures, focal neurologic abnormalities, and other characteristics of viral encephalitis. HSV is the most common viral cause of sporadic encephalitis and results in significant morbidity and mortality, even in patients who receive appropriate treatment. The disease occurs at all ages and at any time of the year. HSV meningitis may be a complication of genital HSV-2 infection; symptoms resolve by themselves.

HSV infection in the neonate is a devastating and often fatal disease caused most often by HSV-2. It may be acquired in utero but more commonly is contracted either during passage of the infant through the vaginal canal, or it is acquired postnatally from family members or hospital personnel. The baby initially appears septic, and vesicular lesions may or may not be present. Because the cell-mediated immune response is not yet developed in the neonate, HSV disseminates to the liver, lung, and other organs, as well as to the central nervous system (CNS). Progression of the infection to the CNS results in death, mental retardation, or neurologic disability, even with treatment.

Laboratory Diagnosis

Cellular Pathological Analysis of a Clinical Sample

Characteristic cytopathologic effects (CPEs) can be identified in a skin scraping smear (a scraping of the base of a lesion), Papanicolaou (Pap) smear, or biopsy specimen. CPEs include syncytia, "ballooning" cytoplasm, and intranuclear inclusions. A definitive diagnosis can be made by demonstrating viral antigen (using immunofluorescence or the immunoperoxidase method) or DNA (using in situ hybridization or PCR) in the tissue sample or vesicle fluid.

Virus Isolation

Virus isolation is the most definitive assay for the diagnosis of HSV infection. Virus can be obtained from vesicles but not crusted lesions. Specimens are collected by aspiration of the lesion fluid or by application of a cotton swab to the vesicles and direct inoculation of the sample into cell cultures. HSV produces CPEs within 1 to 3 days in HeLa cells, human embryonic fibroblasts, and other cells. Infected cells become enlarged and appear ballooned. Some isolates induce fusion of neighboring cells, giving rise to multinucleated giant cells (syncytia).

Genome Detection

HSV type-specific DNA probes, specific DNA primers for PCR and quantitative PCR, are used to detect and differentiate HSV-1 and HSV-2. PCR analysis of cerebrospinal fluid has replaced immunofluorescence analysis of a brain biopsy in the diagnosis for herpes encephalitis. The distinction between HSV-1 or HSV-2 and different strains of either virus can also be made by restriction endonuclease cleavage patterns of the viral DNA.

Serology

Serologic procedures are useful only for diagnosing a primary HSV infection with IgM detection and for epidemiologic studies with IgG detection. They are not useful for diagnosing recurrent disease because a significant rise in antibody titers does not usually accompany recurrent disease.

Treatment, Prevention, and Control

HSV encodes several target enzymes for antiviral drugs. Most antiherpes drugs are nucleoside analogues that inhibit the viral DNA polymerase. Treatment prevents or shortens the course of primary or recurrent disease. None of the drug treatments can eliminate latent infection.

Acyclovir (ACV). Valacyclovir (the valyl ester of ACV), penciclovir, and famciclovir have been used in treating genital herpes and serious HSV diseases (e.g., herpes encephalitis and herpetic keratitis).

HSV is readily inactivated by soap, disinfectants, bleach, and 70% ethanol. Washing with soap readily disinfects the virus. No vaccine is currently available for HSV.

VARICELLA-ZOSTER VIRUS

VZV causes chickenpox (varicella) and, upon recurrence, causes herpes zoster, or shingles. As an alphaherpesvirus, VZV shares many characteristics with HSV, including (1) the ability to establish latent infection of neurons and recurrent disease, (2) the importance of cell-mediated immunity in controlling and preventing serious disease, and (3) the characteristic blister-like lesions. Like HSV, VZV encodes a thymidine kinase and is susceptible to antiviral drugs. Unlike HSV, VZV spreads predominantly by the respiratory route and, after local replication of the virus in the respiratory tract, by viremia to form skin lesions over the entire body.

Structure and Replication

VZV has the smallest genome of the human herpesviruses. VZV replicates in a similar manner but slower and in fewer types of cells than HSV. Human diploid fibroblasts in vitro and activated T cells, epithelial cells, and epidermal cells in vivo support productive VZV replication. Like HSV, VZV establishes a latent infection of neurons, but unlike HSV, several viral RNAs and specific viral proteins can be detected in the cells.

Pathogenesis and Immunity

VZV is generally acquired by inhalation, and primary infection begins in the tonsils and mucosa of the respiratory tract. The virus then progresses via the bloodstream and lymphatic system to the cells of the reticuloendothelial system (Figures 45-7). A secondary viremia occurs after 11 to 13 days and spreads the virus throughout the body and to the skin. The virus infects T cells, and these cells can home to the skin and transfer virus to skin epithelial cells. The virus overcomes inhibition by IFN-α, and vesicles are produced in the skin. The virus remains cell associated and is transmitted on cell-to-cell interaction, except for terminally differentiated epithelial cells in the lungs and keratinocytes of skin lesions, which can release infectious virus. Virus replication in the lung is a major source of contagion. The virus causes a dermal vesiculopustular rash that develops over time in successive crops. Fever and systemic symptoms occur with the rash.

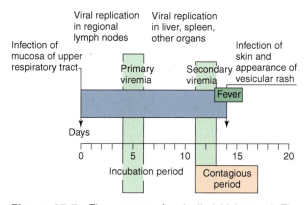

Figure 45-7   Time course of varicella (chickenpox). The course in young children, as presented in this figure, is generally shorter and less severe than that in adults.

The virus becomes latent in the dorsal root or cranial nerve ganglia after the primary infection. The virus can be reactivated in older adults when immunity wanes or in patients with impaired cellular immunity. On reactivation, the virus replicates and is released along the entire neural pathway to infect the skin, causing a vesicular rash along the entire dermatome, known as herpes zoster, or shingles. This damages the neuron and may result in postherpetic neuralgia.

IFN-α, IFN-stimulated protections, and natural killer and T cells limit the spread of the virus in tissue, but antibody is important for limiting the viremic spread of VZV. Cell-mediated immunity is essential for resolving the disease, but cannot prevent the occurrence of herpes zoster.

Epidemiology

VZV is extremely communicable, with rates of infection exceeding 90% among susceptible household contacts. The disease is spread principally by the respiratory route but may also be spread through contact with skin vesicles. Patients are contagious before and during symptoms. More than 90% of adults have the VZV antibody. Herpes zoster results from the reactivation of a patient's latent virus. The disease develops in approximately 10% to 20% of the population infected with VZV, and the incidence rises with age. Herpes zoster lesions contain viable virus and therefore may be a source of varicella infection in a nonimmune person (child).

Clinical Syndromes

Primary Infection

Varicella (chickenpox) is one of the five classic childhood exanthems (along with rubella, roseola, fifth disease, and measles). The disease results from a primary infection with VZV; it is usually a mild disease of childhood and is normally symptomatic, although asymptomatic infection can occur (see Figure 45-7). Varicella characteristics include fever and a maculopapular rash that appear after an incubation period of approximately 14 days (Figure 45-8). Within hours, each maculopapular lesion forms a thin-walled vesicle on an erythematous base ("dewdrop on a rose petal") that measures approximately 2 to 4 mm in diameter. This vesicle is the hallmark of varicella. Within 12 hours, the vesicle becomes pustular and begins to crust, after which scabbed lesions appear. Successive crops of lesions appear for 3 to 5 days, and at any given time, all stages of skin lesions can be observed.

The rash spreads across the entire body but is more prevalent on the trunk and head than on the

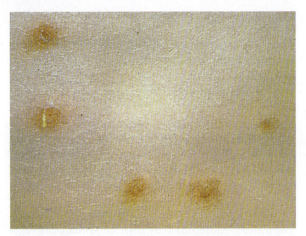

Figure 45-8 Characteristic rash of varicella in all stages of its evolution. (From Hart CA, Broadhead RL: *A color atlas of pediatric infectious diseases*, London, 1992, Wolfe.)

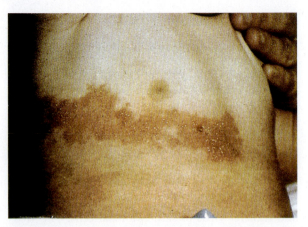

Figure 45-9 Herpes zoster ("shingles") in a thoracic dermatome.

extremities. Its presence on the scalp distinguishes it from many other rashes. The lesions itch and cause scratching, which may lead to bacterial superinfection and scarring. Lesions on the mucous membrane typically occur in the mouth, conjunctivae, and vagina.

Primary infection is usually more severe in adults than in children. Interstitial pneumonia may occur in 20% to 30% of adult patients and may be fatal. The pneumonia results from inflammatory reactions at this primary site of infection.

Recurrence Infection

As noted earlier, herpes zoster (zoster means "belt" or "girdle") is a recurrence of a latent varicella infection acquired earlier in the patient's life. Severe pain in the area innervated by the nerve usually precedes the appearance of the chickenpox-like lesions. The rash is limited to a dermatome and resembles varicella (Figure 45-9). A chronic pain syndrome called postherpetic neuralgia, which can persist for months to years, occurs in as many as 30% of patients in whom herpes zoster develops.

VZV infection in immunocompromised patients or neonates can result in serious, progressive, and potentially fatal disease. Defects of cell-mediated immunity in such patients increase the risk for dissemination of the virus to the lungs, brain, and liver, which may be fatal. The disease may occur in response to a primary exposure to varicella or because of recurrent disease.

Laboratory Diagnosis

The CPEs in VZV-infected cells are similar to those seen in HSV-infected cells and include intranuclear inclusions and syncytia. These cells may be seen in skin lesions, respiratory specimens, or organ biopsy specimens. Syncytia may also be seen in scraping smears from a vesicle's base. A direct fluorescent antibody to membrane antigen (FAMA) test can also be used to examine skin lesion scrapings or biopsy specimens. Antigen and genome detection are sensitive means of diagnosing VZV infection. PCR techniques are especially useful for systemic and neuronal disease.

Isolation of VZV is not routinely done because the virus is labile during transport to the laboratory and replicates poorly in vitro.

Serologic tests that detect antibodies to VZV are used to screen populations for immunity to VZV. However, antibody levels are normally low, so sensitive tests such as immunofluorescence and ELISA must be performed to detect the antibody. A significant increase in antibody level can be detected in people experiencing herpes zoster.

Treatment, Prevention, and Control

Treatment may be appropriate for adults and immunocompromised patients (adults and children) with VZV infections and for people with shingles, but no treatment is usually necessary for children with varicella. ACV, famciclovir, valacyclovir, and IFN have been approved for the treatment of VZV infections.

Immunosuppressed patients susceptible to severe disease may be protected from serious disease through the administration of varicella-zoster immunoglobulin (VZIG). VZIG prophylaxis can prevent viremic spread leading to disease but is ineffective as a therapy for patients already suffering from active varicella or herpes zoster disease.

A live attenuated vaccine for VZV is available for use.

EPSTEIN-BARR VIRUS

EBV is the ultimate B-lymphocyte parasite, and the diseases it causes reflect this association. EBV was discovered by electron-microscopic observation of characteristic herpes virions in biopsy specimens of a B-cell neoplasm, African Burkitt lymphoma (AfBL).

EBV causes heterophile antibody-positive infectious mononucleosis and stimulates the growth and immortalizes B cells in tissue culture. EBV has been causally associated with AfBL (endemic Burkitt lymphoma), Hodgkin disease, and nasopharyngeal carcinoma. EBV has also been associated with B-cell lymphomas in patients with acquired or congenital immunodeficiencies.

Structure and Replication

EBV is a member of the subfamily *Gammaherpesvirinae*, with a very limited host range and a tissue tropism defined by the limited cellular expression of its receptor. The primary receptor for EBV is also the receptor for the C3d component of the complement system (also called CR2 or CD21). It is expressed on B cells of humans and New World monkeys and on some epithelial cells of the oropharynx and nasopharynx.

EBV infection has the following three potential outcomes:

EBV can replicate in B cells or epithelial cells permissive for EBV replication.

EBV can cause latent infection of memory B cells in the presence of competent T cells.

EBV can stimulate and immortalize B cells.

EBV encodes more than 70 proteins, different groups of which are expressed for the different types of infections.

EBV in saliva infects epithelial cells and then naïve resting B cells in the tonsils. The growth of the B cells is stimulated first by virus binding to the C3d receptor, and then by expression of the transformation and latency proteins. These include Epstein-Barr nuclear antigens (EBNAs) 1, 2, 3A, 3B, and 3C; latent proteins (LPs); latent membrane proteins (LMPs) 1 and 2; and two small Epstein-Barr-encoded RNA (EBER) molecules, EBER-1 and EBER-2. The EBNAs and LPs are DNA-binding proteins that are essential for establishing and maintaining the infection (EBNA-1), immortalization (EBNA-2), and other purposes. The LMPs are membrane proteins with oncogene-like activity. The genome becomes circularized; the cells proceed to follicles that become germinal centers in the lymph node, where the infected cells differentiate into memory cells. EBV protein synthesis ceases, and the virus establishes latency in these memory B cells. EBNA-1 will be expressed only at cell division to hold onto and retain the genome in the cells.

Antigen stimulation of the B cells and infection of certain epithelial cells allow the transcription and translation of the ZEBRA (peptide encoded by the Z-gene region) transcriptional activator protein, which activates the immediate early genes of the virus and the lytic cycle. After synthesis of the DNA polymerase and replication of DNA, the structural and other late proteins are synthesized. They include gp350/220 (related glycoproteins of 350,000 and 220,000 Da), which is the viral attachment protein, and other glycoproteins. These glycoproteins bind to CD21 and MHC II molecules, receptors on B cells and epithelial cells, and also promote fusion of the envelope with cell membranes.

The viral proteins produced during a productive infection are serologically defined and grouped as early antigen (EA), viral capsid antigen (VCA), and the glycoproteins of the membrane antigen (MA) (Table 45-2). An early protein mimics a cellular inhibitor of apoptosis, and a late protein mimics the activity of human interleukin-10, which enhances B-cell growth and inhibits Th1 immune responses.

Table 45-2 Markers of Epstein-Barr Virus (EBV) Infection

Name	Abbreviation	Characteristics	Biologic Association	Clinical Association
EBV nuclear antigens	EBNAs	Nuclear	EBNAs are nonstructural antigens and first antigens to appear; EBNAs seen in all infected and transformed cells	Anti-EBNA develops after resolution of infection
Early antigen	EA-R	Only cytoplasmic	EA-R appears before EA-D; appearance is first sign that infected cell has entered lytic cycle	
Viral capsid antigen	VCA	Cytoplasmic	VCA are late proteins; found in virus producing cells	Anti-VCA IgM is transient; anti-VCA IgG is persistent
Membrane antigen	MA	Cell surface	MAs are envelope glycoproteins	Same as VCA
Heterophile antibody		Recognition of Paul-Bunnell antigen on sheep, horse, or bovine erythrocytes	EBV-induced B-cell proliferation promotes production of heterophile antibody	Early symptom occurs in more than 50% of patients

EA, Early antigen; *EBNA,* Epstein-Barr nuclear antigen; *IgG,* immunoglobulin G; *IgM,* immunoglobulin M; *MA,* membrane antigen; *VCA,* viral capsid antigen.

Pathogenesis and Immunity

EBV has adapted to the human B cell and manipulates and uses the different phases of B-cell development to establish a lifelong infection in the individual, and it still promotes its transmission. The diseases of EBV result from either an overactive immune response (infectious mononucleosis) or the lack of effective immune control (lymphoproliferative disease and hairy cell leukoplakia).

The productive infection of B cells and epithelial cells of the oropharynx, such as in the tonsils (Figure 45-10), promotes virus shedding into saliva to transmit the virus to other hosts and establishes a viremia to spread the virus to other B cells in lymphatic tissue and blood.

EBV proteins replace host factors that normally activate B-cell growth and development. In the absence of T cells (e.g., in tissue culture), EBV can immortalize B cells and promote the development of B-lymphoblastoid cell lines.

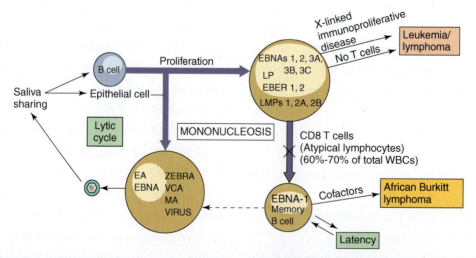

Figure 45-10 Progression of Epstein-Barr virus (EBV) infection. Infection may result in lytic, latent, or immortalizing infection, which can be distinguished on the basis of production of virus and expression of different viral proteins and antigens. T cells limit the outgrowth of the EBV-infected cells and maintain the latent infection. *CD,* Cluster of differentiation; *EA,* early antigen; *EBER,* Epstein-Barr-encoded RNA; *EBNA,* Epstein-Barr nuclear antigen; *LMPs,* latent membrane proteins; *LP,* latent protein; *MA,* membrane antigen; *VCA,* viral capsid antigen; *WBCs,* white blood cells; *ZEBRA,* peptide encoded by the *Z* gene region.

The outgrowth of the B cell is normally controlled by T cells responding to proliferation indicators on the B cell and to EBV antigenic peptides. B cells are excellent antigen-presenting cells and present EBV antigens on both MHC I and MHC II molecules. The activated T cells appear as atypical lymphocytes. They increase in number in the peripheral blood during the second week of infection, accounting for 10% to 80% of the total white blood cell count at this time (hence the "mononucleosis").

Infectious mononucleosis is essentially *a "civil war" between the EBV-infected B cells and the protective T cells.* The classic lymphocytosis (increase in mononuclear cells), swelling of lymphoid organs (lymph nodes, spleen, and liver), and malaise associated with infectious mononucleosis results mainly from the activation and proliferation of T cells. A great amount of energy is required to power the T-cell response, leading to great fatigue. The sore throat of infectious mononucleosis is a response to EBV-infected epithelium and B cells in the tonsils and throat. Children have a less active immune response to EBV infection and therefore have very mild disease.

During productive infection, antibody is first developed against the components of the virion, VCA, and MA, and later against the EA. After resolution of the infection (lysis of the productively infected cells), antibody against the nuclear antigens (EBNAs) is produced. T cells are essential for limiting the proliferation of EBV-infected B cells and controlling the disease (Figure 45-11). EBV counteracts some of the protective action of Th1 CD4 T-cell responses during productive infection by producing an interleukin-10 analogue (BCRF-1) that inhibits the protective Th1 CD4 T-cell responses and also stimulates B-cell growth.

The virus persists in at least one memory B cell per milliliter of blood for the infected person's lifetime. EBV may be reactivated when the memory B cell is activated (especially in the tonsils or oropharynx) and may be shed in saliva.

Epidemiology

EBV is transmitted in saliva. More than 90% of EBV-infected people intermittently shed the virus for

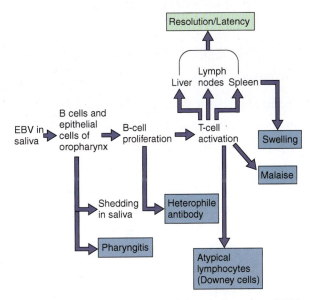

Figure 45-11 Pathogenesis of Epstein-Barr virus *(EBV)*. EBV is acquired by close contact between persons through saliva and infects the B cells. The resolution of the EBV infection and many of the symptoms of infectious mononucleosis result from the activation of T cells in response to the infection.(original Figure 51-14, 7th)

life, even when totally asymptomatic. Children can acquire the virus at an early age by sharing contaminated drinking glasses. *Children generally have subclinical disease.* Saliva sharing between adolescents and young adults often occurs during kissing. Disease in these people may go unnoticed or may manifest in varying degrees of severity.

The geographic distribution of some EBV-associated neoplasms indicates a possible association with cofactors. Malaria appears to be a cofactor in the progression of chronic or latent EBV infection to AfBL. The restriction of nasopharyngeal carcinoma to people living in certain regions of China indicates a possible genetic predisposition to the cancer or the presence of cofactors in the food or environment. More subtle mechanisms may facilitate the role of EBV in 30% to 50% of cases of Hodgkin disease.

Transplant recipients, patients with the acquired immunodeficiency syndrome (AIDS), and genetically immunodeficient people are at high risk for lymphoproliferative disorders initiated by EBV. These disorders may appear as polyclonal and monoclonal B-cell lymphomas. Such people are also at high risk for a productive EBV infection in the form of hairy oral leukoplakia.

Clinical Syndromes

Heterophile Antibody-Positive Infectious Mononucleosis

The triad of classic symptoms for infectious mononucleosis is lymphadenopathy (swollen glands), splenomegaly (large spleen), and exudative pharyngitis accompanied by high fever, malaise, and often hepatosplenomegaly (large liver and spleen). A rash may occur, especially after ampicillin treatment (for the sore throat). The major complaint of people with infectious mononucleosis is fatigue. The disease is rarely fatal in healthy people but can cause serious complications resulting from neurologic disorders, laryngeal obstruction, or rupture of the spleen. Neurologic complications include meningoencephalitis and the Guillain-Barré syndrome. Mononucleosis-like syndromes can also be caused by CMV, HHV-6, *Toxoplasma gondii*, and human immunodeficiency virus (HIV). Similar to infections caused by other herpesviruses, EBV infection in a child is much milder than infection in an adolescent or adult. In fact, infection in children is usually subclinical.

African Burkitt Lymphoma

EBV was first associated with African Burkitt lymphoma (endemic lymphoma) (AfBL) and then Burkitt lymphoma elsewhere in the world, Hodgkin lymphoma, and several other lymphoproliferative diseases. AfBL is a poorly differentiated monoclonal B-cell lymphoma of the jaw and face that is endemic in children living in the malarial regions of Africa. The Burkitt tumors contain EBV DNA sequences but express only the EBNA-1 viral antigen. Virions can occasionally be seen on electron micrographs of infected material.

EBV and Nasopharyngeal Carcinoma

EBV is also associated with nasopharyngeal carcinoma, which is endemic in adults in Southeast Asia, North Africa and North America, especially in Guangdong, Guangxi, Fujian, Hunan, Jiangxi, Zhejiang, and Taiwan of China. The tumor cells contain EBV DNA, but unlike Burkitt lymphoma, in which the tumor cells are derived from lymphocytes, the tumor cells of nasopharyngeal carcinoma are of epithelial origin.

EBV-Induced Lymphoproliferative Diseases

On infection with EBV, people lacking T-cell immunity are likely to suffer life-threatening polyclonal leukemia-like B-cell proliferative disease and lymphoma instead of infectious mononucleosis.

Laboratory Diagnosis

EBV-induced infectious mononucleosis is diagnosed on the basis of the symptoms, the finding of atypical lymphocytes, the presence of lymphocytosis (mononuclear cells constituting 60% to 70% of the white blood cell count, with 30% atypical lymphocytes), heterophile antibody, and antibody to viral antigens. Virus isolation is not practical. PCR and DNA probe analysis for the viral genome and immunofluorescent identification of viral antigens are used to detect evidence of infection.

Atypical lymphocytes are probably the earliest detectable indication of an EBV infection. These cells appear with the onset of symptoms and disappear with resolution of the disease.

Heterophile antibody results from the nonspecific, mitogen-like activation of B cells by EBV and the production of a wide repertoire of antibodies. These antibodies include an IgM heterophile antibody that recognizes the antigen on sheep, horse, and bovine erythrocytes but not that on guinea pig kidney cells. The heterophile antibody response can usually be detected by the end of the first week of illness and lasts for as long as several months. It is an excellent indication of EBV infection in adults but is not as reliable in children or infants.

Serologic tests for antibody to viral antigens are a more dependable method than heterophile antibody to confirm the diagnosis of EBV mononucleosis (Table 45-3). EBV infection is indicated by the finding of any of the following: (1) IgM antibody to the VCA, (2) the presence of VCA antibody and the absence of EBNA antibody, or (3) elevation of antibodies to VCA and early antigen. The finding of both

Table 45-3   Serologic Profile for Epstein-Barr Virus (EBV) Infections

Patient's Clinical Status	Heterophile Antibodies		EBV-Specific Antibodies		Comment
	VCA-IgM	VCA-IgG	EA	EBNA	
Susceptible	–	–	–	–	–	
Acute primary infection	+	+	+	±	–	Anti-VCA and anti-MA present during disease
Chronic primary infection	–	–	+	+	–	Anti-EBNA only present during convalescence
Past infection	–	–	+	–	+	
Reactivation infection	–	–	+	+	+	
Burkitt lymphoma	–	–	+	+	+	
Nasopharyngeal carcinoma	–	–	+	+	+	

EA, Early antigen; *EBNA*, Epstein-Barr nuclear antigen; *IgG*, immunoglobulin G; *IgM*, immunoblobulin M; *VCA*, viral capsid antigen.
Modified from Balows A, et al, editors: *Laboratory diagnosis of infectious diseases: principles and practices*, New York, 1988, Springer-Verlag.

VCA and EBNA antibodies in serum indicates that the person had a previous infection. Generation of antibody to EBNA requires lysis of the infected cell and usually indicates T-cell control of active disease.

Treatment, Prevention, and Control

No effective treatment or vaccine is available for EBV disease. The ubiquitous nature of the virus and the potential for asymptomatic shedding make control of infection difficult. However, infection elicits life-long immunity. Therefore, the best means of preventing infectious mononucleosis is exposure to the virus early in life because the disease is more benign in children.

HUMAN CYTOMEGALOVIRUS

Structure and Replication

CMV is a member of the subfamily *Betaherpesvirinae*. It has the largest genome of the human herpesviruses. In contrast to the traditional definition of a virus, which states that a virion particle contains DNA or RNA, CMV carries specific mRNAs into the cell in the virion particle to facilitate infection. Human CMV replicates only in human cells. Fibroblasts, epithelial cells, granulocytes, macrophages, and other cells are permissive for CMV replication. Virus replication is much slower than for HSV, and CPE may not be seen for 7 to 14 days. This may facil-

itate the establishment of latent infection in myeloid stem cells, monocytes, lymphocytes, the stromal cells of the bone marrow, or other cells.

Pathogenesis and Immunity

The pathogenesis of CMV is similar to that of other herpesviruses in many respects. CMV is an excellent parasite and readily establishes persistent and latent infections rather than an extensive lytic infection. CMV is highly cell associated and is spread throughout the body within infected cells, especially lymphocytes and leukocytes. The virus is reactivated by immunosuppression (e.g., corticosteroids, infection with HIV) and possibly by allogeneic stimulation (i.e., the host response to transfused or transplanted cells).

Cell-mediated immunity is essential for resolving and controlling the outgrowth of CMV infection. However, CMV is an expert at immune evasion and has several means for evading innate and immune responses. CMV infection alters the function of lymphocytes and leukocytes. The virus prevents antigen presentation to both CD8 cytotoxic T cells and CD4 T cells by preventing the expression of MHC I molecules on the cell surface and by interfering with cytokine-induced expression of MHC II molecules on antigen-presenting cells. A viral protein also blocks natural-killer-cell attack of CMV-infected cells. Similar to EBV, CMV also encodes an interleukin-10 analogue that would inhibit Th1 protective immune responses.

Epidemiology and Clinical Syndromes

In most cases, CMV replicates and is shed without causing symptoms. Activation and replication of CMV in the kidney and secretory glands promote its secretion in urine and bodily secretions. CMV can be isolated from urine, blood, throat washings, saliva, tears, breast milk, semen, stool, amniotic fluid, vaginal and cervical secretions, and tissues obtained for transplantation. Virus can be transmitted to other individuals by means of blood transfusions and organ transplants. The congenital, oral, and sexual routes; blood transfusion; and tissue transplantation are the major means by which CMV is transmitted. CMV disease is an opportunistic disorder, rarely causing symptoms in the immunocompetent host but causing serious disease in an immunosuppressed or immunodeficient person, such as a patient with AIDS or a neonate.

Congenital Infection

CMV is the most prevalent viral cause of congenital disease. Approximately 15% of stillborn babies are infected with CMV. A significant percentage (0.5% to 2.5%) of all newborns is infected with CMV before birth, and a large percentage of babies is infected within the first months of life. Disease signs include small size, thrombocytopenia, microcephaly, intracerebral calcification, jaundice, hepatosplenomegaly, and rash (cytomegalic inclusion disease). Unilateral or bilateral hearing loss and mental retardation are common consequences of congenital CMV infection. The risk for serious birth defects is extremely high for infants born to mothers who had primary CMV infections during their pregnancies.

Fetuses are infected by virus in the mother's blood (primary infection) or by virus ascending from the cervix (after a recurrence). The symptoms of congenital infection are less severe or can be prevented by the immune response of a seropositive mother.

Perinatal Infection

The neonates born through an infected cervix can acquire CMV infection and become excreters of the virus at 3 to 4 weeks of age. Neonates may also acquire CMV from maternal milk or colostrum. Perinatal infection causes no clinically evident disease in healthy full-term infants.

Another means by which neonates can acquire CMV is through blood transfusions. Of the seronegative babies who are exposed to blood from seropositive donors. Significant clinical infection may occur in premature infants who acquire CMV from transfused blood, usually resulting in pneumonia and hepatitis.

Infection in Children and Adults

Approximately 40% of adolescents are infected with CMV, but this number increases to 70% to 85% of adults by the age of 40. CMV may be transmitted through sexual contact. The titer of the CMV in semen is the highest of that in any body secretion.

Although most CMV infections acquired in young adulthood are asymptomatic, patients may show a heterophile-negative mononucleosis syndrome. The symptoms of CMV disease are similar to those of EBV infection but with less severe pharyngitis and lymphadenopathy. Although the presence of CMV-infected cells promotes a T-cell outgrowth (atypical lymphocytosis) similar to that seen in EBV infection, heterophile antibody is not present.

Transmission via Transfusion and Transplantation

Transmission of CMV by blood most often results in an asymptomatic infection; if symptoms are present, they typically resemble those of mononucleosis. CMV may also be transmitted by organ transplantation, and CMV infection is often reactivated in transplant recipients during periods of intense immunosuppression.

CMV is also responsible for the failure of many kidney transplants. This may be the result of virus replication in the graft after reactivation in the transplanted kidney or infection from the host.

Infection in the Immunocompromised Host

CMV is a prominent opportunistic infectious agent. In immunocompromised people, it causes symptomatic primary or recurrent disease.

CMV disease of the lung (pneumonia and pneumonitis) is a common outcome in immunosuppressed patients and can be fatal if not treated. CMV often causes retinitis, colitis, or esophagitis in patients who are severely immunodeficient (e.g., patients with AIDS). Interstitial pneumonia and encephalitis may also be caused by CMV but may be difficult to distinguish from infections caused by other opportunistic agents. CMV esophagitis may mimic candidal esophagitis. A smaller percentage of immunocompromised patients may experience CMV infection of the gastrointestinal tract. Patients with CMV colitis usually have diarrhea, weight loss, anorexia, and fever.

Laboratory Diagnosis

Histology

The histologic hallmark of CMV infection is the cytomegalic cell, which is an enlarged cell that contains a dense, central, "owl's eye," basophilic intranuclear inclusion body (Figure 45-12). Such infected cells may be found in any tissue of the body and in urine and are thought to be epithelial in origin. The inclusions are readily seen with Giemsa or HE staining.

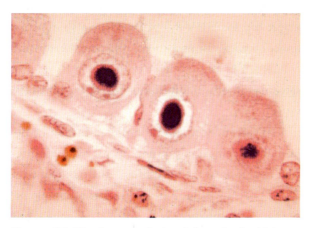

Figure 45-12　Cytomegalovirus-infected cell with basophilic nuclear inclusion body.

Antigen and Genome Detection

A rapid, sensitive diagnosis can be obtained by detection of viral antigen, using immunofluorescence or an ELISA, or the viral genome, using PCR and related techniques in cells of a biopsy, blood, bronchoalveolar lavage, or urine sample.

Culture

CMV is grown in diploid fibroblast cell cultures and normally must be maintained for at least 4 to 6 weeks because the characteristic CPE develops very slowly in specimens with very low titers of the virus. Isolation of CMV is especially reliable in immunocompromised patients, who often have high titers of virus in their secretions.

More rapid results are achieved by centrifuging a patient's sample onto cells grown on a coverslip within a shell vial. Specimens are examined after 1 to 2 days of incubation by indirect immunofluorescence for the presence of one or more of the immediate early viral antigens.

Serology

Seroconversion is usually an excellent marker for primary CMV infection. Titers of CMV-specific IgM antibody may be very high in patients with AIDS. However, CMV-specific IgM antibody may also develop during the reactivation of CMV and is therefore not a dependable indicator of primary infection.

Treatment, Prevention, and Control

Ganciclovir (dihydroxypropoxymethyl guanine), valganciclovir (valyl ester of ganciclovir), cidofovir, and foscarnet (phosphonoformic acid) have been used for the treatment of specific diseases resulting from CMV infections of immunosuppressed patients.

CMV spreads mainly by the sexual, tissue transplantation, and transfusion routes, and spread by these means is preventable. Semen is a major vector for the sexual spread of CMV. The use of condoms or abstinence would limit viral spread. Transmission of the virus can also be reduced through the screening of potential blood and organ donors for CMV seronegativity. Screening is especially important for donors of blood transfusions to be given to infants. Although congenital and perinatal transmission of CMV cannot effectively be prevented, a seropositive mother is least likely to produce a baby with symptomatic CMV disease. No vaccine for CMV is available.

HUMAN HERPESVIRUSES 6 AND 7

The two variants of HHV-6, HHV-6A and HHV-6B, and HHV-7, are members of the genus *Roseolovirus* of the subfamily *Betaherpesvirinae*. HHV-6 was first isolated from the blood of patients with AIDS and grown in T-cell cultures. It was identified as a herpesvirus because of its characteristic morphology within infected cells. Similar to CMV, HHV-6 is lymphotropic and ubiquitous. At least 45% of the population is seropositive for HHV-6 by age 2 years, and almost 100% by adulthood. In 1988, HHV-6 was serologically associated with a common disease of children, exanthem subitum, commonly known as roseola. HHV-7 was isolated in a similar manner from the T cells of a patient with AIDS who was also infected with HHV-6, and later it was also shown to cause exanthem subitum.

Pathogenesis and Immunity

HHV-6 infection occurs very early in life. The virus replicates in the salivary gland, is shed, and transmitted in saliva.

HHV-6 primarily infects lymphocytes, especially CD4 T cells. HHV-6 establishes a latent infection in T cells and monocytes but may replicate on activation of the cells. Cells in which the virus is replicating appear large and refractile and have occasional intranuclear and intracytoplasmic inclusion bodies.

Similar to the replication of CMV, the replication of HHV-6 is controlled by cell-mediated immunity. The virus is likely to become activated in patients with AIDS or other lymphoproliferative and immunosuppressive disorders and cause opportunistic disease.

Clinical Syndromes

Exanthem subitum, or roseola, is caused by either HHV-6B or HHV-7. It is characterized by the rapid onset of high fever of a few days' duration, which is followed by a rash on the trunk and face, and then it spreads and lasts only 24 to 48 hours. The presence of infected T cells or the activation of delayed-type hypersensitivity T cells in the skin may be the cause of the rash. The disease is effectively controlled and resolved by cell-mediated immunity, but the virus establishes a lifelong latent infection of T cells. Although usually benign, HHV-6 is the most common cause of febrile seizures in childhood (age 6 to 24 months).

HHV-6 may also cause a mononucleosis syndrome and lymphadenopathy in adults and may be a cofactor in the pathogenesis of AIDS. Similar to CMV, HHV-6 may reactivate in transplant patients and contribute to the failure of the graft. HHV-6 has also been associated with multiple sclerosis and chronic fatigue syndrome.

Human Herpesvirus 8 (Kaposi Sarcoma-Associated Herpesvirus)

HHV-8 DNA sequences were discovered in biopsy specimens of Kaposi sarcoma, primary effusion lymphoma (a rare type of B-cell lymphoma), and multicentric Castleman disease through the use of PCR analysis. Kaposi sarcoma is one of the characteristic opportunistic diseases associated with AIDS. Genome sequence analysis showed that the virus was unique and a member of the subfamily *Gammaherpesvirinae*. Similar to EBV, the B cell is the primary target cell for HHV-8, but the virus also infects a limited number of endothelial cells, monocytes, and epithelial and sensory nerve cells. Within the Kaposi sarcoma tumors, endothelial spindle cells contain the virus.

HHV-8 encodes several proteins that resemble human proteins and promote the growth and prevent apoptosis of the infected and surrounding cells. These proteins include an interleukin-6 homologue (growth and antiapoptosis), a Bcl-2 analogue (antiapoptosis), chemokines, and a chemokine receptor. These proteins can promote the growth and development of polyclonal Kaposi sarcoma cells in AIDS patients and others. HHV-8 DNA is present and is associated with peripheral blood lymphocytes, most likely B cells, in approximately 10% of immunocompetent people. The virus is most likely a sexually transmitted disease but may be spread by other means.

SUMMARY

Herpesvirus infections are common, and the viruses, except HHV-8, are ubiquitous. Although these viruses usually cause benign disease, especially in children, they can also cause significant morbidity and mortality, especially in immunosuppressed people. All herpesviruses establish lytic, latent, and recurrent infections. HSV and VZV are neurotropic; CMV and EBV are lymphotropic, but unlike EBV, CMV can infect many different cell types. Fortunately, some antiviral agents are available for treatment of herpesviruses, and there is a live vaccine for VZV.

Herpes simplex virus (HSV)

HSV-1 and HSV-2 initially infect, replicate in mucoepithelial cells, cause disease at the site of infection, establish latent infection of the innervating neurons, and can be reactivated by stress or immune suppression. HSV-1 is usually associated with infections in the area of the body above the waist, and HSV-2 with infections where below the waist. Currently, several antiviral drugs, but not vaccine, are applied for HSV infection.

Varicella-zoster virus (VZV)

The primary infection of VZV in children generally begins in the tonsils and mucosa of the respiratory tract and results in chickenpox, and then the virus becomes latent in the dorsal root or cranial nerve ganglia after the primary infection. The virus can be reactivated in older adults and causes herpes zoster (shingles). Antiviral drugs and a live vaccine are available for VZV.

Epstein-Barr Virus (EBV)

EBV is the ultimate B-lymphocyte parasite, and causes heterophile antibody-positive infectious mononucleosis and stimulates the growth and immortalizes B cells in tissue culture. EBV has been causally associated with Burkitt lymphoma, nasopharyngeal carcinoma, and B-cell lymphomas in patients with acquired or congenital immunodeficiencies. EBV in saliva infects epithelial cells and then naïve resting B cells in the tonsils. The growth of In the B cells of EBV-latent infection the transformation and latency proteins including EBNAs and LMPs are expressed, as well as EA, VCA and MA during productive infection period. Some their corresponding antibodies can be detected for use of laboratory diagnosis. There is no vaccine and no true antiviral drug for EBV.

Human Cytomegalovirus (HCMV)

HCMV is a common human pathogen. It is the most common viral cause of congenital and perinatal infections. Although usually causing mild or asymptomatic disease in children and adults, HCMV is particularly important as an opportunistic pathogen in immunocompromised patients. Some antiviral drugs are available, but there is not vaccine for HCMV.

Human Herpesviruses 6 and 7 (HHV-6 and HHV-7)

Similar to CMV, the two variants of HHV-6, HHV-6A and HHV-6B, and HHV-7, are lymphotropic and ubiquitous. HHV-6B, perhaps HHV-7, may be associated with exanthem subitum.

Human Herpesviruses 8 (HHV-8)

Similar to EBV, the B cell is the primary target cell for HHV-8. Virus is associated with Kaposi sarcoma.

KEYWORDS

English	Chinese
herpes simplex viruses types 1 (HSV-1)	单纯疱疹病毒 1 型
herpes simplex viruses types 2 (HSV-2)	单纯疱疹病毒 2 型
gingivostomatitis	龈口炎
cold sore (herpes labialis)	唇疱疹
genital herpes	生殖器疱疹
varicella-zoster virus (VZV)	水痘 - 带状疱疹病毒
varicella (chickenpox)	水痘
herpes zoster (shingles)	带状疱疹
Epstein-Barr virus (EBV)	EB 病毒
infectious mononucleosis	传染性单核细胞增多症
Burkitt lymphoma	伯基特淋巴瘤
nasopharyngeal carcinoma	鼻咽癌
human cytomegalovirus (HCMV)	人巨细胞病毒
human herpesvirus 6 (HHV-6)	人疱疹病毒 6 型

human herpesvirus 7 (HHV-7)	人疱疹病毒 7 型
Exanthem subitum	幼儿急疹
human herpesvirus 8 (HHV-8)	人疱疹病毒 8 型
Kaposi sarcoma	卡波西肉瘤

BIBLIOGRAPHY

1. Boshoff C, Weiss RA. Kaposi sarcoma herpesvirus: new perspectives. Curr Top Microbiol Immunol, vol 312, New York, 2007, Springer-Verlag.

2. Cann AJ. Principles of molecular virology, San Diego, 2005, Academic.

3. Carter J, Saunders V. Virology: principles and applications, Chichester, England, 2007, Wiley.

4. Cohen J, Powderly WG. Infectious diseases, ed 2, St Louis, 2004, Mosby.

5. Collier L, Oxford J. Human virology, ed 3, Oxford, England, 2006, Oxford University Press.

6. Flint SJ, et al. Principles of virology: molecular biology, pathogenesis and control of animal viruses, ed 3, Washington, DC, 2009, American Society for Microbiology Press.

7. Gorbach SL, Bartlett JG, Blacklow NR. Infectious diseases, ed 3, Philadelphia, 2004, WB Saunders.

8. Knipe DM, et al. Fields virology, ed 5, Philadelphia, 2006, Lippincott Williams & Wilkins.

9. Mandell GL, Bennet JE, Dolin R. Principles and practice of infectious diseases, ed 6, Philadelphia, 2004, Churchill Livingstone.

10. McGeoch DJ. The genomes of the human herpesviruses: contents, relationships, and evolution, Annu Rev Microbiol 43: 235-265, 1989.

11. Richman DD, Whitley RJ, Hayden FG. Clinical virology, ed 3, Washington, DC, 2009, American Society for Microbiology Press.

12. Strauss JH, Strauss EG. Viruses and human disease, ed 2, San Diego, 2007, Academic.

13. Voyles BA. The biology of viruses, ed 2, Boston, 2002, McGraw-Hill.

14. White DO, Fenner FJ. Medical virology, ed 4, New York, 1994, Academic.

15. Arbesfeld DM, Thomas I. Cutaneous herpes simplex infections, Am Fam Physician 43: 1655-1664, 1991.

16. Arduino PG, Porter SR. Herpes simplex virus type 1 infection: overview on relevant clinico-pathological features. J Oral Pathol Med 37: 107-121, 2008.

17. Beauman JG. Genital herpes: a review, Am Fam Physician 72: 1527-1534, 2005.

18. Cunningham AL, et al. The cycle of human herpes simplex virus infection: virus transport and immune control, J Infect Dis 194(S1): S11-S18, 2006.

19. Dawkins BJ. Genital herpes simplex infections, Prim Care 17: 95-113, 1990.

20. Kimberlin DW. Neonatal herpes simplex virus infection, Clin Microbiol Rev 17: 1-13, 2004.

21. Landy HJ, Grossman JH. Herpes simplex virus, Obstet Gynecol Clin North Am 16: 495-515, 1989.

22. Rouse BT. Herpes simplex virus: pathogenesis, immunobiology and control, Curr Top Microbiol Immunol, vol 179, Berlin, New York, 1992, Springer-Verlag.

23. Whitley RJ, Kimberlin DW, Roizman B. Herpes simplex virus: state of the art clinical article, Clin Infect Dis 26: 541-555, 1998.

24. Abendroth A, et al. Varicella-zoster virus infections, Curr Top Microbiol Immunol, vol 342, Berlin, Heidelberg, 2010, Springer-Verlag.

25. Chia-Chi Ku V, Besser J, Abendroth A. Varicella-zoster virus pathogenesis and immunobiology: new concepts emerging from investigations with the SCIDhu mouse model, J Virol 79: 2651-2658, 2005.

26. Gnann JW, Whitley RJ. Herpes zoster, N Engl J Med 347: 340-346, 2002.

27. Ostrove JM. Molecular biology of varicella zoster virus, Adv Virus Res 38: 45-98, 1990.

28. White CJ. Varicella-zoster virus vaccine, Clin Infect Dis 24: 753-761, quiz 762-763, 1997.

29. Basgoz N, Preiksaitis JK. Post-transplant lymphoproliferative disorder, Infect Dis Clin North Am 9: 901-923, 1995.

30. Cohen JI. The biology of Epstein-Barr virus: lessons learned from the virus and the host, Curr Opin Immunol 11: 365-370, 1999.

31. Faulkner GC, Krajewski AS, Crawford DH. The ins and outs of EBV infection, Trends Microbiol 8: 185-189, 2000.

32. Hutt-Fletcher L. Epstein Barr virus entry, J Virol 81: 7825-7832, 2007.

33. Sugden B. EBV's open sesame, Trends Biochem Sci 17: 239-240, 1992.

34. Takada K. Epstein-Barr virus and human cancer. Curr Top Microbiol Immunol, vol 258, New York, 2001, Springer-Verlag.

35. Thorley-Lawson DA. Epstein-Barr virus and the B cell: that's all it takes, Trends Microbiol 4: 204-208, 1996.

36. Thorley-Lawson DA, Babcock GJ. A model for persistent infection with Epstein-Barr virus: the stealth virus of human B cells, Life Sci 65: 1433-1453, 1999.

37. Bigoni B, et al. Human herpesvirus 8 is present in the lymphoid system of healthy persons and can reactivate in the course of AIDS, J Infect Dis 173: 542-549, 1996.

38. DeBolle L, et al. Update on human herpesvirus 6 biology, clinical features, and therapy, Clin Microbiol Rev 18: 217-245, 2005.

39. Edelman DC. Human herpesvirus 8—a novel human pathogen, Virol J 2: 78-110, 2005.

40. Flamand L, et al. Review, part 1: human herpesvirus-6—basic biology, diagnostic testing, and antiviral efficacy. J Med V 82: 1560-1568, 2010.

41. Gnann JW, Pellett PE, Jaffe HW. Human herpesvirus 8 and Kaposi sarcoma in persons infected with human immunodeficiency virus, Clin Infect Dis 30: S72-S76, 2000.

42. McDougall JK. Cytomegalovirus, Curr Top Microbiol Immunol, vol 154, Berlin, New York, 1990, Springer-Verlag.

43. Pellet PE, Black JB, Yamamoto Y. Human herpesvirus 6: the virus and the search for its role as a human pathogen, Adv Virus Res 41: 1-52, 1992.

44. Plachter B, Sinzger C, Jahn G. Cell types involved in replication and distribution of human cytomegalovirus, Adv Virus Res 46: 197-264, 1996.

45. Shenk TE, Stinski MF. Human cytomegalovirus, New York, 2008, Springer-Verlag.

46. Stoeckle MY. The spectrum of human herpesvirus 6 infection: from roseola infantum to adult disease, Annu Rev Med 51: 423-430, 2000.

47. Wyatt LS, Frenkel N. Human herpesvirus 7 is a constitutive inhabitant of adult human saliva, J Virol 66: 3206-3209, 1992.

48. Yamanishi K, et al. Identification of human herpesvirus-6 as a causal agent for exanthema subitum, Lancet 1: 1065-1067, 1988.

Poxviruses

Chapter 46

The poxviruses include the human viruses **variola** (**smallpox**) (genus *Orthopoxvirus*) and **molluscum contagiosum** (genus *Molluscipoxvirus*), as well as some viruses that naturally infect animals but can cause incidental infection in humans (**zoonosis**). Many of these viruses share antigenic determinants with smallpox, allowing the use of an animal poxvirus for a human vaccine.

In 18th century England, smallpox accounted for 7% to 12% of all deaths and the deaths of one third of children. However, the development of the first live vaccine in 1796 and the later worldwide distribution of this vaccine led to the eradication of smallpox by 1980.

On a positive note, the vaccinia and canarypox viruses have found a beneficial use as gene delivery vectors and for the development of hybrid vaccines. These hybrid viruses contain and express the genes of other infectious agents, and infection results in immunization against both agents.

STRUCTURE AND REPLICATION

Poxviruses are the largest viruses, almost visible on light microscopy. They measure 230 × 300 nm and are ovoid to brick shaped with a complex morphology. The poxvirus virion particle must carry many enzymes, including a deoxyribonucleic acid (DNA)-dependent ribonucleic acid (RNA) polymerase, to allow viral messenger RNA (mRNA) synthesis to occur in the cytoplasm. The viral genome consists of a large, double-stranded, linear DNA that is fused at both ends. The structure and replication of vaccinia virus is representative of the other poxviruses (Figure 46-1). The genome of vaccinia virus consists of approximately 189,000 base pairs.

The replication of poxviruses is unique among the DNA-containing viruses, in that the entire multiplication cycle takes place within the host cell cytoplasm. Thus, poxviruses must encode the enzymes required for mRNA and DNA synthesis, as well as

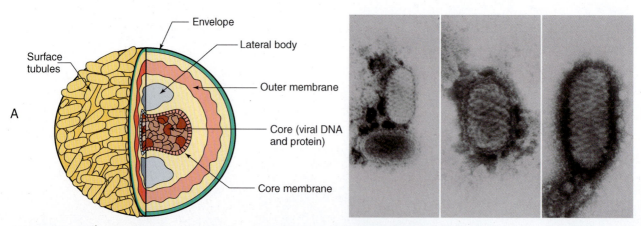

Figure 46-1 **A,** Structure of the vaccinia virus. Within the virion, the core assumes the shape of a dumbbell because of the large lateral bodies. Virions have a double membrane; the "outer membrane" assembles around the core in the cytoplasm, and the virus leaves the cell by exocytosis or upon cell lysis. **B,** Electron micrographs of orf virus. Note its complex structure.

activities other DNA viruses normally obtain from the host cell.

After binding to a cell surface receptor, the poxvirus outer envelope fuses with cellular membranes, either at the cell surface or within the cell. Early gene transcription is initiated on removal of the outer membrane. And then viral DNA liberates into the cell cytoplasm and replicates in electron-dense cytoplasmic inclusions (Guarnieri inclusion bodies). Late viral mRNA for structural, virion, and other proteins is produced after DNA replication. In poxviruses, unlike other viruses, the membranes assemble around the core factories. Different forms of virus are released by exocytosis or upon cell lysis, but both are infectious.

The vaccinia and canarypox viruses are being used as expression vectors to produce live recombinant/hybrid vaccines for more virulent infectious agents.

PATHOGENESIS AND IMMUNITY

After being inhaled, smallpox virus replicates in the upper respiratory tract. Dissemination occurs via lymphatic and cell-associated viremic spread. Internal and dermal tissues are inoculated after a second, more intense viremia, causing the simultaneous eruption of the characteristic "pocks." Molluscum contagiosum and the other poxviruses, however, are acquired through direct contact with lesions and do not spread extensively. Molluscum contagiosum causes a wartlike lesion rather than a lytic infection.

The poxviruses encode many proteins that facilitate their replication and pathogenesis in the host. They include proteins that initially stimulate host cell growth and then lead to cell lysis and viral spread.

Cell-mediated immunity is essential for resolving a poxvirus infection. However, poxviruses encode activities that help the virus evade immune control. These include the cell-to-cell spread of the virus to avoid antibody and proteins that impede the interferon, complement, and inflammatory, antibody, and cell-mediated protective responses.

EPIDEMIOLOGY

Smallpox and molluscum contagiosum are strictly human viruses. In contrast, the natural hosts for the other poxviruses important to humans are vertebrates other than humans (e.g., cow, sheep, and goats). The viruses infect humans only through accidental or occupational exposure (zoonosis).

Smallpox (variola) was very contagious and, as just noted, was spread primarily by the respiratory route. It was also spread less efficiently through close contact with dried virus on clothes or other materials. Despite the severity of the disease and its tendency to spread, several factors contributed to its elimination.

CLINICAL SYNDROMES

The diseases associated with poxviruses are listed in Table 46-1.

Smallpox

The two variants of smallpox were variola major, which was associated with a mortality of 15% to 40%, and variola minor, which was associated with a mortality of 1%. Smallpox was usually initiated by infection of the respiratory tract, with subsequent involvement of local lymph glands, which, in turn, led to viremia.

The characteristic rash of the disease is shown in Figure 46-2. After a 5- to 17-day incubation period, the infected person experienced high fever, fatigue, severe headache, backache, and malaise, followed by

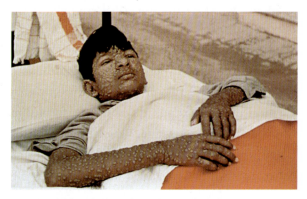

Figure 46-2 Child with smallpox. Note the characteristic rash.

Table 46-1 Diseases Associated with Poxviruses

Virus	Disease	Source	Location
Variola	Smallpox (now extinct)	Humans	Extinct
Vaccinia	Used for smallpox vaccination	Laboratory product	—
Orf	Localized lesion	Zoonosis: sheep, goats	Worldwide
Cowpox	Localized lesion	Zoonosis: rodents, cats, cows	Europe
Pseudocowpox	Milker's nodule	Zoonosis: dairy cows	Worldwide
Monkeypox	Generalized disease	Zoonosis: monkeys, squirrels	Africa
Bovine papular stomatitis virus	Localized lesion	Zoonosis: calves, beef cattle	Worldwide
Tanapox	Localized lesion	Rare zoonosis: monkeys	Africa
Yabapox	Localized lesion	Rare zoonosis: monkeys, baboons	Africa
Molluscum contagiosum	Many skin lesions	Humans	Worldwide

Modified from Balows A, et al, editors: *Laboratory diagnosis of infectious diseases: principles and practice*, vol 2, New York, 1988, Springer-Verlag.

the vesicular rash in the mouth and soon after on the body. Vomiting, diarrhea, and excessive bleeding would quickly follow. The simultaneous outbreak of the vesicular rash distinguishes smallpox from the vesicles of varicella-zoster, which erupt in successive crops.

Smallpox was usually diagnosed clinically but was confirmed by growth of the virus in embryonated eggs or cell cultures. Characteristic lesions (pocks) appeared on the chorioallantoic membrane of embryonated eggs. PCR and rapid DNA sequencing techniques can be used.

Smallpox was the first disease to be controlled by immunization, and its eradication is one of the greatest triumphs of medical epidemiology. Eradication resulted from a massive WHO campaign to vaccinate all susceptible people, especially those exposed to anyone with the disease, and thereby interrupt the chain of human-to-human transmission. The campaign began in 1967 and succeeded. The last case of naturally acquired infection was reported in 1977, and eradication of the disease was acknowledged in 1980.

Variolation, an early approach to immunization, involved the inoculation of susceptible people with the virulent smallpox pus. It was first performed in China and later in England. Variolation was associated with a fatality rate of approximately 1%, a better risk than that associated with smallpox itself. In 1796, Jenner developed and then popularized a vaccine using the less virulent cowpox virus, which shares antigenic determinants with smallpox.

Renewed interest is being paid to antiviral drugs that are effective against smallpox and other poxviruses. Cidofovir, a nucleotide analogue capable of inhibiting the viral DNA polymerase, is effective and approved for treatment of poxvirus infections.

Vaccinia and Vaccine-Related Disease

Vaccinia is the virus used for the smallpox vaccine. Although thought to be derived from cowpox, it may be a hybrid or other poxvirus. The vaccination procedure consisted of scratching live virus into the patient's skin with a bifurcated needle and then observing for the development of vesicles and pustules to confirm a "take." As the incidence of smallpox waned, however, it became apparent that there were more complications related to vaccination than cases of smallpox. Several of these complications were severe and even fatal. They included encephalitis and progressive infection (vaccinia necrosum), the latter occurring occasionally in immunocompromised patients who were inadvertently vaccinated. These individuals are treated with vaccinia immune globulin and antiviral drugs.

Orf, Cowpox, and Monkeypox

Human infection with the orf (poxvirus of sheep and goat) or cowpox (vaccinia) virus is usually an occupational hazard resulting from direct contact with the lesions on the animal. A single nodular lesion usually forms on the point of contact, such as the fingers, hand, or forearm, and is hemorrhagic (cowpox) or granulomatous (orf or pseudocowpox). Vesicular lesions frequently develop and then regress in 25 to 35 days, generally without scar formation. The lesions may be mistaken for anthrax. The virus can be grown in culture or seen directly with electron microscopy but is usually diagnosed from the symptoms and patient history.

The more than 100 cases of illnesses resembling smallpox have been attributed to the monkeypox virus. Except for the outbreak in the USA in 2003, they all have occurred in western and central Africa, especially Zaire. Monkeypox causes a milder version of smallpox disease, including the pocklike rash.

Molluscum Contagiosum

The lesions of molluscum contagiosum differ significantly from pox lesions in being nodular to wartlike. They begin as papules and then become pearl-like, umbilicated nodules that are 2 to 10 mm in diameter and have a central caseous plug that can be squeezed out. They are most common on the trunk, genitalia, and proximal extremities and usually occur in a cluster of 5 to 20 nodules. The incubation period for molluscum contagiosum is 2 to 8 weeks, and the disease is spread by direct contact (e.g., sexual contact, wrestling) or fomites (e.g., towels). The disease is more common in children than adults, but its incidence is increasing in sexually active and immunocompromised individuals.

The diagnosis of molluscum contagiosum is confirmed histologically by the finding of characteristic large, eosinophilic, cytoplasmic inclusions (molluscum bodies) in epithelial cells. These bodies can be seen in biopsy specimens or in the expressed caseous core of a nodule. The molluscum contagiosum virus cannot be grown in tissue culture or animal models.

Lesions of molluscum contagiosum disappear in 2 to 12 months, presumably as a result of immune responses. The nodules can be removed by curettage (scraping) or the application of liquid nitrogen or iodine solutions.

SUMMARY

The poxviruses include the human viruses variola (smallpox) and molluscum contagiosum that cause corresponding human diseases, and some other viruses that naturally infect animals but can cause incidental infection in humans (zoonosis). Smallpox viruses initiated by respiratory tract infection and is spread mainly by the lymphatic system and cell-associated viremia. Molluscum contagiosum virus and other poxviruses are transmitted by contact. Smallpox used to be a terrible disease, also was the first disease to be controlled by immunization.

KEYWORDS

English	Chinese
Variola (smallpox) virus	天花病毒
Molluscum contagiosum virus	传染性软疣病毒
Orf virus (poxvirus of sheep and goat)	绵羊和山羊痘病毒
Cowpox virus	牛痘病毒
Monkeypox virus	猴痘病毒
Vaccinia	牛痘苗

BIBLIOGRAPHY

1. Breman JG, Henderson DA. Diagnosis and management of smallpox, N Engl J Med 346: 1300-1308, 2002.

2. Cann AJ. Principles of molecular virology, San Diego, 2005, Academic.

3. Carter J, Saunders V. Virology: principles and applications, Chichester, England, 2007, Wiley.

4. Cohen J, Powderly WG. Infectious diseases, ed 2, St Louis, 2004, Mosby.

5. Collier L, Oxford J. Human virology, ed 3, Oxford, England, 2006, Oxford University Press.

6. Fenner F. A successful eradication campaign: global eradication of smallpox, Rev Infect Dis 4: 916-930, 1982.

7. Flint SJ, et al. Principles of virology: molecular biology, pathogenesis, and control of animal viruses, ed 3, Washington, DC, 2009, American Society for Microbiology Press.

8. Gorbach SL, Bartlett JG, Blacklow NR. Infectious diseases, ed 2, Philadelphia, 1997, WB Saunders.

9. Knipe DM, et al. Fields virology, ed 5, Philadelphia, 2006, Lippincott Williams & Wilkins.

10. Mandell GL, Bennet JE, Dolin R. Principles and practice of infectious diseases, ed 6, Philadelphia, 2004, Churchill Livingstone.

11. Moyer RW, Turner PC. Poxviruses, Curr Top Microbiol Immunol, vol 163, New York, 1990, Springer-Verlag.

12. Piccini A, Paoletti E. Vaccinia: virus, vector, vaccine, Adv Virus Res 34: 43-64, 1988.

13. Richman DD, Whitley RJ, Hayden FG. Clinical virology, ed 3, Washington, DC, 2009, American Society for Microbiology Press.

14. Strauss JM, Strauss EG: Viruses and human disease, San Diego, 2002, Academic.

15. Voyles BA. Biology of viruses, ed 2, Boston, 2002, McGraw-Hill.

16. White DO, Fenner FJ. Medical virology, ed 4, New York, 1994, Academic.

Chapter 47

Parvoviruses

The *Parvoviridae* are the smallest DNA viruses. Their small size and limited genetic repertoire make them more dependent than any other DNA virus on the host cell, or they require the presence of a helper virus to replicate. **B19** and **bocavirus** are the only parvoviruses known to cause human disease. Other parvoviruses, e.g., feline and canine parvoviruses, have not been shown to cause human disease and are preventable with vaccination of the pet. Adeno-associated viruses (AAVs) are members of the genus *Dependovirus*. They neither cause illness nor modify infection by their helper viruses. The genus *Densovirus* infects only insects.

STRUCTURE AND REPLICATION

The parvoviruses are extremely small (18 to 26 nm in diameter) and have a nonenveloped, icosahedral capsid (Figure 47-1). The B19 virus genome contains one linear, single-stranded DNA molecule with a molecular mass of 1.5 to 1.8×10^6 Da (5500 bases in length). Plus or minus DNA strands are packaged separately into virions. The genome encodes three structural and two major nonstructural proteins.

B19 virus replicates in mitotically active cells and prefers cells of the erythroid lineage, such as fresh human bone marrow cells, erythroid cells from fetal liver, and erythroid leukemia cells. After binding to the erythrocyte blood group P antigen (globoside) and its internalization, the virion is uncoated, and the single-stranded DNA genome is delivered to the nucleus. The single-stranded DNA virion genome is converted to a double-stranded DNA version, which is required for transcription and replication. The two major nonstructural proteins and the VP1 and VP2 structural capsid proteins are synthesized in the cytoplasm, and the structural proteins go to the nucleus, where the virion is assembled. The VP2 protein is cleaved later to produce VP3. The nuclear and cytoplasmic membrane degenerates, and the virus is released on cell lysis.

PATHOGENESIS AND IMMUNITY

B19 targets and is cytolytic for erythroid precursor cells. B19 disease is determined by the direct killing of these cells and the subsequent immune response to the infection (rash and arthralgia).

B19 virus first replicates in the nasopharynx or upper respiratory tract then spreads by viremia to the bone marrow and elsewhere. Bocavirus also initiates infection in the respiratory tract, replicates in the respiratory epithelium, and causes disease.

B19 viral disease has a biphasic course. The initial febrile stage is the infectious stage. During this time,

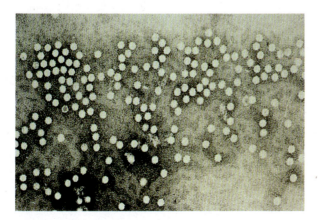

Figure 47-1 Electron micrograph of parvovirus. Parvoviruses are small (18 to 26 nm), nonenveloped viruses with single-stranded DNA. (Courtesy Centers for Disease Control and Prevention, Atlanta.)

401

erythrocyte production is stopped for approximately 1 week because of the viral killing of erythroid precursor cells. A large viremia occurs within 8 days of infection and is accompanied by nonspecific flulike symptoms. Large numbers of virus are also released into oral and respiratory secretions. Antibody stops the viremia and is important for resolution of the disease but contributes to the symptoms. The second, symptomatic, stage is immune mediated. The rash and arthralgia seen in this stage coincide with the appearance of virus-specific antibody, the disappearance of detectable B19 virus, and the formation of immune complexes.

Hosts with chronic hemolytic anemia (e.g., sickle cell anemia) who are infected with B19 are at risk for a life-threatening reticulocytopenia, which is referred to as an aplastic crisis. The reticulocytopenia results from the combination of (1) B19 depletion of the red blood cell precursors and (2) shortened life span of the erythrocytes caused by the underlying anemia.

EPIDEMIOLOGY

Approximately 65% of the adult population has been infected with B19 by 40 years of age. Erythema infectiosum is most common in children and adolescents aged 4 to 15 years, who are a source of contagion. Arthralgia and arthritis are likely to occur in adults. Respiratory droplets and oral secretions most probably transmit the virus. Disease usually occurs in late winter and spring. Parenteral transmission of the virus by a blood-clotting-factor concentrate has also been described.

Bocavirus is found worldwide and causes disease in children younger than 2 years old. The virus is transmitted in respiratory secretions but can also be isolated from stool.

CLINICAL SYNDROMES

B19 Virus Infection

B19 virus, as stated earlier, is the cause of erythema infectiosum. Infection starts with an unremarkable prodromal period of 7 to 10 days, during which the person is contagious. Infection of a normal host may cause either no noticeable symptoms or fever and nonspecific symptoms, such as sore throat, chills, malaise, and myalgia, as well as a slight decrease in hemoglobin levels. This period is followed by a distinctive rash on the cheeks, which appear to have been slapped. The rash then usually spreads, especially to exposed skin such as the arms and legs (Figure 47-2), and then subsides over 1 to 2 weeks. Relapse of the rash is common.

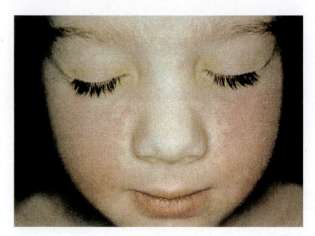

Figure 47-2 A "slapped-cheek" appearance is typical of the rash for erythema infectiosum. (From Hart CA, Broadhead RL: *A color atlas of pediatric infectious diseases*, London, 1992, Wolfe.)

B19 infection in adults causes polyarthritis with or without a rash. B19 infection of immunocompromised people may result in chronic disease.

The most serious complication of parvovirus infection is the aplastic crisis that occurs in patients with chronic hemolytic anemia (e.g., sickle cell anemia). Infection in these people causes a transient reduction in erythropoiesis in the bone marrow. The reduction results in a transient reticulocytopenia.

B19 infection of a seronegative mother increases the risk for fetal death. The virus can infect the fetus and kill erythrocyte precursors, causing anemia and congestive heart failure.

Bocavirus Infection

Bocavirus may cause mild or severe acute respiratory disease. The more severe disease occurs in children younger than 2 years old who may have bronchiolitis with wheezing and with a viremia that extends long beyond the disease. A fatal case of bocavirus bronchiolitis has been reported.

LABORATORY DIAGNOSIS

The diagnosis of erythema infectiosum is usually based on the clinical presentation. For B19 disease to be definitively diagnosed, however, specific IgM or viral DNA must be detected (i.e., to distinguish the rash of B19 from that of rubella in a pregnant woman). ELISAs for B19 IgM and IgG can be used. The PCR is a very sensitive method for detecting the B19 and bocavirus genomes in clinical samples. Virus isolation is not performed.

TREATMENT, PREVENTION, AND CONTROL

No specific antiviral drugs and vaccines are available for B19 virus and bocavirus.

SUMMARY

B19 virus normally causes erythema infectiosum, is also responsible for episodes of aplastic crisis in patients with chronic hemolytic anemia and is associated with acute polyarthritis in adults. Intrauterine infection of a fetus may cause abortion. Bocavirus can cause acute respiratory disease, which may become severe in young children. No antiviral drugs and vaccines are available for infection with both viruses.

KEYWORDS

English	Chinese
B19 virus	B19病毒
erythema infectiosum	传染性红斑
aplastic crisis	再生障碍性危象
hemolytic anemia	溶血性贫血
Bocavirus	博卡病毒

BIBLIOGRAPHY

1. Allander T. Human bocavirus, J Clin Virol 41: 29-33, 2008.

2. Anderson LJ. Human parvoviruses, J Infect Dis 161: 603-608, 1990.

3. Anderson MJ. Parvoviruses. In Belshe RB, editor: Textbook of human virology, ed 2, St Louis, 1991, Mosby.

4. Berns KI. The parvoviruses, New York, 1994, Plenum.

5. Berns KI. Parvovirus replication, Microbiol Rev 54: 316-329, 1990.

6. Brown KE: The expanding range of parvoviruses which infect humans, Rev Med Virol 20: 231-244, 2010.

7. Brown KE, Young NS. Parvovirus B19 in human disease, Annu Rev Med 48: 59-67, 1997.

8. Cann AJ. Principles of molecular virology, San Diego, 2005, Academic.

9. Carter J, Saunders V. Virology: principles and applications, Chichester, England, 2007, Wiley.

10. Chorba T, et al. The role of parvovirus B19 in aplastic crisis and erythema infectiosum (fifth disease), J Infect Dis 154: 383-393, 1986.

11. Cohen J, Powderly WG. Infectious diseases, ed 2, St Louis, 2004, Mosby.

12. Collier L, Oxford J: Human virology, ed 3, Oxford, England, 2006, Oxford University Press.

13. Flint SJ, et al. Principles of virology: molecular biology, pathogenesis and control of animal viruses, ed 3, Washington, DC, 2009, American Society for Microbiology Press.

14. Gorbach SL, Bartlett JG, Blacklow NR. Infectious diseases, ed 3, Philadelphia, 2004, WB Saunders.

15. Knipe DM, et al. Fields virology, ed 5, Philadelphia, 2006, Lippincott Williams & Wilkins.

16. Mandell GL, Bennet JE, Dolin R. Principles and practice of infectious diseases, ed 6, Philadelphia, 2005, Churchill Livingstone.

17. Naides SJ, et al. Rheumatologic manifestations of human parvovirus B19 infection in adults, Arthritis Rheum 33: 1297-1309, 1990.

18. Richman DD, Whitley RJ, Hayden FG. Clinical virology, ed 3, Washington, DC, 2009, American Society for Microbiology Press.

19. Törk TJ. Parvovirus B19 and human disease, Adv Intern Med 37: 431-455, 1992.

20. Ursic T, et al. Human bocavirus as the cause of a life-threatening infection, J Clin Microbiol 49: 1179-1181, 2011.

21. Voyles BA. The biology of viruses, ed 2, Boston, 2002, McGraw-Hill.

22. Ware RE. Parvovirus infections. In Katz SL, et al, editors: Krugman's infectious diseases of children, ed 10, St. Louis, 1998, Mosby.

23. Young NS, Brown KE. Parvovirus B19, N Engl J Med 350: 586-597, 2004.

Picornaviruses

Chapter 48

Picornaviridae is one of the largest families of viruses and includes some of the most important human and animal viruses. As the name indicates, these viruses are **small** (pico) ribonucleic acid (**RNA**) viruses that have a **naked capsid** structure. The family has more than 230 members divided into nine genera, including *Enterovirus*, *Rhinovirus*, *Hepatovirus* (hepatitis A virus, HAV), *Cardiovirus*, and *Aphthovirus*. The enteroviruses are distinguished from the rhinoviruses by the stability of the capsid at pH 3, the optimum temperature for growth, the mode of transmission, and their diseases.

At least 90 serotypes of human enteroviruses exist and are classified as polioviruses, coxsackieviruses A and B, echoviruses, or for the more recently discovered viruses, as numbered enteroviruses (e.g., enterovirus 68). Several different disease syndromes may be caused by a specific serotype of enterovirus. Likewise, several different serotypes may cause the same disease, depending on the target tissue affected.

The capsids of enteroviruses are *very resistant to harsh environmental conditions* (sewage systems) and the conditions in the gastrointestinal tract, which facilitates their transmission by the fecal-oral route. Although they may initiate infection in the gastrointestinal tract, the enteroviruses rarely cause enteric disease. In fact, most infections are usually asymptomatic. The best-known and most-studied picornavirus is poliovirus, of which there are three serotypes.

Coxsackieviruses are named after the town of Coxsackie, New York, where they were first isolated. They are divided into two groups, A and B, on the basis of certain biological and antigenic differences and are further subdivided into numeric serotypes

on the basis of additional antigenic differences.

The name **echovirus** is derived from *e*nteric *c*ytopathic *h*uman *o*rphan because the disease associated with these agents was not initially known. Since 1967, newly isolated enteroviruses have been distinguished numerically.

The human **rhinoviruses** consist of at least 100 serotypes and are the major cause of the common cold. They are sensitive to acidic pH and replicate poorly at temperatures above 33°C. These properties usually limit rhinoviruses to causing upper respiratory tract infections.

STRUCTURE

The plus-strand RNA of the picornaviruses is surrounded by an **icosahedral capsid** that is approximately 30 nm in diameter. The icosahedral capsid has 12 pentameric vertices, each of which is composed of five protomeric units of proteins. The protomers are made of four virion polypeptides (VP1 to VP4). VP2 and VP4 are generated by the cleavage of a precursor, VP0. VP4 in the virion solidifies the structure, but it is not generated until the genome is incorporated into the capsid. This protein is released on binding of the virus to the cellular receptor. The capsids are stable in the presence of heat, acid, and detergent, with the exception of the rhinoviruses, which are labile to acid. The capsid structure is so regular that paracrystals of virions often form in infected cells (Figures 48-1 and 48-2).

The **genome of the picornaviruses resembles a messenger RNA (mRNA)** (Figure 48-3). It is a single strand of plus-sense RNA(+ssRNA) of approximately

7200 to 8450 bases. It has a poly(A) (polyadenosine) sequence at the 3' end and a small protein, VPg (viral protein genome-linked; 22 to 24 amino acids), attached to the 5' end. The poly(A) sequence enhances the infectivity of the RNA, and the VPg is important in packaging the genome into the capsid and initiating viral RNA synthesis. *The naked picornavirus genome is sufficient for infection if microinjected into a cell.*

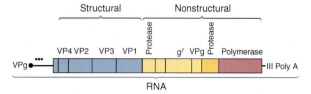

Figure 48-3 Structure of the picornavirus genome. The genome (7200 to 8400 bases) is translated as a polyprotein that is cleaved by viral-encoded proteases into individual proteins. Viral genes: *VP1*, *2*, *3*, *4*, capsid proteins 1, 2, 3, 4; *2A* and *3C^{pro}*, proteases. *2A* cleaves eIF4G to inhibit host protein synthesis; *2B*, *2C*, *3A*, *3B* generate membrane-binding, vesicle-forming proteins that facilitate replication; *3B* also encodes VPg genome-binding protein; *RdRp*, RNA-dependent RNA polymerase (Redrawn from Whitton JL, Cornell CT, Feuer R: Host and virus determinants of picornavirus pathogenesis and tropism, *Nat Rev Microbiol* 3: 765-776, 2005.)

Figure 48-1 Electron micrograph of poliovirus (Curtesy Contents for Disease Control and Prevention, Atlanta).

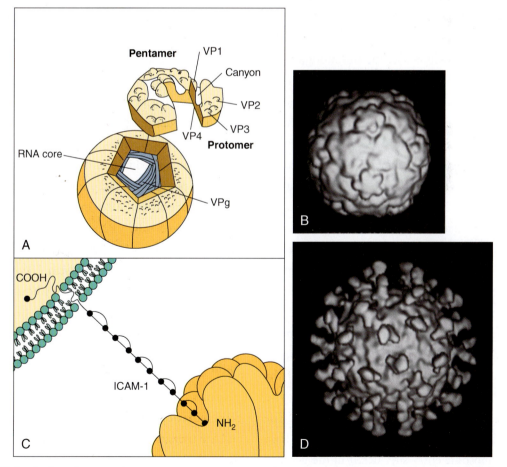

Figure 48-2 **A,** Cryoelectron microscopy computer-generated reconstruction of human rhinovirus 16. **B,** Cryoelectron microscopy reconstruction of the interaction of a soluble form of intercellular adhesion molecule-1 (ICAM-1) with human rhinovirus 16. Note: There is one ICAM-1 per capsomere. **C,** Structure of the human rhinovirus and its interaction with ICAM-1 on the target cell. **D,** Binding of the ICAM-1 molecule within the canyon of the virion triggers the opening of the capsid for release of the genome into the cell. RNA, Ribonucleic acid; *VP1, 2, 3, 4,* viral protein 1, 2, 3, 4; *VPg,* viral protein genome-linked. (**A** and **B,** Courtesy Tim Baker, Purdue University, West Lafayette, Ind.)

The genome encodes a polyprotein that is proteolytically cleaved by viral-encoded proteases to produce the enzymatic and structural proteins of the virus. In addition to the capsid proteins and VPg, the picornaviruses encode at least two proteases (2A and 3C) and an RNA-dependent RNA polymerase (RdRp).

REPLICATION

The specificity of the picornavirus interaction for cellular receptors is the major determinant of the target tissue tropism and disease. The VP1 proteins at the vertices of the virion contain a canyon structure to which the receptor binds. Pleconaril and related antiviral compounds bind to the floor of this canyon and alters its conformation to prevent the uncoating of the virus.

The picornaviruses can be categorized according to their cell surface receptor specificity. The receptors for polioviruses, some coxsackieviruses, and rhinoviruses are members of the immunoglobulin superfamily of proteins. At least 80% of the rhinoviruses and several serotypes of coxsackievirus bind to the intercellular adhesion molecule-1 (ICAM-1) expressed on epithelial cells, fibroblasts, and endothelial cells. Several coxsackieviruses, echoviruses, and other enteroviruses bind to decay accelerating factor (CD55), and coxsackievirus B shares a receptor with adenovirus. Poliovirus binds to a different molecule (PVR/CD155) that is similar to the receptor for HSV. The poliovirus receptor is present on many different human cells, but not all of these cells will replicate the virus.

On binding to the receptor, the genome is injected directly across the membrane through a channel created by the VP1 protein at one of the vertices of the virion. The genome binds directly to ribosomes, despite the lack of a 5'-cap structure. The ribosomes recognize a unique internal RNA loop (internal ribosome entry site, IRES) in the genome that is also present in some cellular mRNAs. A **polyprotein** containing all the viral protein sequences is synthesized within 10 to 15 minutes of infection. This polyprotein is cleaved by viral proteases

encoded in it (see Figure 48-3). Viral proteins tether the genome to endoplasmic reticulum membranes, and the machinery for replication of the genome is collected into a vesicle. The viral RNA-dependent RNA polymerase generates a negative-strand RNA template from which the new mRNA/genome can be synthesized. The amount of viral mRNA increases rapidly in the cell, with the number of viral RNA molecules reaching as many as 400,000 per cell.

Most picornaviruses inhibit cellular RNA and protein synthesis during infection. For example, cleavage of the cell's cap-binding protein (eIF4G) of the ribosome by a poliovirus protease prevents most cellular mRNA from binding to the ribosome. Inhibition of transcription factors decreases cellular mRNA synthesis, and permeability changes induced by picornaviruses reduce the ability of cellular mRNA to bind to the ribosome. In addition, viral mRNA can out-compete cellular mRNA for the factors required in protein synthesis. These activities contribute to the cytopathologic effect of the virus on the target cell.

As the viral genome is being replicated and translated, the structural proteins VP0, VP1, and VP3 are cleaved from the polyprotein by a viral-encoded protease and assembled into subunits. Five **subunits** associate into **pentamers**, and 12 **pentamers** associate to form the **procapsid**. After insertion of the genome, VP0 is cleaved into VP2 and VP4 to complete the **capsid**. As many as 100,000 virions per cell may be produced and released on cell lysis. The entire replication cycle may be as short as 3 to 4 hours.

ENTEROVIRUSES

Pathogenesis and Immunity

Contrary to their name, enteroviruses do not usually cause enteric disease, but they do replicate within and are transmitted by the fecal-oral route. The diseases produced by the enteroviruses are determined mainly by differences in tissue tropism and the cytolytic capacity of the virus (Figure 48-4). The virions are impervious to stomach acid, proteases, and bile. Enteroviruses are acquired through the upper respiratory tract and mouth. Viral replication is initiated in the mucosa and lymphoid tissue of the tonsils and pharynx, and the virus later infects M cells and lymphocytes of the Peyer patches and enterocytes in the intestinal mucosa. Primary viremia spreads the virus to receptor-bearing target tissues, including the reticuloendothelial cells of the lymph nodes, spleen, and liver, to initiate a second phase of viral replication, resulting in a secondary viremia and symptoms.

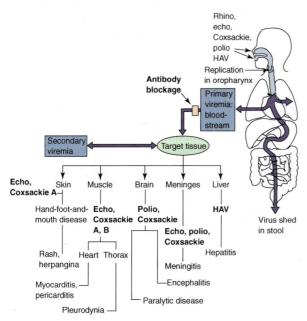

Figure 48-4   Pathogenesis of enterovirus infection. The target tissue infected by the enterovirus determines the predominant disease caused by the virus.

Most enteroviruses are **cytolytic**, replicating rapidly and causing direct damage to the target cell. In the case of poliovirus, the virus gains access to the brain by infecting skeletal muscle and traveling up the innervating nerves to the brain, similar to the rabies virus. The virus is cytolytic for the motor neurons of the anterior horn and brainstem.

Viral shedding from the oropharynx can be detected for a short time before symptoms begin, whereas viral production and shedding from the intestine may last for 30 days or longer, even in the presence of a humoral immune response.

Antibody is the major protective immune response to the enteroviruses. Secretory antibody can prevent the initial establishment of infection in the oropharynx and gastrointestinal tract, and serum antibody pre-

vents viremic spread to the target tissue and therefore disease. The time course for antibody development after infection with a live vaccine is presented in Figure 48-6. Cell-mediated immunity is not usually involved in protection but may play a role in resolution and pathogenesis.

Epidemiology

The enteroviruses are exclusively human pathogens. As the name implies, these viruses primarily spread via the **fecal-oral** route. **Asymptomatic shedding** can occur for up to a month, putting virus into the environment. Poor sanitation and crowded living conditions foster transmission of the viruses. Sewage contamination of water supplies can result in enterovirus epidemics. Outbreaks of enterovirus disease are seen in schools and day-care settings, and summer is the major season for such disease. The coxsackieviruses and echoviruses may also be spread in aerosol droplets and cause respiratory tract infections.

Polioviruses are spread most often during the summer and autumn. With the success of the polio vaccines, the wild-type poliovirus has almost been eliminated from the world. Paralytic polio was never eliminated from Nigeria, Afghanistan, and Pakistan, and the viruses are spreading from these countries to others, including Somalia, Kenya, Ethiopia, Cameroon, Syria, and Israel. A small but significant number of vaccine-related cases of polio result from mutation of one of the three strains in the live vaccine virus, which reestablishes neurovirulence. Change in the receptor-binding VP1 protein gene has occurred by recombination with another enterovirus.

Similar to poliovirus infection, coxsackievirus A-caused disease is generally more severe in adults than in children. Coxsackievirus B and some of the echoviruses (especially echovirus 11) can be particularly harmful to infants.

Clinical Syndromes

The clinical syndromes produced by the enteroviruses are determined by several factors, including (1) viral serotype, (2) infecting dose, (3) tissue tropism, (4) portal

Table 48-1 Summary of Clinical Syndromes Associated with Major Enterovirus Groups

Syndrome	Occurrence	Polioviruses	Coxsackie A Viruses	Coxsackie B Viruses	Echoviruses
Paralytic disease	Sporadic	+	+	+	+
Encephalitis, meningitis	Outbreaks	+	+	+	+
Carditis	Sporadic		+	+	+
Neonatal disease	Outbreaks			+	+
Pleurodynia	Outbreaks			+	
Herpangina	Common		+		
Hand-foot-and-mouth disease	Common		+		
Rash disease	Common		+	+	+
Acute hemorrhagic conjunctivitis	Epidemics		+		
Respiratory tract infections	Common	+	+	+	+
Undifferentiated fever	Common	+	+	+	+
Diarrhea, gastrointestinal disease	Uncommon				+
Diabetes, pancreatitis	Uncommon			+	
Orchitis	Uncommon			+	
Disease in immunodeficient patients	—	+	+	+	+
Congenital anomalies	Uncommon		+	+	

of entry, (5) patient's age, gender, and state of health, and (6) pregnancy (Table 48-1). The incubation period for enterovirus disease varies from 1 to 35 days, depending on the virus, the target tissue, and the person's age. Viruses that affect oral and respiratory sites have the shortest incubation periods.

Poliovirus Infections

There are three poliovirus types (1-3), with 85% of the cases of paralytic polio caused by type 1. Reversion of the attenuated vaccine virus types 2 and 3 to virulence can cause vaccine-associated disease. Poliovirus may cause one of the following four outcomes in unvaccinated people, depending on the progression of the infection (Figure 48-5):

Asymptomatic illness results if the viral infection is limited to the oropharynx and the gut. At least 90% of poliovirus infections are asymptomatic.

Abortive poliomyelitis, the minor illness, is a nonspecific febrile illness occurring in approximately 5% of infected people. Fever, headache, malaise, sore throat, and vomiting occur in such persons within 3 to 4 days of exposure.

Nonparalytic poliomyelitis or **aseptic meningitis**

occurs in 1% to 2% of patients with poliovirus infections. In this disease, the virus progresses into the central nervous system and the meninges, causing back pain and muscle spasms in addition to the symptoms of the minor illness.

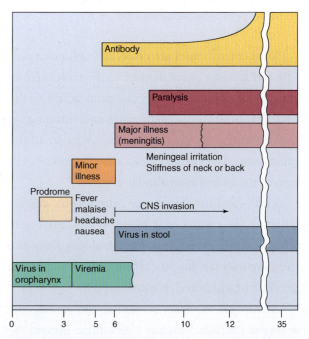

Figure 48-5 Progression of poliovirus infection. Infection may be asymptomatic or may progress to minor or major disease.

Paralytic poliomyelitis, the major illness, occurs in 0.1% to 2.0% of persons with poliovirus infections and is the most severe outcome. In this disease, the virus spreads from the blood to the anterior horn cells of the spinal cord and to the motor cortex of the brain. The severity of paralysis is determined by the extent of the neuronal infection and by which neurons are affected. Paralytic poliomyelitis is characterized by an asymmetric flaccid paralysis with no sensory loss. Spinal paralysis may involve one or more limbs, whereas bulbar (cranial) paralysis may involve a combination of cranial nerves and even the medullary respiratory center.

The paralysis progress over the first few days and may result in complete recovery, residual paralysis, or death. **Bulbar poliomyelitis** can be more severe, may involve the muscles of the pharynx, vocal cords, and respiration, and may result in death in 75% of patients. **Postpolio syndrome** is a sequela of poliomyelitis that may occur much later in life (30 to 40 years later) in 20% to 80% of the original victims. Affected persons suffer a deterioration of the originally affected muscles. Poliovirus is not present, but the syndrome is believed to result from a loss of neurons in the initially affected nerves.

Coxsackievirus and Echovirus Infections

Several clinical syndromes may be caused by either a coxsackievirus or an echovirus (e.g., aseptic meningitis), but certain illnesses are specifically associated with coxsackieviruses. Coxsackievirus A is associated with diseases involving vesicular lesions (e.g., herpangina), whereas coxsackievirus B is most frequently associated with myocarditis and pleurodynia. Coxsackieviruses and enterovirus 68 can also cause a polio-like paralytic disease. The most common result of infection is lack of symptoms or a mild upper respiratory tract or flulike disease.

Herpangina is caused by several types of coxsackievirus A and is not related to a herpesvirus infection. Fever, sore throat, pain on swallowing, anorexia, and vomiting characterize this disease. The classic finding is vesicular ulcerated lesions around the soft palate and uvula. Less typically, the lesions affect the hard palate. The virus can be recovered from the lesions or from feces. The disease is self-limited and requires only symptomatic management.

Hand-foot-and-mouth disease (HFMD) is a vesicular exanthem usually caused by coxsackievirus A16 and enterovirus 71 (EV71). The name is descriptive because the main features of this infection consist of vesicular lesions on the hands, feet, mouth, and tongue. Usually, coxsackievirus A16 causes mild HFMD with a febrile, and the illness subsides in a few days. Enterovirus 71 always causes severe and life-threatening HFMD with central nerve system injury. A high mortality of EV71-related HFMD in neonates has been observed in Asian countries.

Pleurodynia (Bornholm disease) caused by coxsackievirus B is an acute illness in which patients have a sudden onset of fever and unilateral low thoracic, pleuritic chest pain that may be excruciating. Abdominal pain and even vomiting may also occur, and muscles on the involved side may be extremely tender. Pleurodynia lasts an average of 4 days but may relapse after the condition has been asymptomatic for several days.

Myocardial and **pericardial infections** caused by coxsackievirus B occur sporadically in older children and adults but are most threatening in newborns. Neonates with these infections have febrile illnesses and sudden and unexplained onset of heart failure. Cyanosis, tachycardia, cardiomegaly, and hepatomegaly occur. The mortality associated with the infection is high, and autopsy typically reveals involvement of other organ systems, including the brain, liver, and pancreas. Acute benign pericarditis affects young adults but may be seen in older persons. The symptoms resemble those of myocardial infarction with fever.

Viral (aseptic) meningitis is an acute febrile illness accompanied by headache and signs of meningeal irritation, including nuchal rigidity. Petechiae or a rash may occur in patients with enteroviral meningitis. Recovery is usually uneventful unless the illness is associated with encephalitis (meningoencephalitis) or occurs in children younger than 1 year. Outbreaks of picornavirus meningitis (echovirus 11) occur each year during the summer and autumn.

Fever, rash, and **common cold like symptoms** may occur in patients infected with echoviruses or coxsackieviruses. The rash is usually maculopapular but may occasionally be petechial or even vesicular. The petechial type of eruption can be confused with the rash of meningococcemia, which is life threatening and must be treated. Enteroviral disease is usually less intense for the child than meningococcemia. Coxsackie viruses A21 and A24 and echoviruses 11 and 20 can cause rhinovirus-like symptoms resembling the common cold.

Other Enterovirus Diseases

Enterovirus 70 and a variant of coxsackievirus A24 have been associated with an extremely contagious ocular disease, acute hemorrhagic conjunctivitis. The infection causes subconjunctival hemorrhages and conjunctivitis. The disease has a 24-hour incubation period and resolves within 1 or 2 weeks. Some strains of coxsackievirus B and echovirus can be transmitted transplacentally to the fetus. Infection of the fetus or an infant by this or another route may produce severe disseminated disease. Coxsackie virus B infections of the beta cells of the pancreas are a major cause of **type 1 insulin-dependent diabetes** as a result of immune destruction of the islets of Langerhans.

Laboratory Diagnosis

Clinical Chemistry

Cerebrospinal fluid (CSF) from enterovirus aseptic meningitis can be distinguished from bacterial meningitis. The CSF lacks neutrophils, and the glucose level is usually normal or slightly low. The CSF protein level is normal to slightly elevated. The CSF is rarely positive for the virus.

Culture

Polioviruses may be isolated from the patient's pharynx during the first few days of illness, from the feces for as long as 30 days, but only rarely from CSF. The virus grows well in monkey kidney tissue culture. Coxsackie viruses and echoviruses can usually be isolated from the throat and stool during infection and often from CSF in patients with meningitis. Virus is rarely isolated in patients with myocarditis, because the symptoms occur several weeks after the initial infection. Coxsackie virus B can be grown on primary monkey or human embryo kidney cells. Many strains of coxsackie virus A do not grow in tissue culture but can be grown in suckling mice.

Genome and Serology Studies

The exact type of enterovirus can be determined through the use of specific antibody and antigen assays (e.g., neutralization, immunofluorescence, enzyme-linked immunosorbent assay) or RT-PCR detection of viral RNA. RT-PCR of clinical samples has become a rapid and routine method to detect the presence of an enterovirus or distinguish a specific enterovirus, depending upon the primers used. RT-PCR has become especially important for confirming a diagnosis of echovirus 11 meningitis in an infant.

Serology can be used to confirm an enterovirus infection through detection of specific IgM or the finding of a fourfold increase in the antibody titer between the time of the acute illness and the period of convalescence. Because of their many serotypes, this approach may not be practical for detection of echovirus and coxsackie virus unless a specific virus is suspected.

Treatment, Prevention, and Control

Pleconaril is available on a limited basis. The drug inhibits penetration of picornaviruses into the cell. It must be administered early in the course of the infection.

Prevention of paralytic poliomyelitis is one of the triumphs of modern medicine. Similar to smallpox, polio has been targeted for elimination. The two types of poliovirus vaccine are (1) **inactivated polio vaccine (IPV)**, developed by Jonas Salk, and (2) **live attenuated oral polio vaccine (OPV)**, developed by Albert Sabin. Both vaccines incorporate the three strains of polio, are stable, are relatively inexpensive, and induce a protective antibody response (Figure 48-6).

The IPV was proven effective in 1955, but the OPV took its place because it is less expensive, easy to administer, limits production of virus and virus

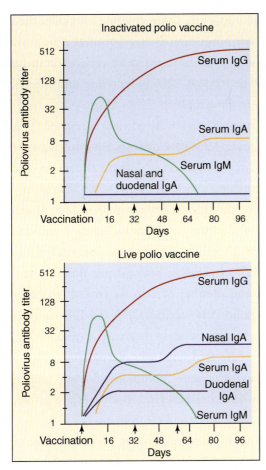

Figure 48-6　Serum and secretory antibody response to intramuscular inoculation of inactivated polio vaccine (IPV) and to oral live attenuated polio vaccine (OPV). Note the presence of secretory IgA induced by the OPV. (Modified from Ogra P, Fishaut M, Gallagher MR: Viral vaccination via the mucosal routes, *Rev Infect Dis* 2: 352-369, 1980. Copyright 1980, University of Chicago Press.)

transmission, and elicits lifelong and mucosal immunity. The OPV was attenuated (i.e., rendered less virulent) by passage in human or monkey cell cultures. Attenuation yielded a virus that can replicate in the oropharynx and intestinal tract but cannot infect neuronal cells. The vaccine elicits IgA and IgG that can stop virus spread in and from the gut as well as spread within the body. The major drawbacks of the live vaccine are that (1) the vaccine virus may infect an immunologically compromised person, and (2) there is a remote potential for the virus to revert to its virulent form and cause paralytic disease. IPV has less potential for vaccine-related disease and is the vaccine of choice for routine vaccination.

There are no vaccines for coxsackieviruses or echoviruses. Enteroviruses are impervious to most common disinfectants and detergents but can be inactivated by formaldehyde, hypo- chlorite, and chlorine.

RHINOVIRUSES

Rhinoviruses are the most important cause of the common cold and upper respiratory tract infections. Such infections are self-limited and do not cause serious disease. More than 100 serotypes of rhinovirus have been identified. At least 80% of the rhinoviruses have a common receptor that is also used by some of the coxsackieviruses. This receptor has been identified as ICAM-1, a member of the immunoglobulin superfamily, which is expressed on epithelial, fibroblast, and B-lymphoblastoid cells.

Pathogenesis

Unlike the enteroviruses, rhinoviruses are **unable to replicate in the gastrointestinal tract**. The rhinoviruses are **labile to acidic pH**. Also, they **grow best at 33°C**, a feature that contributes to their preference for the cooler environment of the nasal mucosa. The virus enters through the nose, mouth, or eyes and initiates infection of the upper respiratory tract, including the throat. Most viral replication occurs in the nose, and the onset and severity of the symptoms correlate with the time of viral shedding and quantity (titer) of virus shed. Infected cells release bradykinin and histamine, which cause a "runny nose."

Rhinoviruses cause at least half of all upper respiratory tract infections. Rhinoviruses can be transmitted by two mechanisms: as aerosols and on fomites (e.g., by hands or on contaminated inanimate objects). Hands appear to be the major vector, and direct person-to-person contact is the predominant mode of spread. Rhinovirus "colds" occur most often in early autumn and late spring in persons living in temperate climates. Rates of infection are highest in infants and children.

Rhinoviruses produce clinical illness in only half of the persons infected. The illness peaks in 3 to 4 days, but the cough and nasal symptoms may persist for 7 to 10 days or longer. Asymptomatic persons are also capable of spreading the virus, even though they may produce less of it.

Immunity to rhinoviruses is transient and unlikely to prevent subsequent infection (because of the numerous serotypes of the virus). Both nasal secretory IgA and serum IgG antibody are induced by a primary rhinovirus infection and can be detected within a week of infection. The secretory IgA response dissipates quickly, and immunity begins to wane approximately 18 months after infection. Cell-mediated immunity is not likely to play an important role in controlling rhinovirus infections.

Laboratory Diagnosis

The clinical syndrome of the common cold is usually so characteristic that laboratory diagnosis is unnecessary. Virus can be obtained from nasal washings. Rhinoviruses are grown in human diploid fibroblast cells (e.g., WI-38) at 33℃. Identification can also be made by genome analysis by RT-PCR. The performance of serologic testing to document rhinovirus infection is not practical.

Treatment, Prevention, and Control

There are many over-the-counter (OTC) remedies for the common cold. Nasal vasoconstrictors may provide relief, but their use may be followed by rebound congestion and a worsening of symptoms.

No antiviral drugs are effective. Rhinovirus is not a good candidate for a vaccine program because of the multiple serotypes. The benefit-to-risk ratio would also be very low because rhinoviruses do not cause significant disease. Handwashing and disinfection of contaminated objects are the best means of preventing viral spread.

SUMMARY

Picornaviridae represents a large family of viruses that can be divided into nine genera, including enterovirus, rhinovirus, hepatovirus, cardiovirus, and aphthovirus. Picornaviruses are small, single-stranded positive RNA viruses with a naked icosahedral capsid structure. The genome of picornaviruses resembles a mRNA which is sufficient for infection if microin-

jected into a cell. Upon entering host cells, the viral genome binds directly to ribosomes which synthesize viral proteins required for replication including RNA-dependent RNA polymerase and then replicates in the cytoplasm.

Enteroviruses are capsid virus spread via the fecal-oral route. Most enteroviruses are cytolytic and their rapid replication cause damage to target cells. For example, poliovirus is cytolytic for the motor neurons of the anterior horn and brainstem, producing one of the four outcomes including asymptomatic illness, abortive poliomyelitis, nonparalytic poliomyelitis or paralytic polio, depending on the location and number of cells destroyed by the virus. The poliovirus vaccines OPV and IPV have greatly brought down disease incidence. Coxsackie virus A viruses are associated with herpangina, hand-foot-and-mouth disease, common cold, and meningitis etc, while coxsackievirus B viruses are associated with myocarditis and pleurodynia.

Rhinoviruses are the most important cause of the common cold and upper respiratory tract infections, transmitted by aerosols and direct contact. Diagnosis can be made by immune assays (ELISA) or RT-PCR genome analysis of blood, CSF, or other relevant sample. Currently there are no antiviral drugs that are effective against Rhinoviruses, while vaccine development is also hindered by the multiple serotypes and antigenic shift in rhinoviral antigens.

KEYWORDS

English	Chinese
Picornavirus	小 RNA 病毒
Enterovirus	肠道病毒
Poliovirus	脊髓灰质炎病毒
Coxsackievirus	柯萨奇病毒
Echovirus	埃可病毒
Rhinovirus	鼻病毒
Poliomyelitis	脊髓灰质炎

BIBLIOGRAPHY

1. Ansardi DC, Porter DC, Anderson MJ, et al: Poliovirus assembly and encapsidation of genomic RNA, *Adv Virus Res* 46: 1-68, 1996.

2. Buenz EJ, Howe CL: Picornaviruses and cell death, *Trends Microbiol* 14: 28-38, 2006.

3. Cann AJ: *Principles of molecular virology*, San Diego, 2005, Academic.

4. Carter J, Saunders V: *Virology: principles and applications*, Chichester, England, 2007, Wiley. Cohen J, Powderly WG: *Infectious diseases*, ed 2, St Louis, 2004, Mosby.

5. Collier L, Oxford J: *Human virology*, ed 4, Oxford, England, 2011, Oxford University Press.

6. Flint SJ, Enquist LW, Racaniello VR, et al: *Principles of virology: molecular biology, pathogenesis and control of animal viruses*, ed 3, Washington, DC, 2009, American Society for Microbiology Press.

7. Knipe DM, Howley PM: *Fields virology*, ed 6, Philadelphia, 2013, Lippincott Williams & Wilkins.

8. Levandowski RA: Rhinoviruses. In Belshe RB, editor: *Textbook of human virology*, ed 2, St Louis, 1991, Mosby.

9. McKinlay MA, Pevear DC, Rossmann MG: Treatment of the picornavirus common cold by inhibitors of viral uncoating and attachment, *Annu Rev Microbiol* 46: 635-654, 1992.

10. Moore M, Morens DM: Enteroviruses including polioviruses. In Belshe RB, editor: *Textbook of human virology*, ed 2, St Louis, 1991, Mosby.

11. Plotkin SA, Vidor E: Poliovirus vaccine—inactive. In Plotkin SA, Orenstein WA, editors: *Vaccines*, ed 4, Philadelphia, 2004, WB Saunders.

12. Racaniello VR: One hundred years of poliovirus pathogenesis, *Virology* 344: 9-16, 2006.

13. Richman DD, Whitley RJ, Hayden FG: *Clinical virology*, ed 3, Washington, DC, 2009, American Society for Microbiology Press.

14. Robbins FC: The history of polio vaccine development. In Plotkin SA, Orenstein WA, editors: *Vaccines*, ed 4, Philadelphia, 2004, WB Saunders.

15. Strauss JM, Strauss EG: *Viruses and human disease*, San Diego, 2002, Academic.

16. Sutter RW, Kew OM, Cochi SL: Poliovirus vaccine—live. In Plotkin SA, Orenstein WA, editors: *Vaccines*, ed 4, Philadelphia, 2004, WB Saunders.

17. Tracy S, Chapman NM, Mahy BWJ: Coxsackie B viruses, *Curr Top Microbiol Immunol* 223: 153-167, 1997.

18. Voyles BA: *The biology of viruses*, ed 2, Boston, 2002, McGraw-Hill. Whitton JL, Cornell CT, Feuer R: Host and virus determinants of picornavirus pathogenesis and tropism, *Nat Rev Microbiol* 3: 765-776, 2005.

Coronaviruses and Noroviruses

CORONAVIRUSES

Coronaviruses are named for the solar corona-like appearance (the surface projections) of their virions when viewed with an electron microscope (Figure 49-1). These viruses are pathogens of the common cold and the severe acute respiratory syndrome (SARS). SARS is caused by SARS-Coronavirus (SARS-CoV).

Structure and Replication

Coronaviruses are **enveloped virions** with the longest **positive (+) RNA** genome. Virions measure 80 to 160 nm in diameter. The glycoproteins on the surface of the envelope appear as club-shaped projections that appear as a halo (corona) around the virus. Unlike most enveloped viruses, the "corona" formed by the glycoproteins allows the virus to endure the conditions in the gastrointestinal tract and be spread by the fecal-oral route.

The large, plus-stranded RNA genome (27,000 to 30,000 bases) associates with the N protein to form a helical nucleocapsid. Protein synthesis occurs in two phases, similar to that of the togaviruses. On infection, the genome is translated to produce a polyprotein that is cleaved to produce an RNA-dependent RNA polymerase (L). The polymerase generates a negative-sense template RNA. The L protein then uses the template RNA to replicate new genomes and produce five to seven individual mRNAs for the individual viral proteins. Generation of the individual mRNAs may also promote recombination events between viral genomes to promote genetic diversity.

Virions contain the glycoproteins E1 and E2 and a core nucleoprotein (N); some strains also contain a hemagglutinin-neuraminidase (E3) (Table 49-1). The E2 glycoprotein is responsible for mediating viral attachment and membrane fusion and is the target of neutralizing antibodies. The E1 glycoprotein is a transmembrane matrix protein. The replication scheme for coronaviruses is shown in Figure 49-2.

Pathogenesis and Clinical Syndromes

Coronaviruses inoculated into the respiratory tracts of human volunteers infect and disrupt the function of ciliated epithelial cells. Infection remains localized to the upper respiratory tract because the *optimum temperature for viral growth is 33℃ to 35℃*. The virus is most likely spread by aerosols and in large droplets (e.g., sneezes). Most human coronaviruses cause an upper respiratory tract infection similar to the colds

Table 49-1 Major Human Coronavirus Proteins

Proteins	Molecular Weight (kDa)	Location	Functions
E2 (peplomeric glycoprotein)	160-200	Envelope spikes (peplomer)	Binding to host cells; fusion activity
H1 (hemagglutinin protein)	60-66	Peplomer	Hemagglutination
N (nucleoprotein)	47-55	Core	Ribonucleoprotein
E1 (matrix glycoprotein)	20-30	Envelope	Transmembrane protein
L (polymerase)	225	Infected cell	Polymerase activity

caused by rhinoviruses but with a longer incubation period (average, 3 days). The infection may exacerbate a preexisting chronic pulmonary disease, such as asthma or bronchitis, and, on rare occasions, may cause pneumonia.

Infections occur mainly in infants and children. Coronavirus disease appears either sporadically or in outbreaks in the winter and spring. Usually, one strain predominates in an outbreak. Findings from serologic studies show that coronaviruses cause approximately 10% to 15% of upper respiratory tract infections in humans. Antibodies to coronaviruses are uniformly present by adulthood, but reinfections are common, despite the preexisting serum antibodies.

SARS is a form of atypical pneumonia characterized by high fever (>38℃), chills, rigors, headache, dizziness, malaise, myalgia, cough, or breathing difficulty, leading to acute respiratory distress syndrome. The virus infects and kills the alveolar epithelium. Up to 20% of patients will also develop diarrhea. Persons with SARS were exposed within the previous 10 days. Mortality is at least 10% of people with

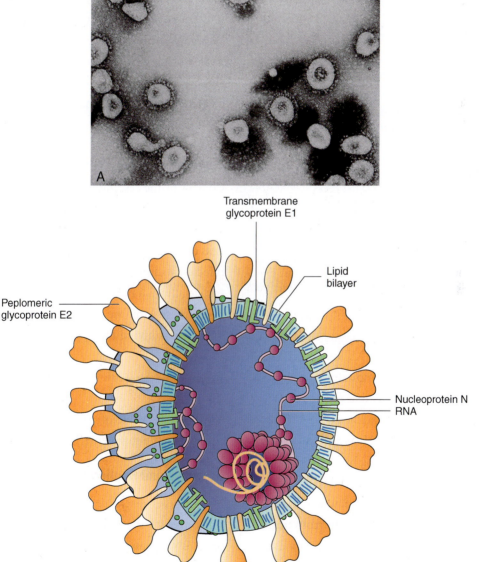

Figure 49-1   A, Electron micrograph of the human respiratory coronavirus (magnification 90,000×). **B,** Model of a coronavirus. The viral nucleocapsid is a long, flexible helix composed of the positive-strand genomic RNA and many molecules of the phosphorylated nucleocapsid protein N. The viral envelope consists of a lipid bilayer derived from the intracellular membranes of the host cell and two viral glycoproteins (*E1* and *E2*). (**A,** Courtesy Centers for Disease Control and Prevention, Atlanta; **B,** Modified from Fields BF, Knipe DM: *Virology,* New York, 1985, Raven.)

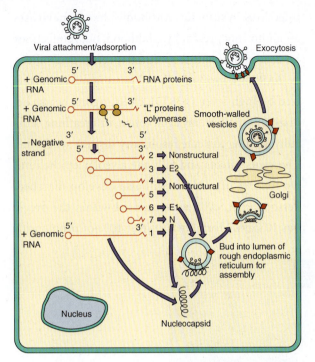

Figure 49-2 Replication of human coronaviruses. The E2 glycoprotein interacts with receptors on epithelial cells, the virus fuses or is endocytosed into the cell, and the genome is released into the cytoplasm. Protein synthesis is divided into early and late phases, similar to that in the togaviruses. The genome binds to ribosomes, and an RNA-dependent RNA polymerase is translated. This enzyme generates a full-length, negative-sense RNA template for the production of new virion genomes and six individual mRNAs for the other coronavirus proteins. The genome associates with rough endoplasmic reticulum membranes modified by virion proteins and buds into the lumen of the rough endoplasmic reticulum. Vesicles that contain virus migrate to the cell membrane, and virus is released by exocytosis. (Modified from Balows A, et al: *Laboratory diagnosis of infectious diseases: principles and practice*, New York, 1988, Springer-Verlag.)

indication of SARS infection. Although SARS-CoV is most likely transmitted in respiratory droplets, it is also present in sweat, urine, and feces.

As already mentioned, the outbreak of SARS started in November 2002 in South China's Guangdong Province, was brought to Hong Kong by a physician working within the original outbreak, and then was brought to Vietnam, Toronto, and other places by travelers. The virus apparently jumped to man from animals (masked-palm civets, raccoon dogs, and Chinese ferret badgers) raised for food. A World Health Organization (WHO) global alert prompted containment measures to control the spread of the virus and limited the outbreak to 8000 known diseased individuals but with at least 784 deaths. Travel restrictions and

public concern resulted in a loss of hundreds of millions of dollars in travel and other business.

Laboratory Diagnosis

Laboratory tests are not routinely performed to diagnose coronavirus infections other than SARS. The method of choice for coronaviruses, including SARS-CoV, is detection of the viral RNA genome in respiratory and stool samples by RT-PCR. Virus isolation of the coronaviruses is difficult and for SARS-CoV requires stringent biosafety level 3 (BSL-3) conditions. Testing of samples suspected of containing SARS-CoV must be performed with appropriate BSL-2 precautions, attainable in many virology laboratories. Serology using enzyme-linked immunosorbent assay (ELISA) can be used to evaluate acute and convalescent sera. Electron microscopy has also been used to detect coronavirus-like particles in stool specimens.

Treatment, Prevention, and Control

Control of the respiratory transmission of the common cold form of coronavirus would be difficult and is probably unnecessary because of the mildness of the infection. Strict quarantine of individuals infected with SARS-CoV and screening for fever in travelers from a region with an outbreak of SARS are necessary to limit the spread of the virus. No vaccine or specific antiviral therapy is available.

NOROVIRUSES

Noroviruses is one of pathogen agents caused epidemic of acute gastroenteritis.

Structure and Replication

Noroviruses resemble and are approximately the same size as the picornaviruses. Their positive-sense RNA genome (approximately 7500 bases) has a VPg protein (viral protein genome-linked) and a 3' terminal polyadenylate (polyA) sequence similar to picornaviruses. The genome is contained in a 27-nm naked capsid consisting of 60,000 Da capsid proteins. Norwalk virions are round with a ragged outline, whereas other calicivirions have cup-shaped indentations or a six-point star shape. The virions of the astroviruses have a five- or six-point star shape on the surface but no indentations. Antibodies from seropositive people can also be used to distinguish these viruses.

Most caliciviruses and astroviruses can be grown in cell culture, but the Norwalk viruses cannot. Expression of the structural protein genes of different Norwalk viruses in tissue culture cells produces Norwalk virus-like particles. These particles were used to show that Norwalk viruses bind to the carbohydrate of the A, B, or O blood group antigen on the cell surface. The noroviruses enter and exit cells similar to the picornaviruses but transcribe an early and late mRNA similar to the togaviruses and coronaviruses. The early mRNA encodes a polyprotein containing the RNA polymerase and other enzymes. The late mRNA encodes the capsid proteins.

Pathogenesis

The norovirus strains that infect humans can only infect humans. As few as 10 virions will initiate disease in humans. Damage to the intestinal brush border prevents proper absorption of water and nutrients and causes a watery diarrhea. Although no histologic changes occur in the gastric mucosa, gastric emptying may be delayed, causing vomiting. Examination of jejunal biopsy specimens from human volunteers infected with noroviruses revealed the existence of blunted villi, cytoplasmic vacuolation, and infiltration with mononuclear cells. Shedding of the virus may continue for 2 weeks after symptoms have ceased. Immunity is generally short lived at best and may not be protective. The large number of strains and high rate of mutation allows reinfection despite antibodies from a previous exposure.

Epidemiology

Norwalk and related viruses typically cause outbreaks of gastroenteritis because of a common source of contamination (e.g., water, shellfish, salad, raspberries, food service). These viruses are transmitted mainly by the fecal-oral route in stool and vomitus. Infected individuals shed large amounts of virus upon onset of symptoms and up to 4 weeks after recovery. During peak shedding, 100 billion virions are released per gram of feces. Up to 30% of infected individuals are asymptomatic but can spread the infection.

Outbreaks in developed countries may occur year-round and have been described in schools, resorts, hospitals, nursing homes, restaurants, and cruise ships. Common-source outbreaks can often be traced to a careless, infected food handler. The Centers for Disease Control and Prevention estimates that nearly 50% (23 million cases in the United States per year) of all foodborne outbreaks of gastroenteritis can be attributed to noroviruses, which is a tribute to the importance of this virus. As many as 70% of children in the United States have antibodies to noroviruses by the age of 7 years.

Clinical Syndromes

Norwalk and related viruses cause symptoms similar to those caused by the rotaviruses. Infection causes an acute onset of diarrhea, nausea, vomiting, and abdominal cramps, especially in children Bloody stools do not occur. Fever may occur in as many as a third of patients. The incubation period is usually 12 to 48 hours, and the illness usually resolves within 1 to 3 days without problems but can last up to 6 days. The below is one of examples of clinical cases.

Outbreak of Norwalk Virus Infection

A group of children got gastroenteritisafter attending a concert. Infection was traced back to contamination of a specific seating area, bathrooms, and other areas visited by one individual. A male concert attendee was ill prior to attending a concert and then vomited four times in the concert hall: once in a waste bin in the corridor, into the toilets, onto the floor of the fire escape, and on a carpeted area in the walkway. His family members showed symptoms within 24 hours. A children's concert for several schools was held the next day. Children sitting in the same section as the incident case and those who traversed the contaminated carpet had the highest incidence of disease, characterized by watery diarrhea and vomiting for approximately

2 days. RT-PCR analysis of fecal samples from two ill children detected Norwalk virus genomic RNA. Infected vomit may have up to a million viruses per milliliter, and only 10 to 100 viruses are required to transmit the disease. Contact with contaminated shoes, hands, clothing, or aerosols may have infected the children. The encapsidated nature of the Norwalk virus makes it resistant to routine cleansers; disinfection usually requires freshly prepared hypochlorite bleach-containing solutions or steam cleaning.

Laboratory Diagnosis

The use of RT-PCR for detection of the Norovirus genome in stool or emesis samples has enhanced the speed and detection of the virus during outbreaks. Immunoelectron microscopy can be used to concentrate and identify the virus from stool. The addition of an antibody directed against the suspected agent causes the virus to aggregate, thereby facilitating recognition. ELISA tests have been developed to detect the virus, viral antigen, and antibody to the virus. Serology can be used to confirm a diagnosis. Antibodies to the other calicivirus-like agents are more difficult to detect.

Treatment, Prevention, and Control

No specific treatment for infection with the calicivirus or other small, round gastroenteritis viruses is available. Bismuth subsalicylate may reduce the severity of the gastrointestinal symptoms. Outbreaks may be minimized by handling food carefully and by maintaining the purity of the water supply. Careful hand washing is also important. More resistant to environmental pressures than polioviruses or rotaviruses, Norwalk virus is resistant to heat (60℃), pH 3, detergent, and even the chlorine levels of drinking water. Contaminated surfaces can be cleaned with a 1:50 to 1:10 dilution of household bleach.

SUMMARY

Coronavirus is the second most prevalent cause of the common cold. The etiological agent of severe acute respiratory syndrome (SARS) is coronavirus (SARS-CoV). SARS-CoV spreads to man from animals (masked-palm civets, raccoon dogs, and Chinese ferret badgers).

Noroviruses, astroviruses and other small round gastroenteritis viruses cause epidemic of acute gastroenteritis. Noroviruses are members of the *Caliciviridae* family. Norwalk virus is the prototypical norovirus.

KEYWORDS

English	Chinese
Coronaviruses	冠状病毒
Severe acute respiratory syndrome, SARS	严重急性呼吸综合征
SARS-CoV	SARS 冠状病毒
Noroviruses	诺如病毒
Caliciviruses	杯状病毒
Astroviruses	星状病毒
Norwalk virus	诺瓦克病毒

BIBLIOGRAPHY

1. Blacklow NR, Greenberg HB: Viral gastroenteritis, N Engl J Med 325: 252-264, 1991.

2. Cann AJ: Principles of molecular virology, San Diego, 2005, Academic.

3. Carter J, Saunders V: Virology: principles and applications, Chichester, England, 2007, Wiley.

4. Christensen ML: Human viral gastroenteritis, ClinMicrobiol Rev 2: 51-89, 1989.

5. Cohen J, Powderly WG: Infectious diseases, ed 2, St Louis, 2004, Mosby.

6. Collier L, Oxford J: Human virology, ed 3, Oxford, England, 2006, Oxford University Press.

7. Flint SJ, et al: Principles of virology: molecular biology, pathogenesis and control of animal viruses, ed 3, Washington, DC, 2009, American Society for Microbiology Press.

8. Hall AJ, et al: Updated norovirus outbreak management and disease prevention guidelines, MMWR Morb Mortal Wkly Rep 60: 1-15, 2011.

9. Knipe DM, et al: Fields virology, ed 5, Philadelphia, 2006, Lippincott Williams & Wilkins.

10. Meulen V, Siddell S, Wege H: Biochemistry and biology of coronaviruses, New York, 1981, Plenum.

11. Patel MM, Hall AJ, Vinjé J, et al: Noroviruses: a comprehensive review, J ClinVirol 44: 1-8, 2009.

12. Perlman S, Netland J: Coronaviruses post-SARS: update on replication and pathogenesis, Nat Rev Microbiol 7: 439-450, 2009.

13. Richman DD, Whitley RJ, Hayden FG: Clinical virology, ed 3, Washington, DC, 2009, American Society for Microbiology Press.

14. Strauss JM, Strauss EG: Viruses and human disease, ed 2, San Diego, 2007, Academic.

15. Tan M, et al: Mutations within the P2 domain of norovirus capsid affect binding to human histo-blood group antigens: evidence for a binding pocket, J Virol 77: 12562-12571, 2003.

16. Voyles BA: The biology of viruses, ed 2, Boston, 2002, McGraw-Hill.

17. Xi JN, et al: Norwalk virus genome cloning and characterization, Science 250: 1580-1583, 1990.

Paramyxoviruses

Chapter 50

The *Paramyxoviridae* include the following genera: *Morbillivirus, Paramyxovirus,* and *Pneumovirus* (Table 50-1). Human pathogens within the *Morbilliviruses* include the **measles** virus; within the *Paramyxoviruses,* the **parainfluenza** and **mumps** viruses; and within the *Pneumoviruses,* the **respiratory syncytial virus (RSV)** and the newly discovered but relatively common **metapneumovirus.** Measles virus causes highly contagious measles. **Mumps virus** is the pathogen of **epidemic mumps.** Respiratory syncytial virus produces fatal acute respiratory tract infection in infants and young children. **Parainfluenza virus** is the cause of severe lower respiratory tract infection in infants and young children (Types 1, 2, and 3) and causes mild upper respiratory tract infection in children and adults (Type 4). **Human metapneumovirus** is a recently recognized member of the *Pneumovirinae* subfamily, which produces common cold-type disease, or serious bronchiolitis and pneumonia. **Hendra virus** discovered in 1994 in Australia and **Nipah virus** isolated from patients after an outbreak of severe encephalitis in Malaysia and Singapore in 1998 are two new members of *Paramyxoviridae* family.

Table 50-1 Paramyxoviridae

Genus	Human Pathogen
Morbillivirus	Measles virus
Paramyxovirus	Parainfluenza viruses 1 to 4 Mumps virus
Pneumovirus	Respiratory syncytial virus Metapneumovirus

STRUCTURE AND REPLICATION

Paramyxoviruses are relatively large viruses with a **negative-sense, single-stranded RNA** (5 to 8 × 10⁶ Da) genome in a helical nucleocapsid surrounded by a pleomorphic **envelope** of approximately 156 to 300 nm (Figure 50-1). They are similar in many respects to orthomyxoviruses but are larger and do not have the segmented genome of the influenza viruses. Although there are similarities in paramyxovirus genomes, the order of the protein-coding regions differs for each genus.

The gene products of the measles virus are listed in Table 50-2. The nucleocapsid consists of the negative-sense, single-stranded RNA associated with the nucleoprotein (**NP**), polymerase phosphoprotein (**P**), and large (**L**) protein. The L protein is the RNA polymerase, the P protein facilitates RNA synthesis, and the NP protein helps maintain genomic structure. The nucleocapsid associates with the matrix (**M**) protein lining the inside of the virion envelope. The envelope contains two glycoproteins, a fusion (**F**) protein, which promotes fusion of the viral and host cell membranes, and a viral attachment protein (hemagglutinin-neuraminidase [**HN**], hemagglutinin [**H**], or glycoprotein [**G**] protein). To express membrane-fusing activity, the F protein must be activated by proteolytic cleavage, which produces F_1 and F_2 glycopeptides held together by a disulfide bond.

Replication of the paramyxoviruses is initiated by the binding of the HN, H, or G protein on the virion envelope to sialic acid on the cell surface glycolipids and glycoproteins. The measles virus can bind to the CD46 (membrane cofactor protein, MCP) present on most cell types and also CD150 signaling lymphocyte-activation molecule (SLAM), which is expressed on activated T and B cells. CD46 protects the cell from complement by regulating complement

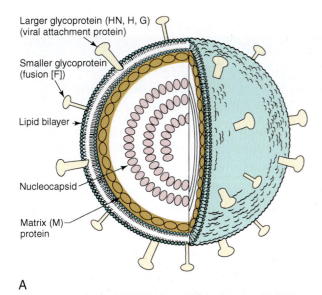

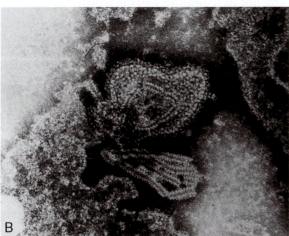

Larger glycoprotein (HN, H, G)
(viral attachment protein)

Smaller glycoprotein
(fusion [F])

Lipid bilayer

Nucleocapsid

Matrix (M)
protein

A

B

Figure 50-1 **A,** Model of paramyxovirus. The helical nucleocapsid—consisting of negative-sense, single-stranded RNA and the P protein, nucleoprotein, and large protein—associates with the matrix *(M)* protein at the envelope membrane surface. The nucleocapsid contains RNA transcriptase activity. The envelope contains the viral attachment glycoprotein (hemagglutinin-neuraminidase *[HN]*, hemagglutinin *[H]*, or G protein *[G]*, depending upon the virus) and the fusion *(F)* protein. **B,** Electron micrograph of a disrupted paramyxovirus, showing the helical nucleocapsid. (**A,** Modified from Jawetz E, Melnick JL, Adelberg EA: *Review of medical microbiology*, ed 17, Norwalk, Conn, 1987, Appleton & Lange. **B,** Courtesy Centers for Disease Control and Prevention, Atlanta.)

The replication of the genome occurs in a manner similar to that of other negative-strand RNA viruses (i.e., rhabdoviruses). The RNA polymerase is carried into the cell as part of the nucleocapsid. Transcription, protein synthesis, and replication of the genome all occur in the host cell's cytoplasm. The genome is transcribed into individual messenger RNAs (mRNAs) and a full-length positive-sense RNA template. New genomes associate with the L, N, and NP proteins to form helical nucleocapsids, which associate with the M proteins on viral glycoprotein-modified plasma membranes. The glycoproteins are synthesized and processed like cellular glycoproteins. Mature virions then bud from the host cell plasma membrane and exit without killing the cell. Replication of the paramyxoviruses is represented by the RSV infectious cycle shown in Figure 50-2.

MEASLES VIRUS

Measles, also known as rubeola, is one of the five classic childhood exanthems, along with rubella, roseola, fifth disease, and chickenpox. Historically, measles was one of the most common and unpleasant viral infections, with serious potential sequelae. Before 1960, more than 90% of the population younger than 20 years had experienced the rash, high fever, cough, conjunctivitis, and coryza of measles. Since the use of the live vaccine, fewer cases have been reported. But measles is still one of the most prominent causes of disease and death worldwide in unvaccinated populations.

Pathogenesis and Immunity

Measles is known for its propensity to cause cell fusion, leading to the formation of giant cells. As a result, the virus can pass directly from cell to cell and escape antibody control. Inclusions occur most commonly in the cytoplasm and are composed of incomplete viral particles. Virus production occurs with eventual cell lysis. Persistent infections without lysis can occur in certain cell types (e.g., human brain cells).

Measles is **highly contagious** and is transmitted from person to person by **respiratory droplets**.

activation and is also the receptor for human herpes virus 6 and some strains of adenovirus. SLAM regulates TH1 and TH2 responses, and measles virus may upset this regulation. The F protein promotes fusion of the envelope with the plasma membrane. Paramyxoviruses are also able to induce cell-to-cell fusion, thereby creating multinucleated giant cells (syncytia).

Table 50-2 Viral-Encoded Proteins of Measles Virus

Gene Products*	Virion Location	Function
Nucleoprotein (NP)	Major internal protein	Protection of viral RNA
Polymerase phosphoprotein (P)	Association with nucleoprotein	Part of transcription complex
Matrix (M)	Inside virion envelope	Assembly of virions
Fusion protein (F)	Transmembranous envelope glycoprotein	Protein promotes fusion of cells, hemolysis, and viral entry
Hemagglutinin (H)	Transmembranous envelope glycoprotein	Viral attachment protein
Large protein (L)	Association with nucleoprotein	Polymerase

Modifi ed from Fields BN: Virology, New York, 1985, Raven.
*In order on the genome.

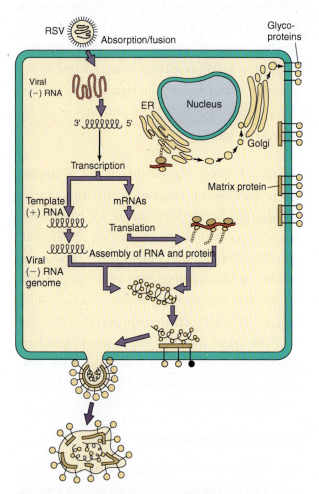

Figure 50-2 Replication of paramyxoviruses. The virus binds to glycolipids or proteins and fuses with the cell surface. Individual messenger RNAs *(mRNAs)* for each protein and a full-length template are transcribed from the genome. Replication occurs in the cytoplasm. Proteins associate with the genome, and the nucleocapsid associates with matrix and glycoprotein-modified plasma membranes. The virus leaves the cell by budding. *(–),* Negative sense; *(+),* positive sense; *ER,* endoplasmic reticulum; *RSV,* respiratory syncytial virus.(Modified from Balows A, et al: *Laboratory diagnosis of infectious diseases: principles and practice*, New York, 1988, Springer-Verlag.)

After local replication of virus in epithelial cells of the respiratory tract, the virus infects monocytes and lymphocytes, and the virus is spread through the lymphatic system and by a cell-associated viremia. The wide dissemination of the virus causes infection of the conjunctiva, respiratory tract, urinary tract, small blood vessels, lymphatic system, and the central nervous system. The characteristic **maculopapular** measles rash is caused by immune T cells targeted to measles-infected endothelial cells lining small blood vessels. Recovery follows the rash in most patients, who then have **lifelong immunity** to the virus. Death can occur because of pneumonia, diarrhea, or encephalitis.

Measles can cause encephalitis in three ways: (1) direct infection of neurons; (2) a postinfectious encephalitis, which is believed to be immune mediated; and (3) subacute sclerosing panencephalitis (SSPE) caused by a defective variant of measles generated during the acute disease. The SSPE virus acts as a slow virus and causes symptoms and cytopathologic effect in neurons many years after acute disease.

Measles and other paramyxoviruses are excellent inducers of interferon-α and -β, which activate natural killer (NK) cells. Cell-mediated immunity is responsible for most of the symptoms and is essential for the control of measles infection. T-cell-deficient children who are infected with measles have an atypical presentation, consisting of **giant cell pneumonia without a rash.** Antibody, including maternal antibody and passive immunization, can block the viremic spread of the virus and prevent or lessen disease. Protection from reinfection is lifelong.

During the incubation period, measles causes a

decrease in eosinophils and lymphocytes, including B and T cells, and a depression of their response to activation (mitogens). The virus depresses the immune response by (1) directly infecting monocytes and T and B cells and (2) by depressing interleukin 12 (IL-12) production and TH1-type T-cell helper responses. Depression of cell-mediated immune and delayed-type hypersensitivity (DTH) responses increases risk to opportunistic and other infections. This immunosuppression lasts for weeks or months after the disease.

Epidemiology

The development of effective vaccine programs has made measles a rare disease. In areas without a vaccine program, epidemics tend to occur in 1- to 3-year cycles, when a sufficient number of susceptible people have accumulated. Many of these cases occur in preschool-age children who have not been vaccinated and live in large urban areas. The incidence of infection peaks in the winter and spring. Measles is still common in people living in some places of developing countries, especially in individuals who refuse immunization or have not received a booster in their teenage years. Immunocompromised and malnourished people with measles may not be able to resolve the infection, resulting in death. It is the most significant cause of death in children 1 to 5 years of age in several countries.

Measles, which can be spread in respiratory secretions before and after the onset of characteristic symptoms, is one of the most contagious infections known. In a household, approximately 85% of exposed susceptible people become infected, and 95% of these people develop clinical disease.

The measles virus has only one serotype, infects only humans, and infection usually manifests as symptoms. These properties facilitated the development of an effective vaccine program. Once vaccination was introduced, the yearly incidence of measles dropped dramatically both in the United States and China.

Despite the effectiveness of vaccination programs, poor compliance and the prevaccinated population (children younger than 2 years) continue to provide susceptible individuals. The virus may surface from within the community or can be imported by immigration from areas of the world lacking an effective vaccine program.

Clinical Syndromes

Measles is a serious febrile illness. The incubation period lasts 7 to 13 days, and the prodrome starts with **high fever** and **"CCC and P"—cough, coryza, conjunctivitis**, and **photophobia.** The disease is most infectious during this time.

After 2 days of prodromal illness, the typical mucous membrane lesions known as **Koplik spots** (Figure 50-3) appear. They are seen most commonly on the buccal mucosa across from the molars, but they may appear on other mucous membranes as well, including the conjunctivae and the vagina. The vesicular lesions, which last 24 to 48 hours, are usually small (1 to 2 mm) and are best described as grains of salt surrounded by a red halo. Their appearance with the other disease signs establishes with certainty the diagnosis of measles.

Within 12 to 24 hours of the appearance of Koplik spots, the **exanthem** of measles starts below the ears and spreads over the body. The **rash is maculo-**

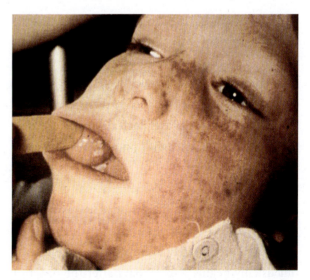

Figure 50-3   Koplik spots in the mouth and exanthem. Koplik spots usually precede the measles rash and may be seen for the first day or two after the rash appears. (Courtesy Dr JI Pugh, St Albans City Hospital, West Hertfordshire, England; from Emond RTD, Rowland HAK: *A color atlas of infectious diseases,* ed 3, London, 1995, Mosby.)

papular, usually very extensive, and often the lesions become confluent. The rash, which takes 1 or 2 days to cover the body, fades in the same order in which it appeared. The fever is highest and the patient is sickest on the day the rash appears (Figure 50-4).

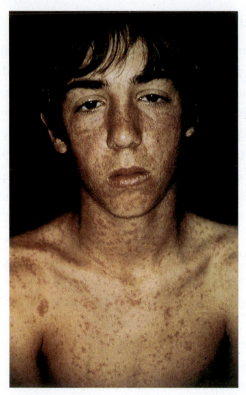

Figure 50-4 Measles rash. (From Habif TP: *Clinical dermatology: color guide to diagnosis and therapy,* St Louis, 1985, Mosby.)

Pneumonia, which can also be a serious complication, accounts for 60% of the deaths caused by measles. Similar to the incidence of the other complications associated with measles, the mortality associated with pneumonia is higher in the malnourished and for the extremes of age. **Bacterial superinfection** is common in patients with pneumonia caused by the measles virus.

One of the most feared complications of measles is **encephalitis,** which occurs in as few as 0.5% of those infected but carries a fatality rate of 15%. Encephalitis may rarely occur during acute disease but usually begins 7 to 10 days after the onset of illness. This **postinfectious encephalitis** is caused by immunopathologic reactions, is associated with demyelination of neurons, and occurs more often in older children and adults.

Atypical measles occurred in people who received the older inactivated measles vaccine and were subsequently exposed to the wild-type measles virus. It may also rarely occur in those vaccinated with the attenuated virus vaccine. Prior sensitization with insufficient protection can enhance the immunopathologic response to the challenge by wild measles virus. The illness begins abruptly and is a more intense presentation of measles.

Subacute sclerosing panencephalitis (SSPE) is an extremely serious, very late neurologic sequela of measles that afflicts approximately seven of every one million patients. The incidence of SSPE has decreased markedly because of measles vaccination programs.

This disease occurs when a defective measles virus persists in the brain and acts as a slow virus. The virus can replicate and spread directly from cell to cell but is not released. SSPE is most prevalent in children who were initially infected when younger than 2 years and occurs approximately 7 years after clinical measles. The patient demonstrates changes in personality, behavior, and memory, followed by myoclonic jerks, blindness, and spasticity. Unusually high levels of measles antibodies are found in the blood and cerebrospinal fluid of patients with SSPE.

The immunocompromised and malnourished child is at highest risk for severe outcome of measles. **Giant cell pneumonia without rash** occurs in children lacking T-cell immunity. Whereas the death rate to measles in the United States is only 0.1%, complications, severe bacterial superinfection, and pneumonia in malnourished children result in up to 60% mortality.

Laboratory Diagnosis

The clinical manifestations of measles are usually so characteristic that it is rarely necessary to perform laboratory tests to establish the diagnosis. The measles virus is difficult to isolate and grow, although it can be grown in primary human- or monkey-cell cultures. Respiratory tract secretions, urine, blood, and brain tissue are the recommended specimens. It is best to collect respiratory and blood specimens during the prodromal stage and until 1 to 2 days after the appearance of the rash.

Measles antigen can be detected in pharyngeal cells or urinary sediment with immunofluorescence; the measles genome can be identified by RT-PCR in either of the aforementioned specimens. Characteristic cytopathologic effects, including multinucleated giant cells with cytoplasmic inclusion bodies, can be seen in Giemsa-stained cells taken from the upper respiratory tract and urinary sediment.

Antibody, especially immunoglobulin M (IgM), can be detected when the rash is present. Measles infection can be confirmed by the finding of seroconversion or by a fourfold increase in the titer of measles-specific antibodies between sera obtained during the acute stage and the convalescent stage.

Treatment, Prevention, and Control

As stated previously, a live attenuated measles vaccine, has been responsible for a significant reduction in the incidence of measles. The Schwartz or Moraten attenuated strains of the original Edmonston B vaccine are currently being used. Live attenuated vaccine is given to all children at 2 years of age, in combination with mumps and rubella (**measles-mumps-rubella [MMR] vaccine**) and the varicella vaccines. Although early childhood immunization is successful in more than 95% of vaccinees, revaccination before grade school or junior high school is required in many states. Misinformation regarding immunization risks caused many parents to refrain from vaccinating their children, putting them at risk of infection and disease. Because of the contagious nature of measles, a decrease in the immunized population to 93% creates a risk of an outbreak of measles.

As noted earlier, a killed measles vaccine introduced in 1963 was not protective; its use was subsequently discontinued because recipients were at risk of the more serious atypical measles presentation on infection. Because measles is strictly a human virus with only one serotype, it is a good candidate for eradication, but this is prevented by difficulties in distributing the vaccine to regions that lack proper

refrigeration facilities (e.g., Africa) and distribution networks.

Hospitals in areas experiencing endemic measles may wish to vaccinate or check the immune status of their employees to decrease the risk of nosocomial transmission. Pregnant women, immunocompromised individuals, people with allergies to gelatin or neomycin (components of the vaccine) should not receive the MMR vaccine. Exposed susceptible people who are immunocompromised should be given immune globulin to lessen the risk and severity of clinical illness. This product is most effective if given within 6 days of exposure. High-dose vitamin A treatment reduces the risk of measles mortality and is recommended by the World Health Organization. No specific antiviral treatment is available for measles.

PARAINFLUENZA VIRUSES

Parainfluenza viruses, which were discovered in the late 1950s, are respiratory viruses that usually cause **mild cold like symptoms** but can also cause **serious respiratory tract disease.** Four serologic types within the parainfluenza genus are human pathogens. Types 1, 2, and 3 are second only to RSV as important causes of severe lower respiratory tract infection in infants and young children. They are especially associated with **laryngotracheobronchitis (croup).** Type 4 causes only mild upper respiratory tract infection in children and adults.

Pathogenesis and Immunity

Parainfluenza viruses infect epithelial cells of the upper respiratory tract. The virus replicates more rapidly than measles and mumps viruses and can cause giant cell formation and cell lysis. Unlike measles and mumps viruses, the parainfluenza viruses rarely cause viremia. The viruses generally stay in the upper respiratory tract, causing only cold like symptoms. In approximately 25% of cases, the virus spreads to the lower respiratory tract, and in 2% to 3%, disease may take the severe form of laryngotracheobronchitis.

The cell-mediated immune response both causes

cell damage and confers protection. IgA responses are protective but short lived. Parainfluenza viruses manipulate cell-mediated immunity to limit development of memory. Multiple serotypes and the short duration of immunity after natural infection make reinfection common, but the reinfection disease is milder, suggesting at least partial immunity.

Epidemiology

Parainfluenza viruses are ubiquitous, and infection is common. The virus is transmitted by person-to-person contact and respiratory droplets. Primary infections usually occur in infants and children younger than 5 years. Reinfections occur throughout life, indicating short-lived immunity. Infections with parainfluenza viruses 1 and 2, the major causes of croup, tend to occur in the autumn, whereas parainfluenza virus 3 infections occur throughout the year. All of these viruses spread readily within hospitals and can cause outbreaks in nurseries and pediatric wards.

Clinical Syndromes

Parainfluenza viruses 1, 2, and 3 may cause respiratory tract syndromes ranging from a **mild cold like upper respiratory tract infection** (coryza, pharyngitis, mild bronchitis, wheezing, and fever) to **bronchiolitis** and **pneumonia.** Older children and adults generally experience milder infections than those seen in young children, although pneumonia may occur in the elderly.

A parainfluenza virus infection in infants may be more severe than infections in adults, causing bronchiolitis, pneumonia, and most notably croup (laryngotracheobronchitis). **Croup** results in subglottal swelling, which may close the airway. Hoarseness, a "seal bark" cough, tachypnea, tachycardia, and suprasternal retraction develop in infected patients after a 2- to 6-day incubation period. Most children recover within 48 hours. The principal differential diagnosis is epiglottitis caused by *Haemophilusinfluenzae.*

Laboratory Diagnosis

Parainfluenza virus is isolated from nasal washings and respiratory secretions and grows well in primary monkey kidney cells. Similar to other paramyxoviruses, the virions are labile during transit to the laboratory. The presence of virus-infected cells in aspirates or in cell culture is indicated by the finding of syncytia and is identified with immunofluorescence. Similar to the hemagglutinin of the influenza viruses, the hemagglutinin of the parainfluenza viruses promotes hemadsorption and hemagglutination. The serotype of the virus can be determined through the use of specific antibody to block hemadsorption or hemagglutination (hemagglutination inhibition). Rapid RT-PCR techniques are becoming the method of choice to detect and identify parainfluenza viruses from respiratory secretions.

Treatment, Prevention, and Control

Treatment of croup consists of the administration of nebulized cold or hot steam and careful monitoring of the upper airway. On rare occasions, intubation may become necessary. No specific antiviral agents are available.

Vaccination with killed vaccines is ineffective, possibly because they fail to induce local secretory antibody and appropriate cellular immunity. No live attenuated vaccine is available.

MUMPS VIRUS

Mumps virus is the cause of acute, benign viral **parotitis** (painful swelling of the salivary glands). Mumps is rarely seen in countries that promote use of the live vaccine, which is administered with the measles and rubella live vaccines.

Mumps virus was isolated in embryonated eggs in 1945 and in cell culture in 1955. The virus is most closely related to parainfluenza virus 2, but there is no cross-immunity with the parainfluenza viruses.

Pathogenesis and Immunity

The mumps virus, of which only one serotype is known, causes a lytic infection of cells. The virus initiates infection in the epithelial cells of the upper respiratory tract and infects the parotid gland, either by way of the Stensen duct or by means of a viremia.

The virus is spread by the viremia throughout the body to the testes, ovary, pancreas, thyroid, and other organs. Infection of the central nervous system, especially the meninges, occurs in as many as 50% of those infected. Inflammatory responses are mainly responsible for the symptoms. Immunity is lifelong.

Epidemiology

Mumps, like measles, is a very communicable disease with only one serotype, and it infects only humans. In the absence of vaccination programs, infection occurs in 90% of people by the age of 15 years. The virus spreads by direct person-to-person contact and respiratory droplets. The virus is released in respiratory secretions from patients who are asymptomatic and during the 7-day period before clinical illness, so it is virtually impossible to control the spread of the virus. Living or working in close quarters promotes the spread of the virus, and the incidence of the infection is greatest in the winter and spring.

Clinical Syndromes

Mumps infections are often asymptomatic. Clinical illness manifests as a parotitis that is almost always bilateral and accompanied by fever. Onset is sudden. Oral examination reveals redness and swelling of the ostium of the Stensen (parotid) duct. The swelling of other glands (epididymoorchitis, oophoritis, mastitis, pancreatitis, and thyroiditis) and meningoencephalitis may occur a few days after the onset of the viral infection but can occur in the absence of parotitis. The swelling that results from mumps orchitis may cause sterility. Mumps virus involves the central nervous system in approximately 50% of patients; 10% of those affected may exhibit mild meningitis with 5 per 1000 cases of encephalitis.

Laboratory Diagnosis

Virus can be recovered from saliva, urine, the pharynx, secretions from the Stensen duct, and cerebrospinal fluid. Virus is present in saliva for approximately 5 days after the onset of symptoms and in urine for as long as 2 weeks. Mumps virus grows well in monkey kidney cells, causing the formation of multinucleated giant cells. The hemadsorption of guinea pig erythrocytes also occurs on virus-infected cells, because of the viral hemagglutinin.

A clinical diagnosis can be confirmed by serologic testing. A fourfold increase in the virus-specific antibody level or the detection of mumps-specific IgM antibody indicates recent infection. Enzyme-linked immunosorbent assay, immunofluorescence tests, and hemagglutination inhibition can be used to detect the mumps virus, antigen, or antibody.

Treatment, Prevention, and Control

Vaccines provide the only effective means for preventing the spread of mumps infection. Since the introduction of the live attenuated vaccine (Jeryl Lynn vaccine) in the United States in 1967 and its administration as part of the MMR vaccine, the yearly incidence of the infection has declined from 76 to 2 per 100,000. Antiviral agents are not available.

RESPIRATORY SYNCYTIAL VIRUS

RSV, first isolated from a chimpanzee in 1956, is a member of the *Pneumovirus* genus. Unlike the other paramyxoviruses, RSV lacks a hemagglutinin and does not bind to sialic acid and therefore does not need or have a neuraminidase. It is the most common cause of **fatal acute respiratory tract infection** in infants and young children. It infects virtually everyone by 2 years of age, and reinfections occur throughout life, even among elderly persons.

Pathogenesis and Immunity

RSV produces an infection that is localized to the respiratory tract. As the name suggests, RSV induces syncytia. The pathologic effect of RSV is mainly caused by direct viral invasion of the respiratory epithelium, which is followed by immunologically mediated cell injury. Necrosis of the bronchi and bronchioles leads to the formation of "plugs" of mucus, fibrin, and necrotic material within smaller airways. The narrow airways of young infants are readily obstructed by such plugs. Natural immunity does not prevent reinfection, and vaccination with killed vaccine appears to enhance the severity of subsequent disease.

Epidemiology

RSV is very prevalent in young children; almost all children have been infected by 2 years of age, with global annual infection rates of 64 million and mortality of 160,000. As many as 25% to 33% of these cases involve the lower respiratory tract, and 1% are severe enough to necessitate hospitalization (occurring in as many as 95,000 children in the United States each year).

RSV infections almost always occur in the winter. Unlike influenza, which may occasionally skip a year, RSV epidemics occur every year.

The virus is very contagious, with an incubation period of 4 to 5 days. The introduction of the virus into a nursery, especially into an intensive care nursery, can be devastating. Virtually every infant becomes infected, and the infection is associated with considerable morbidity and occasionally death. The virus is transmitted in aerosols but also on hands and by fomites.

As already noted, RSV infects virtually all children by the age of 4 years, especially in urban centers. Outbreaks may also occur among the elderly population (e.g., in nursing homes). Virus is shed in respiratory secretions for many days, especially by infants.

Clinical Syndromes

RSV can cause any respiratory tract illness, from a **common cold** to **pneumonia.** Upper respiratory tract infection with prominent rhinorrhea (runny nose) is most common in older children and adults. A more severe lower respiratory tract illness, **bronchiolitis,** may occur in infants. Because of inflammation at the level of the bronchiole, there is air trapping and decreased ventilation. Clinically, the patient usually has low-grade fever, tachypnea, tachycardia, and expiratory wheezes over the lungs. Bronchiolitis is usually self-limited, but it can be a frightening disease to observe in an infant. It may be fatal in premature infants, persons with underlying lung disease, and immunocompromised people.

Laboratory Diagnosis

RSV is difficult to isolate in cell culture. The presence of the viral genome in infected cells and nasal washings can be detected by RT-PCR techniques, and commercially available immunofluorescence and enzyme immunoassay tests are available for detection of the viral antigen. The finding of seroconversion or a fourfold or greater increase in the antibody titer can confirm the diagnosis for epidemiologic purposes.

Treatment, Prevention, and Control

In otherwise healthy infants, treatment is supportive, consisting of the administration of oxygen, intravenous fluids, and nebulized cold steam. **Ribavirin,** a guanosine analogue, is approved for the treatment of patients predisposed to a more severe course (e.g., premature or immunocompromised infants). It is administered by inhalation (nebulization).

Passive immunization with anti-RSV immunoglobulin is available for premature infants. Infected children must be isolated. Infection-control measures are required for hospital staff caring for infected children to avoid transmitting the virus to uninfected patients. These measures include hand washing and wearing gowns, goggles, and masks.

No vaccine is currently available for RSV prophylaxis. A previously available vaccine containing inactivated RSV caused recipients to have more severe RSV disease when subsequently exposed to the live virus. This development is thought to be the result of a heightened immunologic response at the time of exposure to the wild virus.

HUMAN METAPNEUMOVIRUS

Human metapneumovirus is a recently recognized member of the Pneumovirinae subfamily. Use of RT-PCR methods was and remains the means of detecting the pneumoviruses and distinguishing them from other respiratory disease viruses. Its identity was unknown until recently, because it is difficult to grow in cell culture. The virus is ubiquitous, and almost all 5-year-old children have experienced a virus infection and are seropositive.

As with its close cousin RSV, infections by human metapneumovirus may be asymptomatic, cause common cold-type disease, or serious bronchiolitis and pneumonia. Seronegative children, the elderly, and immunocompromised people are at risk for disease. Human metapneumovirus probably causes 15% of common colds in children, especially those which are complicated by otitis media. Signs of disease usually include cough, sore throat, runny nose, and high fever. Approximately 10% of patients with metapneumovirus will experience wheezing, dyspnea, pneumonia, bronchitis, or bronchiolitis. As with other common cold agents, laboratory identification of the virus is not performed routinely but can be performed by RT-PCR. Supportive care is the only therapy available for these infections.

NIPAH AND HENDRA VIRUSES

A new paramyxovirus, Nipah virus, was isolated from patients after an outbreak of severe encephalitis in Malaysia and Singapore in 1998. Nipah virus is more closely related to the Hendra virus, discovered in 1994 in Australia, than to other paramyxoviruses. Both viruses have broad host ranges, including pigs, man, dogs, horses, cats, and other mammals. For Nipah virus, the reservoir is a fruit bat (flying fox). The virus can be obtained from fruit contaminated by infected bats or amplified in pigs and then spread to humans. The human is an accidental host for these viruses, but the outcome of human infection is severe. Disease signs include flulike symptoms, seizures, and coma. Of the 269 cases occurring in 1999, 108 were fatal. Another epidemic in Bangladesh in 2004 had a higher mortality rate.

SUMMARY

The *Paramyxoviridae* include three genera: *Morbillivirus*, *Paramyxovirus*, and *Pneumovirus*. Human pathogens include the measles virus (within the morbilliviruses); the parainfluenza and mumps viruses

(within the paramyxoviruses) the respiratory syncytial virus (RSV)(within the pneumoviruses) and the newly discovered but relatively common metapneumovirus. Nipah virus and Hendra virus, two zoonosis-causing viruses, are two newly identified group of highly pathogenic paramyxoviruses. The virions of paramyxoviruses have similar morphologies and protein components, and they share the capacity to induce cell-to-cell fusion (syncytia formation and multinucleated giant cells). The paramyxoviruses cause some well-known major diseases. Measles virus causes a potentially serious generalized infection characterized by a maculopapular rash (rubeola). Subacute sclerosing panencephalitis (SSPE) is the serious sequelae of measles. Parainfluenza viruses cause upper and lower respiratory tract infections, primarily in children, including pharyngitis, croup, bronchitis, bronchiolitis, and pneumonia. Mumps virus causes a systemic infection whose most prominent clinical manifestation is parotitis. RSV causes mild upper respiratory tract infections in children and adults but can cause life-threatening pneumonia in infants. Measles and mumps viruses have only one serotype, and protection is provided by an effective live vaccine.

KEYWORDS

English	Chinese
Paramyxoviridae	副黏病毒科
Measles	麻疹
Paramyxoviruses	副黏病毒
Respiratory syncytial virus RSV	呼吸道合胞病毒
Measles virus	麻疹病毒
Mumps virus	腮腺炎病毒
Epidemic mumps	流行性腮腺炎
Parainfluenza virus	副流感病毒
Humanmetapneumovirus	人类偏肺病毒
Hendra virus	亨德拉病毒
Nipah virus	尼帕病毒
Subacute sclerosing panencephalitits, SSPE	亚急性硬化性全脑炎
Measles-mumps-rubella (MMR) vaccine	麻疹腮腺炎风疹疫苗

BIBLIOGRAPHY

1. Cann AJ: Principles of molecular virology, San Diego, 2005, Academic.

2. Carter J, Saunders V: Virology: principles and applications, Chichester, England, 2007, Wiley.

3. Centers for Disease Control and Prevention: Public-sector vaccination efforts in response to the resurgence of measles among preschool-aged children: United States, 1989-1991, MMWR Morb Mortal Wkly Rep 41: 522-525, 1992.

4. Cohen J, Powderly WG: Infectious diseases, ed 2, St Louis, 2004, Mosby.

5. Collier L, Oxford J: Human virology, ed 3, Oxford, England, 2006, Oxford University Press.

6. Flint SJ, et al: Principles of virology: molecular biology, pathogenesis and control of animal viruses, ed 3, Washington, DC, 2009, American Society for Microbiology Press.

7. Galinski MS: Paramyxoviridae: transcription and replication, Adv Virus Res 40: 129-163, 1991.

8. Gershon AA, et al: Krugman's infectious diseases of children, ed 11, St Louis, 2004, Mosby.

9. Griffin DE, Oldstone MBA, editors: Measles: pathogenesis and control, vol 330, Heidelberg, Germany, 2009, Springer-Verlag.

10. Hart CA, Broadhead RL: Color atlas of pediatric infectious diseases, St Louis, 1992, Mosby.

11. Hinman AR: Potential candidates for eradication, Rev Infect Dis 4: 933-939, 1982.

12. Knipe DM, Howley PM: Fields virology, ed 4, New York, 2001, Lippincott Williams & Wilkins.

13. Lennette EH: Laboratory diagnosis of viral infections, ed 3, New York, 1999, Marcel Dekker.

14. Meulen V, Billeter MA: Measles virus, Curr Top MicrobiolImmunol, vol 191, Berlin, 1995, Springer-Verlag, pp 1-196.

15. Moss WJ, Griffen DE: Measles, Lancet 379: 153-164, 2012.

16. Strauss JM, Strauss EG: Viruses and human disease, ed 2, San Diego, 2007, Academic.

17. Voyles BA: The biology of viruses, ed 2, Boston, 2002, McGraw-Hill.

Chapter 51

Orthomyxoviruses

Influenza A, B, and C viruses are the only members of the *Orthomyxoviridae* family, and only influenza A and B viruses cause significant human disease. Historically the most famous influenza **pandemic** caused by influenza A is the Spanish influenza that swept the world in 1918 to 1919, killing 20 to 40 million people. The recent pandemic was caused by 2009 H1N1 pandemic influenza virus.

STRUCTURE AND REPLICATION

Influenza virions are pleomorphic, appearing spheric or tubular (Figure 51-1) and ranging in diameter from 80 to 120 nm. The envelope contains two glycoproteins, **hemagglutinin (HA)** and **neuraminidase (NA)**, the **membrane (M_2) protein** and is internally lined by the **matrix (M_1) protein.** The genome of the influenza A and B viruses consists of **eight different helical nucleocapsid segments**, each of which contains a negative-sense RNA associated with the **nucleoprotein (NP)** and the **transcriptase (RNA polymerase components: PB1, PB2, PA)** (Table 57-1). Influenza C has only seven genomic segments.

The genomic segments in the influenza A virus range from 890 to 2340 bases. All the proteins are encoded on separate segments, with the exception of the nonstructural proteins (NS_1 and NS_2) and the M_1 and M_2 proteins, which are transcribed from one segment each.

The **HA** forms a spike-shaped trimer; each unit is activated by a protease and is cleaved into two subunits held together by a disulfide bond. The HA has several functions. It is the viral attachment protein, binding to sialic acid on epithelial cell surface recep-

Table 51-1 Products of Influenza Gene Segments

Segment*	Protein	Function
1	PB2	Polymerase component
2	PB1	Polymerase component
3	PA	Polymerase component
4	HA	Hemagglutinin, viral attachment protein, fusion protein, target of neutralizing antibody
5	NP	Nucleocapsid
6	NA	Neuraminidase (cleaves sialic acid and promotes virus release)
7†	M_1	Matrix protein: viral structural protein (interacts with nucleocapsid and envelope, promotes assembly)
	M_2	Membrane protein (forms membrane channel and target for amantadine, facilitates uncoating and HA production)
8†	NS_1	Nonstructural protein (inhibits cellular messenger RNA translation)
	NS_2	Nonstructural protein (promotes export of nucleocapsid from nucleus)

*Listed in decreasing order of size.
†Encodes two messenger RNAs.

tors; it promotes fusion of the envelope to the cell membrane at acidic pH; it hemagglutinates (binds and aggregates) human, chicken, and guinea pig red blood cells; and it elicits the protective neutralizing antibody response. Mutation-derived changes in HA are responsible for the minor ("drift") and major ("shift") changes in antigenicity. Shifts occur only with influenza A virus, and the different HAs are designated H1, H2…H18.

The **NA** glycoprotein forms a tetramer and has enzyme activity. The NA cleaves the sialic acid on glycoproteins, including the cell receptor. Cleavage of the sialic acid on virion proteins prevents clumping and facilitates the release of virus from infected cells,

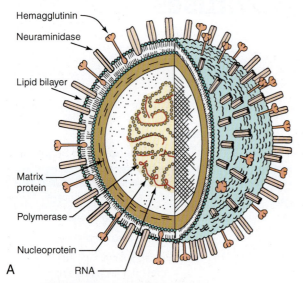

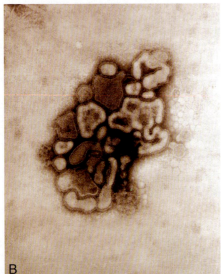

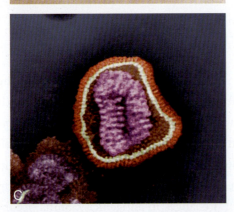

Figure 51-1 **A,** Model of influenza A virus. **B** and **C,** Electron micrographs of influenza A virus. *RNA,* Ribonucleic acid. (**A,** From Kaplan MM, Webster RG: The epidemiology of influenza, *Sci Am* 237: 88-106, 1977. **B,** From Balows A, et al: *Labo*ratory diagnosis of infectious diseases: principles and practice, vol 2, New York, 1988, Springer-Verlag.)

making NA a target for two antiviral drugs, **zanamivir (Relenza),** and **oseltamivir (Tamiflu).** The NA of influenza A virus also undergoes antigenic shift, and major differences acquire the designations N1, N2... N11.

The M_1, M_2, and **NP** proteins are type specific and are therefore used to differentiate influenza A from B or C viruses. The M_1 proteins line the inside of the virion and promote assembly. The M_2 protein forms a proton channel in membranes and promotes uncoating and viral release. The M_2 of influenza A is a target for the antiviral drugs **amantadine** and **rimantadine.**

Viral replication begins with the binding of HA to sialic acid on cell surface glycoproteins (Figure 51-2). The different HAs (HA1-18) bind to different sialic acid structures. The virus is then internalized into a coated vesicle and transferred to an endosome. Acidification of the endosome causes the HA to bend over and expose hydrophobic fusion-promoting regions of the protein. The viral envelope then fuses with the endosome membrane. The proton channel formed

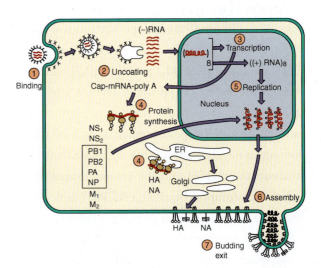

Figure 51-2 Replication of influenza A virus. After binding *(1)* to sialic acid-containing receptors, influenza is endocytosed and fuses *(2)* with the vesicle membrane. Unlike for most other ribonucleic acid (RNA) viruses, transcription *(3)* and replication *(5)* of the genome occur in the nucleus. Viral proteins are synthesized *(4)*, helical nucleocapsid segments form and associate *(6)* with the M_1 protein-lined membranes containing M_2 and the hemagglutinin *(HA)* and neuraminidase *(NA)* glycoproteins. The virus buds *(7)* from the plasma membrane and eventually kills the cell. *(−),* Negative sense; *(+),* positive sense; *ER,* endoplasmic reticulum; *NP,* nucleocapsid; *NS₁, NS₂,* nonstructural proteins 1 and 2; *PA, PB1, PB2,* polymerase A, B1, and B2; *polyA,* polyadenylate.

by the M_2 protein promotes acidification of the envelope contents to break the interaction between the M_1 protein and the NP, allowing uncoating and delivery of the nucleocapsid into the cytoplasm.

Unlike most RNA viruses, the influenza nucleocapsid travels to the nucleus, where it is transcribed into mRNA. The transcriptase (PA, PB1, and PB2) uses host cell mRNA as a primer for viral mRNA synthesis. In so doing, it steals the methylated cap region of the RNA, the sequence required for efficient binding to ribosomes. All the genomic segments are transcribed into 5′-capped, 3′-polyadenylated (polyA) mRNA for individual proteins except the segments for the M_1, M_2 and NS_1, NS_2 proteins, which are each differentially spliced (using cellular enzymes) to produce two different mRNAs. The mRNAs are translated into protein in the cytoplasm. The HA and NA glycoproteins are processed by the endoplasmic reticulum and Golgi apparatus. The M_2 protein inserts into cellular membranes. Its proton channel prevents acidification of Golgi and other vesicles, thus preventing acid-induced folding and inactivation of the HA within the cell. The HA and NA are then transported to the cell surface.

Positive-sense RNA templates for each segment are produced, and the negative-sense RNA genome is replicated in the nucleus. The genomic segments associate with polymerase and NP proteins to form nucleocapsids, and the NS_2 protein facilitates the transport of ribonucleocapsids into the cytoplasm, where they interact with the M_1 protein-lined plasma membrane sections containing M_2, HA, and NA. The virus buds selectively from the apical (airway) surface of the cell as a result of the preferential insertion of the HA in this membrane. Virus is released approximately 8 hours after infection.

PATHOGENESIS AND IMMUNITY

Influenza initially establishes a local upper respiratory tract infection. To do so, the virus first targets and kills mucus-secreting, ciliated, and other epithelial cells, causing the loss of this primary defense system. NA facilitates the development of the infection by cleaving sialic acid (neuraminic acid) residues of the mucus, thereby providing access to tissue. Preferential release of the virus at the apical surface of epithelial cells and into the lung promotes cell-to-cell spread and transmission to other hosts. If the virus spreads to the lower respiratory tract, the infection can cause severe desquamation (shedding) of bronchial or alveolar epithelium down to a single-cell basal layer or to the basement membrane.

In addition to compromising the mucociliary defenses of the respiratory tract, influenza infection promotes bacterial adhesion to the epithelial cells. Pneumonia may result from a viral pathogenesis or from a secondary bacterial infection. Influenza may also cause a transient or low-level viremia but rarely involves tissues other than the lung.

Influenza infection leads to an inflammatory cell response of the mucosal membrane, which consists primarily of monocytes and lymphocytes and few neutrophils. Submucosal edema is present. Lung tissue may reveal hyaline membrane disease, alveolar emphysema, and necrosis of the alveolar walls.

Interferon and cytokine responses, which peak at almost the same time as virus in nasal washes, may be sufficient to control the infection, and are responsible for the systemic "flulike" symptoms. T-cell responses are important for effecting recovery and immunopathogenesis, but antibody, including vaccine-induced antibody, can prevent disease. As for measles, influenza infection depresses macrophage and T-cell function, hindering immune resolution. Of interest, recovery often precedes detection of antibody in serum or secretions.

Protection against reinfection is primarily associated with the development of antibodies to HA, but antibodies to NA are also protective. The antibody response is specific for each strain of influenza, but the cell-mediated immune response is more general and is capable of reacting to influenza strains of the same type (influenza A or B virus). Antigenic targets for T-cell responses include peptides from HA but also from the nucleocapsid proteins (NP, PB2) and M_1 protein. The NP, PB2, and M_1 proteins differ considerably for influenza A and B but minimally between strains of these viruses; hence T-cell memory may provide future protection against infection by different strains of either influenza A or B.

The symptoms and time course of the disease are determined by the extent of viral and immune killing of epithelial tissue and cytokine action. Influenza is normally a self-limited disease that rarely involves organs other than the lung. *Many of the classic "flu" symptoms (e.g., fever, malaise, headache, and myalgia) are associated with interferon and cytokine induction.* Repair of the compromised tissue is initiated within 3 to 5 days of the start of symptoms but may take as long as a month or more, especially for elderly people.

EPIDEMIOLOGY

Strains of influenza A virus are classified by the following four characteristics:

(1) Type (A)

(2) Place of original isolation

(3) Date of original isolation

(4) Antigen (HA and NA)

For example, a current strain of influenza virus might be designated A/Bangkok/1/79 (H3N2), meaning that it is an influenza A virus that was first isolated in Bangkok in January 1979 and contains HA (H3) and NA (N2) antigens.

Strains of influenza B are designated by (1) type, (2) geography, and (3) date of isolation (e.g., B/Singapore/3/64), but without specific mention of HA or NA antigens, because influenza B does not undergo antigenic shift or pandemics as does influenza A.

Minor antigenic changes resulting from mutation of the HA and NA genes are called **antigenic drift**. This process occurs every 2 to 3 years, causing local outbreaks of influenza A and B infection. **Major antigenic changes (antigenic shift)** result from the reassortment of genomes among different strains, including animal strains. *This process occurs only with the influenza A virus.* Such changes are often associated with the occurrence of pandemics. *In contrast to influenza A, influenza B is predominantly a human virus and does not undergo antigenic shift.*

Antigenic shifts occur infrequently, but the pandemics they cause can be devastating (Table 51-2). For example, the prevalent influenza A virus in 1947 was the H1N1 subtype. In 1957, there was a shift in both antigens, resulting in an H2N2 subtype. H3N2 appeared in 1968, and H1N1 reappeared in 1977. The reappearance of H1N1 put the population younger than age 30 years at risk of disease. Prior exposure and an anamnestic antibody response protected the members of the population older than 30 years.

Table 51-2 Influenza Pandemics Resulting from Antigenic Shift.

Year of Pandemic	Influenza A Subtype
1918	H1N1
1947	H1N1
1957	H2N2; Asian flu strain
1968	H3N2; Hong Kong flu strain
1977	H1N1; Russian
1997, 2003	H5N1: China, Avian
2009	H1N1, Swine flu

The genetic diversity of influenza A is fostered by its segmented genomic structure and ability to infect and replicate in humans and many animal species (**zoonose**), including birds and pigs. Hybrid viruses are created by coinfection of a cell with different strains of influenza A virus, allowing the genomic segments to randomly associate into new virions. An exchange of the HA glycoproteins may generate a new virus that can infect an immunologically naïve human population. Figure 51-3 depicts the origins of the pandemic A/California/04/2009/H1N1 virus through multiple reassortments of human, avian, and pig influenza viruses, resulting in a virus that was able to infect humans.

In the spring of 2009, a new amantadine- and rimantadine-resistant reassortant H1N1 virus was detected in a 10-year-old patient in California and proceeded to cause a pandemic. As indicated in Figure 51-3, the virus is a triple-triple reassortant of multiple swine, avian, and human influenza viruses. The virus originated in Mexico and rapidly spread as many cases went unrecognized because of the unseasonal nature of the outbreak. Up to 25,000 deaths have occurred worldwide, primarily in people between the ages of 22 months and 57 years. People with chronic medical conditions, especially pregnant women, were at greatest risk to complications, but unlike other outbreaks, this virus had a tendency to affect younger and healthier individuals. Of interest, many people older than 60 years had cross-reactive antibody resulting from prior exposure to an H1N1 influenza virus. Neuraminidase inhibitors were made available for prophylaxis, but detection of resistant strains became a concern. By September, a vaccine had been developed, approved, manufactured, and available for distribution on a prioritized basis and then was administered with the seasonal influenza vaccine. The pandemic was declared over by August

2010, and the H1N1 virus joined H3N2 and influenza B as a seasonal virus.

Because of its high population density and proximity of humans, pigs, chickens, and ducks, China is often the breeding ground for new reassortant viruses and the source of many of the pandemic strains of influenza. In 1997, a highly pathogenic avian influenza virus (HPAIV) (H5N1) strain was isolated from at least 18 humans and caused six deaths in Hong Kong. The virus was spread by domestic and wild water fowl in their feces and directly from bird to man, with cases occurring around the globe. This avian H5N1 virus is unusual because it is not a reassortant; yet, it can infect and kill cells of the lower human lung. This requires

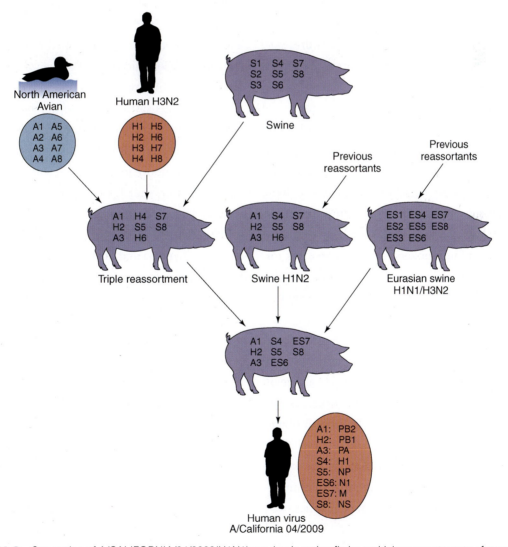

Figure 51-3 Generation of A/CALIFORNIA/04/2009(H1N1) pandemic swine flu by multiple reassortments of genomic segments of influenza A virus. The pandemic H1N1 virus arose from the mixing of a triple reassortment of avian, human and swine viruses with two other swine viruses, each of which were also generated by reassortment between swine, human, and other influenza viruses. This new virus emerged in the spring of 2009 (out of season) in Mexico but was first identified in California.

inhalation of large amounts of virus (shared living environments). Outbreaks of avian influenza require the destruction of all potentially infected birds, such as for the 1.6 million chickens in Hong Kong, to destroy the potential source of the virus.

The changing antigenic nature of influenza ensures a large proportion of immunologically naïve, susceptible people (especially children) in the population. An influenza outbreak can be readily detected from the increased absenteeism in schools and work and the number of emergency department visits. During the winter, influenza outbreaks occur annually in temperate climates. Fortunately, influenza virus is usually present in a community for only a short time (4 to 6 weeks).

Influenza infection is spread readily via small airborne droplets expelled during talking, breathing, and coughing. Low humidity and cool temperatures stabilize the virus, and close proximity during the winter months promotes spread of the virus. The virus can also survive on countertops for as long as a day.

The most susceptible population is children, and school-age children are most likely to spread the infection. Contagion precedes symptoms and lasts for a long time, especially in children. Children, immunosuppressed people (including pregnant women), the elderly, and people with heart and lung ailments (including smokers) are at highest risk for more serious disease, pneumonia, or other complications of infection. More than 90% of mortalities occur in patients who are older than 65 years.

Extensive surveillance of influenza A and B outbreaks is conducted to identify new strains that should be incorporated into new vaccines. The prevalence of a particular strain of influenza A or B virus changes each year and reflects the particular immunologic naïveté of the population at that time. Surveillance also extends into the animal populations because of the possible presence of recombinant animal influenza A strains that can cause human pandemics.

CLINICAL SYNDROMES

Depending on the degree of immunity to the infect-

ing strain of virus and other factors, infection may range from asymptomatic to severe. Patients with underlying cardiorespiratory disease, people with immune deficiency (even that associated with pregnancy), the elderly, and smokers are more prone to have a severe case.

After an incubation period of 1 to 4 days, the "flu syndrome" begins with a brief prodrome of malaise and headache lasting a few hours. The prodrome is followed by the abrupt onset of fever, chills, severe myalgias, loss of appetite, weakness and fatigue, sore throat, and usually a nonproductive cough. The fever persists for 3 to 8 days, and unless a complication occurs, recovery is complete within 7 to 10 days. Influenza in young children (younger than 3 years) resembles other severe respiratory tract infections, causing bronchiolitis, croup, otitis media, vomiting, and abdominal pain, accompanied rarely by febrile convulsions. Complications of influenza include bacterial pneumonia, myositis, and Reye syndrome. The central nervous system can also be involved. Influenza B disease is similar to influenza A disease.

Influenza may directly cause pneumonia, but it more commonly promotes a secondary bacterial superinfection that leads to bronchitis or pneumonia. The tissue damage caused by progressive influenza virus infection of alveoli can be extensive, leading to hypoxia and bilateral pneumonia. Secondary bacterial infection usually involves *Streptococcus pneumoniae*, *Haemophilusinfluenzae*, or *Staphylococcus aureus*. In these infections, sputum usually is produced and becomes purulent.

Although the infection generally is limited to the lung, some strains of influenza can spread to other sites in certain people. For example, myositis (inflammation of muscle) may occur in children. Encephalopathy, although rare, may accompany an acute influenza illness and can be fatal. Postinfluenza encephalitis occurs 2 to 3 weeks after recovery from influenza. These diseases are thought to be autoimmune diseases triggered by influenza.

Reye syndrome is an acute encephalitis that affects children and occurs after a variety of acute febrile viral infections, including varicella and influenza B and A diseases. Children given salicylates (aspirin) are at increased risk for this syndrome. In addition to encephalopathy, hepatic dysfunction is present. The mortality rate may be as high as 40%.

LABORATORY DIAGNOSIS

The diagnosis of influenza is usually based on the characteristic symptoms, the season, and the presence of the virus in the community. Laboratory methods that distinguish influenza from other respiratory viruses and identify its type and strain confirm the diagnosis.

Influenza viruses are obtained from respiratory secretions taken early in the illness. The virus is generally isolated in primary monkey kidney cell cultures or the Madin-Darby canine kidney cell line. Nonspecific cytopathologic effects are often difficult to distinguish but may be noted within as few as 2 days (average, 4 days). Before the cytopathologic effects develop, the addition of guinea pig erythrocytes may reveal **hemadsorption** (the adherence of these erythrocytes to HA-expressing infected cells). The addition of influenza virus-containing media to erythrocytes promotes the formation of a gel-like aggregate resulting from **hemagglutination.** Hemagglutination and hemadsorption are not specific to influenza viruses because parainfluenza and other viruses also exhibit these properties.

More rapid techniques detect and identify the influenza genome or antigens of the virus. Rapid antigen assays (less than 30 minutes) can detect and distinguish influenza A and B. Reverse transcriptase polymerase chain reaction (RT-PCR), using generic influenza primers, can be used to detect and distinguish influenza A and B, and more specific primers can be used to distinguish the different strains, such as H5N1. Enzyme immunoassay or immunofluorescence can be used to detect viral antigen in exfoliated cells, respiratory secretions, or cell culture and are more sensitive assays. Immunofluorescence or inhibition of hemadsorption or hemagglutination (hemagglutination inhibition) with specific antibody can also detect and distinguish different influenza strains.

Laboratory studies are primarily used for epidemiologic purposes.

TREATMENT, PREVENTION, AND CONTROL

Hundreds of millions of dollars are spent on acetaminophen, antihistamines, and similar drugs to relieve the symptoms of influenza. The antiviral drug **amantadine** and its analogue **rimantadine** inhibit an uncoating step of the influenza A virus but do not affect the influenza B and C viruses. The target for their action is the M_2 protein. **Zanamivir** and **oseltamivir** inhibit both influenza A and B as enzyme inhibitors of neuraminidase. Without neuraminidase, the hemagglutinin of the virus binds to sialic acid on other glycoproteins and viral particles to form clumps, thereby preventing virus release. Zanamivir is inhaled, whereas oseltamivir is taken orally as a pill. These drugs are effective for prophylaxis and for treatment during the first 24 to 48 hours after the onset of influenza A illness. Treatment cannot prevent the later host-induced immunopathogenic stages of the disease. Naturally resistant or mutant strains are selected when antiviral prophylaxis is used.

The airborne spread of influenza is almost impossible to limit. However, the best way to control the virus is through immunization. Natural immunization, which results from prior exposure, is protective for long periods. A killed-virus vaccine representing the "strains of the year" and antiviral drug prophylaxis can also prevent infection.

The influenza vaccine is a mixture of extracts or purified HA and NA proteins from three different strains of virus. The vaccines are prepared from virus grown in embryonated eggs and then chemically inactivated. Killed (formalin-inactivated) virion preparations have also been used. Vaccines grown in tissue culture cells or by genetic engineering are being developed. Ideally, the vaccine incorporates antigens of the A and B influenza strains that will be prevalent in the community during the upcoming winter. Vaccination is routinely recommended for all individuals and especially persons older than 50 years, health care workers, pregnant women who will be in their second or third trimester during flu season, people living in a nursing home, people with chronic pulmonary heart disease, and others at high risk. Persons with allergies to eggs should not get the vaccine.

A live vaccine is also available for administration as a nasal spray instead of a "flu shot". The trivalent vaccine consists of reassortants for the HA and NA gene segments of the desired influenza strains, with a master donor virus that is cold adapted to optimum growth at 25℃. This vaccine will elicit a more natural protection, including cell-mediated, serum antibody and mucosal-secretory IgA antibody. Currently, the vaccine is recommended for people ages 2 to 50 years.

SUMMARY

Influenza virus is the only member of the *Orthomyxoviridae* family. The orthomyxoviruses include influenza A, B and C viruses. These viruses are **enveloped and have a segmented negative-sense RNA genome.** Influenza A virus is characterized by the segmented viral genome facilitates the development of new strains through the mutation and reassortment of the gene segments among different human and animal strains of viruses. Therefore, the genetic instability is responsible for the annual epidemics (mutation: drift) and for influenza A, periodic pandemics (reassortment: shift) of influenza infection worldwide. Influenza A and B viruses cause influenza. It is one of the most prevalent viral infections. Influenza viruses cause respiratory symptoms and the classic flulike symptoms of fever, malaise, headache, and myalgias (body aches). Prophylaxis with vaccines and antiviral drugs is now available for people at risk for influenza infections.

KEYWORDS

English	Chinese
Influenza	流行性感冒
Orthomyxoviridae	正黏病毒科
Influenza viruses	流感病毒
Influenza A	甲型流感病毒
Pandemics	世界性大流行
Hemagglutinin (HA)	血凝素
Neuraminidase (NA)	神经氨酸酶
Antigenic drift	抗原漂移
Antigenic shift	抗原转换
Reassortment	重配
Hemagglutination	血凝
Hemagglutination inhibition	血凝抑制

BIBLIOGRAPHY

1. Cann AJ: Principles of molecular virology, San Diego, 2005, Academic.

2. Carr CM, Chaudhry C, Kim PS: Influenza hemagglutinin is spring-loaded by a metastable native conformation, ProcNatlAcadSci U S A 94: 14306-14313, 1997.

3. Carter J, Saunders V: Virology: principles and applications, Chichester, England, 2007, Wiley.

4. Cohen J, Powderly WG: Infectious diseases, ed 2, St Louis, 2004, Mosby.

5. Collier L, Oxford J: Human virology, ed 3, Oxford, England, 2006, Oxford University Press.

6. Cox NJ, Subbarao K: Global epidemiology of influenza: past and present, Annu Rev Med 51: 407-421, 2000.

7. Das K, et al: Structures of influenza A proteins and insights into antiviral drug targets, Nat StructMolBiol 17: 530-538, 2010.

8. Flint SJ, et al: Principles of virology: molecular biology, pathogenesis and control of animal viruses, ed 3, Washington, DC, 2009, American Society for Microbiology Press.

9. Helenius A: Unpacking the incoming influenza virus, Cell 69: 577-578, 1992.

10. Knipe DM, et al: Fields virology, ed 5, Philadelphia, 2006, Lippincott Williams & Wilkins.

11. Laver WG, Bischofberger N, Webster RG: Disarming flu viruses, Sci Am 280: 78-87, 1999.

12. Laver WG, Bischofberger N, Webster RG: The origin and control of pandemic influenza, PerspectBiol Med 43: 173-192, 2000.

13. Poland GA, Jacobson RM, Targonski PV: Avian and pandemic influenza: an overview, Vaccine 25: 3057-3061, 2007.

14. Richman DD, Whitley RJ, Hayden FG: Clinical virology, ed 3, Washington, DC, 2009, American Society for Microbiology Press.

15. Salomon R, Webster RG: The influenza virus enigma, Cell 136: 402-410, 2009.

16. Strauss JM, Strauss EG: Viruses and human disease, ed 2, San Diego, 2007, Academic.

17. Tong S, et al: New world bats harbor diverse influenza A viruses, PLoSPathog 9(10): e1003657, 2013.

18. Webster RG, Govorkova EA: H5N1 Influenza, continuing evolution and spread, N Engl J Med 355: 2174-2177, 2006.

19. Voyles BA: The biology of viruses, ed 2, Boston, 2002, McGraw-Hill.

Rhabdoviruses, Filoviruses, and Bornaviruses

RHABDOVIRUSES

The members of the family Rhabdoviridae (from the Greek word rhabdos, meaning "rod") contain *Vesiculovirus* (vesicular stomatitis viruses, VSVs), *Lyssavirus* (Greek for "frenzy") (rabies and rabies-like viruses), an unnamed genus constituting the plant rhabdovirus group, and other ungrouped rhabdoviruses of mammals, birds, fish, and arthropods. Rabies virus is the most significant pathogen of the rhabdoviruses.

Physiology, Structure, and Replication

Rhabdoviruses are simple viruses encoding only five proteins and appearing as bullet-shaped, enveloped virions with a diameter of 50 to 95 nm and length of 130 to 380 nm (Figure 52-1). Spikes composed of a trimer of the glycoprotein (G) cover the surface of the virus. The viral attachment protein, G protein, generates neutralizing antibodies. The G protein of the vesicular stomatitis virus is a simple glycoprotein with *N*-linked glycan.

Within the envelope, the helical nucleocapsid is coiled symmetrically into a cylindric structure, giving it the appearance of striations (see Figure 52-1). The nucleocapsid is composed of one molecule of single-stranded, negative-sense RNA of approximately 12,000 bases and the nucleoprotein (N), large (L), and nonstructural (NS) proteins. The matrix (M) protein lies between the envelope and the nucleocapsid. The N protein is the major structural protein of the virus. It protects the RNA from ribonuclease digestion and maintains the RNA in a configuration acceptable for transcription. The L and NS proteins constitute the RNA-dependent RNA polymerase.

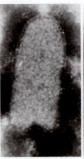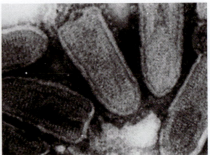

Figure 52-1   Rhabdoviridae seen by electron microscopy: rabies virus *(left)* and vesicular stomatitis virus *(right)*. (From Fields BN: *Virology*, New York, 1985, Raven.)

The replicative cycle of VSV is the prototype for the rhabdoviruses and other negative-strand RNA viruses. The viral G protein attaches to the host cell and is internalized by endocytosis. The viral envelope then fuses with the membrane of the endosome on acidification of the vesicle. This uncoats the nucleocapsid, releasing it into the cytoplasm, where replication takes place. Endosomal vesicles may deliver whole rabies virions along the axon to neuronal cell bodies, where its replication takes place.

The RNA-dependent RNA polymerase associated with the nucleocapsid transcribes the viral genomic RNA, producing five individual mRNAs. For rabies virus, this occurs in the Negri bodies. These mRNAs are then translated into the five viral proteins. The viral genomic RNA is also transcribed into a full-length, positive-sense RNA template that is used to generate new genomes. The G protein is synthesized by membrane-bound ribosomes, processed by the Golgi apparatus, and delivered to the cell surface in membrane vesicles. The M protein associates with the G protein-modified membranes.

The genome associates with the N protein and

then with the polymerase proteins L and NS to form the nucleocapsid. Association of the nucleocapsid with the M protein at the plasma membrane induces coiling into its condensed form and the characteristic bullet shape of the virion. The virus then buds through the plasma membrane and is released when the entire nucleocapsid is enveloped. Cell death and lysis occur after infection with most rhabdoviruses, with the important exception of rabies virus, which produces little discernible cell damage.

Pathogenesis and Immunity

Rabies infection of the animal causes secretion of the virus in the animal's saliva and promotes aggressive behavior ("mad" dog), which in turn promotes transmission of the virus. The virus can also be transmitted through the inhalation of aerosolized virus, in transplanted infected tissue, and by inoculation through intact mucosal membranes.

The virus replicates quietly at the site for days to months (Figure 52-2) before progressing to the central nervous system (CNS). Rabies virus travels by retrograde axoplasmic transport to the dorsal root ganglia and to the spinal cord. Once the virus gains access to the spinal cord, the brain becomes rapidly infected. The virus then disseminates from the CNS via afferent neurons to highly innervated sites, such as the skin of the head and neck, salivary glands, retina, etc. After the virus invades the brain and spinal cord, encephalitis develops and neurons degenerate.

Rabies is fatal once clinical disease is apparent. The length of the incubation period is determined by (1) the concentration of the virus in the inoculum, (2) the proximity of the wound to the brain, (3) the severity of the wound, (4) the host's age, and (5) the host's immune status.

In contrast to other viral encephalitis syndromes, rabies is minimally cytolytic and rarely causes inflammatory lesions. Viral proteins inhibit apoptosis and aspects of interferon action. Neutralizing antibodies are not apparent until after the clinical disease is well established. Cell-mediated immunity appears to play little or no role in protection against rabies virus infection.

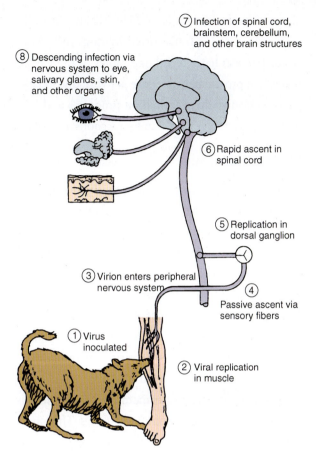

Figure 52-2 Pathogenesis of rabies virus infection. Numbered steps describe the sequence of events. (Modified from Belshe RB: *Textbook of human virology*, ed 2, St Louis, 1991, Mosby.)

The incubation period is usually long enough to allow generation of a therapeutic protective antibody response after active immunization with the killed rabies vaccine.

Epidemiology

Rabies is the classic zoonotic infection spread from animals to humans, and spread in two ways. In urban rabies, dogs are the primary transmitter, and in sylvatic (forest) rabies, many species of wildlife such as bats can serve as transmitters. The principal reservoir for rabies in most of the world is the dog. In Latin America and Asia, unvaccinated dogs and the absence of rabies-control programs are responsible for thousands of rabies cases in dogs each year. Although rare, there are cases of rabies transmission via corneal and organ transplants.

Although underreported, it is estimated that rabies accounts for 70,000 deaths, mostly children, annually worldwide, with at least 25,000 deaths in India, where the virus is transmitted by dogs in 96% of cases. The incidence of human rabies in the United States is approximately one case per year, due in large part to effective dog vaccination programs and limited human contact with skunks, raccoons, and bats.

Clinical Syndromes

Rabies is virtually always fatal unless treated by vaccination. After a long but highly variable incubation period, the prodrome phase of rabies ensues (Table 52-1). The prodrome usually lasts 2 to 10 days, after which the neurologic symptoms specific to rabies appear. Hydrophobia (fear of water), the most characteristic symptom of rabies, occurs in 20% to 50% of patients. Fifteen percent to 60% of patients exhibit paralysis as the only manifestation of rabies. The paralysis may lead to respiratory failure.

The patient becomes comatose after the neurologic phase, which lasts from 2 to 10 days. This phase almost universally leads to death resulting from neurologic and pulmonary complications.

Laboratory Diagnosis

The occurrence of neurologic symptoms in a person who has been bitten by an animal generally establishes the diagnosis of rabies. Unfortunately, *evidence of infection, including symptoms and the detection of antibody, does not occur until it is too late for intervention.* Laboratory tests are usually performed to confirm the diagnosis and to determine whether a suspected individual or animal is rabid (postmortem).

The hallmark diagnostic finding has been the detection of intracytoplasmic inclusions consisting of aggregates of viral nucleocapsids (Negri bodies) in affected neurons. However, Negri bodies are seen in only 70% to 90% of brain tissue from infected humans.

Antigen detection using direct immunofluorescence or genome detection using reverse transcriptase polymerase chain reaction (RT-PCR) are relatively quick and sensitive assays that are the preferred methods for diagnosing rabies. Samples of saliva, serum, spinal fluid, skin biopsy material from the nape of the neck, brain biopsy or autopsy material, and impression smears of corneal epithelial cells can also be examined.

Inoculated cell cultures or brain tissues are subsequently examined with direct immunofluorescence.

Rabies antibody titers in serum and cerebrospinal fluid are usually measured by enzyme-linked immunosorbent assay (ELISA) or a rapid fluorescent focus inhibition test. Antibody usually is not detectable until late in the disease, however.

Treatment and Prophylaxis

Clinical rabies is almost always fatal unless treated with postrabies immunization. Once the symptoms have appeared, little other than supportive care can be given.

Postexposure prophylaxis is the only hope for

Table 52-1 Progression of Rabies Disease

Disease Phase	Symptoms	Time (Days)	Viral Status	Immunologic Status
Incubation phase	Asymptomatic	60-365 after bite	Low titer, virus in muscle	—
Prodrome phase	Fever, nausea, vomiting, loss of appetite, headache, lethargy, pain at site of bite	2-10	Low titer, virus in CNS and brain	—
Neurologic phase	Hydrophobia, pharyngeal spasms, hyperactivity, anxiety, depression CNS symptoms: loss of coordination, paralysis, confusion, delirium	2-7	High titer, virus in brain and other sites	Detectable antibody in serum and CNS
Coma	Coma, hypotension, hypoventilation, secondary infections, cardiac arrest	0-14	High titer, virus in brain and other sites	—
Death	—	—	—	—

CNS, Central nervous system.

preventing overt clinical illness in the affected person. Prophylaxis should be initiated for anyone exposed to the saliva or brain tissue of an suspected animal.

The first protective measure is local treatment of the wound. The wound should be washed immediately with soap and water. The World Health Organization Expert Committee on Rabies also recommends the instillation of antirabies serum around the wound.

Subsequently, immunization with vaccine in combination with administration of one dose of human rabies immunoglobulin (HRIG) or equine antirabies serum is recommended. A series of five vaccinations is then administered over the course of a month.

The rabies vaccine is a killed-virus vaccine prepared through the chemical inactivation of rabies infected-tissue culture human diploid cells (HDCV) or fetal rhesus lung cells. The HDCV is administered intramuscularly on the day of exposure and then on days 3, 7, 14, and 28 or intradermally with a lower dose of vaccine to multiple sites on days 0, 3, 7, 28, and 90. Preexposure vaccination should be performed on animal workers, laboratory workers who handle potentially infected tissue, and people traveling to areas where rabies is endemic. HDCV administered intramuscularly or intradermally in three doses is recommended and provides 2 years of protection.

Ultimately the prevention of human rabies hinges on the effective control of rabies in domestic and wild animals. Its control in domestic animals depends on the removal of stray and unwanted animals and the vaccination of all dogs and cats. A live recombinant vaccinia virus vaccine expressing the rabies virus G protein is injected into bait and parachuted into the forest, successfully immunizes raccoons, foxes, and other animals in the United States.

FILOVIRUSES

The Marburg and Ebola viruses (Figure 52-3) are now classified as filoviruses (Filoviridae). They are filamentous, enveloped, negative-strand RNA viruses, cause severe or fatal hemorrhagic fevers and are endemic in Africa.

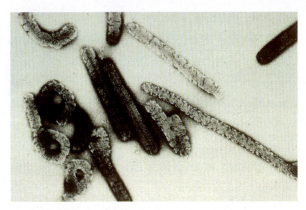

Figure 52-3 Electron micrograph of the Ebola virus. (Courtesy Centers for Disease Control and Prevention, Atlanta.)

Structure and Replication

Filoviruses have a single-stranded RNA genome (4.5×10^6 Da) that encodes seven proteins. The virions form enveloped filaments with a diameter of 80 nm but may also assume other shapes. They vary in length from 800 nm to as long as 1400 nm. The nucleocapsid is helical and enclosed in an envelope containing one glycoprotein. The Ebola virus binds to the Niemann-Pick C1 (NPC1) protein enters the cell and replicates in the cytoplasm like the rhabdoviruses.

Pathogenesis

The filoviruses replicate efficiently, producing large amounts of virus in monocytes, macrophage, dendritic cells, and other cells. Replication in monocytes elicits a cytokine storm of proinflammatory cytokines. Viral cytopathogenesis causes extensive tissue necrosis in parenchymal cells of the liver, spleen, lymph nodes, and lungs. The breakdown of endothelial cells leading to vascular injury can be attributed to the Ebola glycoproteins. The widespread hemorrhage that occurs in affected patients causes edema and hypovolemic shock. A small soluble glycoprotein is shed, can inhibit neutrophil activation, and block antibody action. The viral proteins can also inhibit interferon production and action.

Epidemiology

Marburg virus infection was first detected among laboratory workers in Marburg, Germany, who had been exposed to tissues from apparently healthy African green monkeys.

Ebola virus was named for the river in the Democratic Republic of Congo (formerly Zaire) where it was discovered. Since 1976, when the virus was discovered, approximately 1850 cases and more than 1200 deaths have occurred. However, in rural areas of central Africa, as much as 18% of the population have antibody to this virus, indicating that subclinical infections do occur.

These viruses may be endemic in bats or wild monkeys and can be spread to humans and between humans. Contact with the animal reservoir or direct contact with infected blood or secretions can spread the disease. These viruses have been transmitted by accidental injection and through the use of contaminated syringes. Health care workers tending the sick and monkey handlers may be at risk.

Clinical Syndromes

Marburg and Ebola viruses are the most severe causes of viral hemorrhagic fevers. The illness usually begins with flulike symptoms and diarrhea occurs within a few days; a rash also may develop. Subsequently, hemorrhage from multiple sites (especially the gastrointestinal tract) and death occur in as many as 90% of patients with clinically evident disease.

Laboratory Diagnosis

All specimens from patients with a suspected filovirus infection must be handled with extreme care to prevent accidental infection. Handling of these viruses requires level 4 isolation procedures that are not routinely available. Marburg virus may grow rapidly in tissue culture (Vero cells), but animal (e.g., guinea pig) inoculation may be necessary to recover Ebola virus.

Infected cells have large eosinophilic cytoplasmic inclusion bodies. Viral antigens can be detected in tissue by direct immunofluorescence analysis and in fluids by ELISA. RT-PCR amplification of the viral genome in secretions can be used to confirm the diagnosis and minimize handling of samples.

Treatment, Prevention, and Control

Antibody-containing serum and interferon therapies have been tried in patients with filovirus infections. Infected patients should be quarantined, and contaminated animals should be sacrificed. Handling of the viruses or contaminated materials requires very stringent (level 4) isolation procedures.

BORNA DISEASE VIRUS

Borna disease virus (BDV) is the only member of a family of enveloped, negative-strand RNA viruses. BDV was first associated with infection of horses in Germany. The virus has received considerable recent interest because of its association with specific neuropsychiatric diseases, such as schizophrenia.

Structure and Replication

The 8910-nucleotide-long genome of BDV encodes five detectable proteins, including a polymerase (L), nucleoprotein (N), phosphoprotein (P), matrix protein (M), and envelope glycoprotein (G). Unlike most negative-strand viruses, BDV replicates in the nucleus. Although this is similar to the orthomyxoviruses, BDV differs in that its genome is unsegmented. Also unusual for an RNA virus, one of the positive-strand RNAs that is transcribed from the genome is processed to remove introns to produce three mRNAs for three different proteins.

Pathogenesis

BDV is highly neurotropic and capable of spreading throughout the CNS. BDV also infects parenchymal cells of different organs and peripheral blood mononuclear cells. The virus establishes a persistent infection in the infected individual. T-cell immune responses are important for controlling BDV infections but also contribute to tissue damage leading to disease.

Clinical Syndromes

Many of the outcomes of BDV infection of laboratory animals resemble human neuropsychiatric diseases, including depression, bipolar disorder, schizophrenia, and autism. The presence of antibodies to the virus and/or infected peripheral blood mononuclear cells suggest that BDV either causes or exacerbates these mental illnesses.

Epidemiology

BDV is a zoonose capable of infecting many different mammalian species, including horses, sheep, and humans in central Europe, North America and Asia. Neither the reservoir nor the mode of transmission of BDV is known. Higher levels of infection of humans are present where outbreaks in horses have been observed.

Laboratory Diagnosis

Direct analysis for the viral genome and mRNA in peripheral blood mononuclear cells using RT-PCR and serologic analysis of antibody to the viral proteins are used to identify an association of BDV with human diseases.

Treatment

Ribavirin treatment may be a reasonable treatment approach for some psychoneurologic disorders if BDV was demonstrated as a cofactor.

SUMMARY

Rhabdoviruses

Rhabdoviruses are bullet-shaped, enveloped, negative-sense, single-stranded RNA viruses that encode five proteins. The viral replication occurs in the cytoplasm. Rabies is zoonotic and is usually transmitted in saliva by a rabid animal. Rabies virus is not very cytolytic. Virus replicates in the site of the bite, with no symptoms (incubation phase). Reservoir is wild animals, and vectors are wild animals and unvaccinated dogs and cats. The length of the incubation phase is determined by the infectious dose and the proximity of the infection site to the central nervous system (CNS) and brain (prodrome phase). Infection of the brain causes classic symptoms, coma, and death (neurologic phase). The virus spreads to the salivary glands, from where it is transmitted. Rabies infection does not elicit an antibody response until the virus has spread from the CNS to other sites.

Administration of antibody can block the progression of the virus and disease if given early enough. The long incubation period allows active immunization as a postexposure treatment.

Filoviruses

Filoviruses are filamentous, enveloped, negative-strand RNA viruses, which cause severe or fatal hemorrhagic fevers and are endemic in Africa. The Marburg and Ebola viruses are now classified as filoviruses. Viral cytopathogenesis causes extensive tissue necrosis in parenchymal cells of the liver, spleen, lymph nodes, and lungs. The breakdown of endothelial cells leading to vascular injury can be attributed to the Ebola glycoproteins. They are the most severe causes of viral hemorrhagic fevers. These viruses may be endemic in bats or wild monkeys and can be spread to humans and between humans. Viral antigens can be detected in tissue by direct immunofluorescence analysis and in fluids by ELISA. RT-PCR amplification of the viral genome in secretions can be used to confirm the diagnosis and minimize handling of samples. Antibody-containing serum and interferon therapies have been tried in patients with filovirus infections

Borna disease virus

Borna disease virus is the only member of a family of enveloped, unsegmented negative-strand RNA viruses. Unlike most negative-strand viruses, BDV replicates in the nucleus. BDV is a zoonose capable of infecting many different mammalian species. Higher levels of infection of humans are present where outbreaks in horses have been observed. Viral genome and mRNA detection in PBMC by RT-PCR and serological detection of viral protein by ELISA are often used for diagnosis.

KEYWORDS

English	Chinese
Rhabdoviruses	弹状病毒
Filoviruses	线状病毒
Borna disease virus	博尔纳病病毒
Rabies virus	狂犬病病毒
Ebola virus	埃博拉病毒

| Marburg virus | 马尔堡病毒 |
| Hemorrhagic fevers | 出血热 |

BIBLIOGRAPHY

1. Booth TF, Rabb MJ, Beniac DR: How do filovirus filaments bend without breaking? Trends Microbiol 21(11): 583-593, 2013.

2. Centers for Disease Control and Prevention: Rabies vaccine, absorbed: a new rabies vaccine for use in humans, MMWR Morb Mortal Wkly Rep 37: 217-223, 1988.

3. Cohen J, Powderly WG: Infectious diseases, ed 2, St Louis, 2004, Mosby.

4. Fishbein DB: Rabies, Infect Dis Clin North Am 5: 53-71, 1991.

5. Plotkin SA: Rabies: state of the art clinical article, Clin Infect Dis 30: 4-12, 2000.

6. Richman DD, Whitley RJ, Hayden FG: Clinical virology, ed 3, Washington, DC, 2009, American Society for Microbiology Press.

7. Rupprecht CE: Human infection due to recombinant vaccinia-rabies glycoprotein virus, N Engl J Med 345: 582-586, 2001.

8. Schnell MJ, et al: The cell biology of rabies virus: using stealth to reach the brain. Nat Rev Microbiol 8: 51-61, 2010.

9. Warrell DA, Warrell MJ: Human rabies and its prevention: an overview, Rev Infect Dis 10(Suppl 4): S726-S731, 1988.

10. Winkler WG, Bogel K: Control of rabies in wildlife, Sci Am 266: 86-92, 1992.

11. Wunner WH, et al: The molecular biology of rabies viruses, Rev Infect Dis 10(Suppl 4): S771-S784, 1988.

12. Groseth A, Feldmann H, Strong JE: The ecology of Ebola virus, Trends Microbiol 15: 408-416, 2007.

13. Klenk HD: Marburg and Ebola viruses, Curr Top Microbiol Immunol, vol 235, Berlin, New York, 1999, Springer-Verlag.

14. Mohamadzadeh M, Chen L, Schmaljon AL: How Ebola and Marburg viruses battle the immune system, Nat Rev Immunol 7: 556-567, 2007.

15. Jordan I, Lipkin WI: Borna disease virus, Rev Med Virol 11: 37-57, 2001.

16. Richt JA, et al: Borna disease virus infection in animals and humans, Emerg Infect Dis 3: 343-352, 1997.

Chapter 53

Reoviridae

The *Reoviridae* consist of the orthoreoviruses, rotaviruses, orbiviruses, and coltiviruses (Table 53-1). The name reovirus was proposed in 1959 by Albert Sabin for a group of respiratory and enteric viruses that were not associated with any known disease (**respiratory, enteric, orphan**). The Reoviridae are nonenveloped viruses with **double-layered protein capsids** containing **10 to 12 segments of the double-stranded RNA (dsRNA) genomes.** These viruses are stable in detergents, over wide pH and temperature ranges, and in airborne aerosols. The orbiviruses and coltiviruses are spread by arthropods and are arboviruses. The **orthoreoviruses,** or simply reoviruses, were first isolated in the 1950s from the stools of children, and cause asymptomatic infections in humans. **Rotaviruses** cause **human infantile gastroenteritis,** and account for approximately 50% of all cases of diarrhea in children requiring hospitalization because of dehydration. Rotaviruses are even more of a problem in underdeveloped countries, where before the development of vaccines they were responsible for at least 1 million deaths each year from uncontrolled viral diarrhea in undernourished children.

Table 53-1 Reoviridae Responsible for Human Disease

Virus	Disease
Orthoreovirus*	Mild upper respiratory tract illness, gastrointestinal tract illness, biliary atresia
Orbivirus/Coltivirus	Febrile illness with headache and myalgia (zoonosis)
Rotavirus	Gastrointestinal tract illness, respiratory tract illness (?)

*Reovirus is the common name for the family Reoviridae and for the specific genus *Orthoreovirus.*

The comparisons of rotaviruses and reoviruses are as follows.

STRUCTURE

Rotaviruses and reoviruses share many structural, replicative, and pathogenic features. Reoviruses and rotaviruses have an icosahedral morphology with a double-layered capsid (60 to 80 nm in diameter) and a double-stranded segmented genome ("double:double"). The name rotavirus is derived from the Latin word *rota*, meaning "wheel," which refers to the virion's appearance in negative-stained electron micrographs (Figure 53-1).

The outer capsid is composed of structural proteins (Figure 53-2), which surround a nucleocapsid

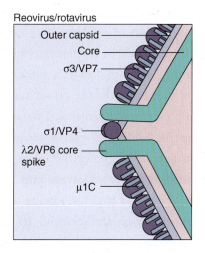

Figure 53-1 Structure of reovirus/rotavirus core and outer proteins. *σ1/VP4*, Viral attachment protein; *σ3/VP7*, major capsid component; *λ2/VP6*, major inner capsid protein; *μ1C*, minor outer capsid protein. (Modified from Sharpe AH, Fields BN: Pathogenesis of viral infections. Basic concepts derived from the reovirus model, *N Engl J Med* 312: 486-497, 1985.)

core that includes enzymes for RNA synthesis and 10 (reo) or 11 (rota) different double-stranded RNA genomic segments. For rotavirus, the outer capsid has two layers, an intermediate layer consisting of the major capsid protein (VP6) and an outer layer that contains the viral attachment protein (VP4) and glycoprotein (VP7). As for the influenza virus, reassortment of gene segments can occur and thus create hybrid viruses.

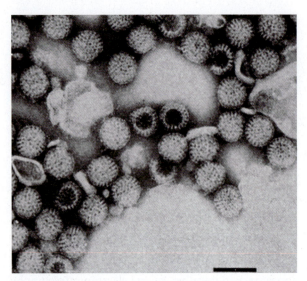

Figure 53-2 Electron micrograph of rotavirus. Bar = 100 nm. (From Fields BN, et al: *Virology*, New York, 1985, Raven.)

The genomic segments of rotaviruses and reoviruses encode structural and nonstructural proteins. Core proteins include enzymatic activities required for the transcription of mRNA. They include a 5′-methyl guanosine mRNA capping enzyme and an RNA polymerase. The σ1 protein (reo) and VP4 (rota) are located at the vertices of the capsid and extend from the surface like spike proteins. They have several functions, including viral attachment and hemagglutination, and they elicit neutralizing antibodies. VP4 is activated by protease cleavage into VP5 and VP8 proteins, exposing a structure similar to that of the fusion proteins of paramyxoviruses. Its cleavage facilitates productive entry of the virus into cells.

REPLICATION

The replication of reoviruses and rotaviruses starts with ingestion of the virus (Figure 53-3). The virion

outer capsid protects the inner nucleocapsid and core from the environment, especially the acidic environment of the gastrointestinal tract. The complete virion is then partially digested in the gastrointestinal tract and activated by protease cleavage and loss of the external capsid proteins (σ3/VP7) and cleavage of the σ1/VP4 protein to produce the intermediate/infectious subviral particle (ISVP). The σ1/VP4 protein at the vertices of the ISVP binds to sialic acid-containing glycoproteins on epithelial and other cells. Additional receptors include the β-adrenergic receptor for reovirus and integrin molecules for rotavirus. The σ1/VP4 of rotavirus also promotes the penetration of the virion into the cell. Whole virions of reovirus and rotavirus can also be taken up by receptor-mediated endocytosis.

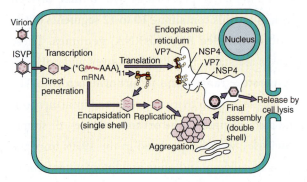

Figure 53-3 Replication of rotavirus. Rotavirus virions can be activated by protease (e.g., in the gastrointestinal tract) to produce an intermediate/infectious subviral particle (ISVP). The virion or ISVP binds, penetrates the cell, and loses its outer capsid. The inner capsid contains the enzymes for messenger ribonucleic acid (mRNA) transcription using the (±) strand as a template. Some mRNA segments are transcribed early; others are transcribed later. Enzymes in the virion cores attach 5′-methyl capped guanosine (*G) and 3′ polyadenylate sequence (poly A [AAA]) to mRNA. (+) RNA is mRNA and is also enclosed into inner capsids as a template to replicate the ± segmented genome. VP7 and NSP4 are synthesized as glycoproteins and expressed in the endoplasmic reticulum. The capsids aggregate and "dock" onto the NSP4 protein in the endoplasmic reticulum, acquiring VP7 and its outer capsid and an envelope. The virus loses the envelope and leaves the cell on cell lysis.

The ISVP releases the core into the cytoplasm, and the enzymes in the core initiate mRNA production. The dsRNA always remains in the core. Transcription of the genome occurs in two phases, early and late. In a manner similar to a negative-sense RNA virus, each of the negative-sense (−) RNA strands is used as a template by virion core enzymes, which synthesize individual mRNAs. Virus-encoded enzymes within the core add a 5'-methyl guanosine cap and a 3'-poly-adenylate tail. The 5'-methyl guanosine cap was first discovered for reovirus mRNA and then shown to occur for celluar mRNA. The mRNA then leaves the core and is translated. Later, virion proteins and posi-tive-sense (+) RNA segments associate together into corelike structures that aggregate into large cytoplas-mic inclusions. The (+) RNA segments are copied to produce (−) RNAs in the new cores, replicating the double-stranded genome. The new cores either gen-erate more (+) RNA or are assembled into virions.

The assembly processes for reovirus and rotavirus differ. In the assembly of reovirus, the outer cap-sid proteins associate with the core, and the virion leaves the cell upon cell lysis. Assembly of rotavirus resembles that of an enveloped virus, in that the rotavirus cores associate with the NSP4 viral protein on the outside of the endoplasmic reticulum (ER); on budding into the ER, they acquire its VP7 outer capsid glycoprotein. The membrane is lost in the ER, and the virus leaves the cell during cell lysis. Reovirus inhibits cellular macromolecular synthesis within 8 hours of infection.

ORTHOREOVIRUSES (MAMMALIAN REOVI-RUSES)

The orthoreoviruses are ubiquitous. The virions are very stable and have been detected in sewage and river water. The mammalian reoviruses occur in three serotypes, referred to as reovirus types 1, 2, and 3; these serotypes are based on neutralization and hemagglutination-inhibition tests. All three serotypes share a common complement-fixing antigen.

Pathogenesis and Immunity

Orthoreoviruses do not cause significant disease in humans. However, studies of reovirus disease in mice have advanced our understanding of the pathogen-esis of viral infections in humans. Depending on the reovirus strain, the virus can be neurotropic or vis-cerotropic in mice.

After ingestion and proteolytic production of the ISVP, the orthoreoviruses bind to M cells in the small intestine, which then transfer the virus to the lym-phoid tissue of Peyer patches lining the intestines. The viruses then replicate and initiate a viremia. Although the virus is cytolytic in vitro, it causes few if any symptoms before entering the circulation and producing infection at a distant site. In the mouse model, the viral attachment protein (δ1) facilitates viral spread to the mesenteric lymph nodes and determines whether the virus is neurotropic.

Epidemiology

As already mentioned, the orthoreoviruses have been found worldwide. Most people are probably infected during childhood because approximately 75% of adults have antiviral antibody.

Clinical Syndromes

Orthoreoviruses infect people of all ages, but linking specific diseases to these agents has been difficult. Most infections are thought to be asymptomatic or are so mild they go undetected. Thus far, these viruses have been linked to common coldlike, mild, upper respiratory tract illness (low-grade fever, rhi-norrhea, and pharyngitis), gastrointestinal tract dis-ease, and biliary atresia.

Laboratory Diagnosis

Human orthoreovirus infection can be detected through assay of the viral antigen or RNA in clinical material, virus isolation, or serologic assays for virus-specific antibody. Throat, nasopharyngeal, and stool specimens from patients with suspected upper respi-ratory tract or diarrheal disease are used as samples. Human orthoreoviruses can be isolated using mouse L-cell fibroblasts, primary monkey kidney cells, and HeLa cells. Serologic assays can be performed for epidemiologic purposes.

Treatment, Prevention, and Control

Orthoreovirus disease is mild and self-limited. For this reason, treatment has not been necessary, and preven-tion and control measures have not been developed.

ROTAVIRUSES

Human and animal rotaviruses are divided into sero-types, groups, and subgroups. Serotypes are distinguished primarily by the VP7 (glycoprotein, G) and VP4 (protease-sensitive protein, P) outer capsid proteins. Groups are determined primarily on the basis of the antigenicity of VP6 and the electrophoretic mobility of the genomic segments. Seven groups (A to G) of human and animal rotaviruses have been identified on the basis of the VP6 inner capsid protein. Human disease is caused by group A rotavirus and occasionally group B and C rotaviruses.

Pathogenesis and Immunity

The rotavirus can survive the acidic environment in a buffered stomach or in a stomach after a meal and is converted to the ISVP by proteases. Viral replication occurs after adsorption of the ISVP to columnar epithelial cells covering the villi of the small intestine. Approximately 8 hours after infection, cytoplasmic inclusions that contain newly synthesized proteins and RNA are seen. As many as 10^{10} viral particles per gram of stool may be released during disease.

Similar to cholera, rotavirus infection prevents the absorption of water, causing a net secretion of water and loss of ions, which together result in a watery diarrhea. The NSP4 protein of rotavirus acts in a toxin-like manner to promote calcium ion influx into enterocytes, release of neuronal activators, and a neuronal alteration in water absorption. The loss of fluids and electrolytes can lead to severe dehydration and even death if therapy does not include electrolyte replacement. Of interest, the diarrhea also promotes spread and transmission of the virus.

Immunity to infection requires the presence of antibody, primarily immunoglobulin A (IgA), in the lumen of the gut. Antibodies to the VP7 and VP4 neutralize the virus. Actively or passively acquired antibody (including antibody in colostrum and mothers' milk) can lessen the severity of disease but does not consistently prevent reinfection.

Epidemiology

Rotaviruses are ubiquitous worldwide, with 95% of children infected by 3 to 5 years of age. Rotaviruses are passed from person to person by the fecal-oral route. Maximal shedding of the virus occurs 2 to 5 days after the start of diarrhea but can occur without symptoms. The virus survives well on fomites (e.g., furniture and toys) and on hands because it can withstand drying. Outbreaks occur in preschools and day-care centers and among hospitalized infants.

Rotaviruses are one of the most common causes of serious diarrhea in young children worldwide, affecting more than 18 million infants and children and accounting for close to 1600 deaths per day resulting from dehydration. Rotavirus diarrhea is a very contagious, severe, life-threatening disease for infants in developing countries, and it occurs year-round. Several outbreaks of group B rotavirus have occurred in China because of contaminated water supplies that affected millions of people.

Clinical Syndromes

Rotavirus is a major cause of gastroenteritis. The incubation period for rotavirus diarrheal illness is estimated to be 48 hours. The major clinical findings in hospitalized patients are vomiting, diarrhea, fever, and dehydration. Neither fecal leukocytes nor blood occurs in stool for this form of diarrhea. Rotavirus gastroenteritis is a self-limited disease. However, the infection may prove fatal in infants who are malnourished and dehydrated before the infection.

Laboratory Diagnosis

Resemble to Norwalk virus, most patients have large quantities of virus in stool. Enzyme immunoassay and latex agglutination are quick, easy, and relatively inexpensive ways to detect rotavirus in stool. Viral particles in specimens can also be readily detected on electron microscopy or by immunoelectron microscopy. Reverse transcriptase polymerase chain reaction is useful to detect and distinguish the genotypes of rotavirus. Because so many people have rotavirus-specific antibody, a fourfold rise in antibody titer is necessary for the diagnosis of recent infection or active disease.

Treatment, Prevention, and Control

Rotaviruses are acquired very early in life. Their ubiquitous nature makes it difficult to limit the spread of the virus and infection. Hospitalized patients with disease must be isolated to limit spread of the infection to other susceptible patients. No specific antiviral therapy is available for a rotavirus infection. The morbidity and mortality associated with rotavirus diarrhea result from dehydration and electrolyte imbalance. The purpose of supportive therapy is to replace fluids so that blood volume and electrolyte and acid-base imbalances are corrected.

Development of a safe rotavirus vaccine was a high priority for protecting children, especially those in underdeveloped countries, from potentially fatal disease. Two new safer rotavirus vaccines have since been developed and are U.S. Food and Drug Administration-approved in the United States and elsewhere. RotaTeq consists of five reassortant bovine rotaviruses containing the VP4 or VP7 of five different human rotaviruses. The RotaRix vaccine is a single-strain attenuated human rotavirus. The vaccines are administered as young as possible, at 2, 4, and 6 months of age.

COLTIVIRUSES AND ORBIVIRUSES

The coltiviruses and orbiviruses infect vertebrates and invertebrates. The coltiviruses cause Colorado tick fever and related human disease. The orbiviruses mainly cause disease in animals, including blue tongue disease of sheep, African horse sickness, and epizootic hemorrhagic disease of deer. Colorado tick fever, an acute disease characterized by fever, headache, and severe myalgia, was originally described in the 19th century and is now believed to be one of the most common tick-borne viral diseases in the United States.

The structure and physiology of the coltiviruses and orbiviruses are similar to those of the other *Reoviridae*, with the following major exceptions:

The outer capsid of the orbiviruses has no discernible capsomeric structure, even though the inner capsid is icosahedral.

The virus causes viremia, infects erythrocyte precursors, and remains in the mature red blood cells, protected from the immune response.

The orbivirus life cycle includes vertebrates and invertebrates (insects).

Colorado tick fever viruses have 12 double-stranded RNA genomic segments, and orbiviruses have 10.

Pathogenesis

Colorado tick fever virus infects erythroid precursor cells without severely damaging them. The virus remains within the cells, even after they mature into red blood cells; this factor protects the virus from clearance. The resulting viremia can persist for weeks or months, even after cessation of symptoms. Both of these factors promote transmission of the virus to the tick vector.

Serious hemorrhagic disease can result from the infection of vascular endothelial and vascular smooth muscle cells and pericytes, thereby weakening capillary structure. The weakness leads to leakage, hemorrhage, and potentially hypotension and shock. Neuronal infection can lead to meningitis and encephalitis.

Epidemiology

Colorado tick fever occurs in western and northwestern areas of the United States and western Canada, where the wood tick *Dermacentor andersoni* is distributed (elevations of 4000 to 10,000 feet). Ticks acquire the virus by feeding on a viremic host and subsequently transmit the virus in saliva when feeding on a new host. Natural hosts of this virus constitute many mammals, including squirrels, chipmunks, rabbits, and deer..

Clinical Syndromes

Colorado tick fever virus generally causes mild or subclinical infection. The symptoms of the acute disease resemble those of dengue fever. After a 3- to 6-day incubation period, symptomatic infections start with the sudden onset of fever, chills, headache, photophobia, myalgia, arthralgia, and lethargy (Figure 53-4). Characteristics of the infection include a biphasic fever, conjunctivitis, and possibly lymph-adenopathy, hepatosplenomegaly, and a maculo-papular or petechial rash. A leukopenia involving both neutrophils and lymphocytes is an important hallmark of the disease. Children occasionally have a more severe hemorrhagic disease.

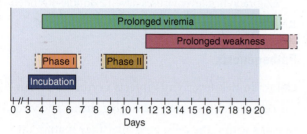

Figure 53-4   Time course of Colorado tick fever.

Laboratory Diagnosis

A diagnosis of Colorado tick fever can be established through the direct detection of viral antigens, virus isolation, or serologic tests. The best, most rapid method is detection of viral antigen on the surfaces of erythrocytes in a blood smear through the use of immunofluorescence.

Specific IgM is present for approximately 45 days after the onset of illness, and its detection is also presumptive evidence of an acute or very recent infection. Immunofluorescence is the best technique, but complement fixation, neutralization, and enzyme immunoassay are also used to detect Colorado tick fever antibody.

Treatment, Prevention, and Control

No specific treatment is available for Colorado tick fever. The disease is generally self-limited, indicating that supportive care is sufficient. The viremia is long lasting, implying that infected patients should not donate blood soon after recovery. Prevention consists of (1) avoiding tick-infested areas, (2) using protective clothing and tick repellents, and (3) removing ticks before they bite. Unlike tick-borne rickettsial disease, in which prolonged feeding is required for the bacteria to be transmitted, the coltivirus from the tick's saliva can enter the bloodstream rapidly.

SUMMARY

Orthoreoviruses

The orthoreoviruses are ubiquitous. The virions are very stable and have been detected in sewage and river water. After ingestion and proteolytic production of the ISVP, the orthoreoviruses infect M cells in the small intestine. Most infections are thought to be asymptomatic or are so mild they go undetected. Throat, nasopharyngeal, and stool specimens from patients with suspected upper respiratory tract or diarrheal disease are used as samples for the viral detection. Orthoreovirus disease is mild and self-limited.

Rotavirus

The rotavirus can survive the acidic environment in a buffered stomach or in a stomach after a meal and is converted to the ISVP by proteases. Rotaviruses are passed from person to person by the fecal-oral route. Rotaviruses are one of the most common causes of serious diarrhea in young children worldwide. Rotavirus is a major cause of gastroenteritis. The incubation period for rotavirus diarrheal illness is estimated to be 48 hours. Hospitalized patients with disease must be isolated to limit spread of the infection to other susceptible patients. No specific antiviral therapy is available for a rotavirus infection.

Coltiviruses and Orbiviruses

The coltiviruses cause Colorado tick fever in human, while orbiviruses mainly cause disease in animals. Both viruses cause viremia by infecting with erythrocyte precursors and being protected from immune responses. A leukopenia involving both neutrophils and lymphocytes is an important hallmark of the Colorado tick fever. Diagnostic detection of viral antigen on the surfaces of erythrocytes in a blood smear by immunofluorescence is often conducted. No specific treatment is available for Colorado tick fever. The disease is generally self-limited.

KEYWORDS

English	Chinese
Reoviruses	呼肠孤病毒
Arboviruses	虫媒病毒

Orthoreoviruses	正呼肠孤病毒
Rotaviruses	轮状病毒
Coltivirus	科罗提病毒
Orbivirus	环状病毒
Colorado tick fever	科罗拉多蜱传热
ISVP	感染性亚病毒颗粒

BIBLIOGRAPHY

1. Bellamy AR, Both GW: Molecular biology of rotaviruses, Adv Virol 38: 1-44, 1990.

2. Blacklow NR, Greenberg HB: Viral gastroenteritis, N Engl J Med 325: 252-264, 1991.

3. Christensen ML: Human viral gastroenteritis, Clin Microbiol Rev 2: 51-89, 1989.

4. Cohen J, Powderly WG: Infectious diseases, ed 2, St Louis, 2004, Mosby.

5. Glass RI: New hope for defeating rotavirus, Sci Am 294: 47-55, 2006.

6. Greenberg HB, Estes MK: Rotaviruses: from pathogenesis to vaccination, Gastroenterology 136: 1939-1951, 2009.

7. McDonald SM, Nelson MI, Turner PE, Patton JT: Reassortment in segmented RNA viruses: mechanisms and outcomes, Nat Rev Microbiol 14(7): 448-460, 2016.

8. Murray PR, et al: Manual of clinical microbiology, ed 9, Washington, DC, 2007, American Society for Microbiology Press.

9. Ramig RF: Systemic rotavirus infection, Expert Rev Anti Infect Ther 5: 591-612, 2007.

10. Richman DD, Whitley RJ, Hayden FG: Clinical virology, ed 3, Washington, DC, 2009, American Society for Microbiology Press.

11. Roy P: Reoviruses: entry, assembly and morphogenesis, *Curr Top Microbiol Immunol*, vol 309, Heidelberg, Germany, 2006, Springer-Verlag.

12. Sharpe AH, Fields BN: Pathogenesis of viral infections: basic concepts derived from the reovirus model, N Engl J Med 312: 486-497, 1985.

13. Strauss JM, Strauss EG: Viruses and human disease, ed 2, San Diego, 2007, Academic.

14. Tyler KL, Oldstone MBA: Reoviruses, *Curr Top Microbiol Immunol*, vol 233, Berlin, 1998, Springer-Verlag.

Togaviruses and Flaviviruses

The *Togaviridae* (togaviruses) can be classified into the following major genera (Table 54-1): *Alphavirus*, *Rubivirus*, and *Arterivirus*. No known arteriviruses cause disease in humans, so this genus is not discussed further. **Rubella** virus is the only member of the *Rubivirus* group; it is discussed separately because its disease manifestation (**German measles**) and its means of spread differ from those of the alphaviruses. The *Flaviviridae* include the flaviviruses, pestiviruses, and hepaciviruses (hepatitis C and G viruses). Hepatitis C and G are discussed in other Chapter.

Table 54-1 Togaviruses and Flaviviruses

Virus Group	Human Pathogens
Togaviruses	
Alphavirus	Arboviruses
Rubivirus	Rubella virus
Arterivirus	None
Flaviviruses	Arboviruses
Hepaciviridae	Hepatitis C virus
Pestivirus	None

ALPHAVIRUSES AND FLAVIVIRUSES

The alphaviruses and flaviviruses are classified as arboviruses because they are usually spread by arthropod vectors. These viruses have a very broad host range, including vertebrates (e.g., mammals, birds, amphibians, reptiles) and invertebrates (e.g., mosquitoes, ticks). Diseases spread by animals or with an animal reservoir are called zoonoses. Examples of pathogenic alphaviruses and flaviviruses are listed in Table 54-2.

Structure and Replication of Alphaviruses

The alphaviruses have an icosahedral capsid and a positive-sense, single-strand RNA genome that resembles mRNA. They are slightly larger than picornaviruses (45 to 75 nm in diameter) and are surrounded by an envelope (Latin toga, "cloak"). The togavirus genome encodes early and late proteins.

Alphaviruses have two or three glycoproteins that associate to form a single spike. The carboxy (COOH) terminus of the glycoproteins is anchored in the capsid, forcing the envelope to wrap tightly ("shrink-wrap") and take on the shape of the capsid. The envelope glycoproteins express unique antigenic determinants that distinguish the different viruses and also express antigenic determinants that are shared by a group, or "complex," of viruses.

The alphaviruses attach to specific receptors expressed on many different cell types from many different species (Figure 54-1) including vertebrates, such as humans, monkeys, horses, birds, reptiles, and amphibians, and invertebrates, such as mosquitoes and ticks with different tissue tropisms. The virus enters the cell by means of receptor-mediated endocytosis (see Figure 54-2). The viral envelope then fuses with the membrane of the endosome on acidification of the vesicle to deliver the capsid and genome into the cytoplasm.

Once released into the cytoplasm, the alphavirus genomes bind to ribosomes as mRNA. The alphavirus genome is translated in early and late phases. The initial two thirds of the alphavirus RNA is translated into a polyprotein, which is subsequently cleaved into four nonstructural early proteins (NSPs 1 through 4).

Table 54-2 Arboviruses

Virus	Vector	Host	Distribution	Disease
Alphaviruses				
Sindbis[*]	*Aedes* and other mosquitoes	Birds	Africa, Australia, India	Subclinical
Semliki Forest[*]	*Aedes* and other mosquitoes	Birds	East and West Africa	Subclinical
Venezuelan equine encephalitis	*Aedes*, *Culex*	Rodents, horses	North, South, and Central America	Mild systemic; severe encephalitis
Eastern equine encephalitis	*Aedes*, *Culiseta*	Birds	North and South America, Caribbean	Mild systemic; encephalitis
Western equine encephalitis	*Culex*, *Culiseta*	Birds	North and South America	Mild systemic; encephalitis
Chikungunya	*Aedes*	Humans, monkeys	Africa, Asia	Fever, arthralgia, arthritis
Flaviviruses				
Dengue[*]	*Aedes*	Humans, monkeys	Worldwide, especially tropics	Mild systemic; break-bone fever, dengue hemorrhagic fever, and dengue shock syndrome
Yellow fever[*]	*Aedes*	Humans, monkeys	Africa, South America	Hepatitis, hemorrhagic fever
Japanese encephalitis	*Culex*	Pigs, birds	Asia	Encephalitis
West Nile encephalitis	*Culex*	Birds	Africa, Europe, Central Asia, North America	Fever, encephalitis, hepatitis
St. Louis encephalitis	*Culex*	Birds	North America	Encephalitis
Russian spring-summer encephalitis	*Ixodes* and *Dermacentor* ticks	Birds	Russia	Encephalitis
Powassan encephalitis	*Ixodes* ticks	Small mammals	North America	Encephalitis

[*]Prototypical viruses.

The protease is part of the polyprotein and precedes the site of cleavage. Each of these proteins is a portion of the RNA-dependent RNA polymerase. A full-length, 42S, negative-sense RNA is synthesized as a template for replication of the genome, and more 42S positive-sense mRNA is produced. In addition, a 26S late mRNA, corresponding to one third of the genome, is transcribed from the template. The 26S RNA encodes the capsid (C) and envelope (E1 through E3) proteins. Late in the replication cycle, viral mRNA can account for as much as 90% of the mRNA in the infected cell. The abundance of late mRNAs allows the production of a large amount of the structural proteins required for packaging the virus.

The structural proteins are produced by protease cleavage of the late polyprotein that was produced from the 26S mRNA. The C protein is translated first and is cleaved from the polyprotein. A signal sequence is then made that associates the nascent polypeptide with the endoplasmic reticulum. Thereafter, envelope glycoproteins are translated, glycosylated, and cleaved from the remaining portion of the polyprotein to produce the E1, E2, and E3 glycoprotein spikes. The E3 is released from most alphavirus glycoprotein spikes. The glycoproteins are processed by the normal cellular machinery in the endoplasmic reticulum and Golgi apparatus and are also acetylated and acylated with long-chain fatty acids. Alphavirus glycoproteins are then transferred efficiently to the plasma membrane.

The C proteins associate with the genomic RNA soon after their synthesis and form an icosahedral capsid. Once this step is completed, the capsid associates with portions of the membrane expressing the viral glycoproteins. The alphavirus capsid has binding sites for the C-terminus of the glycoprotein spike, which pulls the envelope tightly around itself

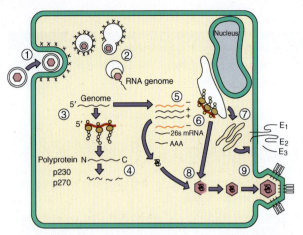

Figure 54-1   Replication of a togavirus. Semliki Forest virus. *1,* Semliki Forest virus binds to cell receptors and is internalized in a coated vesicle. *2,* On acidification of the endosome, the viral envelope fuses with the endosomal membrane to release the nucleocapsid into the cytoplasm. *3,* Ribosomes bind to the positive-sense ribonucleic acid (RNA) genome, and the p230 or p270 (full-length) early polyproteins are made. *4,* The polyproteins are cleaved to produce nonstructural proteins 1 to 4 (NSP1 to NSP4), which include a polymerase to transcribe the genome into a negative-sense RNA template. *5,* The template is used to produce a full-length 42S positive-sense mRNA genome and a late 26S mRNA for the structural proteins. *6,* The capsid (C) protein is translated first, exposing a protease cleavage site and then a signal peptide for association with the endoplasmic reticulum. *7,* The E glycoproteins are then synthesized, glycosylated, processed in the Golgi apparatus, and transferred to the plasma membrane. *8,* The capsid proteins assemble on the 42S genomic RNA and then associate with regions of cytoplasmic and plasma membranes containing the E1, E2, and E3 spike proteins. 9, Budding from the plasma membrane releases the virus. *AAA,* Polyadenylate; *mRNA,* messenger ribonucleic acid.

in a manner like shrink-wrapping (see Figures 54-1). Alphaviruses are released on budding from the plasma membrane.

Structure and Replication of Flaviviruses

The flaviviruses also have a positive-strand RNA genome, an icosahedral capsid, and an envelope but are slightly smaller than an alphavirus (40 to 65 nm in diameter). The E viral glycoprotein folds over, pairs up with another E glycoprotein, and lies flat across the surface of the virion to form an outer protein layer. Most of the flaviviruses are serologically related, and antibodies to one virus may neutralize another virus.

The attachment and penetration of the flaviviruses occur in the same way as described for the alphavi-

ruses. Flaviviruses also enter macrophages, monocytes, and other cells that have Fc receptors, when the virus is coated with antibody. The antibody actually enhances the infectivity of these viruses by providing new receptors for the virus and promoting viral uptake into these target cells.

The major differences between alphaviruses and flaviviruses are in the organization of their genomes and their mechanisms of protein synthesis. The entire flavivirus genome is translated into a single polyprotein in a manner more similar to the process for picornaviruses than for alphaviruses (Figure 54-2). As a result, there is no temporal distinction in the translation of the different viral proteins. The polyprotein produced from the yellow fever genome contains five nonstructural proteins, including a protease and components of the RNA-dependent RNA polymerase, plus the capsid and envelope structural proteins.

Unlike in the alphavirus genome, the structural genes are at the 5'-end of the flavivirus genome. As a result, the portions of the polyprotein containing the structural (not the catalytic) proteins are synthesized first and with the greatest efficiency that may contribute to the lag before detection of their replication.

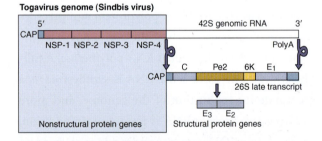

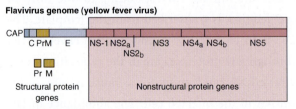

Figure 54-2   Comparison of the togavirus (alphavirus) and flavivirus genomes. *Alphavirus:* The enzymatic activities are translated from the 5'-end of the input genome, promoting their early rapid translation. The structural proteins are translated later from a smaller messenger ribonucleic acid (mRNA) transcribed from the genomic template. *Flavivirus:* The genes for the structural proteins of the flaviviruses are at the 5'-end of the genome/mRNA, and only one species of polyprotein is made, which represents the entire genome. *PolyA,* Polyadenylate.

Unlike the togaviruses, the flaviviruses acquire their envelope by budding into the endoplasmic reticulum rather than at the cell surface. The virus is then released by exocytosis or cell lysis mechanisms. This route is less efficient, and the virus may remain cell-associated.

Pathogenesis and Immunity

The arboviruses can cause lytic or persistent infections of both vertebrate and invertebrate hosts. Infections of invertebrates are usually persistent, with continued virus production.

The large amount of viral RNA produced on the replication and transcription of the genome blocks cellular mRNA from binding to ribosomes. Increased permeability of the target cell membrane and changes in ion concentrations can alter enzyme activities and favor the translation of viral mRNA over cellular mRNA. The displacement of cellular mRNA from the protein synthesis machinery prevents rebuilding and maintenance of the cell and is a major cause of the death of the virus-infected cell.

Female mosquitoes acquire the alphaviruses and flaviviruses by taking a blood meal from a viremic vertebrate host. *A sufficient viremia must be maintained in the vertebrate host to allow acquisition of the virus by the mosquito.* The virus then infects the epithelial cells of the midgut of the mosquito, spreads through the basal lamina of the midgut to the circulation, and infects the salivary glands. The virus sets up a persistent infection and replicates to high titers in these cells. The salivary glands can then release virus into the saliva. Not all arthropod species support this type of infection, however. For example, the normal vector for the WEEV is the *Culex tarsalis* mosquito, but certain strains of virus are limited to the midgut of this mosquito, cannot infect its salivary glands, and therefore cannot be transmitted to humans.

On biting a host, the female mosquito regurgitates virus-containing saliva into the victim's bloodstream. The virus then circulates freely in the host's plasma and comes into contact with susceptible target cells, such as the endothelial cells of the capillaries, monocytes, dendritic cells, and macrophages.

The nature of alphavirus and flavivirus disease is determined primarily by (1) the specific tissue tropisms of the individual virus type, (2) the concentration of infecting virus, and (3) individual responses to the infection. These viruses are associated with mild systemic disease, encephalitis, arthrogenic disease, or hemorrhagic disease.

The initial viremia produces systemic symptoms, such as fever, chills, headaches, backaches, and other flulike symptoms, within 3 to 7 days of infection. The viremia is considered a mild systemic disease, and most viral infections do not progress beyond this point. A secondary viremia can produce sufficient virus to infect target organs, such as the brain, liver, skin, and vasculature, depending on the tissue tropism of the virus (Figure 54-3).

The primary target cells of the flaviviruses are of the monocyte-macrophage lineage that expresses Fc receptors for antibody and release cytokines on challenge. Flavivirus infection is enhanced 200- to 1000-fold by nonneutralizing antiviral antibody that promotes binding of the virus to the Fc receptors and its uptake into the cell.

Immune Response

Both humoral immunity and cellular immunity are elicited and are important to the control of primary infection and the prevention of future infections with the alphaviruses and flaviviruses.

Replication of the alphaviruses and flaviviruses produces a double-stranded RNA replicative intermediate that is a good inducer of interferon-α and interferon-β. The interferon is released into the bloodstream and limits replication of the virus; it also stimulates innate and immune responses but in doing so causes the rapid onset of the flulike symptoms characteristic of mild systemic disease.

Circulating IgM is produced within 6 days of infection, followed by the production of IgG. Due to the common antigens expressed on all viruses in the family, immunity to one flavivirus can provide some protection against infection with other flaviviruses. Cell-mediated immunity is also important in controlling the primary infection.

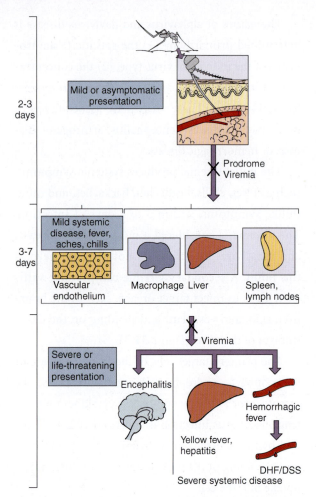

Figure 54-3 Disease syndromes of the alphaviruses and flaviviruses. Primary viremia may be associated with mild systemic disease. Most infections are limited to this. If sufficient virus is produced during the secondary viremia to escape innate and immune protection and to reach critical target tissues, severe systemic disease or encephalitis may result. If antibody is present *(X)*, viremia is blocked. For dengue virus, rechallenge with another strain can result in severe dengue hemorrhagic fever *(DHF)*, which can cause dengue shock syndrome *(DSS)* because of the loss of fluids from the vasculature.

Inflammation resulting from the cell-mediated immune response can destroy tissues and significantly contribute to the pathogenesis of encephalitis. Hypersensitivity reactions initiated by the formation of immune complexes with virions and viral antigens, and the activation of complement, can also occur. They can weaken the vasculature and cause it to rupture, leading to hemorrhagic symptoms. A nonneutralizing antibody can enhance the uptake of flaviviruses into macrophages and other cells that express Fc receptors. Such an antibody can be generated to a related strain of virus in which the neutral-izing epitope is not expressed or is different. Immune responses to a related strain of dengue virus that do not prevent infection can promote immunopathogenesis, leading to dengue hemorrhagic fever or dengue shock syndrome.

Epidemiology

Alphaviruses and most flaviviruses are prototypical arboviruses. To be an arbovirus, the virus must be able to (1) infect both vertebrates and invertebrates, (2) initiate a sufficient viremia in a vertebrate host for a sufficient time to allow acquisition of the virus by the invertebrate vector, and (3) initiate a persistent productive infection of the salivary gland of the invertebrate to provide virus for the infection of other host animals. Humans are usually "dead-end" hosts, in that they cannot spread the virus back to the vector because they do not maintain a persistent viremia. *If the virus is not in the blood, the mosquito cannot acquire it.* A full cycle of infection occurs when the virus is transmitted by the arthropod vector and amplified in a susceptible, immunologically naïve host (reservoir) that allows the reinfection of other arthropods. The vectors, natural hosts, and geographic distribution of representative alphaviruses and flaviviruses are listed in Table 54-2.

These viruses are usually restricted to a specific arthropod vector, its vertebrate host, and their ecologic niche. The most common vector is the mosquito, but ticks and sandflies spread some arboviruses.

Birds and small mammals are the usual reservoir hosts for the alphaviruses and flaviviruses, but reptiles and amphibians can also act as hosts. A large population of viremic animals can develop in these species to continue the infection cycle of the virus. WNV establishes a sufficient viremia in humans to be a risk factor for transmission through blood transfusions. Documentation of two such cases has led to screening blood donors for WNV and rejecting donors who have fever and headache during the week of blood donation.

Arbovirus diseases occur during the summer months and rainy seasons, when the arthropods breed, and the arboviruses are cycled among a host reservoir (birds), an arthropod (e.g., mosquitoes), and human hosts. In the winter, the virus may either (1) persist in arthropod larvae or eggs or in reptiles or amphibians that remain in the locale or (2) migrate with the birds and then return during the summer.

When humans travel into the ecologic niche of the mosquito vector, they risk being infected by the virus. Pools of standing water, drainage ditches, and trash dumps in cities can also provide breeding grounds for mosquitoes such as *Aedes aegypti*, the vector for yellow fever, dengue, and chikungunya. An increase in the population of these mosquitoes therefore puts the human population at risk for infection. Health departments in many areas monitor birds and mosquitoes caught in traps for arboviruses and initiate control measures, such as insecticide spraying, when necessary.

Urban outbreaks of arbovirus infections occur when the reservoirs for the virus are humans or urban animals. Humans can be reservoir hosts for yellow fever, dengue, and chikungunya viruses. These viruses are maintained by *Aedes* mosquitoes in a sylvatic or jungle cycle, in which monkeys are the natural host, and also in an urban cycle, in which humans are the host. *A. aegypti*, a vector for each of these viruses, is a household mosquito. It breeds in pools of water, open sewers, and other accumulations of water in cities.

Clinical Syndromes

More humans are infected with alphaviruses and flaviviruses than show significant, characteristic symptoms. The incidence of arbovirus disease is sporadic. Alphavirus infections are usually asymptomatic or cause low-grade disease, such as flulike symptoms (chills, fever, rash, and aches) that correlate with systemic infection during the initial viremia. EEEV, WEEV, and Venezuelan equine encephalitis virus (VEEV) infections can progress to encephalitis in humans. The equine encephalitis viruses are usually more of a problem to livestock than to humans. An affected human may experience fever, headache, and decreased consciousness 3 to 10 days after infection. Unlike herpes simplex virus encephalitis, the disease generally resolves without sequelae, but there is the possibility of paralysis, mental disability, seizures, and death.

Most flavivirus infections are relatively benign, but serious aseptic meningitis and encephalitic or hemorrhagic disease can occur. The encephalitis viruses include St. Louis, West Nile, Japanese, Murray Valley, and Russian spring-summer viruses. Symptoms and outcomes are similar to those of the togavirus encephalitides.

The hemorrhagic viruses are dengue and yellow fever viruses. Dengue virus is a major worldwide problem, with up to 100 million cases of dengue fever and 300,000 cases of dengue hemorrhagic fever (DHF) occurring per year. The virus and its vector are present in central and northern South America, and cases have occurred in Puerto Rico, Texas, and Florida. The incidence of the more serious DHF has quadrupled since 1985. Dengue fever is also known as break-bone fever; the symptoms and signs consist of high fever, headache, rash, and back and bone pain that last 6 to 7 days. On rechallenge with another of the four related strains, dengue can also cause DHF and dengue shock syndrome (DSS). Nonneutralizing antibody promotes uptake of the virus into macrophages, which causes memory T cells to become activated, release cytokines, and initiate inflammatory reactions. These reactions and the virus result in weakening and rupture of the vasculature, internal bleeding, and loss of plasma, leading to shock symptoms and internal bleeding. In 1981 in Cuba, dengue-2 virus infected a population previously exposed to dengue-1 virus between 1977 and 1980, leading to an epidemic of more than 100,000 cases of DHF/DSS and 168 deaths.

Yellow fever infections are characterized by severe systemic disease, with degeneration of the liver, kidney, and heart, as well as hemorrhage. Liver involvement causes the jaundice from which the disease gets its name, but massive gastrointestinal hemorrhages ("black vomit") may also occur. The mortality rate associated with yellow fever during epidemics is as high as 50%.

Laboratory Diagnosis

The alphaviruses and flaviviruses can be grown in both vertebrate and mosquito cell lines, but most are difficult to isolate. Infection can be detected through the use of cytopathologic studies, immunofluorescence, and the hemadsorption of avian erythrocytes. Detection and characterization can be performed by RT-PCR testing of genomic RNA or viral mRNA in blood or other samples. Monoclonal antibodies to the individual viruses have become a useful tool for distinguishing the individual species and strains of viruses. The presence of specific IgM or a fourfold increase in titer between acute and convalescent sera is used to indicate a recent infection. The serologic cross-reactivity among viruses limits distinction of the actual viral species in many cases.

Treatment, Prevention, and Control

No treatments exist for arbovirus diseases, other than supportive care. *The easiest means of preventing the spread of any arbovirus is elimination of its vector and breeding grounds.* After 1900, when Walter Reed and his colleagues discovered that yellow fever was spread by *A. aegypti*, the number of cases was reduced from 1400 to none within 2 years, purely through control of the mosquito population such as periodical spray.

A live vaccine against yellow fever virus and killed vaccines against EEEV, WEEV, Japanese encephalitis virus, and Russian spring-summer encephalitis virus are available. A live Japanese encephalitis virus vaccine is used in China. These vaccines are meant for people working with the virus or at risk for contact.

The yellow fever vaccine is prepared from the 17D strain isolated from a patient in 1927 and grown for long periods in monkeys, mosquitoes, embryonic tissue culture, and embryonated eggs. The vaccine is administered intradermally and elicits lifelong immunity to yellow fever and possibly other cross-reacting flaviviruses.

RUBELLA VIRUS

Rubella virus has the same structural properties and mode of replication as the other togaviruses. However, unlike the other togaviruses, rubella is a respiratory virus and does not cause readily detectable cytopathologic effects.

Rubella is one of the five classic childhood exanthems, along with measles, roseola, fifth disease, and chickenpox. Rubella, meaning "little red" in Latin, was first distinguished from measles and other exanthems by German physicians. Maternal rubella infection has been correlated with several other severe congenital defects such as congenital cataracts. This finding prompted the development of a unique program to vaccinate children to prevent infection of pregnant women and neonates.

Pathogenesis and Immunity

Rubella virus is not cytolytic but does have limited cytopathologic effects in certain cell lines, such as Vero and RK13. The replication of rubella prevents (in a process known as heterologous interference) the replication of superinfecting picornaviruses. This property allowed the first isolations of rubella virus in 1962.

Rubella infects the upper respiratory tract and then spreads to local lymph nodes, which coincides with a period of lymphadenopathy (Figure 54-4). This stage is followed by establishment of viremia, which spreads the virus throughout the body. Infection of other tissues and the characteristic mild rash occur. The prodromal period lasts approximately 2 weeks (Figure 54-5). The infected person can shed virus in respiratory droplets during the prodromal period and for as long as 2 weeks after the onset of the rash.

Immune Response

Antibody is generated after the viremia, and its appearance correlates with the appearance of the rash. Only one serotype of rubella exists, and natural infection produces lifelong protective immunity. Most important, serum antibody in a pregnant woman prevents spread of the virus to the fetus. *Immune complexes most likely cause the rash and arthralgia associated with rubella infection.*

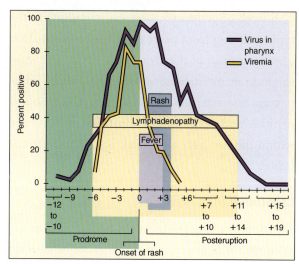

Figure 54-5 Time course of rubella disease. Rubella production in the pharynx precedes the appearance of symptoms and continues throughout the course of the disease. The onset of lymphadenopathy coincides with the viremia. Fever and rash occur later. The person is infectious as long as the virus is produced in the pharynx. (Modified from Plotkin SA: Rubella vaccine. In Plotkin SA, Mortimer EA, editors: *Vaccines*, Philadelphia, 1988, WB Saunders.)

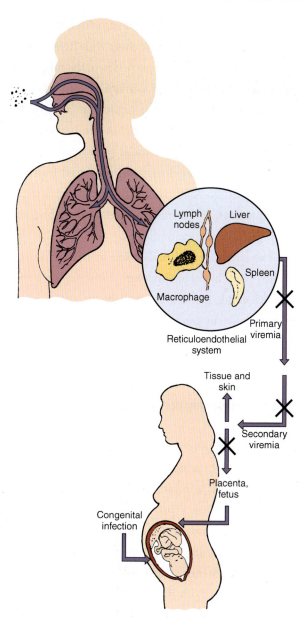

Figure 54-4 Spread of rubella virus within the host. Rubella enters and infects the nasopharynx and lung and then spreads to the lymph nodes and monocyte-macrophage system. The resulting viremia spreads the virus to other tissues and the skin. Circulating antibody can block the transfer of virus at the indicated points *(X)*. In an immunologically deficient pregnant woman, the virus can infect the placenta and spread to the fetus.

Congenital Infection

Rubella infection in a pregnant woman can result in serious congenital abnormalities in the child. If the mother does not have antibody, the virus can replicate in the placenta and spread to the fetal blood supply and throughout the fetus. Rubella can replicate in most tissues of the fetus. The nature of the disorder is determined by (1) the tissue affected and (2) the stage of development disrupted.

Epidemiology

Humans are the only host for rubella. The virus is spread in respiratory secretions and is generally acquired during childhood. Spread of virus, before or in the absence of symptoms, and crowded conditions, such as those in day-care centers, promote contagion.

Clinical Syndromes

Rubella disease is normally benign in children. After a 14- to 21-day incubation period, the symptoms in children consist of a 3-day maculopapular or macular rash and swollen glands. Infection in adults, however, can be more severe and include problems such as bone and joint pain (arthralgia and arthritis) and (rarely) thrombocytopenia or postinfectious encephalopathy. Immunopathologic effects resulting from cell-mediated immunity and hypersensitivity reactions are a major cause of the more severe forms of rubella in adults.

Congenital disease is the most serious outcome of rubella infection. The fetus is at major risk until the

20th week of pregnancy. Maternal immunity to the virus resulting from prior exposure or vaccination prevents spread of the virus to the fetus. The most common manifestations of congenital rubella infection are cataracts, mental retardation, cardiac abnormalities, and deafness. The mortality in utero and within the first year after birth is high for affected babies.

Laboratory Diagnosis

Isolation of the rubella virus is difficult and rarely attempted. The presence of the virus can be detected by RT-PCR detection of viral RNA. The diagnosis is usually confirmed by the presence of antirubella-specific IgM. A fourfold increase in specific IgG antibody titer between acute and convalescent sera is also used to indicate a recent infection. Antibodies to rubella are assayed early in pregnancy to determine the immune status of the woman.

When isolation of the virus is necessary, the virus is usually obtained from urine and is detected as interference with replication of echovirus 11 in primary African green monkey kidney cell cultures.

Treatment, Prevention, and Control

No treatment is available for rubella. The best means of preventing rubella is vaccination with the live cold-adapted RA27/3 vaccine strain of virus. The live rubella vaccine is usually administered with the measles and mumps vaccines (MMR vaccine) at 24 months of age. The triple vaccine is included routinely in well-baby care. Vaccination promotes both humoral and cellular immunity. Because only one serotype for rubella exists, and humans are the only reservoir, vaccination of a large proportion of the population can significantly reduce the likelihood of exposure to the virus.

SUMMARY

The alphaviruses are enveloped, single-stranded positive RNA viruses. Alphavirus enters the cell by receptor-mediated endocytosis. The initial two thirds of the viral genome are translated into an early polyprotein, which is subsequently cleaved into four nonstructural proteins (NSPs 1 through 4) with RNA dependent RNA polymerase property. Then, the full length of minus stranded RNA is synthesized and served as a template for viral genome replication and for the subsequent positive-sense mRNA production. The structural proteins are produced by protease cleavage of the late polyprotein that was produced from the 26S late mRNA. After packaged with the viral structural proteins, alphaviruses are released on budding from the plasma membrane.

The structure and replication of flaviviruses are similar with that of alphaviruses. Unlike in the alphavirus genome, the structural genes are at the 5′-end of the flavivirus genome. The virus is then released by exocytosis or cell lysis mechanisms. The arboviruses can cause lytic or persistent infections of both vertebrate and invertebrate hosts. Infections of invertebrates are usually persistent, with continued virus production.

Female mosquitoes acquire the alphaviruses and flaviviruses by taking a blood meal from a viremic vertebrate host. On biting a host, the female mosquito regurgitates virus-containing saliva into the victim's bloodstream. The infections by alphavirus and flavivirus are associated with mild systemic disease, encephalitis, arthrogenic disease, or hemorrhagic disease. Both humoral immunity and cellular immunity are elicited and are important to the control of primary infection and the prevention of future infections with the alphaviruses and flaviviruses. More humans are infected with alphaviruses and flaviviruses than show significant, characteristic symptoms. No treatments exist for arbovirus diseases, while various vaccines are available for the most of flaviviruses.

Rubella virus has the same structural properties and mode of replication as the other togaviruses. Rubella infects the upper respiratory tract and then spreads to local lymph nodes that is followed by viremia. The infected person can shed virus in respiratory droplets during the prodromal period and for as long as 2 weeks after the onset of the rash. Rubella infection in a pregnant woman can result in serious congenital abnormalities in the child. Humans are the only host for rubella. The virus is spread in respiratory secretions and is generally acquired during childhood. Immunopathologic effects resulting from cell-mediated immunity and hypersensitivity reactions are a major cause of the more severe forms of rubella in adults. The best means of preventing rubella is vaccination with the live vaccine strain of virus.

KEYWORDS

English	Chinese
Togaviruses	披膜病毒
Flaviviruses	黄病毒
Rubella	风疹
Rubivirus	风疹病毒
Alphaviruses	甲病毒属
Arboviruses	虫媒病毒
Encephalitis	脑炎

BIBLIOGRAPHY

1. Chambers TJ, Monath TP: The flaviviruses: detection, diagnosis, and vaccine development, vol 61; The flaviviruses: pathogenesis and immunity, vol 60. In Adv Virus Res, San Diego, 2003, Elsevier Academic.

2. Fernandez-Garcia M-D, et al: Pathogenesis of flavivirus infections: using and abusing the host cell, Cell Host Microbe 5: 318-328, 2009.

3. Gelfand MS: West Nile virus infection. What you need to know about this emerging threat, Postgrad Med 114: 31-38, 2003.

4. Go YY, Balasuriya UB, Lee CK: Zoonotic encephalitides caused by arboviruses: transmission and epidemiology of alphaviruses andflaviviruses, Clin Exp Vaccine Res3(1): 58-77, 2014.

5. Gould EA, Solomon T: Pathogenic flaviviruses, Lancet 371: 500-509, 2008.

6. Hahn CS, et al: Flavivirus genome organization, expression, and replication, Annu Rev Microbiol 44: 663-688, 1990.

7. Koblet H: The "merry-go-round": alphaviruses between vertebrate and invertebrate cells, Adv Virus Res 38: 343-403, 1990.

8. Kuhn RJ, et al: Structure of dengue virus: implications for flavivirus organization, maturation, and fusion, Cell 108: 717-725, 2002.

9. Mackenzie JS, Barrett ADT, Deubel V: Japanese encephalitis and West Nile viruses, Curr Top Microbiol Immunol, vol 267, Berlin, 2002, Springer-Verlag.

10. Monath TP: Yellow fever vaccine. In Plotkin SA, Orenstein WA, editors: Vaccines, ed 4, Philadelphia, 2004, WB Saunders.

11. Mukhopadhyay S, et al: Structure of West Nile virus, Science 302: 248, 2003.

12. Nash D, et al: The outbreak of West Nile virus infection in the New York City area in 1999, N Engl J Med 344: 1807-1814, 2001.

13. Strauss JM, Strauss EG: Viruses and human disease, ed 2, San Diego, 2007, Academic.

14. Tsai TF: Arboviral infections in the United States, Infect Dis Clin North Am 5: 73-102, 1991.

Bunyaviridae and Arenaviridae

Chapter **55**

The Bunyaviridae and Arenaviridae share several similarities. The viruses of these families are negative-strand ribonucleic acid (RNA)-enveloped viruses with similar modes of replication. Both are zoonoses; most of the Bunyaviridae are arboviruses, but the Arenaviridae are not. Many of the viruses from these families cause encephalitis or hemorrhagic disease.

BUNYAVIRIDAE

The Bunyaviridae constitute a "supergroup" of at least 200 enveloped, segmented, negative-strand RNA viruses. The supergroup of mammalian viruses is further broken down into genera on the basis of structural and biochemical features: *Bunyavirus*, *Phlebovirus*, *Nairovirus*, and *Hantavirus* (Table 55-1). Most of the Bunyaviridae are arboviruses (*arthropod-borne*) that are spread by mosquitoes, ticks, or flies and are endemic to the environment of the vector. The hantaviruses are the exception; they are carried by rodents. New viruses are still being discovered, including the tick-borne severe fever with thrombocytopenia syndrome virus (SFTSV) in 2011 in China.

Structure

The bunyaviruses are roughly spheric particles 90 to 120 nm in diameter. The envelope of the virus contains two glycoproteins (G1 and G2) and encloses three unique negative-strand RNAs, the large (L), medium (M), and small (S) RNAs that are associated

Table 55-1   Notable Bunyaviridae Genera*

Genus	Members	Insect Vector	Pathologic Conditions	Vertebrate Hosts
Bunyavirus	Bunyamwera virus, California encephalitis virus, La Crosse virus, Oropouche virus; 150 members	Mosquito	Febrile illness, encephalitis, rash	Rodents, small mammals, primates, marsupials, birds
Phlebovirus	Rift Valley fever virus, sandfly fever virus; 36 members	Fly	Sandfly fever, hemorrhagic fever, encephalitis, conjunctivitis, myositis	Sheep, cattle, domestic animals
Nairovirus	Crimean-Congo hemorrhagic fever virus; 6 members	Tick	Hemorrhagic fever	Hares, cattle, goats, seabirds
Uukuvirus	Uukuniemi virus; 7 members	Tick	—	Birds
Hantavirus	Hantaan virus	None	Hemorrhagic fever with renal syndrome, adult respiratory distress syndrome	Rodents
	Sin Nombre	None	Hantavirus pulmonary syndrome, shock, pulmonary edema	Deer mouse

*Additional viruses possess several common properties with Bunyaviridae but are as yet unclassified.

with protein to form nucleocapsids. The genome segments for the La Crosse and related California encephalitis viruses have complementary ends and form circles. The nucleocapsids include the RNA-dependent RNA polymerase (L protein) and two nonstructural proteins (NS$_s$, NS$_m$) (Figure 55-1). Unlike other negative-strand RNA viruses, the Bunyaviridae do not have a matrix protein.

Replication

The Bunyaviridae replicate in the same way as other enveloped, negative-strand RNA viruses. For most Bunyaviridae, the G1 glycoprotein interacts with β integrins on the cell surface, and the virus is internalized by endocytosis. After fusion of the envelope with endosomal membranes on acidification of the vesicle, the nucleocapsid is released into the cytoplasm, and mRNA and protein synthesis begin. Like influenza, the bunyaviruses steal the 5′-capped portion of mRNAs to prime the synthesis of viral mRNAs; but unlike influenza, this occurs in the cytoplasm.

The M strand encodes the NS$_m$ nonstructural protein and the G1 (viral attachment) and G2 proteins, and the L strand encodes the L protein (polymerase). The S strand of RNA encodes two nonstructural proteins, N and NS$_s$. For the *Phlebovirus* group, the S strand is ambisense, such that one protein is translated from the (+) strand and the other from the (−) RNA template.

Replication of the genome by the L protein also provides new templates for transcription, thereby increasing the rate of mRNA synthesis. The glycoproteins are then synthesized and glycosylated in the endoplasmic reticulum, after which they are transferred to the Golgi apparatus but not translocated to the plasma membrane. Virions are assembled by budding into the Golgi apparatus and are released by cell lysis or exocytosis.

Pathogenesis

Most of the Bunyaviridae are arboviruses and possess many of the same pathogenic mechanisms as the togaviruses and flaviviruses. For example, the viruses are spread by an arthropod vector and are injected into the blood to initiate a viremia. Progression past this stage to secondary viremia and further dissemination of the virus can deliver the virus to target sites typically involved in that particular viral disease, such as the central nervous system, liver, kidney, and vascular endothelium.

Many Bunyaviridae cause neuronal and glial damage and cerebral edema, leading to encephalitis. Like togaviruses, flaviviruses, and arenaviruses, the bunyaviruses are good inducers of type 1 interferons. Bunyavirus disease is due to a combination of immune and viral pathogenesis.

Unlike the other bunyaviruses, rodents are the reservoir and vector for hantaviruses, and humans acquire the virus by breathing aerosols contaminated with infected urine. The virus initiates infection and

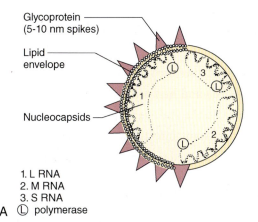

Glycoprotein
(5-10 nm spikes)

Lipid
envelope

Nucleocapsids

1. L RNA
2. M RNA
3. S RNA
A   Ⓛ polymerase

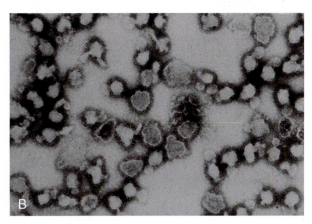

Figure 55-1   A, Model of the bunyavirus particle. **B,** Electron micrograph of La Crosse variant of bunyavirus. Note the spike proteins at the surface of the virion envelope. *RNA,* Ribonucleic acid. (**A,** Modified from Fraenkel-Conrat H, Wagner RR: *Comprehensive virology,* vol 14, New York, 1979, Plenum. **B,** Courtesy of Centers for Disease Control and Prevention, Atlanta.)

remains in the lung, where it causes hemorrhagic tissue destruction and lethal pulmonary disease.

Epidemiology

Most bunyaviruses are transmitted by infected mosquitoes, ticks, or *Phlebotomus* flies to rodents, birds, and larger animals. The animals then become the reservoirs for the virus, thereby continuing the cycle of infection. Humans are infected when they enter the environment of the insect vector (Figure 55-2) but are usually dead-end hosts. Transmission occurs during the summer, but unlike many other arboviruses, many of the Bunyaviridae can survive a winter in the mosquito eggs and remain in a locale.

The hantaviruses do not have an arthropod vector but are maintained in a rodent species specific for each virus. Humans are infected by close contact with rodents or through the inhalation of aerosolized rodent urine.

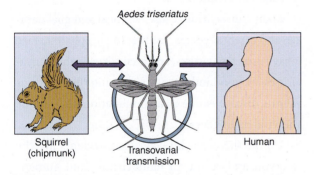

Figure 55-2   Transmission of La Crosse (California) encephalitis virus.

Clinical Syndromes

Bunyaviridae, which are mosquito-borne viruses, usually cause a nonspecific febrile, flulike, viremia-related illness (see Table 55-1) that is indistinguishable from illnesses caused by other viruses. The incubation period for these illnesses is approximately 48 hours, and the fevers typically last 3 days. Most patients with infections, even those infected by agents known to cause severe disease (e.g., Rift Valley fever virus, La Crosse virus), have mild illness.

Laboratory Diagnosis

Detection of viral RNA by RT-PCR has become the accepted method for detecting and identifying bunyaviruses. The Sin Nombre and Convict Creek hantaviruses were initially identified with the RT-PCR test, using primers with characteristic hantavirus sequences.

Serologic tests are generally performed to confirm a diagnosis of bunyavirus infection. Virus neutralization assays can be used to identify the virus. Assays specific for IgM are useful in the documentation of acute infection. Seroconversion or a fourfold increase in the titer of the IgG antibody is used to document recent infection, but cross-reactions within viral genera are common. Enzyme-linked immunosorbent assay (ELISA) may detect antigen in clinical specimens from patients with an intense viremia (e.g., Rift Valley fever, hemorrhagic fever with renal syndrome, Crimean-Congo hemorrhagic fever) or from mosquitoes.

Treatment, Prevention, and Control

No specific therapy for infections of the Bunyaviridae is available. Human disease is prevented by interruption of the contact between humans and the vector, whether arthropod or mammal. Arthropod vectors are controlled by (1) eliminating the growth conditions for the vector, (2) spraying with insecticide, (3) installing netting or screening at windows and doors, (4) wearing protective clothing, and (5) controlling the tick infestation of animals. Rodent control minimizes the transmission of many viruses, especially hantaviruses.

ARENAVIRUSES

The arenaviruses include lymphocytic choriomeningitis (LCM) and hemorrhagic fever viruses, such as the Lassa, Junin, and Machupo viruses. These viruses cause persistent infections in specific rodents and can be transmitted to humans as zoonoses.

Structure and Replication

Arenaviruses are seen in electron micrographs as pleomorphic, enveloped viruses (diameter, 120 nm) that have a sandy appearance (the name comes from the Greek word arenosa, meaning "sandy") because of the ribosomes in the virion. Although functional, the ribosomes do not seem to serve a purpose. Virions contain a nucleocapsid with two single-stranded RNA circles (S, 3400 nucleotides; L, 7200 nucleotides) and a transcriptase. The L strand is a negative-sense RNA and encodes the polymerase. The S strand encodes the nucleoprotein (N protein), and the glycoproteins but is ambisense. Whereas the mRNA for the N protein is transcribed directly from the ambisense S strand, the mRNA for the glycoprotein is transcribed from a full-length template of the S strand. Like togaviruses, the glycoproteins are produced as late proteins after genome replication. Arenaviruses replicate in the cytoplasm and acquire their envelope by budding from the host cell plasma membrane.

Arenaviruses readily cause persistent infections. This may result from inefficient transcription of the glycoprotein genes and thus poor virion assembly.

Pathogenesis

Arenaviruses are able to infect macrophages, induce cytokine and interferon release and promote cell and vascular damage. T-cell-induced immunopathologic effects significantly exacerbate tissue destruction. Persistent infection of rodents results from neonatal infection and the induction of immune tolerance. The incubation period for arenavirus infections averages 10 to 14 days.

Epidemiology

Most arenaviruses, except for the virus that causes LCM, are found in the tropics of Africa and South America. The arenaviruses, like the hantaviruses, infect specific rodents and are endemic to the rodents' habitats. Chronic asymptomatic infection is common in these animals and leads to a chronic viremia and long-term viral shedding in saliva, urine, and feces. Humans may become infected through the inhalation of aerosols, the consumption of contaminated food, or contact with fomites. Bites are not a usual mechanism of spread.

The Lassa fever virus is spread from human to human through contact with infected secretions or body fluids, but the viruses that cause LCM or other hemorrhagic fevers are rarely, if ever, spread in this way.

Clinical Syndromes

Lymphocytic Choriomeningitis

The name of this virus, lymphocytic choriomeningitis, suggests that meningitis is a typical clinical event, but actually, LCM causes a febrile illness with flulike myalgia more often than meningeal illness. Only about 10% of infected persons exhibit clinical evidence of a central nervous system infection. The meningeal illness, if it occurs, will start 10 days after the initial phase of illness, with full recovery. Perivascular mononuclear infiltrates may be seen in neurons of all sections of the brain and in the meninges of an affected patient.

Laboratory Diagnosis

An arenavirus infection is usually diagnosed on the basis of serologic and genomic (RT-PCR) findings. These viruses are too dangerous for isolation. Throat specimens can yield arenaviruses; urine is a source for the Lassa fever virus but not for the LCM virus. The risk of infection is substantial for laboratory workers handling body fluids. Therefore, if the diagnosis is suspected, laboratory personnel should be so warned and the specimens processed only in facilities that specialize in the isolation of contagious pathogens (level 3 for LCM and level 4 for Lassa fever and other arenaviruses).

Treatment, Prevention, and Control

The antiviral drug ribavirin has limited activity against arenaviruses and can be used to treat Lassa fever. However, supportive therapy is usually all that is available for patients with arenavirus infections.

These rodent-borne infections can be prevented by limiting contact with the vector. The incidence of laboratory-acquired cases can be reduced if samples submitted for arenavirus isolation are processed in at least level 3 or 4 biosafety facilities and not in the usual clinical virology laboratory.

SUMMARY

Bunyaviridae

The Bunyaviridae are enveloped negative-strand RNA viruses. Replication of the genome by the L protein also provides new templates for transcription, thereby increasing the rate of mRNA synthesis. Virions are assembled by budding into the Golgi apparatus and are released by cell lysis or exocytosis. Many Bunyaviridae cause neuronal and glial damage and cerebral edema, leading to encephalitis. Most bunyaviruses are transmitted by infected mosquitoes, ticks, or *Phlebotomus* flies to rodents, birds, and larger animals. The animals then become the reservoirs for the virus, thereby continuing the cycle of infection. Humans are infected when they enter the environment of the insect vector but are usually dead-end hosts.

Arenaviruses

Arenaviruses have a sandy appearance because of the ribosomes in the virion. Virions contain a nucleocapsid with two single-stranded RNA circles (S and L) and a transcriptase. L strand encodes polymerase, while S strand is an ambisense for both N and G proteins. Arenaviruses replicate in the cytoplasm and acquire their envelope by budding from the host cell plasma membrane. The incubation period for arenavirus infections averages 10 to 14 days. Chronic asymptomatic infection is common in these animals and leads to a chronic viremia and long-term viral shedding in saliva, urine, and feces. Humans may become infected through the inhalation of aerosols, the consumption of contaminated food, or contact with fomites.

KEYWORDS

English	Chinese
Bunyaviridae	布尼亚病毒科
Arenaviridae	沙粒病毒科
lymphocytic choriomeningitis	淋巴细胞性脉络丛脑膜炎
Machupo viruses	马丘波病毒
Lassa fever	拉沙热
Ribavirin	利巴韦林
Hantaviruses	汉坦病毒
Phlebovirus	白蛉热病毒
Nairovirus	内罗病毒
Rift Valley fever	里夫特裂谷热

BIBLIOGRAPHY

1. Bishop DHL, Shope RE: Bunyaviridae, New York, 1979, Plenum.

2. Cohen J, Powderly WG: Infectious diseases, ed 2, St Louis, 2004, Mosby.

3. Flint SJ, et al: Principles of virology: molecular biology, pathogenesis and control of animal viruses, ed 3, Washington, DC, 2009, American Society for Microbiology Press.

4. Gonzalez JP, et al: Arenaviruses, *Curr Top Microbiol Immunol*, vol 315, Berlin, 2007, Springer-Verlag, pp 253-288.

5. Gorbach SL, Bartlett JG, Blacklow NR: Infectious diseases, ed 3, Philadelphia, 2004, WB Saunders.

6. Knipe DM, et al: Fields virology, ed 5, Philadelphia, 2006, Lippincott Williams & Wilkins.

7. Kolakofsky D: Bunyaviridae, *Curr Top Microbiol Immunol*, vol 169, Berlin, 1991, Springer-Verlag.

8. Oldstone MBA: Arenaviruses I and II, *Curr Top Microbiol Immunol*, vols 262-263, Berlin, 2002, Springer-Verlag.

9. Peters CJ, Simpson GL, Levy H: Spectrum of hantavirus infection: hemorrhagic fever with renal syndrome and hantavirus pulmonary syndrome, Annu Rev Med 50: 531-545, 1999.

10. Schmaljohn CS, Nichol ST: Hantaviruses, *Curr Top Microbiol Immunol*, vol 256, Berlin, 2001, Springer-Verlag.

11. Smith DR, Holbrook MR, Gowen BB: Animal models of viral hemorrhagic fever, Antiviral Res 112: 59-79, 2014.

12. Strauss JM, Strauss EG: Viruses and human disease, ed 2, San Diego, 2007, Academic.

13. Tsai TF: Arboviral infections in the United States, Infect Dis Clin North Am 5: 73-102, 1991.

14. Walter CT, Barr JN: Recent advances in the molecular and cellular biology of bunyaviruses, J Gen Virol 92: 2467-2484, 2011.

15. Wrobel S: Serendipity, science, and a new hantavirus, FASEB J 9: 1247-1254, 1995.

Chapter 56

Retroviruses

The retroviruses are **enveloped positive-strand RNA** viruses with a unique morphology and means of replication. In 1970, Baltimore and Temin showed that the retroviruses encode an **RNA-dependent DNA polymerase (reverse transcriptase, RT)** and replicate through a DNA intermediate. The DNA copy of the viral genome is then integrated into the host chromosome to become a cellular gene. This discovery, which earned Baltimore, Temin, and Dulbecco the 1975 Nobel Prize, contradicted what had been the central dogma of molecular biology—that genetic information passed from DNA to RNA and then to protein.

The first retrovirus to be isolated was the Rous sarcoma virus, shown by Peyton Rous to produce solid tumors (sarcomas) in chickens. Like most retroviruses, the Rous sarcoma virus proved to have a very limited host and species range. Cancer-causing retroviruses have since been isolated from other animal species and are classified as RNA tumor viruses or **oncornaviruses.** Many of these viruses alter cellular growth by expressing analogs of cellular growth-controlling genes (**oncogenes**). Not until 1981, however, when Robert Gallo and his associates isolated human T-cell lymphotropic virus 1 (HTLV-1) from a person with adult human T-cell leukemia, was a human retrovirus associated with human disease.

In the late 1970s and early 1980s, an unusual number of young homosexual men, Haitians, heroin addicts, and hemophiliacs in the United States (the initial "4H club" of risk groups) were noted to be dying of normally benign opportunistic infections. Their symptoms defined a new disease, the **acquired immunodeficiency syndrome (AIDS).** However, as is now known, AIDS is not limited to these groups but can occur in anyone exposed to the virus. Now approximately 34 million men, women, and children around the world are living with the virus that causes AIDS. Montagnier and associates in Paris, and Gallo and colleagues in the United States, reported the isolation of the **human immunodeficiency virus** (HIV-1) from patients with lymphadenopathy and AIDS. A closely related virus, designated HIV-2, was isolated later and is prevalent in West Africa. HIV appears to have been acquired by humans from chimpanzees and then rapidly spread through Africa and the world by an increasingly mobile population. Although a devastating disease that cannot be completely cured, the development of antiviral drug cocktails (highly active antiretroviral therapy [HAART]) has allowed many HIV patients to resume a normal life.

Endogenous retroviruses, the ultimate parasites, have integrated, are transmitted vertically, and may take up as much as 8% of the human chromosome. Although they may not produce virions, they may still contribute to or influence functions of the body.

Our understanding of the retroviruses has paralleled progress in molecular biology and immunology. In turn, the retroviruses have provided a major tool for molecularbiology, the RT enzyme, and through the study of viral oncogenes have also provided a means of advancing our understanding of cell growth, differentiation, and oncogenesis.

The three subfamilies of human retroviruses are the **Oncovirinae** (HTLV-1, HTLV-2, HTLV-5), the **Lentivirinae** (HIV-1, HIV-2), and the **Spumavirinae** (Table 56-1). Although a spumavirus was the first human retrovirus to be isolated, no such virus has been associated with human disease.

469

Table 56-1   Classification of Retroviruses

Subfamily	Characteristics	Examples
Oncovirinae	Are associated with cancer and neurologic disorders	—
B	Have eccentric nucleocapsid core in mature virion	Mouse mammary tumor virus
C	Have centrally located nucleocapsid core in mature virion	Human T-cell lymphotropic virus* (HTLV-1, HTLV-2, HTLV-5), Rous sarcoma virus (chickens)
D	Have nucleocapsid core with cylindric form	Mason-Pfizer monkey virus
Lentivirinae	Have slow onset of disease; cause neurologic disorders and immunosuppression; are viruses with D-type, cylindric nucleocapsid core	Human immunodeficiency virus* (HIV-1, HIV-2), visna virus (sheep), caprine arthritis/encephalitis virus (goats)
Spumavirinae	Cause no clinical disease but cause characteristic vacuolated "foamy" cytopathology	Human foamy virus*
Endogenous viruses	Have retrovirus sequences that are integrated into human genome	Human placental virus

*Also classified as complex retroviruses because of the requirement for accessory proteins for replication.

CLASSIFICATION

The retroviruses are classified by the diseases they cause, tissue tropism and host range, virion morphology, and genetic complexity (Table 56-1). The **oncoviruses** include the only retroviruses that can **immortalize** or **transform target cells**. These viruses are also categorized by the morphology of their core and capsid as type A, B, C, or D, as seen in electron micrographs (Table 56-1). The **lentiviruses are slow viruses associated with neurologic and immunosuppressive diseases**. The spumaviruses, represented by a foamy virus, cause a distinct cytopathologic effect but, as already noted, do not seem to cause clinical disease.

STRUCTURE

The retroviruses are roughly spherical, enveloped, RNA viruses with a diameter of 80 to 120 nm (Figure 56-1). The envelope contains viral glycoproteins and is acquired by budding from the plasma membrane. e envelope surrounds a capsid that contains two identical copies of the positive-strand RNA genome inside an electron-dense core. The virion also contains 10 to 50 copies of the reverse transcriptase and integrase enzymes and two cellular transfer RNA (tRNAs). These tRNAs are base-paired to each copy of the genome to be used as a primer for the RT. The morphology of the core differs for different viruses

and is used as a means of classifying the retroviruses. The HIV virion core resembles a truncated cone (Figure 56-2).

The retrovirus genome has a 5'-cap and is polyadenylated at the 3'-end (Figure 56-3 and Table 56-2). Although the genome resembles a messenger RNA (mRNA), it is not infectious because it does not encode a polymerase that can directly generate more mRNA.

The genome of the simple retroviruses *consists of three major genes that encode polyproteins* for the

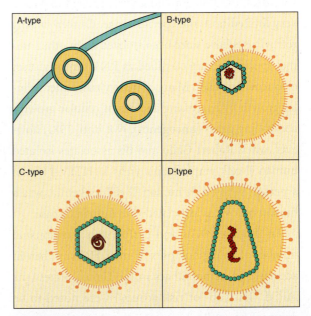

Figure 56-1   Morphologic distinction of retrovirions. The morphology and position of the nucleocapsid core are used to classify the viruses. A-type particles are immature intracytoplasmic forms that bud through the plasma membrane and mature into B-type, C-type, and D-type particles.

following enzymatic and structural proteins of the virus: **Gag** (group-specific antigen, *capsid, matrix,* and *nucleic acid-binding proteins*), **Pol** (*polymerase, protease,* and *integrase*), and **Env** (envelope, *glycoproteins*). At each end of the genome are **long terminal repeat (LTR)** sequences. The LTR sequences contain promoters, enhancers, and other gene sequences used for binding different cellular transcription factors. Oncogenic viruses may also contain a growth-promoting **oncogene**. The **complex retroviruses,** including HTLV and HIV and other lentiviruses, express early and late proteins and encode several virulence-enhancing proteins that require more complex transcriptional processing (splicing) than the simple retroviruses.

The viral glycoproteins are produced by proteolytic cleavage of the polyprotein encoded by the *env* gene. The size of the glycoproteins differs for each group of viruses. For example, the (glycoprotein) gp62 of HTLV-1 is cleaved into gp46 and p21, and

Table 56-2   Retrovirus Genes and Their Function

Gene	Virus	Function
gag	All	Group-specific antigen: core and capsid proteins
int	All	Integrase
pol	All	Polymerase: reverse transcriptase, protease, integrase
pro	All	Protease
env	All	Envelope: glycoproteins
tax	HTLV	Transactivation of viral and cellular genes
tat	HIV-1	Transactivation of viral and cellular genes
rex	HTLV	Regulation of RNA splicing and promotion of export to cytoplasm
rev	HIV-1	Regulation of RNA splicing and promotion of export to cytoplasm
nef	HIV-1	Decreases cell surface CD4; facilitates T-cell activation; progression to AIDS (essential)
vif	HIV-1	Virus infectivity, promotion of assembly, blocks a cellular antiviral protein
vpu	HIV-1	Facilitates virion assembly and release, induces degradation of CD4
vpr (vpx*)	HIV-1	Transport of complementary DNA to nucleus, arresting of cell growth; replication in macrophages
LTR	All	Promoter, enhancer elements

AIDS, Acquired immunodeficiency syndrome; *DNA,* deoxyribonucleic acid; *HIV,* human immunodeficiency virus; *HTLV,* human T-cell lymphotropic virus; *LTR,* long terminal repeat (sequence); *RNA,* ribonucleic acid.
*In HIV-2.

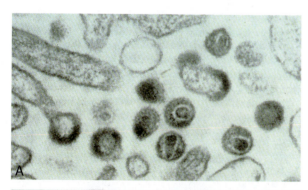
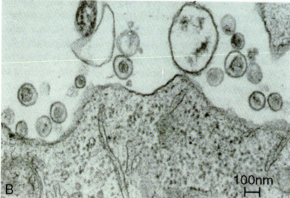

Figure 56-2   Electron micrographs of two retroviruses. **A,** Human immunodeficiency virus. Note the cone-shaped nucleocapsid in several of the virions. **B,** Human T-cell lymphotropic virus. Note the C-type morphology characterized by a central symmetric nucleocapsid. (From Belshe RB: *Textbook of human virology,* ed 2, St Louis, 1991, Mosby.)

the *gp160 of HIV is cleaved into gp41 and gp120.* These glycoproteins form lollipop-like trimer spikes that are visible on the surface of the virion. The larger of the HIV glycoproteins (gp120), which binds to cell surface receptors, initially determines the tissue tropism of the virus and is recognized by neutralizing antibody. The smaller subunit (gp41 in HIV) forms the lollipop stick and promotes cell-to-cell fusion. The gp120 of HIV is extensively glycosylated, and *its antigenicity can drift and receptor specificity can shift by mutations that occur during the course of a chronic HIV infection.* These factors impede antibody clearance of the virus.

The genes are defined in Table 56-2 and Figure 56-2. Unlike the other genes of these viruses, production of

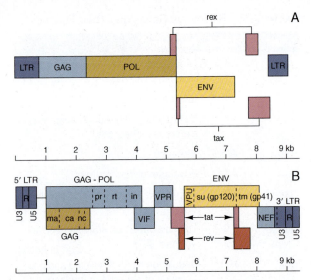

Figure 56-3 Genomic structure of human retroviruses. **A,** Human T-cell lymphotropic virus (HTLV-1). **B,** Human immunodeficiency virus (HIV-1). The genes are defined in Table 62-2 and Figure 62-3. Unlike the other genes of these viruses, production of the messenger RNA for *tax* and *rex* genes (HTLV-1) and *tat* and *rev* genes (HIV) requires excision of two intron units. HIV-2 has a similar genome map. The *vpu* gene for HIV-2 is termed the *vpx* gene. *ENV*, Envelope glycoprotein gene; *GAG*, group antigen gene; *LTR*, long terminal repeat; *POL*, polymerase gene. Protein nomenclature for HIV: *ca*, Capsid protein; *in*, integrase; *ma*, matrix protein; *nc*, nucleocapsid protein; *pr*, protease; *rt*, reverse transcriptase; *su*, surface glycoprotein component; *tm*, transmembrane glycoprotein component. (Modified from Belshe RB: *Textbook of human virology*, ed 2, St Louis, 1991, Mosby.)

the mRNAs for *tax* and *rex* genes (HTLV-1) and *tat* and *rev* genes (HIV) requires excision of two intron units. HIV-2 has a similar genome map but has a *vpx* but not a *vpu* gene. *ENV*, Envelope glycoprotein gene; *GAG*, group antigen gene; *LTR*, long terminal repeats; *POL*, polymerase gene. Protein nomenclature for HIV: *ca*, Capsid protein; *in*, integrase; *ma*, matrix protein; *nc*, nucleocapsid protein; *pr*, protease; *rt*, reverse transcriptase; *su*, surface glycoprotein component; *tm*, transmembrane glycoprotein component. (Modified from Belshe RB: *Textbook of human virology*, ed 2, St Louis, 1991, Mosby.)

REPLICATION

Replication of HIV will serve as an example for the other retroviruses unless noted. Infection starts with binding of the viral glycoprotein spikes (trimer of gp120 and gp41 molecules) to the primary recep-

tor, the **CD4 protein**, and then a second receptor, a 7-transmembrane G-protein-coupled chemokine receptor (Figure 56-4). *Binding to the receptor is the initial and major determinant of tissue tropism and host range for a retrovirus.* The co-receptor used upon initial infection by HIV is **CCR5**, which is expressed on **myeloid and peripheral, activated, central memory, intestinal, and other subsets of CD4 T cells (mac-**

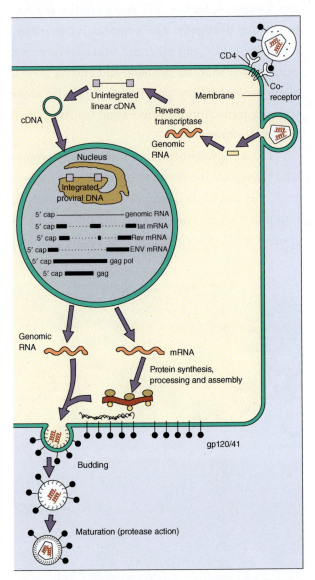

Figure 56-4 The life cycle of human immunodeficiency virus (HIV). HIV binds to CD4 and chemokine co-receptors and enters by fusion. The genome is reverse transcribed into deoxyribonucleic acid (DNA) in the cytoplasm and integrated into the nuclear DNA. Transcription and translation of the genome occur in a fashion similar to that of human T-cell lymphotropic virus (see Figure 62-7). The virus assembles at the plasma membrane and matures after budding from the cell. *cDNA,* Complementary DNA; *mRNA,* messenger ribonucleic acid. (Modifed from Fauci AS: The human immunodeficiency virus: infectivity and mechanisms of pathogenesis, *Science* 239: 617-622, 1988.)

rophages, [M]-tropic virus). Later, during chronic infection of a person, the *env* gene mutates so that the gp120 binds to a different chemokine receptor (**CXCR4**), which is expressed primarily on T cells (**T-tropic virus**) (Figure 56-5). Binding to the chemokine receptor activates the cell and brings the viral envelope and cell plasma membrane close together, allowing the gp41 to interact with and promote fusion of the two membranes. Binding to CCR5 and gp41-mediated fusion are targets for antiviral drugs. HIV can also bind to a cellular adhesion molecule, α-4 β-7 integrin (also known as VLA-4 [very late anti-

gen-4] and the gut homing receptor for T cells), and DC-SIGN (dendritic cell-specific intercellular adhesion molecule-3-grabbing nonintegrin) on dendritic and other cells.

Once the genome is released into the cytoplasm, the early phase of replication begins. The RT, encoded by the pol gene, uses the tRNA in the virion as a primer and synthesizes a **complementary** negative-strand DNA (**cDNA**). The RT also acts as a ribonuclease H, degrades the RNA genome, and then synthesizes the positive strand of DNA (Figure 56-6). The RT is the major target for antiviral drugs. During the synthesis of the virion DNA (**provirus**), sequences from each end of the genome (U3 and U5) are duplicated, thus attaching the LTRs to both ends. This process creates sequences necessary for integration and creates enhancer and promoter sequences within the LTR for regulation of transcription. The DNA copy of the genome is larger than the original RNA.

RT is very error prone. For example, the error rate for the RT from HIV is one error per 2000 bases, or approximately five errors per genome (HIV, 9000 base pairs), the equivalent of at least one typo on every page of this text but different errors for every book. This genetic instability of HIV is responsible for promoting the generation of new strains of virus during a person's disease, a property that may alter the pathogenicity of the virus and promote immune escape.

Unlike other retroviruses, the double-stranded cDNA of HIV and other lentiviruses can enter the nucleus through nuclear pores of resting T cells. Dissolution of the nuclear envelope upon cell division is required by other retroviruses. The cDNA is then spliced into the host chromosome with the aid of a virus-encoded, virion-carried enzyme, integrase. Integration requires cell growth, but the cDNA of HIV and other lentiviruses can remain in the nucleus and cytoplasm in a nonintegrated circular DNA form until the cell is activated. Integrase is a target for an antiviral drug.

Once integrated, the late phase begins and viral DNA provirus is transcribed as a cellular gene by the host RNA polymerase II. Transcription of the genome produces a full-length RNA, which for

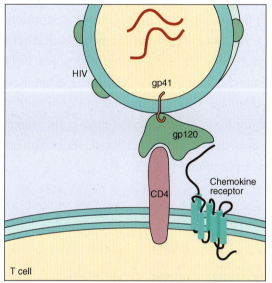

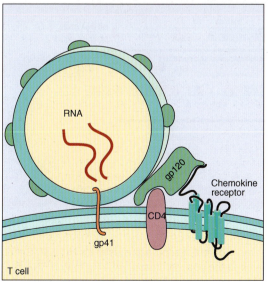

Figure 56-5 Target cell binding of human immunodeficiency virus *(HIV)*. The CCR5 chemokine receptor is used upon initial infection of an individual, and after mutation of the *env* gene, the CXCR4 receptor is also used. *RNA*, Ribonucleic acid.(Modified from Balter M: New hope in HIV disease, *Science* 274: 1988, 1996.)

simple retroviruses is processed to produce several mRNAs that contain the *gag*, *gag-pol*, or *env* gene sequences. The full-length transcripts of the genome can also be assembled into new virions.

Because the provirus acts as a cellular gene, its replication depends on the extent of methylation of the viral DNA and on the cell's growth rate, but mostly on the ability of the cell to recognize the enhancers and promoter sequences encoded in the LTR region. Stimulation of the cell by cytokines or mitogens produced in response to other infections generates transcription factors that bind to the LTR and for HIV are required to activate transcription of the integrated genome. If the virus encodes viral oncogenes, these proteins promote cell growth and stimulate transcription and hence viral replication. *The ability of a cell to transcribe the retroviral genome is also a major determinant of tissue tropism and host range for a retrovirus.*

HTLV and HIV are **complex retroviruses** and undergo two phases of transcription. During the early phase, HTLV-1 expresses two proteins, **Tax** and **Rex**, which regulate viral replication. Unlike the other viral mRNAs, the mRNA for Tax and Rex requires more than one splicing step. The *rex* gene encodes two proteins that bind to a structure on the viral mRNA and thereby prevents further splicing and pro- motes mRNA transport to the cytoplasm. The doubly spliced tax/rex mRNA is expressed early (at a low concentration of Rex), and structural proteins are expressed late (high concentration of Rex). Late in the infection, Rex selectively enhances expression of the singly spliced structural genes, which are required in abundance. The tax protein is **a transcriptional activator** and enhances transcription of the viral genome from the promoter gene sequence in the 5' LTR. Tax also activates other genes, including those for interleukin (IL)-2, IL-3, granulocyte-macrophage colony-stimulating factor, and the receptor for IL-2. Activation of these genes promotes the growth of the infected T cell, which enhances virus replication.

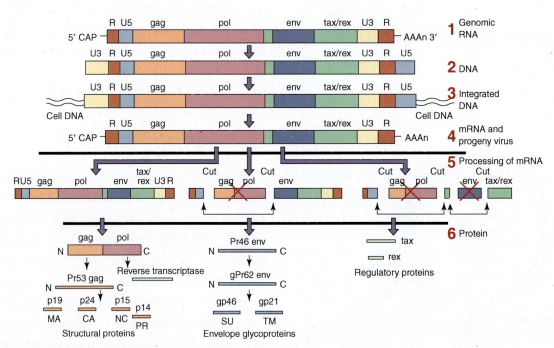

Figure 56-6 Transcription and translation of HTLV. (A similar but more complex approach is used for HIV.) *(1)* Genomic RNA is reverse transcribed and *(2)* circularized and then *(3)* integrated into the host chromatin. *(4)* A full-length RNA and *(5)* individual mRNAs are processed from this RNA. The mRNA for *tax* and *rex* requires excision of two sequences *(red X)*, the *gag-pol* and *env* sequences. The other mRNAs, including the *env* mRNA, require excision of one sequence. (6) Translation of these mRNAs produces polyproteins, which are subsequently cleaved. *AAAn*, Polyadenylate. Gene nomenclature: *env*, Envelope glycoprotein; *gag*, group antigen gene; *pol*, polymerase; *rex*, regulator of splicing; *tax*, transactivator. Protein nomenclature: *C*, Carboxyl terminus of peptide; *CA*, capsid; *MA*, matrix; *N*, amino terminus; *NC*, nucleocapsid; *PR*, protease; *SU*, surface component; *TM*, transmembrane component of envelope glycoprotein. Prefixes: *gp*, glycoprotein; *gPr*, glycosylated precursor polyprotein; *p*, protein; *PR*, precursor polyprotein.

HIV replication is regulated by as many as six "**accessory**" gene products (see Table 54-2). The Tat protein, like **Tax**, is a transactivator of the transcription of viral and cellular genes. The **Rev** protein acts like the Rex protein to regulate and promote transport of viral mRNA into the cytoplasm. The **Nef** protein reduces cell surface expression of CD4 and major histocompatibility class I (MHC I) molecules, alters T-cell signaling pathways, regulates the cytotoxicity of the virus, and is required to maintain high viral loads. The Nef protein appears to be essential for causing the infection to progress to AIDS. The **Vif** protein promotes assembly and maturation and binds to an antiviral cellular protein (APOBEC-3G) to prevent it from hypermutating the cDNA and helps the virus replicate in myeloid and other cells. The **Vpu** protein reduces cell surface CD4 expression and enhances virion release. The **Vpr** protein (Vpx in HIV-2) is important for transport of the cDNA into the nucleus. Vpr protein also arrests the cell in the G2 phase of the growth cycle, which is likely to be optimal for HIV replication. Vpx facilitates virus replication in dendritic cells and macrophages. Interestingly, this facilitates antigen presentation on MHC-1 antigens, which promotes CD8 cytotoxic T-cell production, which can limit HIV-2 disease progression.

The proteins translated from the *gag*, *gag-pol*, and *env* mRNAs are synthesized as polyproteins and are subsequently cleaved to functional proteins (see Figure 56-6). The viral glycoproteins are synthesized, glycosylated, and processed by the endoplasmic reticulum and Golgi apparatus. These glycoproteins are then cleaved, associate to form trimers, and migrate to the plasma membrane.

The Gag and Gag-Pol polyproteins are acylated and then bind to the plasma membrane containing the envelope glycoprotein. The association of two copies of the genome and cellular transfer RNA molecules promotes budding of the virion. After envelopment and release from the cell, the viral protease cleaves the Gag and Gag-Pol polyproteins to release the RT and form the virion core, thus ensuring inclusion of these components into the virion. The protease step is required for the production of infectious virions and is a target for antiviral drugs.

Envelopment and release of retroviruses occur at the cell surface. The HIV envelope picks up cellular proteins, including MHC molecules, upon budding. Replication and budding of the retrovirus does not necessarily kill the cell. HIV can also spread from cell to cell through the production of multinucleated giant cells, or syncytia. Syncytia are fragile, and their formation enhances the cytolytic activity of the virus.

Human Immunodeficiency Virus

There are four genotypes of HIV-1, designated M (main), N, O, and P. Most HIV-1 is of the M subtype, and this is divided into 11 subtypes, or clades, designated A to K (for HIV-2, A to F). The designations are based on differences in the sequence of their *env* (7% to 12% difference) and *gag* genes and hence the antigenicity and immune recognition of the gp120 and capsid proteins of these viruses.

Pathogenesis and Immunity

The major determinant in the pathogenesis and disease caused by HIV is the virus **tropism for CD4-expressing T cells** and **myeloid cells** (Figure 56-7). HIV-induced immunosuppression (AIDS) results from a reduction in the number of CD4 T cells, which decimates the ability to activate and control innate and immune responses.

During sexual transmission, HIV infects a mucosal surface, enters, and rapidly infects cells of the mucosa-associated lymphoid tissue (MALT), including the intestine. The initial stages of infection are mediated by M-tropic viruses that bind to CD4 and the CCR5 chemokine receptors on dendritic and other monocyte-macrophage lineage cells, as well as memory, Th1, most intestine-associated T cells, and other CD4 T cells. Individuals who are deficient in the CCR5 receptor are also resistant to HIV infection, and CCR5 binding is a target for an antiviral drug. The CCR5-delta 32 mutation that prevents surface expression of this co-receptor is prevalent in northern Europeans (1% are homozygous and 10% to 15% are heterozygous for the mutation).

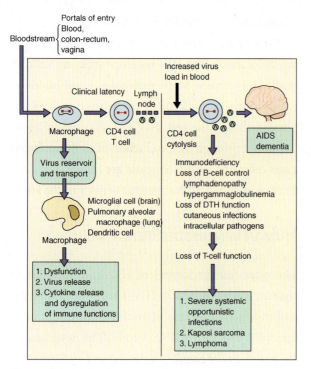

Figure 56-7 Pathogenesis of human immunodeficiency virus (HIV). HIV causes lytic and latent infection of CD4 T cells and persistent infection of monocytes, macrophages, and dendritic cells and disrupts neuron function. The outcomes of these actions are immunodeficiency and acquired immunodeficiency syndrome (AIDS) dementia. DTH, Delayed-type hypersensitivity. (Modifed from Fauci AS: The human immunodeficiency virus: infectivity and mechanisms of pathogenesis, *Science* 239: 617-622, 1988.)

Targeting of CCR5 or α-4 β-7 integrin-expressing CD4 T cells rapidly depletes the intestinal lymphoid tissue of CD4 T cells. Depletion of the intestinal CD4 Tcell population wreaks havoc on immune regulation of normal gut flora and maintenance of the intestinal mucosal epithelium, leading to leakage and diarrhea.

Macrophages, DCs, memory T cells, and hematopoietic stem cells are persistently infected with HIV and are the major reservoirs and means of distribution of HIV (Trojan horse). HIV can bind to the

DC-SIGN lectin molecule and remain on the surface of dendritic cells (including follicular DCs). CD4 T cells can be infected with the cell-bound HIV or by cell-to-cell transmission of virus upon binding to the DC. Late in the disease progression, mutation in the *env* gene for the gp120 occurs for some of the virus, and this shifts its tropism from M-tropic (R5) to T-tropic (X4 virus). The gp120 of the T-tropic virus binds to CD4 and the CXCR4 chemokine receptor. Some viruses may use both receptors (R5X4 viruses). This expands the viral target range to include almost all CD4 T cells.

Killing of CD4 T cells may result from direct HIV-induced cytolysis (including syncytia formation) (Table 56-3) and cytotoxic T-cell-induced immune cytolysis, but large numbers of nonpermissive resting T cells commit a type of inflammatory cell suicide (pyroptosis) induced by the presence of large amounts of nonintegrated circular DNA copies of the genome. Pyroptosis is an inflammatory form of cell death that may lure more unactivated T cells to the site to be infected and also succumb to pyroptosis.

The course of HIV disease parallels the reduction in CD4 T-cell numbers and the amount of virus in the blood (Figure 56-8). HIV infects and depletes the intestinal CCR5-expressing CD4 T cells very soon after infection. During the subsequent acute phase of the infection, there is a large burst of virus production (10^7 particles/ml of plasma). T-cell proliferation in response to antigen presentation by infected dendritic cells, macrophages, and even activated CD4 T cells promotes a **mononucleosis-like syndrome**. CD8 T cells kill many infected cells and limit virus production. Virus levels in the blood decrease and the individual is asymptomatic (latent period), but viral replication continues in the lymph nodes, caus-

Table 56-3 Means of Human Immunodeficiency Virus Escape from the Immune System.

Characteristic	Function
Infection of lymphocytes and macrophages	Inactivation of key element of immune defense
Inactivation of CD4 helper cells	Loss of activator and controller of the immune system
Antigenic drift (via mutation) of gp120	Evasion of antibody detection
Heavy glycosylation of gp120	Evasion of antibody detection
Direct cell to cell spread and syncytia formation	Evasion of antibody detection

ing disruption of structure and function, and CD4 T-cell numbers continue to drop. Late in the disease, CD4 levels decrease to the point that they cannot maintain the antiviral action of CD8 T cells, and then virus levels in the blood increase greatly, T-tropic virus rises, CD4 T-cell numbers drop faster, the structure of the lymph nodes is destroyed, and the patient becomes immunodeficient.

The central role of the CD4 helper T cells in the initiation and control of innate and immune responses is indicated by the onset of opportunistic diseases after HIV infection. Activated CD4 T cells initiate immune responses by the release of cytokines required for the activation of epithelial cells, neutrophils, macrophages, other T cells, B cells, and natural killer cells. The CD4 Th17 responses that activate neutrophils and protect the mucoepithelium are the first to be depleted (CD4 numbers < 500/μl), increasing susceptibility to fungal and bacterial infections. As the CD4 T cells decrease (CD4 numbers < 200/μl), Th1 responses dissipate and cannot activate sufficient numbers of CD8 T cells and macrophages to control latent and new infections of intracellular bacteria and viruses (e.g., herpesviruses and JC polyomavirus progressive multifocal leukoencephalopathy [PML] and EBV and HHV8-associated cancers [Hodgkin and non-Hodgkin lymphomas, Kaposi sarcoma]).

In addition to immunodepression, HIV can also cause neurologic abnormalities. The microglial cell and macrophage are the predominant HIV-infected cell types in the brain. Infected monocytes and microglial cells release neurotoxic substances or chemotactic factors that promote inflammatory responses and neuronal death in the brain. Immunosuppression also puts the individual at risk of opportunistic infections of the brain.

The innate and immune response attempts to restrict viral infection but also contributes to pathogenesis. The infected cells have enzymes that restrict retrovirus replication (including endogenous retroviruses), but HIV can override their actions. The presence of unintegrated HIV cDNA triggers type 1 interferon production but also inflammatory cell

suicide (pyroptosis). CD8 T cells are critical to limiting HIV disease progression. CD8 T cells can kill infected cells by direct cytotoxic action and can produce suppressive factors that restrict viral replication, including chemokines that also block the binding of virus to its co-receptor. Individuals with certain MHC types (human leukocyte antigen [HLA] B27 or B57) will preferentially bind HIV peptides rather than cellular peptides to make infected cells better targets for CD8 T-cell killing, and these individuals are more resistant to HIV disease. Neutralizing antibodies are generated against gp120. Antibody-coated virus can be infectious, however, and is taken up by macrophages.

HIV has several ways of escaping immune control. Most significant is the virus's ability to undergo mutation and hence alter its antigenicity and escape antibody clearance. Persistent infection of macrophages and resting CD4 T cells maintains the virus in an immune-privileged cell and cells in immune-privileged tissues (e.g., central nervous system and genital organs) (see Table 56-3). Ultimately, infection of CD4 T cells compromises the entire immune system.

Epidemiology

HIV-1 is genetically most similar to a chimpanzee immunodeficiency virus. HIV-2 is more similar to simian immunodeficiency virus. The initial human infection occurred in Africa before the 1930s but went unnoticed in rural areas. The migration of infected people to the cities and increased nonsterile use of syringes after the 1960s brought the virus into population centers.

HIV-1 infections are spreading worldwide, with the largest number of AIDS cases in sub-Saharan Africa but with a growing number of cases in the rest of the world. HIV-2 is prevalent in Africa (especially West Africa). HIV-2 produces a disease similar to but less severe than AIDS.

Although rare, there are cases of long-term survivors. Some of these result from infection with HIV strains that lack a functional Nef protein. The Nef protein is necessary to promote the progression of HIV infection to AIDS. Resistance to the virus also correlates with a lack of or mutation of the CCR5 chemokine co-receptor for the virus or specific HLA types that promote more vigorous cytotoxic T-cell responses.

Transmission

The presence of HIV in the **blood, semen,** and **vaginal secretions** of infected people and the long asymptomatic period of infection are factors that have promoted spread of the disease through sexual contact and exposure to contaminated blood and blood products (Table 56-4). The fetus and newborn are likely to acquire the virus from an infected mother. Tattoo needles and contaminated inks are other potential means by which HIV can be transmitted. HIV is not, however, transmitted by casual contact, touching, hugging, kissing, coughing, sneezing, insect bites, water, food, utensils, toilets, swimming pools, or public baths.

Sexually active people (men who have sex with men [MSM] and heterosexual men and women), intravenous drug abusers and their sexual partners, and the newborns of HIV-positive mothers are at highest risk for HIV infections.

People receiving blood transfusions or organ transplants and hemophiliacs receiving clotting factors from pooled blood were at high risk for HIV infection. Proper screening of the blood supply and transplant tissue has practically eliminated the danger of HIV being transmitted in blood transfusions.

Health care workers are at risk for HIV infection from accidental needlesticks or cuts or through the exposure of broken skin and mucosal membranes to contaminated blood.

Clinical Syndromes

AIDS is one of the most devastating epidemics ever recorded. Most HIV-infected people will become symptomatic, and the overwhelming majority of them will ultimately succumb to the disease without treatment. HIV disease progresses from an asymptomatic nonspecific disease to profound immunosuppression, referred to as **AIDS** (Figure 56-8). The diseases related to AIDS mainly consist of opportunistic infections, cancers, and the direct effects of HIV on the central nervous system (Table 56-5).

The initial symptoms following HIV infection (acute phase, 2 to 4 weeks after infection) may resemble those of influenza or infectious mononucleosis, with "aseptic" meningitis or a rash occurring up to 3 months after infection, and are followed by a period of asymptomatic infection or a persistent generalized lymphadenopathy that may last for several years. During this period, the virus is replicating in the lymph nodes.

Deterioration of the immune response is indicated by increased susceptibility to opportunistic pathogens. The onset of symptoms correlates with a reduction in the number of CD4 T cells to less than $500/\mu l$ and increased levels of virus (as determined by PCR-related techniques) and protein p24 in the blood. Full-blown AIDS occurs when **CD4 T-cell counts are less than $200/\mu l$** (oftentimes to $50/\mu l$ or undetectable) and **virus load is greater than 75,000 copies/ml** and involves the onset of more significant diseases, including HIV wasting syndrome (weight loss and diarrhea for > 1 month) and opportunistic infections, malignancies, and dementia (Table 56-5).

AIDS may be manifested in several different ways,

Table 56-4 Transmission of Human Immunodeficiency Virus Infection.

Routes	Specific Transmission
Known Routes of Transmission	
Inoculation in blood	Transfusion of blood and blood products
	Needle sharing among intravenous drug abusers
	Needlestick, open wound, and mucous membrane exposure in health care workers
	Tattoo needles
Sexual transmission	Anal and vaginal intercourse
Perinatal transmission	Intrauterine transmission
	Peripartum transmission
	Breast milk
Routes Not Involved in Transmission	
Close personal contact	Household members
	Health care workers not exposed to blood

Table 56-5   Indicator Diseases of Acquired Immu-nodeficiency Syndrome[*]

Infection	Disease (Selected)
Opportunistic Infections	
Protozoal	Toxoplasmosis of the brain
	Cryptosporidiosis with diarrhea
	Isosporiasis with diarrhea
Fungal	Candidiasis of the esophagus, trachea, and lungs
	Pneumocystis jirovecii (previously called *Pneumocystis carinii*) pneumonia
	Cryptococcosis (extrapulmonary)
	Histoplasmosis (disseminated)
	Coccidioidomycosis (disseminated)
Viral	Cytomegalovirus disease
	Herpes simplex virus infection (persistent or disseminated)
	Progressive multifocal leukoencephalopathy (JC virus)
	Hairy leukoplakia caused by Epstein-Barr virus
Bacterial	*Mycobacterium avium-intracellulare* complex (disseminated)
	Any "atypical" mycobacterial disease
	Extrapulmonary tuberculosis
	Salmonella septicemia (recurrent)
	Pyogenic bacterial infections (multiple or recurrent)
Opportunistic Neoplasias	Kaposi sarcoma
	Primary lymphoma of the brain
	Other non-Hodgkin lymphomas
Others	HIV wasting syndrome
	HIV encephalopathy
	Lymphoid interstitial pneumonia

HIV, Human immunodeficiency virus.
[*]Manifestations of HIV infection—defining AIDS according to criteria of Centers for Disease Control and Prevention.
Modified from Belshe RB: *Textbook of human virology*, ed 2, St Louis, 1991, Mosby.

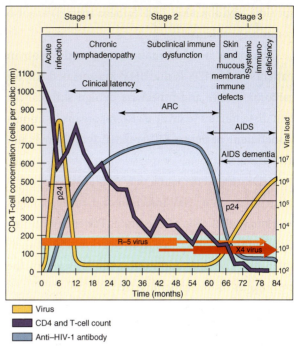

Figure 56-8   Time course and stages of human immunodeficiency virus *(HIV)* disease. A long clinical latency period follows the initial mononucleosis-like symptoms. Initial infection is with the R5-M-tropic virus, and later the X4-T-tropic virus arises. The progressive decrease in the number of CD4 T cells, even during the latency period, allows opportunistic infections to occur. The stages in HIV disease are defined by the CD4 T-cell levels and occurrence of opportunistic diseases. *ARC*, Acquired immunodeficiency syndrome (AIDS)-related complex.(Modified from Redfield RR, Burke DS: HIV infection: the clinical picture, *Sci Am* 259: 90-98, 1988; updated 1996.)

including lymphadenopathy and fever, opportunistic infections, malignancies, and AIDS-related dementia.

Lymphadenopathy and fever develop insidiously and may be accompanied by weight loss and malaise. These findings may persist indefinitely or progress.

Normally opportunistic benign infections caused by agents such as *Candida albicans* and other fungi, DNA viruses capable of recurrent disease, parasites, and intracellularly growing bacteria cause significant

disease after HIV depletion of CD4 T cells and subsequent reduction of CD8 T cells (see Table 56-5). *Pneumocystis jirovecii*-induced *Pneumocystis* pneumonia (PCP) is a major sign of AIDS. Oral candidiasis (thrush), cerebral toxoplasmosis, and cryptococcal meningitis also often occur, as do prolonged and severe viral infections, including molluscum contagiosum poxvirus, papovaviruses (JC virus, causing progressive multifocal leukoencephalopathy), and recurrences of the herpesviruses (e.g., herpes simplex virus, varicella-zoster virus, Epstein-Barr virus [EBV; hairy leukoplakia of the mouth, EBV-associated lymphomas], cytomegalovirus [especially retinitis, pneumonia, and bowel disease]). Tuberculosis and other mycobacterial diseases and diarrhea caused by common pathogens (*Salmonella*, *Shigella*, and *Campylobacter species*) and uncommon agents (cryptosporidia, mycobacteria, and Amoeba species) are also common problems.

The most notable malignancy to develop in patients with AIDS is the HHV-8-associated Kaposi sarcoma, a rare and otherwise benign skin cancer that disseminates to involve visceral organs in immunodeficient patients. EBV-related lymphomas are also prevalent.

AIDS-related dementia may result from opportunistic infection or HIV infection of the macrophages and microglial cells of the brain. Patients with this condition may undergo a slow deterioration of their intellectual abilities and exhibit similar signs of the early stages of Alzheimer disease.

Laboratory Diagnosis

Tests for HIV infection are performed for one of four reasons: (1) to identify those with the infection so that antiviral drug therapy can be initiated, (2) to identify carriers who may transmit infection to others (specifically blood or organ donors, pregnant women, and sex partners), (3) to follow the course of disease and confirm the diagnosis of AIDS, or (4) to evaluate the efficacy of treatment (Table 56-6).

The chronic nature of the disease allows use of serologic tests to document HIV infection, as supplemented by genome detection and quantitation with PCR-related techniques. Unfortunately, serologic tests cannot identify recently infected people. HIV is very difficult to grow in tissue culture, and virus isolation is not performed. Recent infection or late-stage disease are indicated by the presence of large quantities of viral RNA in blood samples, the p24 viral antigen, or the RT enzyme (see Figure 54-9).

Genomics

Newer methods for detection and quantitation of HIV genomes in blood have become a mainstay for following the course of an HIV infection and the efficacy and patient compliance with antiviral therapy. After converting viral RNA into DNA with a RT (laboratory provided), the cDNA of the genome can be detected by PCR and quantitated by real-time PCR, branched-chain DNA amplification, and other methods. Determination of the viral load (amount of genome in blood) is an excellent indicator of the course of disease and efficacy of therapy.

Serology

Screening of blood and organ donors is performed by serology, despite its inability to detect a recent infection. HIV antibody may develop slowly, taking 4 to 8 weeks in most patients; however, it may take 6 months or more in as many as 5% of those infected. ELISA assays or agglutination procedures are used for routine screening. The ELISA test, however, can yield false-positive results. Western blot analysis is used to confirm seropositive results. The Western blot assay demonstrates the presence of antibody to the viral antigens (p24 or p31) and glycoproteins (gp41 and gp120/160). Rapid screening tests are available that detect the p24 antigen and/or anti-HIV antibodies in blood.

Immunologic Studies

The status of an HIV infection can be inferred from an analysis of the T-cell subsets. The absolute number of CD4 lymphocytes and the ratio of CD4 to CD8 lymphocytes are abnormally low in HIV-infected people. The particular concentration of CD4 lymphocytes

Table 56-6   Laboratory Analysis for Human Immunodeficiency Virus (HIV).

Test	Purpose
Serology	
Enzyme-linked immuno-sorbent assay	Initial screening
Latex agglutination	Initial screening
Rapid oral antibody test	Initial screening
Western blot analysis (for antibody)	Confirmation test
Immunofluorescence	Confirmation test
Virion RNA RT-PCR	Detection of virus in blood
Real-time RT-PCR	Quantitation of virus in blood
Branched-chain DNA	Quantitation of virus in blood
p24 antigen	Early marker of infection
Isolation of virus	Test not readily available
CD4:CD8 T-cell ratio	Correlate of HIV disease

DNA, Deoxyribonucleic acid; *RNA,* ribonucleic acid; *RT-PCR,* reverse transcriptase polymerase chain reaction.

identifies the stage of AIDS. The choice to initiate therapy is usually based on CD4 T-cell counts.

Treatment

Antiretroviral therapy should be initiated for individuals showing symptoms of AIDS, AIDS-defining illnesses, or if CD4 T cells drop to less than 350/μl. Therapy may also be considered if viral loads are high (>100,000), even if CD4 numbers are above 350/μl. Therapy is also suggested for postexposure prophylaxis (e.g., needlestick) if HIV is detected in the individual.

The anti-HIV drugs can be classified as inhibitors of **binding, fusion-penetration, integrase or protease or nucleoside analog reverse transcriptase inhibitors, or nonnucleoside reverse transcriptase inhibitors.**

Inhibition of binding to the CCR5 co-receptor with a receptor agonist (maraviroc) or fusion of the viral envelope and cell membrane with a peptide (T-20: enfuvirtide) that blocks the action of the gp41 molecule will prevent the initial infection event. Inhibition of the integrase prevents all subsequent events in the replication of the virus. Inhibition of the RT prevents the initiation of virus replication by blocking cDNA synthesis. Azidothymidine (AZT) and the other nucleotide analogs are phosphorylated by cellular enzymes and incorporated into cDNA by the RT to cause DNA chain termination. Nonnucleoside RT inhibitors (nevirapine) inhibit the enzyme by other mechanisms. Protease inhibitors block the morphogenesis of the virion by inhibiting cleavage of the Gag and Gag-Pol polyproteins. The viral proteins and resulting virion are inactive. Most anti-HIV drugs have significant side effects, and the search continues for new anti-HIV drugs. Each of the replicative steps and all of the viral proteins are being targeted for development of new anti-HIV drugs.

Single use of antiretroviral drug is not recommended. Anti-HIV therapy is currently given as a cocktail of several antiviral drugs termed **highly active antiretroviral treatment (HAART)**. Use of a mixture of drugs with different mechanisms of action has less potential to select for resistance. Multidrug therapy can reduce blood levels of virus to nearly zero and reduce morbidity and mortality in many patients with advanced AIDS. These drugs are often difficult to tolerate, and each drug has its own side effects. Customization of HAART for each patient can minimize the drug side effects, ease the pill-taking regimen, and allow the patient to return to nearly normal health and lifestyle. HAART is expensive and may require taking many pills during the day.

Prevention, and Control

The principal way HIV infection can be controlled is by educating the population about the methods of transmission and the measures that may curtail viral spread. For instance, monogamous relationships, the practice of safe sex, and use of condoms reduce the possibility of exposure. Because contaminated needles are a major source of HIV infection in intravenous drug abusers, people must be taught that needles must not be shared.

Potential blood and organ donors are screened before they donate blood, tissue, and blood products. People testing positive for HIV must not donate blood.

The infection-control procedures for HIV infection are the same as those for hepatitis B virus. They include use of universal blood and body fluid precautions, which are based on the assumption that all patients are infectious for HIV and other bloodborne pathogens. Precautions include wearing protective clothing (e.g., gloves, mask, gown) and using other barriers to prevent exposure to blood products. Syringes and surgical instruments should never be reused unless carefully disinfected. Contaminated surfaces should be disinfected with 10% household bleach, 70% ethanol or isopropanol, 2% glutaraldehyde, and 4% formaldehyde, or 6% hydrogen peroxide. Washing laundry in hot water with detergent should be sufficient to inactivate HIV.

There are many difficulties in development of a vaccine against HIV. The primary target of neutralizing antibody, the gp120, is different for the different HIV clades and even within a clade; there are many antigenically distinct mutants that change during the infection of the individual. HIV can be spread through cell-to-cell bridges and remains latent, thereby hiding from antibody.

Several different approaches have been tried for developing an HIV vaccine. Live attenuated vaccines (e.g., deletion of the *nef* gene) were too dangerous because they still cause disease in infants and may establish chronic infection. Protein subunit vaccines with gp120 or its precursor, gp160, by themselves, elicit only antibody to a single strain of HIV and have not been successful. The most recent HIV vaccines prime T-cell responses with a vaccinia, canarypox, or defective adenovirus vector or with a DNA vaccine also failed.

Incorporation of an anti-HIV drug into contraceptive creams has demonstrated some ability to reduce transmission of HIV. Circumcision of males reduces their risk of infection.

HUMAN T-CELL LYMPHOTROPIC VIRUS AND OTHER ONCOGENIC RETROVIRUSES

The Oncovirinae were originally called the **RNA tumor viruses** and have been associated with the development of leukemias, sarcomas, and lymphomas in many animals. These viruses are not cytolytic.

Members of this family are distinguished by their mechanism of cell transformation (immortalization) and the length of the latency period between infection and development of disease: (1) The **sarcoma and acute leukemia viruses** have incorporated modified versions of cellular genes (protooncogenes) encoding growth-controlling factors into their genome (*v-onc*). At least 35 different viral oncogenes have been identified, including genes that encode growth hormones, growth hormone receptors, protein kinases, guanosine triphosphate-binding proteins (G-proteins), and nuclear DNA-binding proteins. These viruses can cause transformation of cells relatively rapidly and are highly oncogenic. *No human virus of this type has been identified.* (2) The **leukemia viruses**, including HTLV-1, are competent in terms of replication but cannot transform cells in vitro. They cause cancer after a **long latency period** of at least 30 years. The leukemia viruses promote

cell growth in more indirect ways than the oncogene-encoding viruses. For HTLV-1, a transcriptional regulator, Tax, is produced and is capable of activating promoters in the LTR region and specific cellular genes (including growth-controlling and cytokine genes, such as those encoding IL-2 and granulocyte-macrophage colony-stimulating factor) to promote the outgrowth of that cell. These viruses are also associated with nonneoplastic neurologic disorders and other diseases. For example, HTLV-1 causes **adult acute T-cell lymphocytic leukemia (ATLL)** and **HTLV-1-associated myelopathy (tropical spastic paraparesis)**, a nononcogenic neurologic disease.

The human oncoviruses include HTLV-1, HTLV-2, and HTLV-5, but only HTLV-1 has been definitively associated with disease (i.e., ATLL). HTLV-2 was isolated from atypical forms of hairy cell leukemia, and HTLV-5 was isolated from a malignant cutaneous lymphoma.

Pathogenesis and Immunity

HTLV-1 is transmitted and acquired by the same routes as HIV. It is endemic in southern Japan, the Caribbean, Central Africa, and among African Americans in the southeastern United States. In the endemic regions of Japan, the children acquire HTLV-1 at birth and in breast milk from their mothers, whereas the adults are infected sexually. The number of seropositive people in some regions of Japan may be as high as 35% (Okinawa), with twice the mortality rate from leukemia compared to other regions. Intravenous drug abuse and blood transfusion are becoming the most prominent means of transmitting the virus in the United States, where the high-risk groups for HTLV-1 infection are the same as those for HIV infection. Upon serological survey, only a few persons were identified as HTLV-1-positive in China.

HTLV infection is usually asymptomatic but can progress to ATLL in approximately 1 in 20 persons over a 30- to 50-year period. There is a long latency period ($\approx$30 years) before the onset of leukemia. ATLL caused by HTLV-1 is a neoplasia of the CD4 helper T cells that can be acute or chronic. ATLL is usually fatal within a year of diagnosis, regardless of treatment. HTLV-1 can also cause other diseases, including uveitis, HTLV-associated infectious dermatitis, and other inflammatory disorders.

HTLV-1 is spread in cells after blood transfusion, sexual intercourse, or breastfeeding. The virus enters the bloodstream and infects the CD4 helper T cells. In addition to blood and lymphatic organs, these T cells have a tendency to reside in the skin, thus contributing to the symptoms of ATLL. Neurons also express a receptor for HTLV-1.

HTLV is competent for replication, with the *gag*, *pol*, and *env* genes transcribed, translated, and processed as described earlier. In addition to its action on viral genes, the Tax protein transactivates the cellular genes for the T-cell growth factor IL-2 and its receptor (IL-2R), which activates growth in the infected cell. The virus may remain latent or may replicate slowly for many years but may also induce the clonal outgrowth of particular T-cell clones. HTLV-1-induced adult T-cell leukemia is usually monoclonal. A cellular protein, HBZ, limits Tax activity, promoting cell survival.

Antibodies are elicited to the gp46 and other proteins of HTLV-1. HTLV-1 infection also causes immunosuppression.

Laboratory Diagnosis

HTLV-1 infection is detected using ELISA to find virus-specific antigens in blood, using RT-PCR for viral RNA, or using ELISA to detect specific antiviral antibodies.

Treatment, Prevention, and Control

A combination of AZT and interferon-α has been effective in some patients with ATLL. However, no particular treatment has been approved for the management of HTLV-1 infection.

The measures used to limit the spread of HTLV-1 are the same as those used to limit transmission of HIV. Sexual precautions, screening of the blood supply, and increased awareness of the potential risks and diseases are ways to prevent transmission of the virus. Maternal infection of children is very difficult to control.

ENDOGENOUS RETROVIRUSES

Different retroviruses have integrated into and become a part of the chromosomes of humans and animals. In fact, retrovirus sequences may make up at least 8% of the human genome. Complete and partial provirus sequences with gene sequences similar to those of HTLV, mouse mammary tumor virus, and other retroviruses can be detected in humans. These endogenous viruses generally lack the ability to replicate because of deletions or the insertion of termination codons or because they are poorly transcribed. One such retrovirus can be detected in placental tissue and is activated by pregnancy. This virus produces syncytin, necessary to facilitate placental function. Another endogenous retrovirus is associated with prostate cancer.

SUMMARY

Retroviruses are enveloped positive-strand RNA viruses of medium size. The genome of simple retroviruses encompass three genes: *gag, pol, env*, while that of complex retroviruses (HIV, HTLV) contain *gag, pol, env*, and other important genes. The retroviral virion carries RNA-dependent DNA polymerase (reverse transcriptase), integrase, and protease enzymes, and replicates through *provirus*, a DNA intermediate that integrates randomly into the host chromosome.

Human immunodeficiency virus is so named due to its being able to incapacitate and escape host immune control. HIV primarily infects CD4 T cells, causing syncytia formation and subsequent lysis of those cells. The human immunodeficiency virus is transmitted via body fluids including blood and semen, thus rendering intravenous drug abusers, people with multiple sexual partners, newborns of HIV-positive mothers, etc at relatively high risk of HIV infections. Diagnosis of HIV infection relies on genomic, serological, and immunological studies by means of RT-PCR, ELISA, etc. HIV infection is treated with antiviral agents including nucleoside analogue reverse transcriptase inhibitors (NRTI), nonnucleoside reverse transcriptase inhibitors (NNRTI), protease inhibitors (PI), binding and fusion inhibitors, and integrase inhibitors; meanwhile, disease transmission should be properly controlled by education, blood product screening and appropriate control measures.

Oncovirinae have been associated with the development of a group of cancers, among which human T-cell lymphocytic virus-1 is thought to be related to acute T-cell lymphocytic leukemia and tropical spastic paraparesis. The routes of transmission, diagnostic means, and prevention methods of HTLV are the same as HIV.

Endogenous retroviruses refer to those integrated into the chromosomes of humans and animals. Retrovirus sequences may make up at least 8% of the human genome.

KEYWORDS

English	Chinese
Retrovirus	逆转录病毒
Acquired immunodeficiency syndrome (AIDS)	获得性免疫缺陷综合征（AIDS）
Human immunodeficiency virus (HIV)	人类免疫缺陷病毒（HIV）
Reverse transcriptase	逆转录酶
RNA-dependent deoxyribonucleic acid (DNA) polymerase	依赖 RNA 的 DNA 聚合酶
Integrase	整合酶
Lentivirus	慢病毒
Endogenous retrovirus	内源性逆转录病毒
Provirus	前病毒
Long terminal repeat	长末端重复序列
Co-receptor	辅助受体
Pneumocystis jirovecii	耶氏肺孢菌
Pneumocystis carinii	卡氏肺孢菌
Pneumocystis pneumonia (PCP)	肺孢菌肺炎
Pyroptosis	细胞凋亡
Nucleoside analog	核苷类似物
Nonnucleoside reverse transcriptase inhibitor (NNRTI)	非核苷类似物逆转录酶抑制剂
Protease inhibitor	蛋白酶抑制剂
Highly active antiretroviral treatment (HAART)	高效抗逆转录病毒治疗
Human T-cell lymphotropic virus (HTLV)	人类嗜 T 细胞病毒
Oncogene	癌基因
RNA tumor virus	RNA 肿瘤病毒
Adult T-cell lymphocytic leukemia (ATLL)	成人 T 淋巴细胞白血病

BIBLIOGRAPHY

1. Caldwell JC, Caldwell P: The African AIDS epidemic, *Sci Am* 274: 62-68, 1996.

2. Centers for Disease Control and Prevention: Updated U.S. Public Health Service guidelines for the management of exposures to HBV, HCV, and HIV and recommendations for postexposure prophylaxis, *MMWR Morb Mortal Recomm Rep* 50(RR-11): 1-42, 2001.

3. Cohen J, Powderly WG: *Infectious diseases*, ed 2, St Louis, 2004, Mosby.

4. Doltch G, Cavrois M, Lassen KG, et al: Abortive HIV infection mediates CD4 T cell depletion and inflammation in human lymphoid tissue, Cell 143: 789-801, 2010.

5. Flint SJ, Enquist LW, Racaniello VR, et al: *Principles of virology: molecular biology, pathogenesis and control of animal viruses*, ed 3, Washington, DC, 2009, American Society for Microbiology Press.

6. Knipe DM, Howley PM: *Fields virology*, ed 6, Philadelphia, 2013, Lippincott Williams & Wilkins.

7. Kräusslich HG: *Morphogenesis and maturation of retroviruses*, Berlin, 1996, Springer-Verlag.

8. Levy JA: *HIV and the pathogenesis of AIDS*, ed 7, Washington, DC, 2007, American Society for Microbiology Press.

9. Morse SA, Ballard RC, Holmes KK, et al: *Atlas of sexually transmitted diseases and AIDS*, ed 3, St Louis, 2003, Mosby.

10. Ng VL, McGrath MS: Human T-cell leukemia virus involvement in adult T-cell leukemia, *Cancer Bull* 40: 276-280, 1988.

11. Oldstone MBA, Vitkovic L: *HIV and dementia*, Berlin, 1995, Springer-Verlag.

12. Ryan FP: Human endogenous retroviruses in health and disease: a symbiotic perspective, *J R Soc Med* 97: 560-565, 2004.

13. Stine GJ: *AIDS update* 2011, New York, 2011, McGraw-Hill.

14. Strauss JM, Strauss EG: *Viruses and human disease*, ed 2, San Diego, 2007, Academic.

Hepatitis Viruses

The hepatitis alphabet of viruses includes at least six viruses, A through E, and G (Table 57-1). Although the target organ for each of these viruses is the liver and the basic hepatitis symptoms are similar, they differ greatly in their structure, mode of replication, mode of transmission, and in the time course and sequelae of the disease they cause. **Hepatitis A virus (HAV)** and **hepatitis B virus (HBV)** are the classic hepatitis viruses, and **hepatitis C, G, E, and hepatitis D virus (HDV)**, the delta agent, are called **non-A, non-B hepatitis (NANBH) viruses.** Other viruses can also cause hepatitis.

Each of the hepatitis viruses infects and damages the liver, causing the classic **icteric symptoms of jaundice and the release of liver enzymes.** The specific virus causing the disease can be distinguished by the course, nature, and serology of the disease. These viruses are readily spread because infected people are contagious before, or even without, showing symptoms.

Table 57-1 Comparative Features of Hepatitis Viruses.

Feature	Hepatitis A	Hepatitis B	Hepatitis C	Hepatitis D	Hepatitis E
Common name	"Infectious"	"Serum"	"Non-A, non-B posttransfusion"	"Delta agent"	"Enteric non-A, non-B"
Virus structure	Picornavirus; capsid, RNA	Hepadnavirus; envelope, DNA	Flavivirus; envelope, RNA	Viroid-like; envelope, circular RNA	Calicivirus-like capsid, RNA
Transmission	Fecal-oral	Parenteral, sexual	Parenteral, sexual	Parenteral, sexual	Fecal-oral
Onset	Abrupt	Insidious	Insidious	Abrupt	Abrupt
Incubation period (days)	15-50	45-160	14-180+	15-64	15-50
Severity	Mild	Occasionally severe	Usually subclinical; 70% chronicity	Co-infection with HBV occasionally severe; superinfection with HBV often severe	Normal patients, mild; pregnant women, severe
Mortality	<0.5%	1%-2%	≈4%	High to very high	Normal patients, 1%-2%; pregnant women, 20%
Chronicity/carrier state	No	Yes	Yes	Yes	No
Other disease associations	None	Primary hepatocellular carcinoma, cirrhosis	Primary hepatocellular carcinoma, cirrhosis	Cirrhosis, fulminant hepatitis	None
Laboratory diagnosis	Symptoms and anti-HAV IgM	Symptoms and serum levels of HBsAg, HBeAg, and anti-HBc IgM	Symptoms and anti-HCV ELISA	Anti-HDV ELISA	—

Hepatitis A, which is sometimes known as **infectious hepatitis,** (1) is caused by a picornavirus, a RNA virus; (2) is spread by the fecal-oral route; (3) has an incubation period of approximately 1 month, after which icteric symptoms start abruptly; (4) does not cause chronic liver disease; and (5) rarely causes fatal disease.

Hepatitis B, previously known as **serum hepatitis,** (1) is caused by a hepadnavirus with a DNA genome; (2) is spread parenterally by blood or needles, by sexual contact, and perinatally; (3) has a median incubation period of approximately 3 months, after which icteric symptoms start insidiously; (4) is followed by chronic hepatitis in 5% to 10% of patients; and (5) is causally associated with primary hepatocellular carcinoma (PHC). More than one third of the world's population has been infected with HBV, resulting in 1 to 2 million deaths per year. The incidence of HBV is decreasing, however, especially in infants, because of the development and use of the HBV subunit vaccine.

Hepatitis C virus (HCV) is also widely prevalent, with more than 170 million carriers of the disease. HCV is spread by the same routes as HBV but is more prone to cause chronic disease. HCV also increases risk for PHC. HCV is a flavivirus with an RNA genome. **Hepatitis G virus (HGV)** is also a flavivirus and causes chronic infections. **Hepatitis E virus (HEV)** is an enteric encapsidated virus with an RNA genome in its own family, and its disease resembles HAV.

Hepatitis D, or **delta hepatitis,** is unique in that it requires actively replicating HBV as a "helper virus" and occurs only in patients who have active HBV infection. HBV provides an envelope for HDV RNA and its antigens. HDV exacerbates the symptoms caused by HBV.

HEPATITIS A VIRUS

HAV causes infectious hepatitis and is spread by the fecal-oral route. HAV infections often result from consumption of contaminated water, shellfish, or other food. HAV is a **picornavirus** and was formerly called enterovirus 72, but it has been placed into a

new genus, *Heparnavirus*, on the basis of its unique genome.

Structure

HAV has a 27-nm, **naked, icosahedral capsid** surrounding a **positive-sense, single-stranded RNA** genome consisting of approximately 7470 nucleotides (Figure 57-1). The HAV genome has a VPg protein attached to the 5′ end and a polyadenylate sequence attached to the 3′ end. The capsid is even more stable than other picornaviruses to acid and other treatments. There is only one serotype of HAV.

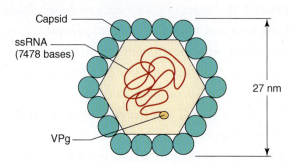

Capsid
ssRNA
(7478 bases)
27 nm
VPg

Figure 57-1 The picornavirus structure of hepatitis A virus. The icosahedral capsid is made up of four viral polypeptides (VP1 to VP4). Inside the capsid is a single-stranded, positive-sense ribonucleic acid *(ssRNA)* that has a genomic viral protein *(VPg)* on the 5′ end.

Replication

HAV replicates like other picornaviruses. It interacts specifically with the HAV cell receptor 1 glycoprotein (HAVCR-1), also known as T-cell immunoglobuluin and mucin domain protein (TIM-1), expressed on liver cells and T cells. The structure of HAVCR-1 can vary for different individuals, and specific forms correlate with severity of disease. Unlike other picornaviruses, however, HAV is not cytolytic and is released by exocytosis. Laboratory isolates of HAV have been adapted to grow in primary and continuous monkey kidney cell lines, but clinical isolates are difficult to grow in cell culture.

Pathogenesis

HAV is ingested and probably enters the bloodstream through the epithelial lining of the oropharynx or the intestines to reach its target, the parenchymal cells of the liver (Figure 57-2). The virus replicates in hepatocytes and Kupffer cells. Virus is produced in these cells and is released into the bile and from there into the stool. Virus is shed in large quantity into the stool approximately 10 days before symptoms of jaundice appear or antibody can be detected.

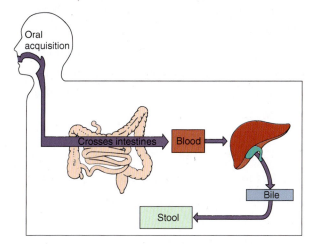

Figure 57-2   Spread of hepatitis A virus within the body.

HAV replicates slowly in the liver without producing apparent cytopathic effects. Although interferon limits viral replication, natural killer cells and cytotoxic T cells are required to eliminate infected cells. Antibody, complement, and antibody-dependent cellular cytotoxicity also facilitate clearance of the virus and induction of immunopathology. Icterus, resulting from damage to the liver, occurs when cell-mediated immune responses and antibody to the virus can be detected. Antibody protection against reinfection is lifelong.

The liver pathology caused by HAV infection is indistinguishable histologically from that caused by HBV. It is most likely caused by immunopathology and not virus-induced cytopathology. However, unlike HBV, HAV cannot initiate a chronic infection and is not associated with hepatic cancer.

Epidemiology

Approximately 40% of acute cases of hepatitis are caused by HAV (Box 57-2). The virus spreads readily in a community because most infected people are contagious 10 to 14 days before symptoms occur, and 90% of infected children and 25% to 50% of infected adults have **inapparent but productive** infections.

The virus is released into stool in high concentra-

tions and is spread via the **fecal-oral** route. Virus is spread in contaminated water, in food, and by dirty hands. HAV is resistant to detergents, acid (pH of 1), and temperatures as high as 60℃, and it can survive for many months in fresh water and salt water. Raw or improperly treated sewage can taint the water supply and contaminate shellfish. Shellfish, especially clams, oysters, and mussels, are important sources of the virus because they are efficient filter feeders and can therefore concentrate the viral particles, even from dilute solutions. This is exemplified by an epidemic of HAV that occurred in Shanghai, China in 1988, when 300,000 people were infected with the virus as the result of eating clams obtained from a polluted river.

HAV outbreaks usually originate from a common source (e.g., water supply, restaurant, day-care center). Asymptomatic shedding and a long (15 to 40 days) incubation period make it difficult to identify the source. Day-care settings are a major source for spread of the virus among classmates and their parents.

A relatively high incidence of HAV infection is directly related to poor hygienic conditions and overcrowding. Most people infected with HAV in developing countries are children who have mild illness and then lifelong immune protection against reinfection. In the populations of more highly developed countries, infection occurs later in life. The seropositivity rate of adults ranges from a low of 13% of the adult population in Sweden to highs of 88% in Taiwan and 97% in Yugoslavia, with a 41% to 44% rate in the United States.

Clinical Syndromes

The symptoms caused by HAV are very similar to those caused by HBV and stem from immune-mediated damage to the liver. As already noted, disease in children is generally milder than that in adults and is usually asymptomatic. The **symptoms occur abruptly** 15 to 50 days after exposure and intensify for 4 to 6 days before the icteric (jaundice) phase (Figure 57-3). Initial symptoms include fever, fatigue, nausea, loss of appetite, and abdominal pain. Dark urine (bilirubinuria), pale stool, and then jaundice may be accompanied by abdominal pain and itch. Jaundice is observed in 70% to 80% of adults but in only 10% of children (<6 years of age). Symptoms generally wane during the jaundice period. Viral shedding in the stool precedes the onset of symptoms by approximately 14 days but stops before the cessation of symptoms. Complete recovery occurs 99% of the time within 2 to 4 weeks of onset.

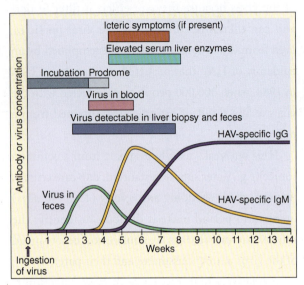

Figure 57-3 Time course of hepatitis A virus *(HAV)* infection. *IgG,* Immunoglobulin G; *IgM,* immunoglobulin M.

Fulminant hepatitis in HAV infection occurs in one to three persons per 1000 and is associated with an 80% mortality rate. Unlike HBV, immune complex-related symptoms (e.g., arthritis, rash) rarely occur in people with HAV disease.

Laboratory Diagnosis

The diagnosis of HAV infection is generally made on the basis of the time course of the clinical symptoms, the identification of a known infected source, and most reliably, the results yielded by specific serologic tests. The best way to demonstrate an acute HAV infection is by finding anti-HAV IgM, as measured by an enzyme-linked immunosorbent assay (ELISA) or radioimmunoassay. Virus isolation is not performed because efficient tissue culture systems for growing the virus are not available.

Treatment, Prevention, and Control

The spread of HAV is reduced by interrupting the

fecal-oral spread of the virus. This is accomplished by avoiding potentially contaminated water or food, especially uncooked shellfish. Proper hand washing, especially in day-care centers, mental hospitals, and other care facilities, is vitally important. Chlorine treatment of drinking water is generally sufficient to kill the virus.

Prophylaxis with immune serum globulin given before or early in the incubation period (i.e., less than 2 weeks after exposure) is 80% to 90% effective in preventing clinical illness.

Killed HAV vaccines are available for all children and for adults at high risk for infection, especially travelers to endemic regions. The vaccine is administered to infants at 2 years of age and can be administered with the HBV vaccine to adults. A live HAV vaccine is in use in China. There is only one serotype of HAV, and HAV infects only humans, factors that help ensure the success of an immunization program.

HEPATITIS B VIRUS

HBV is the major member of the hepadnaviruses. Other members of this family include woodchuck, ground squirrel, and duck hepatitis viruses. These viruses have limited tissue tropisms and host ranges. HBV infects the liver and, to a lesser extent, the kidneys and pancreas of only humans and chimpanzees. Advances in molecular biology have made it possible to study HBV despite the limited host range of the virus and difficult cell-culture systems in which to grow it.

Structure

HBV is a small, enveloped DNA virus with several unusual properties (Figure 57-4). Specifically, the genome is a small, circular, partly double-stranded DNA of only 3200 bases. Although a DNA virus, it encodes a reverse transcriptase and replicates through an RNA intermediate.

The virion, also called the Dane particle, is 42 nm in diameter. The virions are unusually stable for an enveloped virus. They resist treatment with ether, low pH, freezing, and moderate heating. These char-

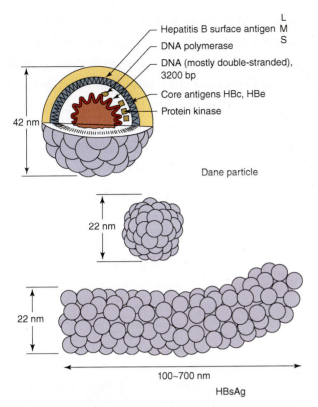

Figure 57-4 Hepatitis B virus (Dane particle) and hepatitis B surface antigen *(HBsAg)* particles. The spheric HBsAg consists mainly of the S form of HBsAg, with some M. The filamentous HBsAg has S, M, and L forms. *bp*, Base pair; *L*, gp42; *M*, gp36; *S*, gp27.

acteristics assist transmission from one person to another and hamper disinfection.

The HBV virion includes a protein kinase and a polymerase with reverse transcriptase and ribonuclease H activity, as well as a P protein attached to the genome. All of this is surrounded by an icosahedral capsid formed by the hepatitis B core antigen (HBcAg) and an envelope containing three forms of the glycoprotein hepatitis B surface antigen (HBsAg). A hepatitis Be antigen (HBeAg) protein shares most of its protein sequence with HBcAg but is processed differently by the cell, is primarily secreted into serum, does not self-assemble (like a capsid antigen), and expresses different antigenic determinants.

HBsAg-containing particles are released into the serum of infected people and outnumber the actual virions. These particles can be spheric (but smaller than the Dane particle) or filamentous (see Figure 57-4). They are immunogenic and were processed into the first commercial vaccine against HBV.

HBsAg, originally termed the Australia antigen,

includes three glycoproteins (L, M, and S) encoded by the same gene and read in the same frame but translated into protein from different AUG (adenine, uracil, guanine) start codons. The S (gp27; 24 to 27 kDa) glycoprotein is completely contained in the M (gp36; 33 to 36 kDa) glycoprotein, which is contained in the L (gp42; 39 to 42 kDa) glycoprotein; all share the same C-terminal amino acid sequences. All three forms of HBsAg are found in the virion. The S glycoprotein is the major component of HBsAg particles; it self-associates into 22-nm spheric particles that are released from the cells. The filamentous particles of HBsAg found in serum contain mostly S but also small amounts of the M and L glycoproteins and other proteins and lipids. The glycoproteins of HBsAg contain the group-specific (termed a) and type-specific determinants of HBV (termed d or y and w or r). Combinations of these antigens (e.g., ady and adw) result in eight subtypes of HBV that are useful epidemiologic markers.

Replication

The replication of HBV is unique for several reasons. First, HBV has a distinctly defined tropism for the liver. Its small genome also necessitates economy, as illustrated by the pattern of its transcription and translation. In addition, HBV replicates through an RNA intermediate and produces and releases antigenic decoy particles (HBsAg) (Figure 57-5).

The attachment of HBV to hepatocytes is mediated by the HBsAg glycoproteins. Several liver cell receptors have been suggested, including the transferrin receptor, the asialoglycoprotein receptor, and human liver annexin V. The mechanism of entry is not known, but HBsAg binds to polymerized human serum albumin and other serum proteins, and binding and uptake of these proteins may facilitate virus uptake by the liver.

On penetration into the cell, the partial DNA strand of the genome is completed by being formed into a complete double-stranded DNA circle, and the genome is delivered to the nucleus. Transcription of the genome is controlled by cellular transcription elements found in hepatocytes. The DNA is transcribed from different starting points on the circle but have the same 3′ end. There are three major classes (2100, 2400, and 3500 bases) and two minor classes (900 bases) of overlapping mRNAs (Figure 57-6). The 3500-base mRNA is larger than the genome. It encodes the HBc and HBe antigens, the polymerase, and a protein primer for DNA replication and acts as the template for replication of the genome. The HBe and HBc are related proteins that are translated from different in-phase start codons of closely related mRNA. This causes differences in their pro-

cessing and structure, with shedding of the HBe and incorporation of HBc into the virion. Similarly, the 2100-base mRNA encodes the small and medium glycoproteins from different in-phase start codons. The 2400-base mRNA, which encodes the large glycoprotein, overlaps the 2100-base mRNA. The 900-base mRNA encodes the X protein, which promotes viral replication as a transactivator of transcription and as a protein kinase.

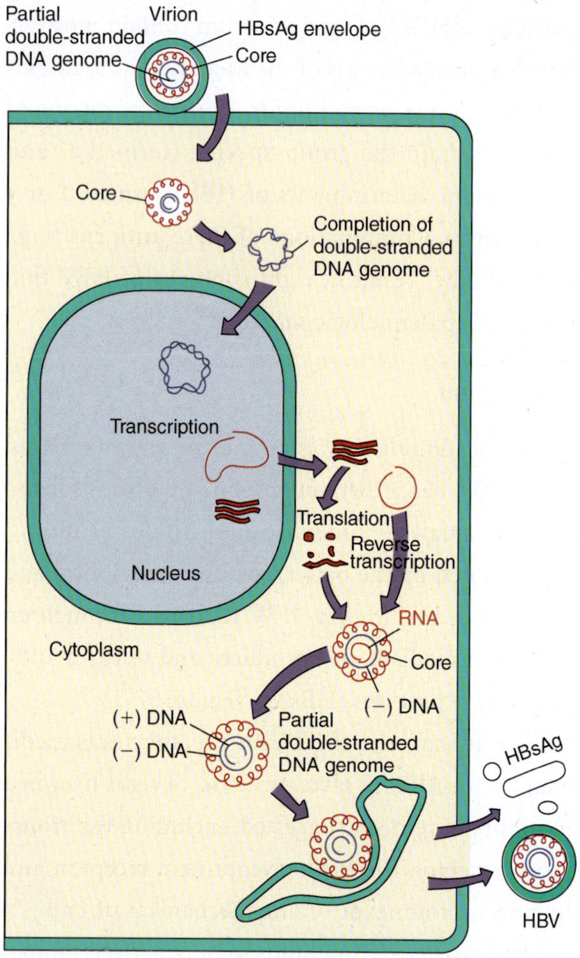

Figure 57-5 Replication of hepatitis B virus. After entry into the hepatocyte and uncoating of the nucleocapsid core, the partially double-stranded *DNA* genome is completed by enzymes in the core and then delivered to the nucleus. Transcription of the genome produces four mRNAs, including an mRNA larger than the genome (3500 bases). The mRNA then moves to the cytoplasm and is translated into protein. Core proteins assemble around the 3500-base mRNA, and negative-sense DNA is synthesized by a reverse transcriptase activity in the core. The RNAis then degraded as a positive-sense (+) DNA is synthesized. The core is enveloped before completion of the positive-sense DNA and then released by exocytosis. *HBsAg*, hepatitis B surface antigen.

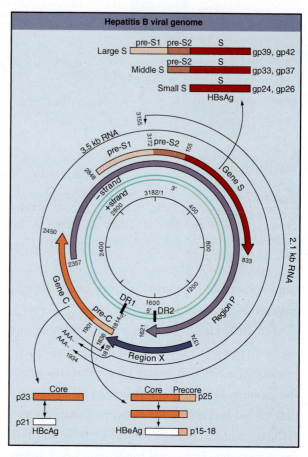

Figure 57-6 DNA, RNA, mRNA, and proteins of hepatitis B virus. The inner green circles represent the DNA genome with the nucleotide number at the center. DR1 and DR2 are direct repeat sequences of DNA and are important for replication and integration of the genome. The 3500-base transcript *(outer black thin-line circle)* is larger than the genome and is the template for replication of the genome. Bold arcs represent mRNA for viral proteins. Note that several proteins are translated from the same mRNA but from different AUG codons and that different mRNAs overlap. *AAA,* 3′ polyA (polyadenylate) at end of mRNA; *AUG,* adenine, uracil, guanine; *C,* C mRNA (hepatitis B core antigen, HBcAg); *E,* E mRNA (hepatitis B e antigen, HBeAg); *HBsAg,* hepatitis B surface antigen; *l,* large glycoprotein; *m,* medium glycoprotein; *P,* polymerase-protein primer for replication; *s,* small glycoprotein; *S,* S mRNA (HBsAg); *X,* X mRNA. (Modified from Armstrong D, Cohen J: *Infectious diseases,* St Louis, 1999, Mosby.)

Replication of the genome utilizes the larger-than-genome 3500-base mRNA. This is packaged into the core nucleocapsid that contains the RNA-dependent DNA polymerase (P protein). This polymerase has reverse transcriptase and ribonuclease H (RNase H) activity, but HBV lacks the integrase activity of the retroviruses. The 3500-base RNA acts as a template, and negative-strand DNA is synthesized using a protein primer from the P protein, which remains covalently attached to the 5′ end. After this, the RNA is degraded by the RNase H activity as the positive-strand DNA is synthesized from the negative-sense DNA template. However, this process is interrupted by envelopment of the nucleocapsid at HBsAg-containing intracellular membranes, thereby capturing genomes containing RNA-DNA circles with different lengths of RNA. Continued degradation of the remainder of the RNA in the virion yields a partly double-stranded DNA genome. The virion is then released from the hepatocyte by exocytosis without killing the cell, not by cell lysis.

The entire genome can also be integrated into the host cell chromatin. HBsAg, but not other proteins, can often be detected in the cytoplasm of cells containing integrated HBV DNA. The significance of the integrated DNA in the replication of the virus is not known, but integrated viral DNA has been found in hepatocellular carcinomas.

Pathogenesis and Immunity

HBV can cause acute or chronic, symptomatic or asymptomatic disease. Which of these occurs seems to be determined by the person's immune response to the infection (Figure 57-7). Detection of both the HBsAg and the HBeAg components of the virion in the blood indicates the existence of an ongoing active infection. HBsAg particles continue to be released into the blood, even after virion release has ended and until the infection is resolved.

The major source of infectious virus is blood, but HBV can be found in semen, saliva, milk, vaginal and menstrual secretions, and amniotic fluid. The most efficient way to acquire HBV is through injection of the virus into the bloodstream (Figure 57-8). Com-

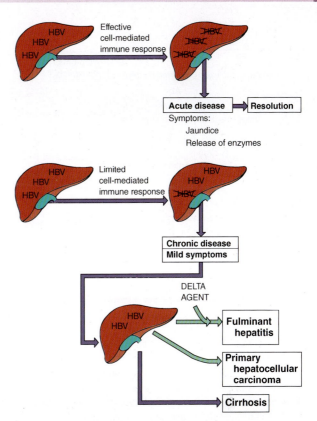

Figure 57-7   Major determinants of acute and chronic hepatitis B virus infection. HBV infects the liver but does not cause direct cytopathology. Cell-mediated immune lysis of infected cells produces the symptoms and resolves the infection. Insufficient immunity can lead to chronic disease. Chronic HBV disease predisposes a person to more serious outcomes. Purple arrows indicate symptoms; green arrows indicate a possible outcome.

mon but less efficient routes of infection are sexual contact and birth.

The virus starts to replicate in the liver within 3 days of its acquisition, but as already noted, symptoms may not be observed for 45 days or longer, depending on the infectious dose, the route of infection, and the person. The virus replicates in hepatocytes with minimal cytopathic effect. Infection proceeds for a relatively long time without causing liver damage (i.e., elevation of liver enzyme levels) or symptoms. During this time, copies of the HBV genome integrate into the hepatocyte chromatin and remain latent. Intracellular buildup of filamentous forms of HBsAg can produce the ground-glass hepatocyte cytopathology characteristic of HBV infection.

Cell-mediated immunity and inflammation are responsible for causing the symptoms and effecting resolution of the HBV infection by eliminating the

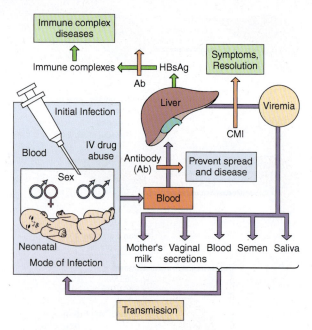

Figure 57-8   Spread of hepatitis B virus in the body. Initial infection with HBV occurs through injection, heterosexual and homosexual sex, and birth. The virus then spreads to the liver, replicates, induces a viremia, and is transmitted in various body secretions in addition to blood to start the cycle again. Symptoms are caused by cell-mediated immunity *(CMI)* and immune complexes between antibody and HBsAg. *IV,* Intravenous.

infected hepatocyte. Epitopes from the HBc antigen are prominent T-cell antigens. An insufficient T-cell response to the infection generally results in the occurrence of mild symptoms, an inability to resolve the infection, and the development of chronic hepatitis (see Figure 57-7). Chronic infection also exhausts CD8 T cells preventing them from killing infected cells. Antibody (as generated by vaccination) can protect against initial infection by preventing delivery of the virus to the liver. Later in the infection, the large amount of HBsAg in serum binds to and blocks the action of neutralizing antibody, which limits the antibody's capacity to resolve an infection. Immune complexes formed between HBsAg and anti-HBs contribute to the development of hypersensitivity reactions (type III), leading to problems such as vasculitis, arthralgia, rash, and renal damage.

Antibody to HBc is present in serum but is nonprotective. The HBeAg protein, like HBsAg, is released into serum, and, during its production, anti-HBeAg is bound to the antigen and undetectable.

Infants and young children have an immature cell-mediated immune response and are less able to resolve the infection, but they suffer less tissue damage and milder symptoms. As many as 90% of infants infected perinatally become chronic carriers. Viral replication persists in these people for long periods.

During the acute phase of infection, the liver parenchyma shows degenerative changes consisting of cellular swelling and necrosis, especially in hepatocytes surrounding the central vein of a hepatic lobule. The inflammatory cell infiltrate is mainly composed of lymphocytes. Resolution of the infection allows the parenchyma to regenerate. Fulminant infections, activation of chronic infections, or co-infection with the delta agent can lead to permanent liver damage and cirrhosis.

Epidemiology

In the United States, more than 12 million people have been infected with HBV (1 out of 20), with 5000 deaths per year. In the world, one out of three people have been infected with HBV, with approximately a million deaths per year. More than 350 million people worldwide have chronic HBV infection, and 120 million people have chronic HBV infection in China. In developing nations, as many as 15% of the population may be infected during birth or childhood. High rates of seropositivity are observed in Italy, Greece, Africa, and Southeast Asia (Figure 57-9). In some areas of the world (southern Africa and southeastern Asia), the seroconversion rate is as high as 50%. Primary hepatocellular carcinoma (HCC), a long-term sequela of the infection, is also endemic in these regions.

The many asymptomatic chronic carriers with virus in blood and other body secretions foster the spread of the virus. In the United States, 0.1% to 0.5% of the general population are chronic carriers, but this is very low in comparison with many areas of the world. Carrier status may be lifelong.

The virus is spread by sexual, parenteral, and perinatal routes. Transmission occurs through contaminated blood and blood components by transfusion, needle sharing, acupuncture, ear piercing, or tattooing, and through very close personal contact

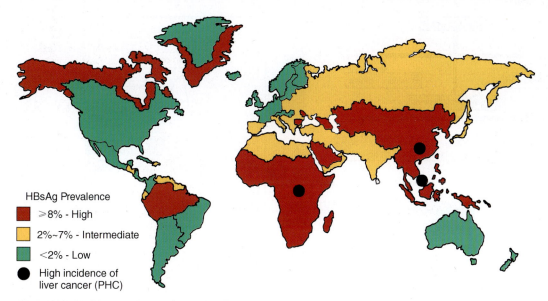

Figure 57-9   Worldwide prevalence of hepatitis B carriers and primary hepatocellular carcinoma *(PHC)*. (Courtesy Centers for Disease Control and Prevention, Atlanta.)

involving the exchange of semen, saliva, and vaginal secretions (e.g., sex, childbirth) (see Figure 57-8). Medical personnel are at risk in accidents involving needlesticks or sharp instruments. People at particular risk are listed in Box 57-4. Sexual promiscuity and drug abuse are major risk factors for HBV infection. HBV can be transmitted to babies through contact with the mother's blood at birth and in the mother's milk. Babies born to chronic HBV-positive mothers are at highest risk for infection. Serologic screening of donor units in blood banks has greatly reduced the risk of acquisition of the virus from contaminated blood or blood products. Safer sex habits adopted to prevent human immunodeficiency virus (HIV) transmission and the administration of the HBV vaccine have also been responsible for decreasing the transmission of HBV.

One of the major concerns about HBV is its association with PHC. This type of carcinoma probably accounts for 250,000 to 1 million deaths per year worldwide.

Clinical Syndromes

Acute Infection

As already noted, the clinical presentation of HBV in children is less severe than that in adults, and infection may even be asymptomatic. Clinically apparent

illness occurs in as many as 25% of those infected with HBV (Figures 57-10 to 57-12).

HBV infection is characterized by a long incubation period and an insidious onset. Symptoms during the prodromal period may include fever, malaise, and anorexia, followed by nausea, vomiting, abdominal discomfort, and chills. The classic icteric symptoms of liver damage (e.g., jaundice, dark urine, pale stools) follow soon thereafter. Recovery is indicated by a decline in the fever and renewed appetite.

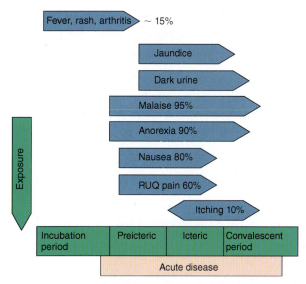

Figure 57-10   Symptoms of typical acute viral hepatitis B infection are correlated with the four clinical periods of this disease. *RUQ,* Right upper quadrant.(Modified from Hoofnagle JH: Type A and type B hepatitis, *Lab Med* 14: 705-716, 1983.)

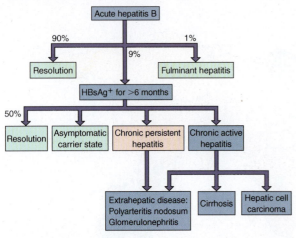

Figure 57-11 Clinical outcomes of acute hepatitis B infection. (Modified from White DO, Fenner F: *Medical virology,* ed 3, New York, 1986, Academic.)

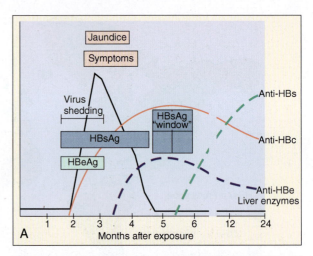

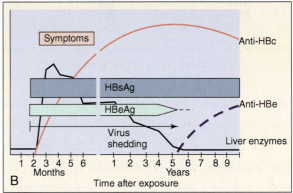

Figure 57-12 **A,** The serologic events associated with the typical course of acute hepatitis B disease. **B,** Development of the chronic hepatitis B virus carrier state. Routine serodiagnosis is difficult during the HBsAg window, when HBs and anti-HBs are undetectable. *Anti-HBc,* Antibody to HBcAg; *Anti-HBe,* antibody to HBeAg; *Anti-HBs,* antibody to HBsAg.(Modified from Hoofnagle JH: Serologic markers of hepatitis B virus infection, *Annu Rev Med* 32: 1-11, 1981.)

Fulminant hepatitis occurs in approximately 1% of icteric patients and may be fatal. It is marked by more severe symptoms and indications of severe liver damage, such as ascites and bleeding.

HBV infection can promote hypersensitivity reactions that are caused by immune complexes of HBsAg and antibody. These may produce rash, polyarthritis, fever, acute necrotizing vasculitis, and glomerulonephritis.

Chronic Infection

Chronic hepatitis occurs in 5% to 10% of people with HBV infections, usually after mild or inapparent initial disease. Approximately one third of these people have chronic active hepatitis with continued destruction of the liver leading to scarring of the liver, cirrhosis, liver failure, or PHC. The other two thirds have chronic passive hepatitis and are less likely to have problems. Chronic hepatitis may be detected accidentally by finding elevated liver enzyme levels on a routine blood chemistry profile. Chronically infected people are the major source for spread of the virus and are at risk for fulminant disease if they become co-infected with HDV.

Primary Hepatocellular Carcinoma

The World Health Organization (WHO) estimates that 80% of all cases of HCC can be attributed to chronic HBV infections. The HBV genome is inte-

grated into these HCC cells, and the cells express HBV antigens. HCC is usually fatal and is one of the three most common causes of cancer mortality in the world. In Taiwan, at least 15% of the population are carriers of HBV, and nearly half die of HCC or cirrhosis. HCC, like cervical cancer, is a vaccine-preventable human cancer.

HBV may induce HCC by promoting continued liver repair and cell growth in response to inflammation and tissue damage or by integrating into the host chromosome and stimulating cell growth directly. Such integration could stimulate genetic rearrangements or juxtapose viral promoters next to cellular growth-controlling genes. Alternatively, a protein encoded by the HBV X gene may transactivate (turn on) the transcription of cellular proteins and stimulate cell growth. The presence of the HBV genome may allow a subsequent mutation to promote carcinogenesis. The latency period between HBV infection and HCC may be as short as 9 years or as long as 35 years.

Laboratory Diagnosis

The initial diagnosis of hepatitis can be made on the basis of the clinical symptoms and the presence of liver enzymes in the blood (see Figure 57-12). However, the serology of HBV infection describes the course and the nature of the disease (Table 57-2). Acute and chronic HBV infections can be distinguished by the presence of HBsAg and HBeAg in the serum and the pattern of antibodies to the individual HBV antigens.

HBsAg and HBeAg are secreted into the blood during viral replication. The detection of HBeAg is the best correlate to the presence of infectious virus. A chronic infection can be distinguished by the continued finding of HBeAg, HBsAg, or both, and a lack of detectable antibody to these antigens. Antibody to HBsAg indicates resolution of infection or vaccination.

Antibody to HBcAg indicates current or prior infection by HBV and IgM anti-HBc is the best way to diagnose a recent acute infection, especially during the period when neither HBsAg nor anti-HBs can be detected (the window). Detection of antibodies to HBeAg and HBsAg is obscured during infection because the antibody is complexed with antigen in the serum.

The amount of virus in blood can be determined by quantitative genome assays using PCR and related techniques. Knowing the virus load can help in following the course of chronic HBV infection and antiviral drug efficacy.

Treatment, Prevention, and Control

Hepatitis B immune globulin may be administered within a week of exposure and to newborn infants of HBsAg-positive mothers to prevent and ameliorate disease. Chronic HBV infection can be treated with drugs targeted at the polymerase—for example, lamivudine (2'3'dideoxy-3'-thiacytidine), which is also an HIV reverse transcriptase inhibitor—or the nucleoside analogues, adefovir dipivoxil and famciclovir. These FDA-approved treatments are taken for 1 year. Unfortunately, antiviral drug resistance can develop. Pegylated interferon-α can also be effective and is taken for at least 4 months.

Transmission of HBV in blood or blood products has been greatly reduced by screening donated blood for the presence of HBsAg and anti-HBc. Additional efforts to prevent transmission of HBV consist of avoiding sex with a carrier of HBV and avoiding the lifestyles that facilitate spread of the virus. Household contacts and sexual partners of HBV carriers are at increased risk, as are patients undergoing hemodialysis, recipients of pooled plasma products, health care workers exposed to blood, and babies born to HBV-carrier mothers.

Vaccination is recommended for infants, children, and especially people in high-risk groups. For new-

Table 57-2　Interpretation of Serologic Markers of Hepatitis B Virus Infection

Serologic Reactivity	Disease State					Healthy State	
	Early (Presymptomatic)	Early Acute	Acute	Chronic	Late Acute	Resolved	Vaccinated
Anti-HBc	−	−	−*	+	+/−	+	−
Anti-HBe	−	−	−	−	+/−	+/−†	−
Anti-HBs	−	−	−	−	−	+	+
HBeAg	−	+	+	+	−	−	−
HBsAg	+	+	+	+	+	−	−
Infectious virus	+	+	+	+	+	−	−

*Anti-HBc immunoglobulin M should be present.
†Anti-HBe may be negative after chronic disease.

borns of HBsAg-positive mothers and people accidentally exposed either percutaneously or permucosally to blood or secretions from an HBsAg-positive person, vaccination is useful even after exposure. Immunization of mothers should decrease the incidence of transmission to babies and older children, also reducing the number of chronic HBV carriers. Prevention of chronic HBV will reduce the incidence of HCC.

The HBV vaccines form virus-like particles. The initial HBV vaccine was derived from the 22-nm HBsAg particles in human plasma obtained from chronically infected people. The current vaccine was genetically engineered by the insertion of a plasmid containing the S gene for HBsAg into a yeast, *Saccharomyces cerevisiae*. The protein self-assembles into particles, which enhances its immunogenicity.

The vaccine must be given in a series of three injections, with the second and third given 1 and 6 months after the first. The single serotype and limited host range (humans) help ensure the success of an immunization program.

Universal blood and body fluid precautions are used to limit exposure to HBV. It is assumed that all patients are infected. Gloves are required for handling blood and body fluids; wearing protective clothing and eye protection may also be necessary. Special care should be taken with needles and sharp instruments. HBV-contaminated materials can be disinfected with 10% bleach solutions, but unlike most enveloped viruses, HBV is not readily inactivated by detergents.

HEPATITIS C AND G VIRUSES

HCV was identified in 1989 after isolation of a viral RNA from a chimpanzee infected with blood from a person with NANBH. The viral RNA obtained from blood was converted to DNA with reverse transcriptase, its proteins were expressed, and antibodies from people with NANBH were then used to detect the viral proteins. These studies led to the development of ELISA and genomic and other tests for detection of the virus, which still cannot be grown in tissue culture.

HCV is the predominant cause of NANBH virus infections and was the major cause of posttransfusion hepatitis before routine screening of the blood supply for HCV. There are more than 170 million carriers of HCV in the world and more than 4 million in the United States. HCV is transmitted by means similar to HBV but has an even greater potential for establishing persistent, chronic hepatitis. Many HCV infected individuals are also infected with HBV or HIV. The chronic hepatitis often leads to cirrhosis and potentially to hepatocellular carcinoma. The significance of the HCV epidemic has become more apparent with the development of laboratory screening procedures.

Structure and Replication

HCV is the only member of the *Hepacivirus* genus of the Flaviviridae family. It is 30 to 60 nm in diameter, has a positive-sense RNA genome, and is enveloped. The genome of HCV (9100 nucleotides) encodes 10 proteins, including two glycoproteins (E1, E2). The viral RNA-dependent RNA polymerase is error prone and generates mutations in the glycoprotein and other genes. This generates antigenic variability. Such variability makes the development of a vaccine very difficult. There are six major groups of variants (clades), which differ in their worldwide distribution.

HCV infects only humans and chimpanzees. HCV binds to CD81 (tetraspanin) surface receptors, which is expressed on hepatocytes and B lymphocytes, and can also coat itself with low-density lipoprotein or very-low-density lipoprotein and then use the lipoprotein receptor to facilitate uptake into hepatocytes. The virus replicates like other flaviviruses. The virion assembles at and buds into the endoplasmic reticulum, becoming cell associated. HCV proteins inhibit apoptosis and interferon-α action by binding to the tumor necrosis factor receptor and to protein kinase R. These actions prevent the death of the host cell and promote persistent infection.

Pathogenesis

The ability of HCV to remain cell associated and prevent host cell death promotes persistent infection but results in liver disease later in life. Cell-mediated immune responses are responsible for both the resolution of infection and tissue damage. As for HBV, chronic infection can exhaust CD8 cytotoxic T cells to prevent resolution of infection. The extent of lymphocytic infiltration, inflammation, portal and periportal fibrosis, and lobular necrosis in liver biopsies can be used to grade the severity of disease. It has been suggested that the cytokines of inflammation and continual liver repair and induction of cell growth occurring during chronic HCV infection are predisposing factors in the development of PHC. Antibody to HCV is not protective.

Epidemiology

HCV is transmitted primarily in infected blood and sexually. Intravenous drug abusers, tattoo recipients, transfusion and organ recipients, and hemophiliacs receiving factors VIII or IX are at highest risk for infection. Almost all (>90%) HIV-infected people who are or were intravenous drug users are infected with HCV. HCV is especially prevalent in southern Italy, Spain, central Europe, Japan, and parts of the Middle East (e.g., almost 20% of Egyptian blood donors are HCV positive). More than 40 million people are infected with HCV in China. The high incidence of chronic asymptomatic infections promotes the spread of the virus in the population. Screening procedures have led to a reduction in the levels of transmission by blood transfusion and organ donation, but transmission by other routes is prevalent.

Clinical Syndromes

HCV causes three types of disease (Figure 57-13): (1) acute hepatitis with resolution of the infection and recovery in 15% of cases, (2) chronic persistent infection with possible progression to disease much later in life for 70% of infected persons, and (3) severe rapid progression to cirrhosis in 15% of patients. A viremia can be detected within 1 to 3 weeks of a transfusion of HCV-contaminated blood. The viremia lasts 4 to 6 months in people with an acute infection and longer than 10 years in those

with a persistent infection. In its acute form, HCV infection is similar to acute HAV and HBV infection, but the inflammatory response is less intense, and the symptoms are usually milder. More commonly (>70% of cases), the initial disease is asymptomatic but establishes chronic persistent disease. The predominant symptom is chronic fatigue. The chronic, persistent disease often progresses to chronic active hepatitis within 10 to 15 years and to cirrhosis (20% of chronic cases) and liver failure (20% of cirrhotic cases) after 20 years. HCV-induced liver damage may be exacerbated by alcohol, certain medications, and other hepatitis viruses to promote cirrhosis. HCV promotes the development of hepatocellular carcinoma after 30 years in up to 5% of chronically infected patients.

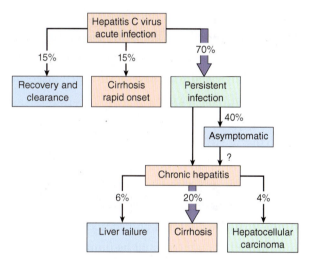

Figure 57-13 Outcomes of hepatitis C virus infection.

Laboratory Diagnosis

The diagnosis and detection of HCV infection are based on ELISA recognition of anti-HCV antibody or detection of the RNA genome. Seroconversion occurs within 7 to 31 weeks of infection. ELISA is used for screening the blood supply from normal donors. As for HIV, results can be confirmed by Western immunoblot procedures. Antibody is not always detectable in viremic people, in immunocompromised patients, or in those receiving hemodialysis. Genome detection and quantitation by RT-PCR, branched-chain DNA, and related techniques is the gold standard for confirming a diagnosis of HCV and for following the success of antiviral drug therapy. Genetic assays are less strain specific and can detect HCV RNA in sero-negative people.

Treatment, Prevention, and Control

Recombinant interferon-α or pegylated interferon (treated with polyethylene glycol to enhance its biologic lifetime), alone or with ribavirin, were the only known treatments for HCV. Treatment with pegylated interferon and ribavirin for extended periods may yield up to 50% recovery rates. This therapy can now be supplemented with either of two protease inhibitors, boceprevir or telaprevir. As for HIV, the addition of a protease inhibitor to the previous antiviral protocol is expected to make a significant difference in therapeutic efficacy.

Sofosbuvir, Harvoni, Epclusa which can inhibit the polymerase in HCV are newly discovered antiviral drugs, the recovery rates after medication are relatively high and they have been widely used in treatment of HCV infection.

The precautions for transmission of HCV are similar to that of HBV and other blood-borne pathogens. The blood supply and organ donors are screened for HCV. Persons with HCV should not share any personal care items and syringe needles that may get contaminated with blood and should practice safe sex. Alcohol drinking should be limited because it exacerbates the liver damage caused by HCV.

HEPATITIS G VIRUS

HGV (also known as GB virus-C, GBV-C) resembles HCV in many ways. HGV is a flavivirus, is transmitted in blood and has a predilection for chronic hepatitis infection. It is identified by detection of the genome by RT-PCR or other RNA detection methods.

HEPATITIS D VIRUS

Approximately 15 million people in the world are infected with HDV (delta agent), and the virus is responsible for causing 40% of fulminant hepatitis

infections. HDV is unique in that it uses HBV and target cell proteins to replicate and produce its one protein. It is a viral parasite, proving that "even fleas have fleas." HBsAg is essential for packaging the virus. The delta agent resembles plant virus satellite agents and viroids in its size, genomic structure, and requirement for a helper virus for replication (Figure 57-14).

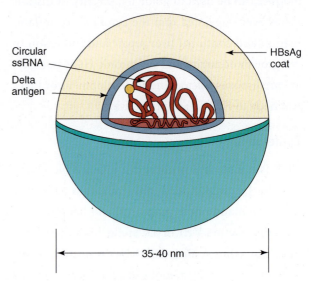

Figure 57-14 The delta hepatitis virion. *HBsAg*, Hepatitis B surface antigen; *ssRNA*, single-stranded RNA.

Structure and Replication

The HDV RNA genome is very small (approximately 1700 nucleotides), and unlike other viruses, the single-stranded RNA is circular and forms a rod shape as a result of its extensive base pairing. The virion is approximately the same size as the HBV virion (35 to 37 nm in diameter). The genome is surrounded by the delta antigen core, which in turn is surrounded by an HBsAg-containing envelope. The delta antigen exists as a small (24 kDa) or large (27 kDa) form; the small form is predominant.

The delta agent binds to and is internalized by hepatocytes in the same manner as HBV because it has HBsAg in its envelope. The transcription and replication processes of the HDV genome are unusual. The host cell's RNA polymerase II makes an RNA copy to replicate the genome. The genome then forms an RNA structure called a ribozyme, which cleaves the RNA circle to produce an mRNA for the small delta antigen. The gene for the delta antigen is mutated by a cellular enzyme (double-stranded RNA-activated adenosine deaminase) during infection, thereby allowing production of the large delta antigen. Production of this antigen limits replication of the virus but also promotes association of the genome with HBsAg to form a virion, and the virus is then released from the cell.

Pathogenesis

Similar to HBV, the delta agent is spread in blood, semen, and vaginal secretions. However, it can replicate and cause disease only in people with active HBV infections. Because the two agents are transmitted by the same routes, a person can be co-infected with HBV and the delta agent. A person with chronic HBV can also be superinfected with the delta agent. More rapid, severe progression occurs in HBV carriers superinfected with HDV than in people co-infected with HBV and the delta agent because, during co-infection, HBV must first establish its infection before HDV can replicate (Figure 57-15), whereas superinfection of an HBV-infected person allows the delta agent to replicate immediately.

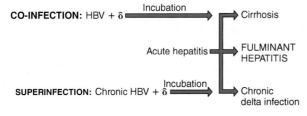

Figure 57-15   Consequences of delta virus infection. Delta virus *(δ)* requires the presence of hepatitis B virus infection. Superinfection of a person already infected with HBV (carrier) causes more rapid, severe progression than co-infection *(shorter arrow)*.

Replication of the delta agent results in cytotoxicity and liver damage. Persistent delta agent infection is often established in HBV carriers. Although antibodies are elicited against the delta agent, protection probably stems from the immune response to HBsAg because it is the external antigen and viral attachment protein for HDV. Unlike HBV disease, damage to the liver occurs as a result of the direct cytopathic effect of the delta agent combined with the underlying immunopathology of the HBV disease.

Epidemiology

The delta agent infects children and adults with underlying HBV infection, and people who are persistently infected with both HBV and HDV are a source for the virus. The agent has a worldwide distribution, infecting approximately 5% of the 3×10^8 HBV carriers and is endemic in southern Italy, the Amazon Basin, parts of Africa, and the Middle East. Epidemics of HDV infection occur in North America and Western Europe, usually in illicit drug users. HDV is spread by the same routes as HBV, and the same groups are at risk for infection, with parenteral drug abusers, hemophiliacs, and others receiving blood products at highest risk. Screening of the blood supply has reduced the risk for recipients of blood products.

Clinical Syndromes

The delta agent increases the severity of HBV infections. Fulminant hepatitis is more likely to develop in people infected with the delta agent than in those infected with the other hepatitis viruses. This very severe form of hepatitis causes altered brain function (hepatic encephalopathy), extensive jaundice, and massive hepatic necrosis, which is fatal in 80% of cases. Chronic infection with the delta agent can occur in people with chronic HBV.

Laboratory Diagnosis

The presence of the agent can be noted by detecting the RNA genome, the delta antigen, or anti-HDV antibodies. ELISA and radioimmunoassay procedures are available for detection. The delta antigen can be detected in the blood during the acute phase of disease in a detergent-treated serum sample. RT-PCR techniques can be used to detect the virion genome in blood.

Treatment, Prevention, and Control

There is no known specific treatment for HDV hepatitis. Because the delta agent depends on HBV for replication and is spread by the same routes, prevention of infection with HBV prevents HDV infection.

Immunization with HBV vaccine protects against subsequent delta virus infection. If a person has already acquired HBV, delta agent infection may be prevented by halting illicit intravenous drug use and avoiding HDV-contaminated blood products.

HEPATITIS E VIRUS

HEV (E-NANBH) (the E stands for enteric or epidemic) is predominantly spread by the fecal-oral route, especially in contaminated water. HEV is unique but resembles the caliciviruses, based on its size (27 to 34 nm) and structure. Although HEV is found throughout the world, it is most problematic in developing countries. Epidemics have been reported in India, Pakistan, Nepal, Burma, North Africa, and Mexico.

The symptoms and course of HEV disease are similar to those of HAV disease; it causes only acute disease. However, the symptoms for HEV may occur later than those of HAV disease. The mortality rate associated with HEV disease is 1% to 2%, approximately 10 times that associated with HAV disease. HEV infection is especially serious in pregnant women (mortality rate of approximately 20%).

SUMMARY

Hepatitis A is caused by hepatitis A virus (HAV) which is unenveloped RNA virus belonging to the *Picornaviridae* family, genus *Heparnavirus*. It is spread by the fecal-oral route and has an incubation period of approximately one month, after which icteric symptoms start abruptly. HAV does not cause chronic liver disease and rarely causes fatal disease.

Hepatitis B is caused by hepatitis B virus (HBV) which is a hepadnavirus with a partially double stranded DNA genome. HBV is spread parenterally by blood or needles, by sexual contact, and perinatally. Hepatitis B has a median incubation period of approximately three months, after which icteric symptoms start insidiously. It is followed by chronic hepatitis in 5% to 10% of patients; and is causally associated with primary hepatocellular carcinoma (HCC).

More than one third of the world's population has been infected with HBV, resulting in 1 to 2 million deaths per year. The incidence of HBV is decreasing, however, especially in infants, because of the development and use of the HBV subunit vaccine.

Hepatitis C is caused by hepatitis C virus (HCV), a flavivirus with an RNA genome. HCV is also widely prevalent. HCV is spread by the same routes as HBV but is more prone to cause chronic disease. HCV also increases risk for HCC.

Hepatitis D virus (HDV), or delta hepatitis virus, is unique in that it requires actively replicating HBV as a "helper virus" and occurs only in patients who have active HBV infection. HBV provides an envelope for HDV RNA and its antigens. HDV exacerbates the symptoms caused by HBV.

Hepatitis E is caused by hepatitis E virus (HEV), which is an enteric encapsidated virus with an RNA genome in its own family, and its disease resembles HAV.

KEYWORDS

English	Chinese
Hepatitis	肝炎
Hepadnavirus	嗜肝 DNA 病毒
Hepatitis B surface antigen	乙肝表面抗原
Hepatitis B core antigen	乙肝核心抗原
Hepatitis B e antigen	乙肝 e 抗原
Superinfection	重叠感染
Hepatocellular carcinoma	肝细胞癌

BIBLIOGRAPHY

1. Blum HE, Gerok W, Vyas GN: The molecular biology of hepatitis B virus, Trends Genet 5: 154-158, 1989.
2. Cann AJ: Principles of molecular virology, San Diego, 2005, Academic.
3. Carter J, Saunders V: Virology: principles and applications, Chichester, England, 2007, Wiley.
4. Casey JL: Hepatitis delta virus, *Curr Top Microbiol Immunol*, vol 307, Heidelberg, Germany, 2006, Springer-Verlag.
5. Catalina G, Navarro V: Hepatitis C: a challenge for the generalist, Hosp Pract 35: 97-108, 2000.
6. Cohen J, Powderly WG: Infectious diseases, ed 2, St Louis, 2004, Mosby.

7. Collier L, Oxford J: Human virology, ed 3, Oxford, England, 2006, Oxford University Press.

8. Fallows DA, Goff AP: Hepadnaviruses: current models of RNA encapsidation and reverse transcription, Adv Virus Res 46: 167-196, 1996.

9. Flint SJ, et al: Principles of virology: molecular biology, pathogenesis and control of animal viruses, ed 3, Washington, DC, 2009, American Society for Microbiology Press.

10. Ganem D, Prince AM: Hepatitis B virus infection—natural history and clinical consequences, N Engl J Med 350: 1118-1119, 2004.

11. Hagedorn CH, Rice CM: The hepatitis C viruses, *Curr Top Microbiol Immunol*, vol 242, Berlin, 2000, Springer-Verlag.

12. Hoofnagle JH: Type A and type B hepatitis, Lab Med 14: 705-716, 1983.

13. Knipe DM, et al: Fields virology, ed 5, Philadelphia, 2006, Lippincott Williams & Wilkins.

14. Lauer GM, Walker BD: Medical progress: hepatitis C virus infection, N Engl J Med 345: 41-52, 2001.

15. Lok ASF: Chronic hepatitis B, N Engl J Med 346: 1682-1683, 2002.

16. Mason WS, Seeger C: Hepadnaviruses: molecular biology and pathogenesis, *Curr Top Microbiol Immunol*, vol 162, Berlin, 1991, Springer-Verlag.

17. Murray PR, et al: Manual of clinical microbiology, ed 9, Washington, DC, 2007, American Society for Microbiology Press.

18. Plageman PGW: Hepatitis C virus, Arch Virol 120: 165-180, 1991.

19. Robinson W, Koike K, Will H: Hepadnavirus, New York, 1987, Liss.

20. Strauss JM, Strauss EG: Viruses and human disease, ed 2, San Diego, 2007, Academic.

21. Tam AW, et al: Hepatitis E virus: molecular cloning and sequencing of the full-length viral genome, Virology 185: 120-131, 1991.

22. Taylor JM: Hepatitis delta virus, Virology 344: 71-76, 2006.

23. Voyles BA: The biology of viruses, ed 2, Boston, 2002, McGraw-Hill.

Prions

Prion causes spongiform encephalopathies, which are slow neurodegenerative diseases. These disorders include the human diseases kuru, Creutzfeldt-Jakob disease (CJD), variant CJD (vCJD), Gerstmann-Sträussler-Scheinker (GSS) syndrome, fatal familial insomnia (FFI), and sporadic fatal insomnia. The animal diseases include scrapie, bovine spongiform encephalopathy (BSE) (mad cow disease), chronic wasting disease (in mule, deer, and elk), and transmissible mink encephalopathy.

Prion, known as **a small proteinaceous infectious particle,** is a mutant or conformationally distinct form of a host protein. Prion is filterable and can transmit disease but otherwise do not conform to the standard definition of a virus (Table 58-1). Unlike viruses, prion has no virion structure or genome, elicit no immune response, and are extremely resistant to inactivation by heat, disinfectants, and radiation.

After long incubation periods, prion causes damage to the central nervous system, leading to a subacute spongiform encephalopathy. The long incubation period, which can last 30 years in humans, has made study of these agents difficult. Carlton Gajdusek won the Nobel Prize for showing that kuru has an infectious etiology and for developing a method for analyzing the agent. Stanley Prusiner won the Nobel Prize in 1997 for developing a hamster infection model for the scrapie agent. He and his coworkers were able to purify, characterize, and then clone the genes for the scrapie and other prion agents and show that the disease-related prion protein is sufficient to cause disease.

STRUCTURE AND PHYSIOLOGY

Unlike conventional viruses, the prion agents are resistant to a wide range of chemical and physical treatments, such as formaldehyde, ultraviolet radiation, and heat up to 80℃.

The prion, which lacks detectable nucleic acids, consists of aggregates of a protease-resistant, hydrophobic glycoprotein termed PrP^{Sc} (scrapie-like prion protein) (27,000 to 30,000 Da). Humans and other animals encode a protein PrP^{C} (cellular prion protein) of unknown function that is held in the cell membrane by a linkage between its terminal serine and a special lipid, glycophosphatidylinositol (GPI-linked protein). The PrP^{C} is closely related or can be identical to PrP^{Sc} in its protein sequence but differs in tertiary structure because of differences in the folding

Table 58-1 Comparison of Classic Viruses and Prions.

	Virus	Prion
Filterable, infectious agents	Yes	Yes
Presence of nucleic acid	Yes	No
Defined morphology (electron microscopy)	Yes	No
Presence of protein	Yes	Yes
Disinfection by:		
Formaldehyde	Yes	No
Proteases	Some	No
Heat (80℃)	Most	No
Ionizing and ultraviolet radiation	Yes	No
Disease		
Cytopathologic effect	Yes	No
Incubation period	Depends on virus	Long
Immune response	Yes	No
Interferon production	Yes	No
Inflammatory response	Yes	No

of the proteins (Table 58-2). PrP^{Sc} is protease resistant, aggregates into amyloid rods (fibrils) and is cell free. The normal PrP^C, on the other hand, is protease sensitive and appears on the cell surface.

Table 58-2 Comparison of Scrapie Prion Protein (PrP^{Sc}) and (Normal) Cellular Prion Protein (PrP^C)

	PrP^{Sc}	PrP^C
Structure	Multimeric	Monomeric
Protease resistance	Yes	No
Presence in scrapie fibrils	Yes	No
Location in or on cells	Cytoplasmic vesicles and extracellular milieu	Plasma membrane
Turnover	Days	Hours

The current theory to explain how an aberrant protein could cause disease is called template-mediated protein refolding. A linear aggregate of PrP^{Sc} binds to an anionic structure on the cell surface, such as a glycosaminoglycan and the normal PrP^C on the cell surface. This causes the PrP^C to refold, acquire the structure of PrP^{Sc}, and join the chain. The alpha helical structure of the PrP^C is changed to a more beta-pleated sheet structure of the PrP^{Sc}. When the string of PrP^{Sc} breaks, it creates new primers upon which more prions can be built. The PrP^C continue to be made by the cell, and as they bind to the PrP^{Sc} primers, the cycle continues. The fact that these plaques consist of host protein may explain the lack of an immune response to these agents in patients with the spongiform encephalopathies.

Different strains of PrP^{Sc} occur because of mutations in the PrP^C or because of self-perpetuating alternative folding patterns of the protein. Specific mutations at codon 129 determine the severity of vCJD disease. Conformational, rather than genetic, mutation is another property that distinguishes prions from viruses. When the PrP^{Sc} aggregates, the PrP^{Sc} acts as a template to transmit its conformation onto each new PrP^{Sc}, analogous to a genetic template (DNA or RNA) transmitting its sequence onto a new viral genome. The different conformational strains can have different properties and varying disease aspects (e.g., incubation period).

PATHOGENESIS

Spongiform encephalopathy describes the appearance of the vacuolated neurons, as well as their loss of function and the lack of an immune response or inflammation. Vacuolation of the neurons, the formation of amyloid-containing plaques and fibrils, a proliferation and hypertrophy of astrocytes, and the vacuolation of neurons and adjacent glial cells are observed (Figure 58-1). The PrP^{Sc} is taken up by neurons and phagocytic cells but is difficult to degrade, a feature that may contribute to the vacuolation of the brain tissue. A protein marker (14-3-3 brain protein) can be detected in the cerebrospinal fluid of symptomatic persons, but this is not specific for prion disease.

The incubation period for CJD and kuru may be as long as 30 years, but once the symptoms become evident, disease progresses rapidly, and death usually occurs within a year.

EPIDEMIOLOGY

CJD is transmitted predominantly by (1) injection, (2) transplantation of contaminated tissue (e.g., corneas), (3) contact with contaminated medical devices (e.g., brain electrodes), and (4) food. CJD usually affects persons older than 50 years. CJD, FFI, and GSS syndrome are also inheritable, and families with genetic histories of these diseases have been identified. The diseases are rare but occur worldwide.

Kuru was limited to a very small area of the New Guinea highlands. The name of the disease means "shivering" or "trembling," and the disease was related to the cannibalistic practices of the Fore tribe of New Guinea. Before Gajdusek intervened, it was the custom of these people to eat the bodies of their deceased kinsmen. Their risk for infection was higher because they handled the contaminated tissue, making it possible for the agent to be introduced through the conjunctiva or cuts in the skin. Cessation of this cannibalistic custom has stopped the spread of kuru.

An epidemic of BSE (mad cow disease) in 1980 in the United Kingdom and the unusual incidence of

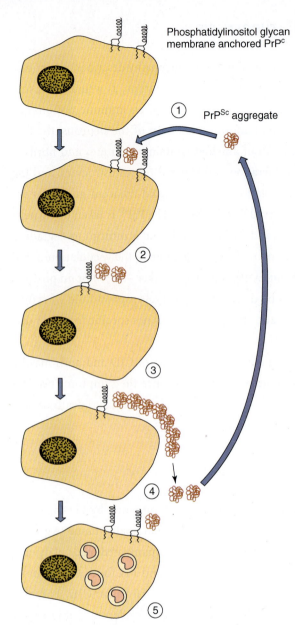

Figure 58-1 Template-mediated protein refolding model for proliferation of prions. PrP^C is a normal cellular protein that is anchored in the cell membrane by phosphatidylinositol glycan. PrP^Sc is a hydrophobic globular protein that aggregates with itself and with PrP^C on the cell surface *(1)*. PrP^C acquires the conformation of PrP^Sc *(2)*. The cell synthesizes new PrP^C *(3)*, and a chain is built along cell surface anionic glycosaminoglycans *(4)*. The chain breaks upon phagocytosis or from shear forces and releases PrP^Sc aggregates that act like seed crystals to start the cycle over. A form of PrP^Sc is internalized by neuronal cells and accumulates *(5)*. Other models have been proposed.

a more rapidly progressing CJD in younger people (younger than 45 years) in 1996 prompted concern that contaminated beef was the source of this new variant of CJD. Infection of cattle is most likely caused by the use of contaminated animal byprod-

ucts (e.g., sheep entrails, brains) as a protein supplement in cattle feed.

In addition to infection, prion diseases can also be familial (genetic) or sporadic, with no known history of exposure. GSS syndrome and FFI are familial prion diseases.

CLINICAL SYNDROMES

As already noted, the slow virus agents cause a progressive, degenerative neurologic disease with a long incubation period but with rapid progression to death after the onset of symptoms (Figure 58-2). The spongiform encephalopathies are characterized by a loss of muscle control, shivering, myoclonic jerks and tremors, loss of coordination, rapidly progressive dementia, and death.

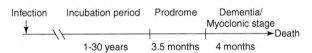

Figure 58-2 Progression of transmissible Creutzfeldt-Jakob disease.

LABORATORY DIAGNOSIS

There are no methods for directly detecting prions in tissue through the use of electron microscopy, antigen detection, or nucleic acid probes. Also, no serologic tests can detect antiprion antibody. The initial diagnosis must be made on clinical grounds. Confirmation of the diagnosis can be made by detection of a proteinase K-resistant form of PrP in a Western blot using antibody to PrP in a tonsil biopsy.

TREATMENT, PREVENTION, AND CONTROL

No treatment exists for kuru or CJD. The causative agents are also impervious to the disinfection procedures used for other viruses, including formaldehyde, detergents, and ionizing radiation. Autoclaving at 15 psi for 1 hour (instead of 20 minutes) or treatment with 5% hypochlorite solution or 1.0 M sodium hydroxide can be used for decontamination. Because these agents can be transmitted on instruments and brain electrodes, such items should be carefully disinfected before being reused.

The outbreak of BSE and vCJD in the United Kingdom promoted legislation to ban animal products in livestock feed and encouraged more careful monitoring of cattle.

SUMMARY

Prion is composed entirely of a mutant or structurally distinct form of a host protein, called PrP^{Sc} (scrapie-like prion protein), which is extremely resistant to inactivation by heat, disinfectants, and radiation, leading to a subacute spongiform encephalopathy. Human prion diseases include Kuru, Creutzfeldt-Jakob disease (CJD), Variant CJD (vCJD), Gerstmann-Sträussler-Scheinker (GSS) syndrome, fatal familial insomnia (FFI) and sporadic fatal insomnia. Animal prion diseases include Scrapie (sheep and goats), transmissible mink encephalopathy, bovine spongiform encephalopathy (BSE; mad cow disease) and chronic wasting disease (mule, deer, and elk). No treatment exists for prion diseases so far. Since these agents can be transmitted on instruments and brain electrodes, such items should be carefully disinfected before being reused.

KEYWORDS

English	Chinese
Bovine spongiform encephalo-pathy, BSE	牛海绵状脑病
Cellular prion protein, PrP^{c}	细胞朊蛋白
Creutzfeldt-Jakob disease, CJD	克-雅病
Fatal familial insomnia, FFI	致死性家族失眠症
Gerstmann-Sträussler-Scheinker, GSS	格斯特曼综合征
Glycophosphatidylinositol, GPI	磷脂酰肌醇
Kuru	库鲁病
Prion	朊粒
Proteinaceous infectious particle	传染性蛋白粒子
Scrapie-like prion protein, PrP^{Sc}	类羊瘙痒症朊粒蛋白
Template-mediated protein refolding	模板介导的蛋白折叠
Transmissible spongiform encephalopathy	传染性海绵状脑病

BIBLIOGRAPHY

1. Belay ED: Transmissible spongiform encephalopathies in humans, Annu Rev Microbiol 53: 283-314, 1999.

2. Brown P, et al: Diagnosis of Creutzfeldt-Jakob disease by Western blot identification, N Engl J Med 314: 547-551, 1986.

3. Cohen J, Powderly WG: Infectious diseases, ed 2, St Louis, 2004, Mosby.

4. Flint SJ, et al: Principles of virology: molecular biology, pathogenesis and control of animal viruses, ed 3, Washington, DC, 2009, American Society for Microbiology Press.

5. Halfmann R, Alberti S, Lindquist S: Prions, protein homeostasis, and phenotypic diversity, Trends Cell Biol 20: 125-133, 2010.

6. Hsich G, et al: The 14-3-3 brain protein in cerebrospinal fluid as a marker for transmissible spongiform encephalopathies, N Engl J Med 335: 924-930, 1996.

7. Knipe DM, et al: Fields virology, ed 5, Philadelphia, 2006, Lippincott Williams & Wilkins.

8. Lee KS, Caughey B: A simplified recipe for prions, Proc Natl Acad Sci U S A 104: 9551-9552, 2007.

9. Manson JC: Understanding transmission of the prion diseases, Trends Microbiol 7: 465-467, 1999.

10. Prusiner SB: Molecular biology and genetics of neurodegenerative diseases caused by prions, Adv Virus Res 41: 241-280, 1992.

11. Prusiner SB: Prions, prions, prions, *Curr Top Microbiol Immunol*, vol 207, Berlin, 1996, Springer-Verlag.

12. Richman DD, Whitley RJ, Hayden FG: Clinical virology, ed 3, Washington, DC, 2009, American Society for Microbiology Press.

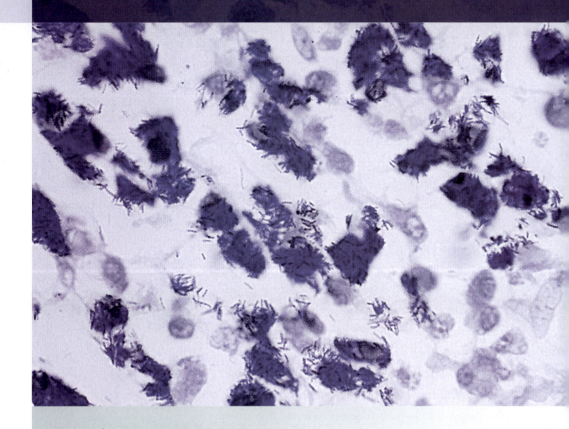

Mycology

Fungal Classification, Structure, and Replication

Chapter

59

This chapter provides an overview of fungal classification, structure, and reproduction. The very basic aspects of fungal cell organization and morphology are discussed.

THE IMPORTANCE OF FUNGI

The fungi represent a ubiquitous and diverse group of organisms, the main purpose of which is to degrade organic matter. All fungi lead a heterotrophic existence as saprobes (organisms that live on dead or decaying matter), symbionts (organisms that live together and in which the association is of mutual advantage), commensals (organisms living in a close relationship in which one benefits from the relationship and the other neither benefits nor is harmed), or as parasites (organisms that live on or within a host from which they derive benefits without making any useful contribution in return; in the case of pathogens, the relationship is harmful to the host).

Fungi have emerged in the past two decades as major causes of human disease (Table 59-1), especially among those individuals who are immunocompromised or hospitalized with serious underlying diseases. Among these patient groups, fungi serve as opportunistic pathogens, causing considerable morbidity and mortality. The overall incidence of specific invasive mycoses continues to increase with time, and the opportunistic fungal pathogens likewise increases each year. In short, *there are no non-pathogenic fungi!* This increase in fungal infections can be attributed to the ever-growing number of immunocompromised patients, including transplant patients, individuals with acquired immunodefi-

ciency syndrome (AIDS), patients with cancer and undergoing chemotherapy, and those individuals who are hospitalized with other serious underlying conditions and who undergo a variety of invasive procedures.

Table 59-1 Incidence and Case-Fatality Ratios of Selected Invasive Fungal Infections,

Pathogen	No. of Cases per Million per Year Incidence	Case-Fatality Ratio (%) for First Episode
Candida species	72.8	33.9
Cryptococcus neoformans	65.5	12.7
Coccidioides immitis	15.3	11.1
Aspergillus species	12.4	23.3
Histoplasma capsulatum	7.1	21.4
Agents of mucormycosis	1.7	30.0
Agents of hyalohyphomycosis	1.2	14.3
Agents of phaeohyphomycosis	1.0	0
Sporothrix schenckii	<1	20.0
Malassezia furfur	<1	0
Total	178.3	22.4

Modified from Rees JR, et al: The epidemiological features of invasive mycotic infections in the San Francisco Bay Area, 1992-1993: results of population-based laboratory active surveillance, *Clin Infect Dis* 27: 1138-1147, 1998.

FUNGAL TAXONOMY AND STRUCTURE

The fungi are classified in their own separate kingdom, Kingdom Fungi. They are eukaryotic organisms that are distinguished from other eukaryotes by a rigid cell wall composed of chitin and glucan and a

508

cell membrane in which ergosterol is substituted for cholesterol as the major sterol component (Figure 59-1).

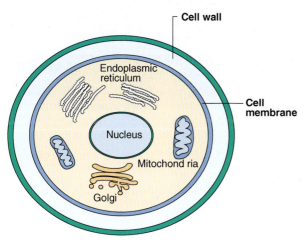

Figure 59-1   Diagram of a fungal cell.

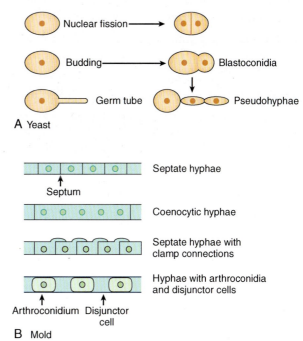

Figure 59-2   Fungal cell morphology. **A,** Yeast cells reproducing by nuclear fission and by blastoconidia formation. The elongation of budding yeast cells to form pseudohyphae is shown, as is the formation of a germ tube. **B,** Types of hyphae seen with various molds.

Classic fungal taxonomy relies heavily on morphology and mode of spore production. Fungi may be unicellular or multicellular. The most simple grouping, based on morphology, lumps fungi into either yeasts or molds. A yeast can be defined morphologically as a cell that reproduces by budding or by fission (Figure 59-2), where a progenitor or "mother" cell pinches off a portion of itself to produce a progeny or "daughter" cell. The daughter cells may elongate to form sausage-like pseudohyphae. Yeasts are usually unicellular and produce round, pasty, or mucoid colonies on agar. Molds, on the other hand, are multicellular organisms consisting of threadlike tubular structures, called hyphae (see Figure 59-2), that elongate at their tips by a process known as apical extension. Hyphae are either coenocytic (hollow and multinucleate) or septate (divided by partitions or cross-walls) (see Figure 59-2).

The hyphae form together to produce a matlike structure called a mycelium. The colonies formed by molds are often described as filamentous, hairy, or woolly. When growing on agar or other solid surfaces, molds produce hyphae, termed vegetative hyphae, that grow on or beneath the surface of the culture medium, and also hyphae that project above the surface of the medium, so-called aerial hyphae. The aerial hyphae may produce specialized structures known as conidia (asexual reproductive elements) (Figure 59-3). The conidia may be produced by either a blastic (budding) process or a thallic process, where hyphal segments fragment into individual cells or arthroconidia. The conidia are easily airborne and serve to disseminate the fungus. The size, shape, and certain developmental features of conidia are used as a means of identifying fungi to genus and species. Many fungi of medical importance are termed dimorphic, because they may exist in both a yeast form and a mold form.

Of the estimated several hundred thousand different fungi, only about 200 are known to cause human disease, although this number appears to be increasing. The major classes of fungi causing disease in humans are the Mucormycetes, the Basidiomycetes, the Pneumocystidiomycetes, the Hemiascomycetes, and the Euascomycetes (Table 59-2).

FUNGAL REPLICATION

Most fungi exhibit aerobic respiration, although some are facultatively anaerobic (fermentative), and others are strictly anaerobic. Metabolically fungi are heterotrophic and biochemically versatile, producing both primary (e.g., citric acid, ethanol, glycerol) and secondary (e.g., antibiotics [penicillin], amanitens, aflatoxins) metabolites. Relative to the bacteria, fungi are slow growing, with cell doubling times in terms of hours rather than minutes.

Table 59-2   Medically Important Fungi (Kingdom Fungi)

Taxonomic Designation	Representative Genera	Human Disease
Subphyla Mucoromycotina and Entomophthoromycotina (Mucormycetes)		
Order: Mucorales	*Rhizopus, Mucor, Lichtheimia, Saksenaea*	Mucormycosis: opportunistic in patients with diabetes, leukemia, severe burns, or malnutrition; rhinocerebral infections
Order: Entomophthorales	*Basidiobolus, Conidiobolus*	Mucormycosis: subcutaneous and gastro-intestinal infections
Phylum: Basidiomycota (Basidiomycetes)	Teleomorphs of *Cryptococcus, Malassezia,* and *Trichosporon* species	Cryptococcosis and numerous mycoses
Phylum: Ascomycota		
Class: Pneumocystidiomycetes	*Pneumocystis jirovecii*	*Pneumocystis* pneumonia
Class: Saccharomycetes	Teleomorphs of *Candida* species; *Saccharomyces*	Numerous mycoses
Subphylum: Euascomycotina		
Order: Onygenales	*Arthroderma* (teleomorphs of *Trichophyton* and *Microsporum*); *Ajellomyces* (teleomorphs of *Blastomyces* and *Histoplasma* species)	Dermatophytoses; systemic mycoses
Order: Eurotiales	Teleomorphs of *Aspergillus* species	Aspergillosis
Order: Sordariales	Teleomorphs of *Fusarium* species	Keratitis and other invasive mycoses
Order: Microascales	*Pseudallescheria* (teleomorph of *Scedosporium* species)	Pneumonia, mycetoma, and invasive mycoses

Modified from Brandt ME, Warnock DW: Taxonomy and classification of fungi. In Versalovic J, et al, editors: *Manual of clinical microbiology*, ed 10, Washington, DC, 2011, American Society for Microbiology Press.

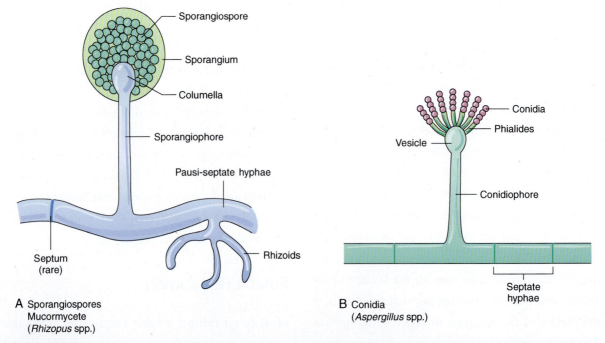

A   Sporangiospores Mucormycete (*Rhizopus* spp.)

B   Conidia (*Aspergillus* spp.)

Figure 59-3   Examples of asexual spore formation and associated structures seen with a Mucorales **(A)** and an *Aspergillus* spp. **(B)**.

Fungi reproduce by the formation of spores that may be sexual (involving meiosis, preceded by fusion of the protoplasm and nuclei of two compatible mating types) or asexual (involving mitosis only). The form of the fungus producing sexual spores is termed the teleomorph, and the form producing asexual spores is termed the anamorph. The fact that the teleomorph and anamorph of the same fungus have different names (e.g., *Ajellomyces capsulatum* [teleomorph] and *Histoplasma capsulatum* [anamorph]) is a source of confusion for nonmycologists.

Irrespective of the ability of a given fungus to produce sexual spores, in clinical situations, it is common to refer to the organisms by their asexual designations. This is because the anamorphic (asexual) state is isolated from clinical specimens, and the sexual or teleomorphic phase occurs only under very specialized conditions in the laboratory.

Asexual spores consist of two general types: sporangiospores and conidia. Sporangiospores are asexual spores produced in a containing structure or sporangia (see Figure 59-3) and are characteristic of genera belonging to the Mucorales, such as *Rhizopus* and *Mucor* spp. Conidia are asexual spores that are borne naked on specialized structures as seen in *Aspergillus* spp.

reproduce by the formation of spores that may be sexual or asexual. Many fungi of medical importance are termed dimorphic, because they may exist in both a yeast form and a mold form.

KEYWORDS

English	Chinese
Fungi	真菌
Yeasts	酵母
Molds	霉菌
Pseudohyphae	假菌丝
Hyphae	菌丝
Mycelium	菌丝体
Vegetative hyphae	营养菌丝
Aerial hyphae	气生菌丝
Conidia	分生孢子
Arthroconidia	关节孢子
Dimorphic	二相性
Teleomorph	有性型
Anamorph	无性型
Sporangiospore	孢子囊孢子

SUMMARY

Fungi are eukaryotic organisms that are distinguished from other eukaryotes by a rigid cell wall composed of chitin and glucan and a cell membrane in which ergosterol is substituted for cholesterol as the major sterol component. Fungi can be lumped into either yeasts or molds. Yeasts are usually unicellular and produce round, pasty, or mucoid colonies on agar and reproduce by budding or by fission. Molds are multicellular organisms consisting hyphae and spores. The colonies formed by molds are often described as filamentous, hairy, or woolly. Fungi

BIBLIOGRAPHY

1. Brandt ME, Warnock DW: Taxonomy and classification of fungi. In Versalovic J, et al, editors: Manual of clinical microbiology, ed 10, Washington, DC, 2011, American Society for Microbiology Press.

2. Pfaller MA, Diekema DJ: The epidemiology of invasive candidiasis: a persistent public health problem, Clin Microbiol Rev 20: 133-163, 2007.

3. Rees JR, et al: The epidemiological features of invasive mycotic infections in the San Francisco Bay Area, 1992-1993: results of population-based laboratory active surveillance, Clin Infect Dis 27: 1138-1147, 1998.

4. Reingold AL, et al: Systemic mycoses in the United States, 1980-1982, J Med Vet Mycol 24: 433-436, 1986.

5. Wilson LS, et al: The direct cost and incidence of systemic fungal infections, Value Health 5: 26-34, 2002.

Pathogenesis of Fungal Disease

Although a great deal is known regarding the molecular and genetic basis for bacterial and viral pathogenesis, our understanding of the pathogenesis of fungal infections is limited. Relatively few fungi are sufficiently virulent to be considered **primary pathogens** (Table 60-1) and most fungi are **opportunists** producing disease in individuals who are compromised in their innate and/or acquired immune defenses.

PRIMARY FUNGAL PATHOGENS

Primary pathogens are capable of initiating infection in a normal, apparently immunocompetent host. They are able to colonize the host, find a suitable microenvironmental niche with sufficient nutritional substrates, avoid or subvert the normal host defense mechanisms, and then multiply within the microenvironmental niche. Among the acknowledged primary fungal pathogens are four ascomycetous fungi, the endemic dimorphic pathogens *Blastomyces dermatitidis*, *Coccidioides immitis* (and *Coccidioides posadasii*), *Histoplasma capsulatum*, and *Paracoccidioides brasiliensis*. Each of these organisms possesses putative virulence factors that allow them to actively breach host defenses that ordinarily restrict the invasive growth of other microbes. When large numbers of conidia of any of these four fungi are inhaled by humans, even if these individuals are healthy and immunocompetent, infection and colonization, tissue invasion, and systemic spread of the pathogen commonly occur. As with most primary microbial pathogens, these fungi may also serve as opportunistic pathogens, given that the more severe forms of

each mycosis are seen most often in individuals who are compromised in their innate and/or acquired immune defenses.

All of the primary systemic fungal pathogens are agents of respiratory infections, and none are obligate parasites. Each has a saprobic phase characterized by filamentous septate hyphae, typically found in soil or decaying vegetation, that produce the airborne infectious cells. Likewise, the parasitic phase of each fungus is adapted to grow at 37°C and to reproduce asexually in the alternative environmental niche of the host respiratory mucosa. This ability to exist in alternate morphogenic forms (dimorphism) is one of several special characteristics (virulence factors) that allow these fungi to cope with the hostile environmental conditions of the host (see Table 60-1).

Opportunistic Pathogens

In general, healthy immunocompetent individuals have a high innate resistance to fungal infection, despite the fact that they are constantly exposed to the infectious forms of various fungi present as part of the normal commensal flora (endogenous) or in the environment (exogenous). The opportunistic fungal pathogens, such as *Candida* spp., *Cryptococcus neoformans*, and *Aspergillus* spp., generally only cause infection when there are disruptions in the protective barriers of the skin and mucous membranes or when defects in the host immune system allow them to penetrate, colonize, and reproduce in the host. However, even with these opportunists, there are factors associated with the organism rather than the host that contribute to the ability of the fungus to cause disease.

The state of the host is of primary importance in determining the pathogenicity of opportunistic fungal pathogens, such as *Candida* spp., *C. neoformans*, and *Aspergillus* spp. In most instances, these organisms may exist as benign colonizers or as environmental saprobes and only cause serious infection when there is a breakdown of host defenses. There are factors associated with these organisms, however, that may be considered "virulence factors," in that they contribute to the disease process and in some instances may explain the differences in pathogenicity of the various organisms.

Table 60-1 Characteristics of Primary and Opportunistic Fungal Pathogens.

	Habitat/Infection	Pathogenesis	Putative Virulence Factors	Clinical Forms of Mycosis
Primary Pathogens				
Blastomyces dermatitidis Saprobic phase • Septate mycelium and conidia Parasitic phase • Large, broad-based, budding yeast	Saprobic habitat • Soil and organic debris • Endemic area southeastern United States and Ohio-Mississippi River Valley Mode of infection • Inhalation of conidia	Inhaled conidia convert to yeast; localized yeast invasion of host invokes inflammatory reaction; yeast escapes recognition by macrophages and disseminates via bloodstream	• Growth at 37℃ • Thermal dimorphism • Modulation of yeast-host immune system interactions • Generation of TH2 response Shedding of WI-1	• Primary pulmonary blastomycosis • Chronic pulmonary blastomycosis • Disseminated blastomycosis • Cutaneous • Bone, genitourinary tract, and brain
Coccidioides immitis (posadasii) Saprobic phase • Septate hyphae and arthroconidia Parasitic phase • Spherules with endospores	Saprobic habitat • Desert soil: southwestern United States, Mexico, regions of Central and South America Mode of infection • Inhalation of arthroconidia • Percutaneous inoculation (rare)	Inhaled arthroconidia reach alveoli; convert to spherule that gives rise to endospores; endospores phagocytosed but survive; large (60-100 μm) spherules escape phagocytosis; alkaline environment allows survival within phagosome	• Growth at 37℃ • Thermal dimorphism • Resistance of conidia to phagocytic killing • Stimulation of ineffective TH2 response • Urease production • Extracellular proteinase production • Molecular mimicry	• Initial pulmonary infection • Chronic pulmonary coccidioidomycosis • Disseminated coccidioidomycosis • Meningitis • Bone and joints • Genitourinary • Cutaneous • Ophthalmic
Histoplasma capsulatum Saprobic phase • Septate hyphae, microconidia, and tuberculate macroconidia Parasitic phase • Small, intracellular, budding yeast	Saprobic habitat • Soil enriched with bird/bat guano • Eastern half of United States, most of Latin America, parts of Asia, Europe, Middle East; var. *duboisii* occurs in Africa Mode of infection • Inhalation of conidia	Inhaled conidia convert to yeast; yeast ingested by macrophages; survive and proliferate within phagosome; some yeast forms remain dormant within macrophage, others proliferate and kill macrophages, releasing daughter cells	• Growth at 37℃ • Thermal dimorphism • Survival in macrophages • Modulate pH of phagosome • Iron and calcium uptake • Alteration of cell wall composition	• Clinically asymptomatic pulmonary and "cryptic dissemination" • Acute pulmonary histoplasmosis • Mediastinitis and pericarditis • Chronic pulmonary histoplasmosis • Mucocutaneous • Disseminated
Paracoccidioides brasiliensis Saprobic phase • Septate hyphae, conidia Parasitic phase • Yeast with multiple buds	Saprobic habitat • Soil and vegetation • Central and South America Mode of infection • Inhalation of conidia	Inhaled conidia convert to large multipolar budding yeast; ingested but not cleared by macrophages; may be dormant for up to 40 years. Disseminate to oral and nasopharyngeal mucosa	• Growth at 37℃ • Thermal dimorphism • Intracellular survival • Hormonal influences • Alteration of cell wall • Ineffective TH2 response to gp43	• Diverse clinical manifestations • Chronic single organ involvement • Chronic multifocal involvement (lungs, mouth, nose) • Juvenile progressive disease: lymph nodes, skin and visceral involvement

Table 60-1　Characteristics of Primary and Opportunistic Fungal Pathogens. (Continued)

	Habitat/Infection	Pathogenesis	Putative Virulence Factors	Clinical Forms of Mycosis
Opportunistic Pathogens				
Candida species Saprobic and parasitic phases are the same: budding yeast, hyphae, pseudohyphae	Saprobic habitat • Gastrointestinal mucosa, vaginal mucosa, skin, nails Mode of infection • Gastrointestinal translocation • Intravascular catheters	Mucosal overgrowth with subsequent invasion; usually impaired mucosal barrier; hematogenous dissemination. Transfer from hands of health care worker to catheter hub; catheter colonization and hematogenous dissemination	• Growth at 37℃ • Bud-hyphae transition • Adherence • Cell surface hydrophobicity • Cell wall mannans • Proteases and phospholipases • Phenotypic switching	• Simple mucosal colonization • Mucocutaneous candidiasis • Oral/vaginal thrush • Hematogenous dissemination • Hepatosplenic candidiasis • Endophthalmitis
Cryptococcus neoformans Saprobic and parasitic phases are the same: encapsulated budding yeast	Saprobic habitat • Soil enriched with bird (pigeon) guano Mode of infection • Inhalation of aerosolized yeast • Percutaneous inoculation	Inhaled yeast cells ingested by macrophages; survive intracellularly; capsule inhibits phagocytosis; capsule and melanin protect from oxidative injury; hematogenous and lymphatic dissemination to brain	• Growth at 37℃ • Polysaccharide capsule • Melanin • Alpha-mating type	• Primary cryptococcal pneumonia • Meningitis • Hematogenous dissemination • Genitourinary (prostatic) cryptococcosis • Primary cutaneous cryptococcosis
Aspergillus species Saprobic phase • Septate mycelium, conidial heads, and conidia Parasitic phase • Septate mycelium; conidia, and conidial heads usually only seen in cavitary lesions	Saprobic habitat • Soil, plants, water, pepper, air Mode of infection • Inhalation of conidia • Transfer to wounds via contaminated tape/bandages	Inhaled conidia bind to fibrinogen and laminin in alveolus; conidia germinate, and hyphal forms secrete proteases and invade epithelium; vascular invasion results in thrombosis and infarction of tissue; hematogenous dissemination	• Growth at 37℃ • Binding to fibrinogen and laminin • Secretion of elastase and proteases • Catalase • Gliotoxin (?)	• Allergic bronchopulmonary aspergillosis • Sinusitis • Aspergilloma • Invasive aspergillosis • Lung • Brain • Skin • Gastrointestinal • Heart

From Cole GT: Fungal pathogenesis. In Anaissie EJ, McGinnis MR, Pfaller MA, editors: *Clinical mycology*, New York, 2003, Churchill Livingstone.

Hypersensitivity Responses

Hypersensitivity reactions are responsible for many of the symptoms associated with fungal infections. Once activated, the immune response is sometimes difficult to control and causes tissue damage. These hypersensitivity reactions are mainly caused by inhalation or ingestion of cetain fungal hypha and/or spore such as *Penicilluim, Fusarium, and Alternaria.*

Mycotoxicoses

Mycotoxicoses caused by ingested toxins. Ergotism, for example, is caused by *Claviceps purpura* which infects grains and produces alkaloids that cause vascular and neurologic effects. Aflatoxins are ingested with spoiled grains and peanets, the toxins are produced by *Aspergillus flavus* that cause liver damage and are suspected of causing hepatic carcinoma in humans.

SUMMARY

Relatively few fungi are sufficiently virulent to be considered primary pathogens which are capable of initiating infection in a normal, apparently immunocompetent host. Otherwise, most fungi are opportunists producing disease in individuals who are compromised in their innate and/or acquired immune defenses. In addition to infections, there are two other types of fungal disease: allergies and mycotoxicoses.

KEYWORDS

English	Chinese
Saprobic phase	腐生阶段
Parasitic phase	寄生阶段
Opportunistic fungal pathogens	机会致病性真菌
Hypersensitivity	超敏反应
Mycotoxicoses	真菌中毒
Aflatoxins	黄曲霉素

BIBLIOGRAPHY

1. Cramer RA Jr, Perfect JR: Recent advances in understanding human opportunistic fungal pathogenesis mechanisms. In Annaisie EJ, McGinnis MR, Pfaller MA, editors: Clinical mycology, ed 2, New York, 2009, Churchill Livingstone.

2. Dignani MC, et al: Candida. In Annaisie EJ, McGinnis MR, Pfaller MA, editors: Clinical mycology, ed 2, New York, 2009, Churchill Livingstone.

3. Nemecek JC, et al: Global control of dimorphism and virulence in fungi, Science 312: 583-588, 2006.

4. Rosenthal KS: Are microbial symptoms "self-inflicted"? The consequences of immunopathology, Infect Dis Clin Pract 13: 306-310, 2005.

Immune Responses to Fungi

We live in a microbial world, and our bodies are constantly being exposed to fungi and other infectious agents. Human beings have three basic lines of protection against infection by fungi to block entry, spread in the body, and inappropriate colonization.

NATURAL BARRIERS

The initial defense mechanisms are **natural barriers**, such as skin, mucus, and ciliated epithelium that inactivate and prevent entry of fungi. If these barriers are compromised or the agent gains entry in another way, the local militia of innate responses must quickly rally to the challenge and prevent expansion of the invasion. **Innate, antigen-non-specific immune defenses.** The primary protective responses to fungal infection are initiated by fungal cell wall carbohydrates binding to **Toll-like receptors (TLRs)** and the dectin-1 lectin and is delivered by neutrophils, macrophages, and antimicrobial peptides produced by the neutrophils, epithelial, and other cells. Defensins and other cationic peptides may be important for some fungal infections (e.g., mucormycosis, aspergillus), and **nitric oxide** may be important against *Cryptococcus* and other fungi.

C-reactive protein complexes with fungi and activates the complement pathway, facilitating removal of these organisms from the body through greater phagocytosis. The acute-phase proteins reinforce the innate defenses against infection.

ADAPTIVE, ANTIGEN-SPECIFIC IMMUNE RESPONSES

CD4 T-cell **TH17** and **TH1 responses** stimulate the neutrophil and macrophage responses. Patients deficient in neutrophils or these CD4 T cell-mediated responses (e.g., patients with AIDS) are most susceptible to fungal (opportunistic) infections. Antibody, as an opsonin, may facilitate clearance of the fungi.

IMMUNOPATHOGENESIS

Once activated, the immune response is sometimes difficult to control and causes tissue damage. **Hypersensitivity reactions** are responsible for many of the symptoms associated with fungal infections. Hypersensitivity reactions occur to people who have already established immunity to the antigen. For example, Type IV hypersensitivity responses are TH1-mediated **delayed-type hypersensitivity (DTH)** inflammatory responses. It usually takes 24 to 48 hours for antigen to be presented to circulating CD4 T cells, for them to move to the site, and then activate macrophages to induce the response. Although essential for the control of fungal infections, DTH is also responsible for contact dermatitis (e.g., cosmetics, nickel) and the response to poison ivy.

SUMMARY

Human beings have three basic lines of protection against infection by fungi to block entry, spread in the body, and inappropriate colonization: (1) natural barriers, such as skin, mucus, and ciliated epithelium,

(3) innate, antigen-nonspecific immune defenses, such as neutrophils, macrophages and cationic peptides and (3) adaptive, antigen-specific immune responses, such as CD4 T-cell TH17 and TH1 responses. Sometimes the immune response also can cause tissue damage such as Type IV hypersensitivity responses.

KEYWORDS

English	Chinese
Natural barriers	天然屏障
Toll-like receptors	Toll 样受体
Macrophages	巨噬细胞
Dectin-1 lectin	模式识别受体植物凝集素
Neutrophils	中性粒细胞
Antimicrobial peptides	抗菌肽
Nitric oxide	一氧化氮
Delayed-type hypersensitivity (DTH)	迟发型超敏反应

BIBLIOGRAPHY

1. DeFranco AL, Locksley RM, Robertson M: Immunity: the immune response in infectious and inflammatory disease, Sunderland, Mass, 2007, Sinauer Associates.

2. Janeway CA, et al: Immunobiology: the immune system in health and disease, ed 6, New York, 2004, Garland Science.

3. Kindt TJ, Goldsby RA, Osborne BA: Kuby immunology, ed 6, New York, 2007, WH Freeman.

4. Mims C, et al: Medical microbiology, ed 3, London, 2004, Elsevier.

Laboratory Diagnosis of Fungal Diseases

This chapter provides a general description of the principles of specimen collection and processing necessary for the diagnosis of most fungal infections. An overview of direct microscopy, culture, immunologic, and molecular diagnostic testing is also provided (Box 62-1).

CLINICAL RECOGNITION OF FUNGAL INFECTIONS

Clinical suspicion, thorough history and physical examination, including a search for cutaneous and mucosal lesions, inspection of all implanted devices (catheters, etc.), a careful ophthalmologic examination, diagnostic imaging studies, and, finally, procurement of appropriate specimens for laboratory diagnosis are all essential steps that must be taken to optimize the diagnosis and treatment of fungal infections.

CONVENTIONAL LABORATORY DIAGNOSIS

Specimen Collection and Processing

As with all types of infectious processes, the laboratory diagnosis of fungal infection is directly dependent on the proper collection of appropriate clinical material and prompt delivery of the specimens to the clinical laboratory. Selection of specimens for culture and microscopic examination is based not only on information obtained from clinical examination and radiographic studies but also on consideration of the most likely fungal pathogen that may cause a specific type of infection. Specimens should be collected aseptically or after proper cleaning and decontamination of the site to be sampled. An adequate amount of clinical material must be submitted promptly for culture and microscopy (Table 62-1). Specimens should be submitted whenever possible in a sterile leak-proof container and be accompanied by a relevant clinical history.

Transportation of specimens to the laboratory should be prompt; however, delayed processing of specimens for fungal culture may not be as detrimental as with specimens for bacteriologic, virologic, or parasitologic examination. In general, if processing is delayed, the specimens for fungal culture may be stored at 4℃ for a short time without loss of organism viability.

Table 62-1 Body Sites, Specimen Collection, and Diagnostic Procedures for Selected Fungal Infections.

Infection Site and Infecting Organism	Specimen Options	Collection Methods	Diagnostic Procedure
Blood			
Candida, Cryptococcus neoformans, Histoplasma capsulatum, Fusarium, Aspergillus terreus, Penicillium marneffei, Trichosporon	Whole blood	Venipuncture (sterile)	Culture, broth, culture, lysis-centrifugation
	Serum	Venipuncture (sterile)	Antigen (Candida, Cryptococcus, and Histoplasma), nucleic acid amplification
	Urine	Sterile	Antigen (Histoplasma)
Bone Marrow			
Histoplasma capsulatum, Penicillium marneffei	Aspirate	Sterile	Microscopic examination, culture
	Serum	Venipuncture (sterile)	Serology, (Histoplasma) antigen, antibody
	Urine	Sterile	Antigen (Histoplasma)
Central Nervous System			
Candida, Cryptococcus neoformans/gattii, Aspergillus, Scedosporium, dematiaceous molds, Mucormycetes, Histoplasma, Coccidioides	Spinal fluid	Sterile	Microscopic examination, culture, antigen (Cryptococcus)
	Biopsy	Sterile, nonsterile to histopathology	Microscopic examination, culture (do not grind tissue)
	Serum	Sterile	Antigen (Aspergillus, Cryptococcus, and Histoplasma)
Bone and Joint			
Candida, Fusarium, Aspergillus, Histoplasma capsulatum, Coccidioides immitis/posadasii, Blastomyces dermatitidis, Penicillium marneffei, Sporothrix schenckii	Aspirate	Sterile	Microscopic examination, culture
	Biopsy	Sterile, nonsterile to histopathology	Microscopic examination, culture (do not grind tissue)
	Serum	Venipuncture	Serology, antigen, antibody
Eye			
Fusarium, Candida, Cryptococcus neoformans, Aspergillus, Mucormycetes	Cornea	Scraping or biopsy	Microscopic examination, culture
	Vitreous fluid	Sterile aspirate	Microscopic examination, culture
Urogenital System			
Candida, Cryptococcus neoformans, Trichosporon, Rhodotorula	Urine	Sterile	Microscopic examination, culture
Rarely: Histoplasma capsulatum, Blastomyces dermatitidis, Coccidioides immitis/posadasii	Vaginal, urethral, prostatic secretions or discharge	Saline swab	Microscopic examination, wet mount, calcofluor white/KOH, culture
	Serum	Venipuncture	Serology (antibody)
	Biopsy	Sterile, nonsterile to histopathology	Microscopic examination, culture (do not grind tissue)
Respiratory Tract			
Cryptococcus neoformans/gattii, Aspergillus, Fusarium, Mucormycetes, Scedosporium apiospermum, dematiaceous molds, endemic dimorphic fungi, Pneumocystis jirovecii	Sputum	Induced, no preservative	Microscopic examination, culture
	Lavage	No preservative	Microscopic examination, culture, galactomannan (Aspergillus)
	Transbronchial	Aspirate or biopsy	Microscopic examination, culture
	Open lung biopsy	Sterile, nonsterile to histopathology	Microscopic examination, culture (do not grind tissue)
	Serum	Venipuncture	Serology, antigen, antibody, nucleic acid amplification
	Urine	Sterile	Antigen (Histoplasma)

Table 62-1   Body Sites, Specimen Collection, and Diagnostic Procedures for Selected Fungal Infections. (Continued)

Infection Site and Infecting Organism	Specimen Options	Collection Methods	Diagnostic Procedure
Skin and Mucous Membranes			
Candida, Cryptococcus neoformans, Trichosporon, Aspergillus, Mucormycetes, *Fusarium,* dematiaceous molds, endemic dimorphic fungi, *Sporothrix schenckii*	Biopsy	Sterile, nonsterile to histopathology	Microscopic examination, culture (do not grind tissue)
	Mucosal	Saline swab	Microscopic examination, wet mount, calcofluor white/KOH, culture
	Skin scraping	Nonsterile	Calcofluor white/KOH
	Serum	Venipuncture	Serology, antigen, antibody, nucleic acid amplification
	Urine	Sterile	Antigen *(Histoplasma)*
Multiple Systemic Sites			
Candida, Cryptococcus neoformans/gattii, Trichosporon, hyaline molds, dematiaceous molds, endemic dimorphic fungi	Whole blood	Venipuncture (sterile)	Culture, broth, or lysis-centrifugation
	Serum	Venipuncture (sterile)	Serology, antigen, antibody, nucleic acid amplification
	Urine	Sterile	Antigen *(Histoplasma)*
	Biopsy	Sterile, nonsterile to histopathology	Microscopic examination, culture (do not grind tissue)

KOH, Potassium hydroxide.

Stains and Direct Microscopic Examination

Direct microscopic examination of tissue sections and clinical specimens is generally considered to be among the most rapid and cost-effective means of diagnosing fungal infections. Microscopic detection of yeasts or hyphal structures in tissue may be accomplished in less than an hour, whereas culture results may not be available for days or even weeks. In certain instances, the fungus may not only be detected but identified by microscopy because it possesses a distinctive morphology. Microscopic detection of fungi in tissue serves to guide the laboratory in selecting the most appropriate means to culture the specimen and also is helpful in determining the significance of culture results. The latter is especially true when the organism isolated in culture is a known component of the normal flora or is frequently found in the environment.

A number of different stains and microscopic techniques may be used to detect and characterize fungi directly in clinical material. The approaches used most often in the clinical mycology laboratory include the fluorescent reagent calcofluor white or staining of smears (Figure 62-1) and touch preparations with either Gram (Figures 62-2 and 62-3) or Giemsa stains (Figures 62-4 and 62-6). The more fungus-specific stains are the Gomori methenamine silver (GMS) stain (Figures 62-5 and 62-7) and periodic acid-Schiff (PAS) stains. These stains are useful in detecting small numbers of organisms and for clearly defining characteristic features of fungal morphology.

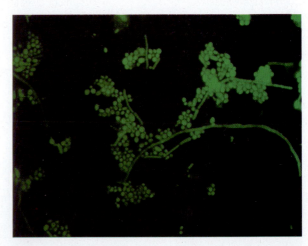

Figure 62-1   Calcofluor white stain demonstrating budding yeasts and pseudohyphae of *Candida albicans.*

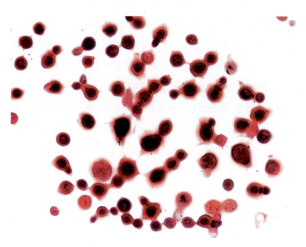

Figure 62-2   Gram stain of *Cryptococcus neoformans*. Variable-sized, encapsulated, budding yeasts showing a stippled pattern resulting from uneven retention of crystal violet stain.

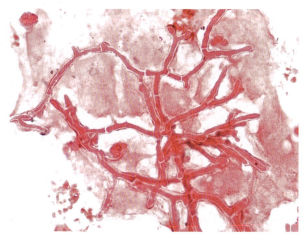

Figure 62-3   Gram stain of *Aspergillus*. This specimen did not retain the crystal violet stain and appears gram-negative.

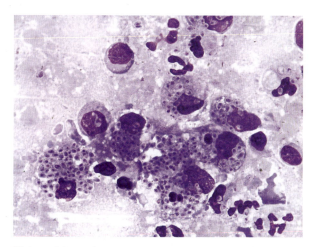

Figure 62-4   Giemsa stain showing intracellular yeast forms of *Histoplasma capsulatum*.

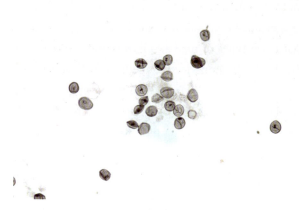

Figure 62-5   Silver stain of *Pneumocystis jirovecii* cysts.

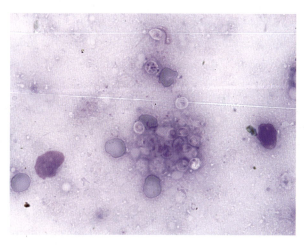

Figure 62-6   Giemsa stain showing intracystic and trophic forms of *Pneumocystis jirovecii*.

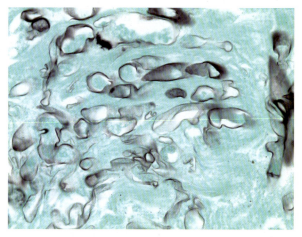

Figure 62-7   Silver stain of *Rhizopus*.

Culture

The most sensitive means of diagnosing a fungal infection is usually considered to be isolation of the fungus in culture. Culture is also necessary, in most instances, to identify the etiologic agents. No single culture medium is sufficient to isolate all medically important fungi, and it is generally accepted that at least two types of media, selective and nonselective, be used. The nonselective medium will permit the growth of rapidly growing yeasts and molds, as well as the more slowly growing fastidious fungi. Fungi will grow in most media used for bacteria; however, growth may be slow, and a more enriched medium, such as brain heart infusion (BHI) agar or SABHI (Sabouraud dextrose and BHI) agar, is recommended. Specimens that may be contaminated with bacteria should be inoculated onto selective media, such as SABHI or BHI supplemented with antibiotics (penicillin plus streptomycin is often used). Specific fungi may require specialized media. Once inoculated, fungal cultures should be incubated in air at a proper temperature and for a sufficient period of time to ensure the recovery of fungi from clinical specimens. Most fungi grow optimally at 25℃ to 30℃, although most species of *Candida* can be recovered from blood cultures incubated at 35℃ to 37℃. Culture dishes should be sealed with gas-permeable tape to prevent dehydration. Specimens submitted for fungal culture are generally incubated for 2 weeks; however, most blood cultures become positive within 5 to 7 days.

Identifying Characteristics of Various Fungi

Distinguishing yeastlike fungi from molds is the first step in identifying a fungal isolate. Gross colony morphology usually provides a good clue: yeastlike fungi form pasty, opaque colonies, and molds form large, filamentous colonies that vary in texture, color, and topography. Microscopic examination provides further delineation and often is all that is required for identification of many fungi. Identification to genus and species, depending on the fungus, requires more detailed microscopic study to delineate characteristic structures. Yeast identification usually requires additional biochemical and physiologic testing, whereas the identification of both yeasts and molds may be enhanced by specialized immunologic and molecular characterization.

The identification of yeastlike fungi to the spe-

cies level often requires the determination of the biochemical and physiologic profile of the organism in addition to the assessment of the microscopic morphology; however, the definitive identification of a mold is based almost entirely on its microscopic morphology. The important features include the shape, method of production, and arrangement of conidia or spores and the size and appearance of the hyphae. Immunologic and/or nucleic acid probe-based tests are often used to identify the endemic dimorphic pathogens, and nucleic acid sequencing is being applied as an aid in the identification of a variety of molds.

IMMUNOLOGIC, MOLECULAR, AND BIO-CHEMICAL MARKERS FOR DIRECT DETECTION OF INVASIVE FUNGAL INFECTIONS

Rapid, sensitive, and specific diagnostic tests for serious fungal infections would allow more timely and focused application of specific therapeutic measures. As such, tests for the detection of antibodies and antigens, metabolites, and fungus-specific nucleic acids have great appeal. Considerable progress has been made in several of these areas in recent years, although with few exceptions, such testing still remains confined to reference laboratories or the research setting.

Determination of antibody (Ab) and/or antigen (Ag) titers in serum may be useful in diagnosing fungal infections. When performed in a serial fashion, Ab/Ag titers also provide a means of monitoring the progression of disease and the patient's response to therapy.

Detection of fungal cell wall and cytoplasmic antigens and metabolites in serum or other body fluids represents the most direct means of providing a serologic diagnosis of invasive fungal infection. The best examples of this approach are the commercially available tests for the detection of polysaccharide antigens of *C. neoformans* and *H. capsulatum*. These tests have proven to be of great value in the rapid diagnosis of cryptococcal meningitis and disseminated histoplasmosis, respectively.

The application of the polymerase chain reaction (PCR) to directly detect fungal-specific nucleic acids in clinical material offers great promise for the rapid diagnosis of fungal infections. A variety of target sequences have been investigated and found to be of potential diagnostic value for most of the more common opportunistic and systemic fungal pathogens. Recent developments, such as real-time PCR and gene chip technology, will facilitate the broad use of this technology, although it is not yet available in most mycology laboratories.

molecular characterization. Immunologic, molecular, and biochemical markers also can be used for direct detection of invasive fungal infections.

KEYWORDS

English	Chinese
Fungal pathogen	病原性真菌
Microscopy	显微镜检查
Fungal culture	真菌培养
Brain heart infusion (BHI) agar	脑心浸液培养基
CHROMagar	科马嘉培养基
SABHI (Sabouraud dextrose and BHI) agar	沙保培养基

SUMMARY

Conventional laboratory diagnosis of fungal infections include specimen collection and processing which dependent on the proper collection of appropriate clinical material and prompt delivery of the specimens to the clinical laboratory. A number of different stains and microscopic techniques may be used to detect and characterize fungi directly in clinical material. And the most sensitive means of diagnosing a fungal infection is usually considered to be isolation of the fungus in culture, specimens that may be contaminated with bacteria should be inoculated onto selective media, such as SABHI or BHI supplemented with antibiotics. Identifying characteristics of various fungi depend on gross colony morphology, microscopic examination, and additional examination such as biochemical and physiologic testing, specialized immunologic and

BIBLIOGRAPHY

1. Alexander BD, Pfaller MA: Contemporary tools for the diagnosis and management of invasive mycoses, Clin Infect Dis 43(Suppl 1): S15-S27, 2006.

2. Avini T, et al: PCR diagnosis of invasive candidiasis: systematic review and meta-analysis, J Clin Microbiol 49: 665-670, 2011.

3. Guarner J, Brandt ME: Histopathologic diagnosis of fungal infections in the 21st century, Clin Microbiol Rev 24: 247-280, 2011.

4. Murray PR: Rapid identification of clinical yeast isolates by mass spectrometry, Curr Fungal Infect Rep 4: 145-150, 2011.

5. Pfaller MA, McGinnis MR: The laboratory and clinical mycology. In Anaissie EJ, McGinnis MR, Pfaller MA, editors: Clinical mycology, ed 2, New York, 2009, Churchill Livingstone.

Antifungal Agents

Chapter 62

Antifungal therapy has undergone a tremendous transformation in recent years. Once the sole domain of the agents amphotericin B and 5-fluorocytosine (flucytosine, 5-FC), which were toxic and difficult to use, the treatment of mycotic disease has now been advanced by the availability of several new, systemically active agents and new formulations of other older agents that provide comparable if not superior efficacy with significantly less toxicity.

In this chapter, we will review the antifungal agents, both systemic and topical (Table 63-1). We will discuss their spectrum, potency, mode of action, and clinical indications for use as therapeutic agents. Furthermore, we will discuss the mechanisms of resistance to the various classes of antifungal agents and the in vitro methods for determining the susceptibility and resistance of fungi to the available agents.

The terminology appropriate for this discussion is summarized in Box 63-1 and Figure 63-1, respectively.

SYSTEMICALLY ACTIVE ANTIFUNGAL AGENTS

Amphotericin B and its lipid formulations are polyene macrolide antifungals used in the treatment of serious life-threatening mycoses (see Table 63-1). Another polyene, nystatin, is a topical agent. A lipid formulation of nystatin has been developed for systemic use but remains investigational.

The basic structure of polyenes consists of a large lactone ring, a rigid lipophilic chain containing three to seven double bonds, and a flexible hydrophilic portion bearing several hydroxyl groups (Figure 63-2). Amphotericin B contains seven conjugated double bonds and may be inactivated by heat, light, and

---

Box 63-1

Terminology

Antifungal spectrum: Range of activity of an antifungal agent against fungi. A broad-spectrum antifungal agent inhibits a wide variety of fungi, including both yeastlike fungi and molds, whereas a narrow-spectrum agent is active only against a limited number of fungi.

Fungistatic activity: Level of antifungal activity that **inhibits** the growth of an organism. This is determined in vitro by testing a standardized concentration of organisms against a series of antifungal dilutions. The lowest concentration of the drug that inhibits the growth of the organism is referred to as the **minimum inhibitory concentration (MIC).**

Fungicidal activity: The ability of an antifungal agent to **kill** an organism in vitro or in vivo. The lowest concentration of the drug that kills 99.9% of the test population is called the **minimum fungicidal concentration (MFC).**

Antifungal combinations: Combinations of antifungal agents that may be used (1) to enhance efficacy in the treatment of a refractory fungal infection, (2) to broaden the spectrum of empiric antifungal therapy, (3) to prevent the emergence of resistant organisms, and (4) to achieve a synergistic killing effect.

Antifungal synergism: Combinations of antifungal agents that have enhanced antifungal activity when used together compared with the activity of each agent alone.

Antifungal antagonism: Combination of antifungal agents in which the activity of one of the agents interferes with the activity of the other agent.

Efflux pumps: Families of drug transporters that serve to actively pump antifungal agents out of the fungal cells, thus decreasing the amount of intracellular drug available to bind to its target.

---

extremes of pH. It is poorly soluble in water and is not absorbed by the oral or intramuscular route of administration. The conventional formulation of amphotericin B for intravenous administration is amphotericin B deoxycholate. The lipid formulations of amphotericin B were developed in an effort to circumvent the nephrotoxic nature of conventional amphotericin B and in many instances have replaced the deoxycholate form.

Table 63-1   Systemic and Topical Antifungal Agents in Use and in Development

Antifungal Agents	Route	Mechanism of Action	Comments
Allylamines			
Naftifine Terbinafine	Topical Oral, topical	Inhibition of squalene epoxidase	Terbinafine has very broad spectrum and acts synergistically with other antifungals
Antimetabolite			
Flucytosine	Oral	Inhibition of DNA and RNA synthesis	Used in combination with amphotericin B and fluconazole; toxicity and secondary resistance are problems
Imidazoles			
Ketoconazole, bifonazole, clotrimazole, econazole, miconazole, oxiconazole, sulconazole, terconazole, tioconazole	Oral, topical	Inhibits lanosterol 14-α-demethylase cytochrome P450-dependent enzymes	Ketoconazole has modest broad-spectrum activity and toxicity problems
Triazoles			
Fluconazole	Oral, IV	Same as imidazoles but more specific binding to target	Limited spectrum (yeasts); good central nervous system penetration; good in vivo activity; primary and secondary resistance seen with *Candida krusei* and *Candida glabrata*, respectively
Itraconazole	Oral	Same as imidazoles but more specific binding to target enzyme	Broad-spectrum activity; erratic absorption; toxicity and drug interactions are problems
Voriconazole	Oral, IV	Same as imidazoles but more specific binding to target enzyme	Broad spectrum, including yeasts and molds; active vs. *Candida krusei*; many drug interactions
Posaconazole	Oral	Same as imidazoles but more specific binding to target enzyme	Broad spectrum including activity vs. Mucormycetes
Ravuconazole	Oral, IV	Same as imidazoles but more specific binding to target enzyme	Investigational; broad spectrum, including yeasts and molds
Albaconazole, isavuconazole		Same as other azoles	Investigational; broad spectrum, including yeasts and molds
Echinocandins			
Caspofungin, anidulafungin, micafungin	IV	Inhibition of fungal cell wall glucan synthesis	Caspofungin is approved for treatment of invasive candidiasis and aspergillosis; anidulafungin is approved for treatment of invasive candidiasis; micafungin is approved for treatment of invasive candidiasis; fungicidal activity against *Candida*
Aminocandin		Same as other echinocandins	Investigational
Polyenes			
Amphotericin B	IV, topical	Binds to ergosterol, causing direct oxidative membrane damage	Established agent; broad spectrum; toxic
Lipid formulations (amphotericin B lipid complex or colloidal dispersion, liposomal amphotericin B)	IV	Same as amphotericin B	Broad spectrum; less toxic, expensive
Nystatin	Oral suspension, topical	Same as amphotericin B	Liposomal formulation (IV) under investigation

Table 63-1 Systemic and Topical Antifungal Agents in Use and in Development (Continued)

Antifungal Agents	Route	Mechanism of Action	Comments
Chitin Synthesis Inhibitor			
Nikkomycin Z	IV	Inhibition of fungal cell wall chitin synthesis	Investigational agent; possibly useful in combination with other antifungals
Sordarin and azasordarin derivatives		Inhibition of elongation factor 3	Investigational agent; broad-spectrum activity, including *Pneumocystis jirovecii*
Other			
Amorolfine	Topical	Miscellaneous, varied	
Butenafine HC	Topical		
Ciclopirox olamine	Topical		
Griseofulvin	Oral		
Haloprogin	Topical		
Tolnaftate	Topical		
Undecylenate	Topical		

IV, Intravenous.

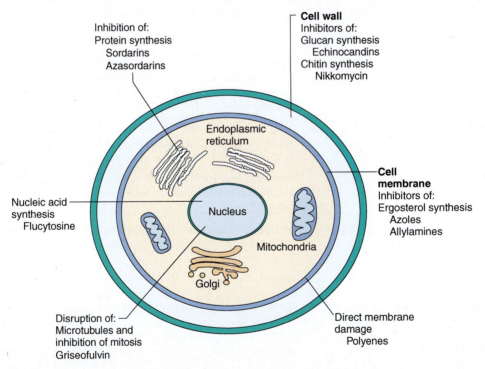

Figure 63-1 Sites of action of antifungals.

Amphotericin B (and its lipid formulations) exerts its antifungal action by at least two different mechanisms. The primary mechanism involves the binding of amphotericin B to ergosterol, the principal membrane sterol of fungi. This binding produces ion channels, which destroy the osmotic integrity of the fungal cell membrane and lead to leakage of intracellular constituents and cell death (Figure 63-3). Amphotericin B also binds to cholesterol, the main membrane sterol of mammalian cells, but does so less avidly than to ergosterol. The binding of amphotericin B to cholesterol accounts for most of the toxicity observed when amphotericin B is administered to humans. An additional mechanism of action of amphotericin B involves direct membrane damage resulting from the generation of a cascade of oxidative reactions triggered by the oxidation of amphotericin B itself. This process may be a major contributor to the rapid fungicidal activity of amphotericin B via the generation of toxic free radicals.

Amphotericin B (polyene)

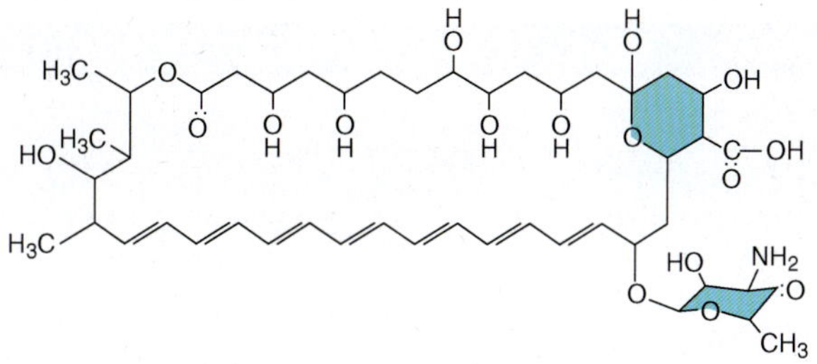

Ketoconazole (imidazole)

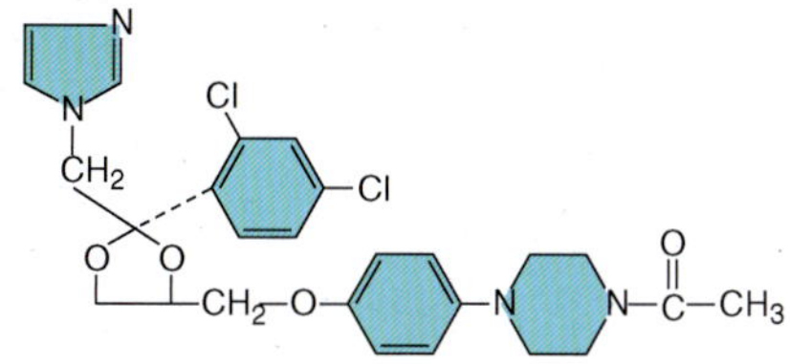

Fluconazole (triazole)

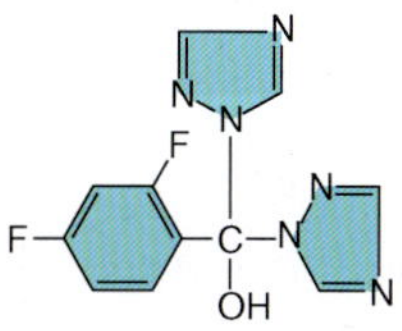

5-Fluorocystine (nucleotide)

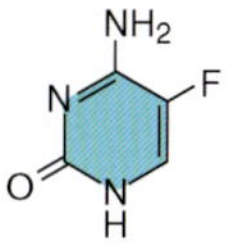

Caspofungin (echinocandin)

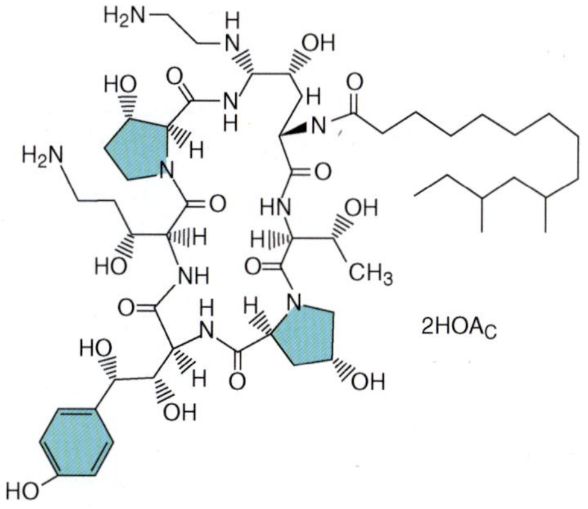

2HOAc

Figure 63-2 Chemical structures of antifungals representing five different classes.

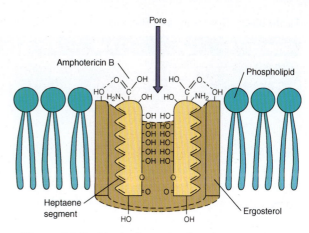

Figure 63-3 Mechanisms of action of amphotericin B.

latum, Paracoccidioides brasiliensis, and *Penicillium marneffei* (Table 63-2). *Aspergillus terreus, Fusarium* spp., *Pseudallescheria boydii, Scedosporium prolificans, Trichosporon* spp., and certain dematiaceous fungi may be resistant to amphotericin B. Likewise, reduced susceptibility to amphotericin B has been noted among some strains of *Candida guilliermondii, Candida glabrata, Candida krusei, Candida lusitaniae,* and *Candida rugosa.* Resistance to amphotericin B has been associated with alterations in membrane sterols, usually a reduction in ergosterol.

Amphotericin B is widely distributed in various tissues and organs, including liver, spleen, kidney, bone marrow, and lung. Although negligible concentrations of amphotericin B can be found in the cerebrospinal fluid, it is generally effective in treating fungal infections of the central nervous system. Amphotericin B is considered to be fungicidal against most fungi.

The primary clinical indications for amphotericin B include invasive candidiasis, cryptococcosis, aspergillosis, mucormycosis, blastomycosis, coccidioidomycosis, histoplasmosis, paracoccidioidomycosis, penicilliosis marneffei, and sporotrichosis. The lipid formulations of amphotericin B offer an improved efficacy-to-toxicity profile and are primarily recommended for the treatment of documented fungal infections in individuals failing conventional amphotericin B or with impaired renal function.

The main adverse effects of amphotericin B include nephrotoxicity, as well as infusion-related side effects, such as fever, chills, myalgias, hypoten-

The spectrum of activity of amphotericin B is broad and includes most strains of *Candida, Cryptococcus neoformans, Aspergillus* spp., the Mucormycetes, and the endemic dimorphic pathogens (*Blastomyces dermatitidis, Coccidioides immitis, Histoplasma capsu-*

Table 63-2 Spectrum and Relative Activity of Systemically Active Antifungal Agents.

Organism	AMB	FC	KTZ	ITZ	FCZ	VCZ	ECH
Candida spp.							
C. albicans	++++	++++	+++	++++	++++	++++	++++
C. glabrata	+++	++++	++	++	++	+++	++++
C. parapsilosis	++++	++++	+++	++++	++++	++++	+++
C. tropicalis	+++	++++	+++	+++	++++	++++	++++
C. krusei	++	+	+	++	0	++++	++++
Cryptococcus neoformans/gattii	++++	+++	+	++	+++	++++	0
Aspergillus spp.	++++	0	+	++++	0	++++	+++
Fusarium spp.	+++	0	0	+	0	+++	0
Mucormycetes	++++	0	0	0	0	0	+
Endemic Dimorphic							
Blastomyces dermatitidis	++++	0	++	++++	+	++++	++
Coccidioides immitis	++++	0	++	++++	++++	++++	++
Histoplasma capsulatum	++++	0	++	++++	++	++++	++
Penicillium marneffei	++++	0	++	++++	++	++++	
Sporothrix schenckii	++++	0	++	++++	++		
Dematiaceous molds	++++	+	++	++++	+	++++	0

AMB, Amphotericin B; *ECH*, echinocandins (anidulafungin, caspofungin, and micafungin); *FC*, flucytosine; *FCZ*, fluconazole; *ITZ*, itraconazole; *KTZ*, ketoconazole; *VCZ*, voriconazole.
0, Inactive or not recommended; +, occasional activity; ++, moderate activity with resistance noted; +++ reliable activity with occasional resistance; ++++ very active, resistance rare or not described.

sion, and bronchospasm. The major advantage of the lipid formulations of amphotericin B are the significantly reduced side effects, especially nephrotoxicity. The lipid formulations are not superior to conventional amphotericin B in terms of efficacy and are much more expensive.

Azoles

The azole class of antifungals may be divided in terms of structure into the imidazoles (two nitrogens in the azole ring) and the triazoles (three nitrogens in the azole ring) (see Figure 63-2). Among the imidazoles, only ketoconazole has systemic activity. The triazoles all have systemic activity and include fluconazole, itraconazole, voriconazole, and posaconazole (see Table 63-1). Ravuconazole, albaconazole, and isavuconazole are also triazoles and are currently investigational (see Table 63-1).

Both imidazoles and triazoles act by inhibiting the fungal cytochrome P450-dependent enzyme lanosterol 14-α-demethylase (Figure 63-4). This enzyme is involved in the conversion of lanosterol to ergosterol,

and its inhibition disrupts membrane synthesis in the fungal cell. Depending on the organism and specific azole, inhibition of ergosterol synthesis results in inhibition of fungal cell growth (fungistatic) or cell death (fungicidal). In general, the azoles exhibit

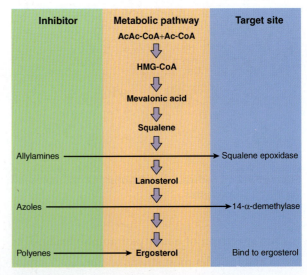

Figure 63-4 Metabolic pathway for the synthesis of ergosterol, showing sites of inhibition by allylamine, azole, and polyene antifungal agents. *Ac-CoA*, Acetyl-coenzyme A; *HMG-CoA*, hydroxymethyl glutaryl-coenzyme A.

fungistatic activity against yeastlike fungi, such as *Candida* spp. and *C. neoformans*; however, itraconazole, voriconazole, posaconazole, and ravuconazole appear to be fungicidal against *Aspergillus* spp.

Ketoconazole is an orally absorbed, lipophilic member of the imidazole class of antifungal agents. Its spectrum of activity includes the endemic dimorphic pathogens, *Candida* spp., *C. neoformans*, and *Malassezia* spp., although it is generally less active than the triazole antifungal agents (see Table 63-2). It is variably active against *P. boydii* and has little or no useful clinical activity against the Mucormycetes, *Aspergillus* spp., *S. prolificans*, or *Fusarium* spp.

The absorption of ketoconazole by the oral route of administration is erratic and requires an acid gastric pH. Its lipophilicity ensures penetration and concentration into fatty tissues and purulent exudates; however, because it is highly (>99%) protein bound, it penetrates poorly into the central nervous system.

Ketoconazole may cause serious adverse effects, including gastric and hepatic toxicity, nausea, vomiting, and rash. At high doses, significant endocrine side effects have been observed secondary to suppression of testosterone and cortisol levels.

Because of the availability of more potent and less toxic agents, the clinical indications for use of ketoconazole are quite limited. It is at best a second-line agent for the treatment of non-life-threatening, non-meningeal forms of histoplasmosis, blastomycosis, coccidioidomycosis, and paracoccidioidomycosis in immunocompetent individuals. Similarly, it may be used in the treatment of mucocutaneous candidiasis and lymphocutaneous sporotrichosis.

Fluconazole is a first-generation triazole with excellent oral bioavailability and low toxicity. Fluconazole is used extensively and is active against most species of *Candida*, *C. neoformans*, dermatophytes, *Trichosporon* spp., *H. capsulatum*, *C. immitis*, and *P. brasiliensis* (see Table 63-2). Among *Candida* spp., decreased susceptibility is seen with *C. krusei* and *C. glabrata*. Whereas *C. krusei* must be considered intrinsically resistant to fluconazole, infections with *C. glabrata* may be treated successfully with high doses (e.g., 800 mg/day) of fluconazole. Resistance

may develop when fluconazole is used to treat histoplasmosis, and it has only limited activity against *B. dermatitidis*. Fluconazole is not active against the opportunistic molds, including *Aspergillus* spp., *Fusarium* spp., and the Mucormycetes.

Fluconazole is a water-soluble agent and may be administered orally or intravenously. Protein binding is low, and the drug is distributed to all organs and tissues, including the central nervous system. Severe side effects such as exfoliative dermatitis or liver failure are uncommon.

Because of its low toxicity, ease of administration, and fungistatic activity against most yeastlike fungi, fluconazole has an important role in the treatment of candidiasis, cryptococcosis, and coccidioidomycosis. It is used as primary therapy for candidemia and mucosal candidiasis and as prophylaxis in selected high-risk populations. It is used in maintenance therapy of cryptococcal meningitis in patients with acquired immunodeficiency syndrome (AIDS) and is the agent of choice in the treatment of meningitis caused by *C. immitis*. Fluconazole is a second-line agent in the treatment of histoplasmosis, blastomycosis, and sporotrichosis.

Itraconazole is a lipophilic triazole that may be administered orally in capsule or in solution. Itraconazole has a broad spectrum of antifungal activity, including against *Candida* spp., *C. neoformans*, *Aspergillus* spp., dermatophytes, dematiaceous molds, *P. boydii*, *Sporothrix schenckii*, and the endemic dimorphic pathogens (see Table 63-2). Itraconazole has activity against some, but not all, fluconazole-resistant strains of *C. glabrata* and *C. krusei*. Itraconazole-resistant strains of *Aspergillus fumigatus* have been reported; however, they are uncommon. The Mucormycetes, *Fusarium*, and *S. prolificans* are resistant to itraconazole.

As with ketoconazole, the oral absorption of itraconazole is erratic and requires an acid gastric pH. Absorption is enhanced with the oral solution when given in the fasting state. Itraconazole is highly protein bound and exhibits fungistatic activity against yeastlike fungi and fungicidal activity against *Aspergillus* spp.

The efficacy of itraconazole in the treatment of hematogenous candidiasis has not been adequately assessed, although it is useful in the treatment of cutaneous and mucosal forms of candidiasis. Itraconazole is often used in the treatment of dermatophytic infections and is the treatment of choice for lymphocutaneous sporotrichosis and non-life-threatening, nonmeningeal forms of histoplasmosis, blastomycosis, and paracoccidioidomycosis. It may be useful in nonmeningeal coccidioidomycosis, for maintenance treatment of cryptococcal meningitis, and for some forms of phaeohyphomycosis (see Table 63-2). Itraconazole is considered a second-line agent for the treatment of invasive aspergillosis; however, it is not useful in the treatment of infections caused by *Fusarium* spp., the Mucormycetes, or *S. prolificans*.

In contrast to fluconazole, drug interactions are common with itraconazole. Severe hepatotoxicity is rare, and other side effects, such as gastrointestinal intolerance, hypokalemia, edema, rash, and elevated transaminases, occur infrequently.

Voriconazole is a new broad-spectrum triazole with activity against *Candida* spp., *C. neoformans*, *Trichosporon* spp., *Aspergillus* spp., *Fusarium* spp., dematiaceous fungi, and the endemic dimorphic pathogens (see Table 63-2). Among the *Candida* species, voriconazole is active against *C. krusei* and some but not all strains of *Candida albicans* and *C. glabrata* with reduced susceptibility to fluconazole. Although voriconazole has no activity against the Mucormycetes, it is active against fungi that are resistant to amphotericin B, including *A. terreus* and *P. boydii*.

Voriconazole is available in both oral and intravenous formulations. It has excellent penetration into the central nervous system, as well as other tissues. Voriconazole exhibits fungistatic activity against yeast-like fungi and is fungicidal against *Aspergillus* spp.

Voriconazole has a primary indication for the treatment of invasive aspergillosis. It is also approved for treatment of infections caused by *P. boydii* and *Fusarium* spp. in patients intolerant of, or with infections refractory to, other antifungal agents. Voriconazole has proven efficacy in the treatment of various forms of candidiasis and has been used successfully in the treatment of a variety of infections caused by emerging or refractory pathogens, including brain abscesses caused by *Aspergillus* spp. and *P. boydii*.

Voriconazole is generally well tolerated, although approximately one third of patients experience transient visual disturbances. Other adverse effects include liver enzyme abnormalities, skin reactions, and hallucinations or confusion. Interactions with other drugs that are metabolized by the hepatic P450 enzyme system are common.

Posaconazole is a triazole derivative with a chemical structure similar to itraconazole. Posaconazole demonstrates potent activity against *Candida*, *Cryptococcus*, dimorphic fungi, and filamentous fungi, including *Aspergillus* as well as the Mucormycetes.

Posaconazole is available only as an immediate-release oral suspension containing polysorbate 80 as an emulsifying agent. In contrast to voriconazole, posaconazole absorption is enhanced with food intake and is greatest with a concomitant fatty meal. There is a relatively wide patient-to-patient variability in peak serum concentrations, suggesting that posaconazole therapeutic drug monitoring may be important in optimizing the use of this agent. Similar to voriconazole, posaconazole exhibits fungistatic activity against yeastlike fungi and is fungicidal against *Aspergillus* spp.

Posaconazole has U.S. Food and Drug Administration (FDA) approval for prophylaxis of invasive fungal infection in hematopoietic stem cell transplant (HSCT) recipients with graft-versus-host disease (GVHD) and patients with hematologic malignancies and prolonged neutropenia. It is also FDA approved for treatment of oropharyngeal candidiasis. In Europe, posaconazole is additionally approved for the following fungal infections refractory to amphotericin B and/or itraconazole: aspergillosis, fusariosis, chromoblastomycosis, mycetoma, and coccidioidomycosis.

Posaconazole is generally well tolerated. The most common adverse events are mild and include gastrointestinal complaints, rash, facial flushing, dry mouth, and headache. As with other azoles, hepatic toxicity has been described, and monitoring of liver function tests is recommended before and during treatment with posaconazole. Interactions with other drugs that are metabolized by the hepatic P450 enzyme system are common.

Echinocandins

The echinocandins are a novel, highly selective, class of semisynthetic lipopeptides (see Figure 63-2) that inhibit the synthesis of 1,3-β-glucans, important constituents of the fungal cell wall (Figure 63-5; see Table 63-1 and Figure 63-1). Because mammalian cells do not contain 1,3-β-glucans, this class of agents is selective in its toxicity for fungi in which the glucans play an important role in maintaining the osmotic integrity of the fungal cell. Glucans are also important in cell division and cell growth. Inhibition of the glucan synthesis enzyme complex results in fungicidal activity against *Candida* spp. and fungistatic activity against *Aspergillus* spp. At the present time, there are three echinocandins (anidulafungin, caspofungin, and micafungin) approved for use in treatment or prevention of various mycoses (see Table 63-1).

The spectrum of activity of the echinocandins is limited to those fungi in which 1,3-β-glucans constitute the dominant cell wall glucan component. As such, they are active against *Candida* and *Aspergillus*

spp. and have variable activity against the dematiaceous fungi and the endemic dimorphic pathogens (see Table 63-2). They are inactive against *C. neoformans*, *Trichosporon* spp., *Fusarium* spp. and other hyaline molds, and the Mucormycetes. The echinocandins have excellent activity against fluconazole-resistant strains of *Candida* spp. Primary or acquired resistance to this class of agents appears to be uncommon among clinical isolates of *Candida* spp. and *Aspergillus* spp.

The echinocandins must be administered intravenously and are highly (>95%) protein bound. They are distributed to all major organs, although concentrations in cerebrospinal fluid are low. All of the echinocandins are very well tolerated and have few drug-drug interactions.

Among the three echinocandins, all have similar spectrum and potency against *Candida* and *Aspergillus* species. Caspofungin is approved for the treatment of invasive candidiasis, including candidemia, and for treatment of patients with invasive aspergillosis refractory to or intolerant of other approved antifungal therapies. Anidulafungin is approved for the treatment of esophageal candidiasis and candidemia, and micafungin is approved for treatment of esophageal candidiasis and candidemia, and for prevention of invasive candidiasis.

Antimetabolites

Flucytosine (5-fluorocytosine [5-FC]) is the only available antifungal agent that functions as an antimetabolite. It is a fluorinated pyrimidine analogue that exerts antifungal activity by interfering with the synthesis of deoxyribonucleic acid (DNA), ribonucleic acid (RNA), and proteins in the fungal cell (see Figure 63-1). Flucytosine enters the fungal cell via cytosine permease and is deaminated to 5-fluorouracil (5-FU) in the cytoplasm. The 5-FU is converted to 5-fluorouridylic acid, which then competes with uracil in the synthesis of RNA, with resultant RNA miscoding and inhibition of DNA and protein synthesis.

The antifungal spectrum of flucytosine is limited to *Candida* spp., *C. neoformans*, *Rhodotorula* spp., *Saccharomyces cerevisiae*, and selected dematiaceous

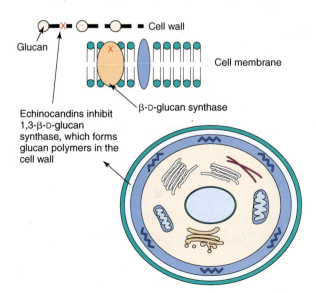

Echinocandins

Glucan — Cell wall

Cell membrane

β-D-glucan synthase

Echinocandins inhibit 1,3-β-D-glucan synthase, which forms glucan polymers in the cell wall

Figure 63-5   Mechanism of action of the echinocandins.

molds (see Table 63-2). Although primary resistance to flucytosine is rare among isolates of *Candida* spp., resistance may develop among *Candida* and *C. neoformans* during flucytosine monotherapy. Flucytosine is not active against *Aspergillus* spp., the Mucormycetes, or other hyaline molds.

Flucytosine is water soluble and has excellent bioavailability when administered orally. High concentrations of flucytosine may be achieved in serum, cerebrospinal fluid, and other body fluids. Major toxicities are observed when flucytosine serum concentrations exceed 100 µg/ml and include bone marrow suppression, hepatotoxicity, and gastrointestinal intolerance. Monitoring of serum concentrations of flucytosine is important in avoiding toxicity.

Flucytosine is not used as monotherapy, because of the propensity for secondary resistance. Combinations of flucytosine with either amphotericin B or fluconazole have been shown to be efficacious in treating both cryptococcosis and candidiasis.

Allylamines

The allylamine class of antifungal agents includes terbinafine, which has systemic activity, and naftifine, which is a topical agent (see Table 63-1). These agents inhibit the enzyme squalene epoxidase, which results in a decrease in ergosterol and an increase in squalene within the fungal cell membrane (see Figures 63-1 and 63-4).

Terbinafine is a lipophilic antifungal agent with a broad spectrum of activity that includes dermatophytes, *Candida* spp., *Malassezia furfur*, *C. neoformans*, *Trichosporon* spp., *Aspergillus* spp., *S. schenckii*, and *P. marneffei* (see Table 63-2). It is available in oral and topical formulations and achieves high concentrations in fatty tissues, skin, hair, and nails.

Terbinafine is efficacious in the treatment of virtually all forms of dermatomycoses, including onychomycosis, and exhibits few side effects. It has shown clinical effectiveness in the treatment of sporotrichosis, aspergillosis, and chromoblastomycosis and has shown promise for the treatment of infections caused by fluconazole-resistant *Candida* spp. when used in combination with fluconazole.

Griseofulvin

Griseofulvin is an oral agent used in the treatment of infections caused by the dermatophytes. It is thought to inhibit fungal growth by interaction with microtubules within the fungal cell, resulting in inhibition of mitosis (see Table 63-1 and Figure 63-1).

Griseofulvin is considered a second-line agent in the treatment of dermatophytoses. Newer agents, such as itraconazole and terbinafine, are more rapid acting and provide greater efficacy. Griseofulvin is also associated with a number of mild side effects, including nausea, diarrhea, headache, hepatotoxicity, rash, and neurologic side effects.

TOPICAL ANTIFUNGAL AGENTS

A wide variety of topical antifungal preparations is available for the treatment of superficial cutaneous and mucosal fungal infections (see Table 63-1). Topical preparations are available for most classes of antifungal agents, including polyenes (amphotericin B, nystatin, pimaricin), allylamines (naftifine and terbinafine), and numerous imidazoles and miscellaneous agents (see Table 63-1). Creams, lotions, ointments, powders, and sprays are available for use in the treatment of cutaneous infections and onychomycosis, whereas mucosal infections are best treated with suspensions, tablets, troches, or suppositories.

Whether one uses topical or systemic therapy for treatment of cutaneous or mucosal fungal infections usually depends on the status of the host and the type and extent of infection. Whereas most cutaneous dermatophytic infections and oral or vaginal candidiasis will respond to topical therapy, the refractory nature of infections, such as onychomycosis or tinea capitis ("ringworm" of the scalp), usually calls for long-term systemic therapy.

COMBINATIONS OF ANTIFUNGAL AGENTS IN THE TREATMENT OF MYCOSES

The high mortality of opportunistic fungal infections has spurred the development of new antifungal agents, including some with novel mechanisms of action (see Table 63-1). In addition to aggressive use of new antifungal agents, such as voriconazole and caspofungin, as monotherapy, the use of azole-, echinocandin-, and polyene-based combinations for treatment of the more difficult-to-treat mycoses, such as opportunistic mold infections, is the focus of intense interest and discussion. The rationale behind combination therapy is that by using combinations of antifungal agents, one may achieve a better clinical outcome than with monotherapy. The push toward the use of combination antifungal therapy is especially strong for those infections such as invasive aspergillosis, where the associated mortality is unacceptably high.

In considering combination therapy, one seeks to achieve **synergy** and avoid **antagonism. Synergy** is achieved when the outcome obtained with the combination of agents is significantly better than that obtained with either drug alone. Conversely, **antagonism** is when the combination is less active or efficacious than either drug alone. In the case of antifungal therapy, there are several mechanisms that one may consider in developing an effective combination treatment strategy: (1) Different stages of the same biochemical pathway can be inhibited. This is a classic approach for achieving synergy with antiinfective agents. An example of this approach to antifungal therapy would be the combination of terbinafine with an azole, where both agents attack the sterol pathway at different points (see Figure 63-4), resulting in inhibition of ergosterol synthesis and disruption of the fungal cell membrane. (2) Increased penetration of one agent into the cell by virtue of the permeabilizing action of another agent on the fungal cell wall or cell membrane can be achieved. The combination of amphotericin B (cell membrane disruption) and flucytosine (inhibition of nucleic acid synthesis intracellularly) is a classic example of this interaction. (3) Inhibition of the transport of one agent out of the cell by another agent can be achieved. Many fungi employ energy-dependent efflux pumps to actively pump antifungal agents out of the cell, thereby avoiding the toxic effects of the antifungal. Inhibition

of these pumps by agents such as reserpine has been shown to enhance the activity of the azole antifungal agents against *Candida* spp. (4) Simultaneous inhibition of different fungal cell targets can be achieved. Inhibition of fungal cell wall synthesis by an agent such as caspofungin, coupled with disruption of cell membrane function by amphotericin B or azoles, is an example of this type of combination.

Although the potential value of combination antifungal therapy is appealing, there are several possible downsides to this strategy that must be considered. Antagonism among antifungal agents when used in combination is also a distinct possibility and may occur via several different mechanisms: (1) The action of one agent results in a decrease in the target of another agent. The action of azole antifungal agents depletes the cell membrane of ergosterol, which is the primary target for amphotericin B. (2) The action of one antifungal agent results in the modification of the target of another agent. The inhibition of ergosterol synthesis by azole antifungal agents results in the accumulation of methylated sterols, to which amphotericin B binds less well. (3) Blocking of the target site of one agent by another may occur. Lipophilic agents, such as itraconazole, may adsorb to the fungal cell surface and inhibit the binding of amphotericin B to membrane sterols.

Despite these possible positive and negative scenarios, the data supporting the achievement of synergy when various combinations are used clinically are limited. Likewise, antagonism may be demonstrated in the laboratory, but significant antagonism has not been observed clinically with antifungal combinations. By considering all of the laboratory and clinical data for antifungal combination therapy, one arrives at a very limited number of instances where combination therapy has been shown to be beneficial in the treatment of invasive mycoses (Table 63-3).

The strongest data exists for the treatment of cryptococcosis, where the combination of amphotericin B and flucytosine has been shown to be beneficial in the treatment of cryptococcal meningitis. The data are less strong for the combination of flucytosine with fluconazole or amphotericin B with

Table 63-3 Summary of Potentially Useful Antifungal Combinations for Treatment of Common Mycoses.

Infection	Antifungal Combination	Comments
Candidiasis	AMB + FCZ	Good clinical success in humans with candidemia
	AMB + FC	Clinical success in humans with peritonitis
Cryptococcosis	AMB + FC	Good clinical success in humans with cryptococcal meningitis
	AMB + FCZ	Clinical success in humans with cryptococcal meningitis
	FC + FCZ	Clinical success in humans with cryptococcal meningitis
Aspergillosis	AMB + FC	In vivo benefit (animal model); minimal human data
	AMB + azoles	No benefit in animals
	AMB + echinocandins	In vivo benefit (animal model); minimal human data
	Triazoles + echinocandins	In vivo benefit (animal model); minimal human data

AMB, Amphotericin B; *FC*, flucytosine; *FCZ*, fluconazole.

triazoles; however, these combinations appear to be beneficial in treating cryptococcosis as well.

Candidiasis is generally treated adequately with a single antifungal agent, such as amphotericin B, caspofungin, or fluconazole; however, combination therapy may be useful in selected situations. The combination of amphotericin B and fluconazole has proven benefits in treating candidemia. Likewise, the combination of terbinafine plus an azole is promising in the treatment of refractory oropharyngeal candidiasis. Flucytosine in combination with either amphotericin B or triazoles has positive effects on survival and tissue burden of infection in animal models of candidiasis. Currently, combination therapy of candidiasis should be reserved for specific individual settings such as meningitis, endocarditis, hepatosplenic infection, and candidiasis that are recurrent or refractory to single-agent therapy.

Although the clinical setting of invasive aspergillosis is where combination therapy is most attractive, the data to support its use are lacking. At the present time, there are no clinical trials published that evaluate the use of combination therapy in the treatment of invasive aspergillosis. Studies in vitro and in animals have produced variable results. Combinations of echinocandins with azoles or amphotericin B have yielded positive results. Likewise, amphotericin B plus rifampin appears synergistic. Studies with flucytosine or rifampin plus amphotericin B or azoles have been inconsistent. Despite the desperate need for better treatment options for invasive aspergillo-

sis, there is little evidence that combination therapy will improve clinical outcome. Combination therapy should be used with caution until more clinical data is available.

MECHANISMS OF RESISTANCE TO ANTIFUNGAL AGENTS

Given the prominent role of *Candida* spp. as etiologic agents of invasive mycoses, it is not surprising that most of our understanding of the mechanisms of resistance to antifungal agents comes from studies of *C. albicans* and other species of *Candida*. Much less is known of resistance mechanisms in *Aspergillus* spp. and *C. neoformans*, and almost no information on antifungal resistance mechanisms is available for other opportunistic fungal pathogens.

In contrast to mechanisms of resistance to antibacterial agents, there is no evidence that fungi are capable of destroying or modifying antifungal agents as a means of achieving resistance. Likewise, antifungal resistance genes are not transmissible from cell to cell in the manner that occurs with many bacterial resistance genes. It is apparent, however, that multidrug efflux pumps, target alterations, and reduced access to drug targets are important mechanisms of resistance to antifungal agents, just as they are for antibacterial resistance (Table 63-4). In contrast to the rapid emergence and spread of high-level multidrug resistance that occurs in bacteria, antifungal resistance usually develops slowly and involves the

Table 63-4   Mechanisms Involved in the Development of Resistance to Antifungal Agents in Pathogenic Fungi.

Fungus	Amphotericin B	Flucytosine	Itraconazole	Fluconazole	Echinocandins
Aspergillus fumigatus			Altered target enzyme, 14-α-demethylase Decreased azole accumulation		
Candida albicans	Decrease in ergosterol Replacement of poly-ene-binding sterols Masking of ergosterol	Loss of permease activity Loss of cytosine deaminase activity Loss of uracil phosphoribosyl-transferase activity		Overexpression or mutation of 14-α-demethylase Overexpression of efflux pumps, CDR and MDR genes	Mutation in fks1 gene
Candida glabrata	Alteration or decrease in ergosterol content	Loss of permease activity		Overexpression of efflux pumps (CgCDR genes)	Mutation in fks1 and/or fks2 gene
Candida krusei	Alteration or decrease in ergosterol content			Active efflux Reduced affinity for target enzyme, 14-α-demethylase	Mutation in fks1 gene
Candida lusitaniae	Alteration or decrease in ergosterol content Production of modified sterols				
Cryptococcus neoformans	Defects in sterol synthesis Decreased ergosterol Production of modified sterols			Alterations in target enzyme Overexpression of MDR efflux pump	

emergence of intrinsically resistant species or a gradual, stepwise alteration of cellular structures or functions that results in resistance to an agent to which there has been prior exposure.

Clinical Factors Contributing to Resistance

Antifungal therapy may fail clinically, despite the fact that the drug employed is active against the infecting fungus. The complex interaction of the host, the drug, and the fungal pathogen may be influenced by a wide variety of factors, including the immune status of the host, the site and severity of the infection, presence of a foreign body (e.g., catheter, vascular graft), the activity of the drug at the site of infection, the dose and duration of therapy, and patient compliance with the antifungal regimen. It must be recognized that the presence of neutrophils, use of immunomodulating drugs, concomitant infections (e.g., human immunodeficiency virus), surgical procedures, age, and nutritional status of the host all

may be more important in determining the outcome of the infection than the ability of the antifungal agent to inhibit or kill the infecting organism.

Antifungal Susceptibility Testing

In vitro susceptibility testing of antifungal agents is designed to determine the relative activity of one or more agents against the infecting pathogen in hopes of selecting the best option for treatment of the infection. Thus antifungal susceptibility tests are performed for the same reasons that tests with antibacterial agents are performed. Antifungal susceptibility tests will (1) provide a reliable estimate of the relative activity of two or more antifungal agents against the tested organism, (2) correlate with in vivo antifungal activity and predict the likely outcome of therapy, (3) provide a means with which to monitor the development of resistance among a normally susceptible population of organisms, and (4) predict the therapeutic potential of newly developed investigational agents.

Standardized methods for performing antifungal susceptibility testing are reproducible, accurate, and available for use in clinical laboratories. Antifungal susceptibility testing is now increasingly and appropriately used as a routine adjunct to the treatment of fungal infections. Guidelines for the use of antifungal testing as a complement to other laboratory studies have been developed. Selective application of antifungal susceptibility testing, coupled with broader identification of fungi to the species level, is especially useful in difficult-to-manage fungal infections. One must keep in mind, however, that the in vitro susceptibility of an infecting organism to the antimicrobial agent is only one of several factors that may influence the likelihood that therapy for an infection will be successful (see Clinical Factors Contributing to Resistance).

SUMMARY

Antifungal spectrum is a range of activity of an antifungal agent against fungi. A broad-spectrum antifungal agent inhibits a wide variety of fungi, including both yeastlike fungi and molds, whereas a narrow-spectrum agent is active only against a limited number of fungi.

Fungistatic activity is the level of antifungal activity that **inhibits** the growth of an organism. This is determined in vitro by testing a standardized concentration of organisms against a series of antifungal dilutions. The lowest concentration of the drug that inhibits the growth of the organism is referred to as the **minimum inhibitory concentration (MIC).**

Fungicidal activity is the ability of an antifungal agent to **kill** an organism in vitro or in vivo. The lowest concentration of the drug that kills 99.9% of the test population is called the **minimum fungicidal concentration (MFC).**

Antifungal combinations are combinations of antifungal agents that may be used (1) to enhance efficacy in the treatment of a refractory fungal infection, (2) to broaden the spectrum of empiric antifungal therapy, (3) to prevent the emergence of resistant organisms, and (4) to achieve a synergistic killing effect.

Antifungal synergism means the combinations of antifungal agents that have enhanced antifungal activity when used together compared with the activity of each agent alone.

Antifungal antagonism is the combination of antifungal agents in which the activity of one of the agents interferes with the activity of the other agent.

Efflux pumps are families of drug transporters that serve to actively pump antifungal agents out of the fungal cells, thus decreasing the amount of intracellular drug available to bind to its target.

KEYWORDS

English	Chinese
Amphotericin B	两性霉素 B
Azoles	氮唑类（抗真菌药）
Ketoconazole	酮康唑
Fluconazole	氟康唑
Itraconazole	伊曲康唑
Voriconazole	伏立康唑
Echinocandins	棘白菌素类（抗真菌药）
Flucytosine	氟胞嘧啶
Allylamines	烯丙胺（抗真菌药）
Terbinafine	特比萘芬
Griseofulvin	灰黄霉素

BIBLIOGRAPHY

1. Gubbins PO, Anaissie EJ: Antifungal therapy. In Anaissie EJ, McGinnis MR, Pfaller MA, editors: Clinical mycology, ed 2, New York, 2009, Churchill Livingstone.

2. Howard SJ, Arendrup MC: Acquired antifungal drug resistance in *Aspergillus fumigatus*: epidemiology and detection, Med Mycol 49(Suppl 1): S90-S95, 2011.

3. Johnson EM, Espinel-Ingroff AV, Pfaller MA: Susceptibility test methods: yeasts and filamentous fungi. In Versalovic J, et al, editors: Manual of clinical microbiology, ed 10, Washington, DC, 2011, American Society for Microbiology Press.

4. Johnson MD, et al: Combination antifungal therapy, Antimicrob Agents Chemother 48: 693-715, 2004.

5. Kanafani ZA, Perfect JR: Resistance to antifungal agents: mechanisms and clinical impact, Clin Infect Dis 46: 120-128, 2008.

6. Perlin DS: Resistance to echinocandin-class antifungal drugs, Drug Resist Updates 10: 121-130, 2007.

Superficial and Cutaneous Mycoses

Fungal infections of the skin and skin structures are extremely common. These infections are generally categorized by the structures that the fungi colonize or invade:

Superficial mycoses, limited to the outmost layers of the skin and hair

Cutaneous mycoses, infections that involve the deeper layers of the epidermis and its integuments, the hair and nails

Subcutaneous mycoses, involving the dermis, subcutaneous tissues, muscle, and fascia. The subcutaneous mycoses will be discussed separately in Chapter 66. This chapter will deal with the superficial and cutaneous mycoses.

SUPERFICIAL MYCOSES

Agents of superficial mycoses are fungi that colonize the keratinized outer layers of the skin, hair, and nails. Infections caused by these organisms elicit little or no host immune response and are nondestructive and thus asymptomatic. They are usually of cosmetic concern only and are easy to diagnose and treat.

Pityriasis (Tinea) Versicolor

Pityriasis versicolor is a common superficial fungal infection that is seen worldwide. In certain tropical environments, it may affect up to 60% of the population. It is caused by the lipophilic yeast *Malassezia furfur*.

Morphology

When viewed in skin scrapings, *M. furfur* appears as clusters of spherical or oval, thick-walled yeastlike

cells, 3 to 8 μm in diameter (Figure 64-1). The yeast cells may be mixed with short, infrequently branched hyphae that tend to orient end to end. The yeastlike cells represent phialoconidia and show polar bud formation with a "lip" or collarette around the point of bud initiation on the parent cell (Figure 64-2). In

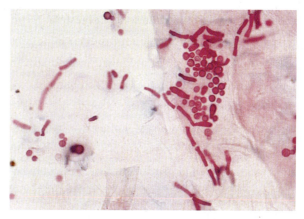

Figure 64-1 Pityriasis versicolor. Periodic acid-Schiff-stained skin scraping showing yeastlike cells and short, infrequently branched hyphae that are often oriented end to end (×100). (From Connor DH, et al: *Pathology of infectious diseases*, Stamford, Conn, 1997, Appleton & Lange.)

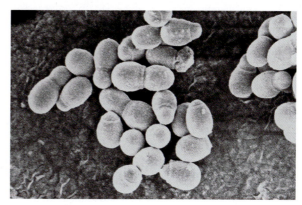

Figure 64-2 Scanning electron micrograph of *Malassezia furfur* demonstrating the liplike collarette around the point of bud initiation on the parent cell. (Courtesy S.A. Messer.)

culture on standard media containing or overlaid with olive oil, *M. furfur* grows as cream-colored to tan yeastlike colonies composed of budding yeastlike cells; hyphae are infrequently produced.

Epidemiology

Pityriasis versicolor is a disease of healthy persons that occurs worldwide, but it is most prevalent in tropical and subtropical regions.

Clinical Syndromes

The lesions of pityriasis versicolor are small hypopigmented or hyperpigmented macules. The upper trunk, arms, chest, shoulders, face, and neck are most often involved, but any part of the body may be affected (Figure 64-3). The lesions are irregular, well-demarcated patches of discoloration that may be raised and covered by a fine scale. Because *M. furfur* tends to interfere with melanin production, lesions are hypopigmented in dark-skinned individuals. In light-skinned individuals, the lesions are pink to pale brown and become more obvious when they fail to tan after exposure to sunlight. Little or no host reaction occurs, and the lesions are asymptomatic, with the exception of mild pruritus in severe cases. Infection of the hair follicles, resulting in folliculitis, perifolliculitis, and dermal abscesses, is a rare complication of this disease.

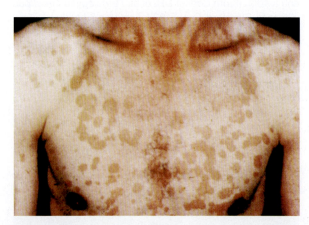

Figure 64-3 Pityriasis versicolor. Multiple, pale brown, hyperpigmented patches on chest and shoulders. (From Chandler FW, Watts JC: *Pathologic diagnosis of fungal infections*, Chicago, 1987, American Society for Clinical Pathology Press.)

Laboratory Diagnosis

The laboratory diagnosis of pityriasis versicolor is made by the direct visualization of the fungal elements on microscopic examination of epidermal scales in 10% potassium hydroxide (KOH) with or without calcofluor white. The organisms are usually numerous and may also be visualized with hematoxylin and eosin (H&E) or periodic acid-Schiff (PAS) stains (see Figure 64-1). The lesions will also fluoresce with a yellowish color upon exposure to a Wood lamp.

Although not usually necessary for establishing the diagnosis, culture may be performed using synthetic mycologic media supplemented with olive oil as a source of lipid. Growth of yeastlike colonies appear after incubation at 30°C for 5 to 7 days. Microscopically, the colonies are comprised of budding yeastlike cells with occasional hyphae.

Treatment

Although spontaneous cure has been reported, the disease is generally chronic and persistent. Treatment consists of the use of topical azoles or selenium sulfide shampoo. For more widespread infection, oral ketoconazole or itraconazole may be used.

White Piedra

White piedra is a superficial infection of hair caused by yeastlike fungi of the genus *Trichosporon*: *T. inkin*, *T. asahii*, or *T. mucoides*.

Morphology

Microscopic examination reveals hyphal elements, arthroconidia (rectangular cells resulting from the fragmentation of hyphal cells), and blastoconidia (budding yeast cells).

Epidemiology

This condition occurs in tropical and subtropical regions and is related to poor hygiene.

Clinical Syndromes

White piedra affects the hairs of the groin and axillae. The fungus surrounds the hair shaft and forms a white to brown swelling along the hair strand. The swellings are soft and pasty and may be easily removed by running a section of the hair between the thumb and forefinger. The infection does not damage the hair shaft.

Laboratory Diagnosis

When microscopic examination reveals hyphal elements, arthroconidia, and/or budding yeast cells, infected hair should be placed on mycologic media without cycloheximide (cycloheximide will inhibit *Trichosporon* spp.). *Trichosporon* spp. will form cream-colored, dry, wrinkled colonies within 48 to 72 hours upon incubation at room temperature. The various species of *Trichosporon* can be identified in the same manner as other yeast isolates. Sugar assimilations, potassium nitrate (KNO_3) assimilation (negative), urease production (positive), and morphology on cornmeal agar (both arthroconidia and blastoconidia are present) should be determined.

Treatment

Treatment may be accomplished by the use of topical azoles; however, improved hygiene and shaving of the infected hair are also effective and usually negate the necessity of medical treatment.

Black Piedra

Another condition affecting the hair, primarily the scalp, is black piedra. The causative agent of black piedra is *Piedraia hortae*.

Morphology

The organism grows as pigmented (brown to reddish-black) mold. As the culture ages, spindle-shaped ascospores are formed within specialized structures (asci). These structures (asci and ascospores) are also produced within the rock-hard hyphal mass that surrounds the hair shaft.

Epidemiology

Black piedra is uncommon and has been reported from tropical areas in Latin America and Central Africa. It is thought to be a condition of poor hygiene.

Clinical Syndromes

Black piedra presents as small, dark nodules that surround the hair shafts. It is asymptomatic and generally involves the scalp. The hyphal mass is held together by a cement-like substance and contains asci and ascospores, the sexual phase of the fungus.

Laboratory Diagnosis

Examination of the nodule reveals branched, pigmented, hyphae held together by a cement-like substance. *P. hortae* can be cultured on routine mycologic media. Very slow growth may be observed at 25℃ and may begin as a yeastlike colony, later becoming velvety as hyphae develop. Asci may be observed microscopically, usually ranging from 4 to 30 μm and containing up to eight ascospores.

Treatment

Treatment of black piedra is easily accomplished by a haircut and proper, regular washings.

CUTANEOUS MYCOSES

The cutaneous mycoses include infections caused by dermatophytic fungi (dermatophytosis) and non-dermatophytic fungi (dermatomycosis) (Table 64-1). Because of the overwhelming importance of dermatophytes as etiologic agents of cutaneous mycoses, the majority of this section will deal with those fungi. The nondermatophytic fungi will be discussed regarding their role in onychomycosis. The superficial and cutaneous infections caused by *Candida* spp. will be discussed in Chapter 67.

Dermatophytoses

The term **dermatophytosis** refers to a complex of diseases caused by any of several species of taxonomically related filamentous fungi in the genera *Trichophyton*, *Epidermophyton*, and *Microsporum* (Tables 64-1). These fungi are known collectively as **the dermatophytes**, and all possess the ability to cause disease in humans and/or animals. All have in common the ability to invade the skin, hair, or nails. In each case,

Table 64-1 Common and Uncommon Agents of Superficial and Cutaneous Dermatomycoses and Dermatophytoses.

Fungus	TP	TCO	TCR	TCA	TBA	TVR	O	TN	BP	WP
Dermatophytic										
Trichophyton rubrum	X	X	X				X			
T. mentagrophytes	X	X	X	X			X			
T. tonsurans		X		X			X			
T. verrucosum		X		X	X					
T. equinum				X						
T. violaceum				X						
T. schoenleinii				X						
T. megnini							X			
Epidermophyton floccosum	X		X				X			
Microsporum canis		X		X						
M. audouinii				X						
Nondermatophytic										
Scopulariopsis brevicaulis							X			
Scytalidium spp.	X						X			
Malassezia spp.						X				
Candida albicans	X		X				X			
Aspergillus terreus							X			
Acremonium spp.							X			
Fusarium spp.							X			
Trichosporon spp.										X
Piedraia hortae									X	
Hortaea werneckii								X		

BP, Black piedra; O, onychomycosis; TBA, tinea barbae; TCA, tinea capitis; TCO, tinea corporis; TCR, tinea cruris; TN, tinea nigra; TP, tinea pedis; TVR, tinea versicolor; WP, white piedra; X, etiologic agents of dermatomycoses or dermatophycoses.

these fungi are keratinophilic and keratinolytic and so are able to break down the keratin surfaces of these structures. In the case of skin infections, the dermatophytes invade only the upper, outermost layer of the epidermis, the stratum corneum. Penetration below the granular layer of the epidermis is rare. Likewise with hair and nails, being part of the skin, only the keratinized layers are invaded. The various forms of dermatophytosis are referred to as "tineas" or ringworm. Clinically, the tineas are classified according to the anatomic site or structure affected: (1) tinea capitis of the scalp, eyebrows, and eyelashes; (2) tinea barbae of the beard; (3) tinea corporis of the smooth or glabrous skin; (4) tinea cruris of the groin; (5) tinea pedis of the foot; (6) tinea unguium of the nails (also known as **onychomycosis**). The clinical signs and symptoms of **dermat**ophytosis vary according to the etiologic agents, the host reaction, and the site of infection.

Morphology

Each genus of dermatophytic mold is characterized by a specific pattern of growth in culture and by the production of macroconidia and microconidia. Further identification to species level requires consideration of colony morphology, spore production, and nutritional requirements in vitro.

Microscopically, the genus *Microsporum* is identified by observation of its macroconidia, whereas microconidia are the characteristic structures of the genus *Trichophyton*. *Epidermophyton floccosum* does not produce microconidia, but its smooth-walled macroconidia borne in clusters of two or three are quite distinctive (Figure 64-4). *Microsporum canis* produces characteristic large, multicellular (five to eight cells per conidium), thick- and rough-walled macroconidia (Figure 64-5). *Trichophyton rubrum* produces microconidia that are teardrop or peg shaped and borne along the sides of hyphae (Figure 64-6), whereas *Trichophyton mentagrophytes* produces both single, cigar-shaped macroconidia and grapelike clusters of spherical microconidia (Figure 64-7).

In skin biopsies, all of the dermatophytes are morphologically similar and appear as hyaline septate hyphae, chains of arthroconidia, or dissociated chains of arthroconidia that invade the stratum corneum, hair follicles, and hairs. When the hair is infected, the pattern of fungal invasion can be either **ectothrix, endothrix,** or **favic** depending on the dermatophytic species (Figure 64-8). Septate hyphae may be seen within the hair shaft in all three patterns. In the **ectothrix** pattern, **arthroconidia** are formed on the outside of the hair (Figure 64-9; see Figure 64-8); in the **endothrix** pattern, arthroconidia are formed inside the hair (see Figure 64-8); and in the **favic** pattern, hyphae, arthroconidia, and empty spaces resembling air bubbles ("honeycomb" pattern) are formed inside the hair (see Figure 64-8). The dermatophytes can usually be seen on H&E stain; however, they are best visualized with special stains for fungi, such as Gomori methenamine silver (GMS) and PAS (see Figure 64-9).

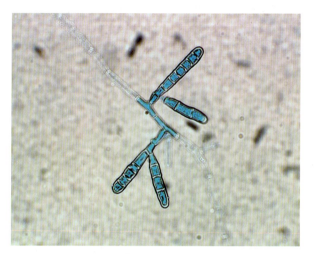

Figure 64-4   *Epidermophyton floccosum.* Lactophenol cotton blue showing smooth-walled macroconidia.

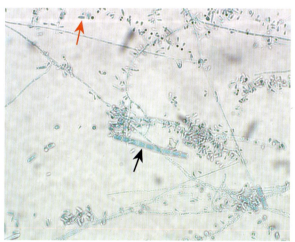

Figure 64-6   *Trichophyton rubrum.* Lactophenol cotton blue showing multicelled macroconidia *(black arrow)* and teardrop- and peg-shaped microconidia *(red arrow).*

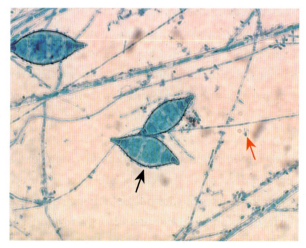

Figure 64-5   *Microsporum canis.* Lactophenol cotton blue showing rough-walled macroconidia *(black arrow)* and microconidia *(red arrow).*

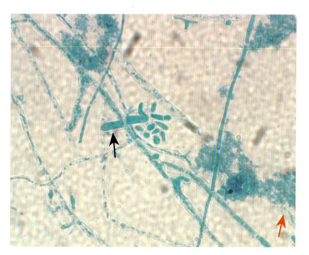

Figure 64-7   *Trichophyton mentagrophytes.* Lactophenol cotton blue showing cigar-shaped macroconidia *(black arrow)* and grapelike clusters of microconidia *(red arrow).*

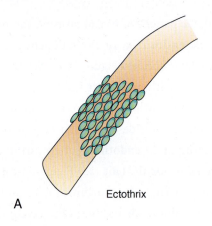

A — Ectothrix

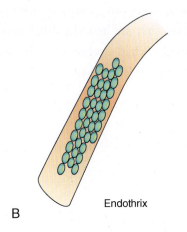

B — Endothrix

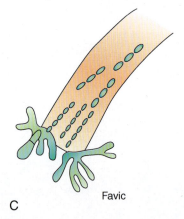

C — Favic

Figure 64-8 Schematic of **(A)** ectothrix hair infection, **(B)** endothrix hair infection, and **(C)** favic hair infection.

Ecology and Epidemiology

Dermatophytes can be classified into three different categories based on their natural habitat: (1) geophilic, (2) zoophilic, and (3) anthropophilic. The geophilic dermatophytes live in the soil and are occasional pathogens of both animals and humans. Zoophilic dermatophytes normally parasitize the hair and skin of animals but can be transmitted to

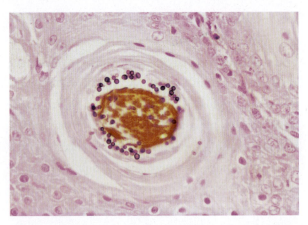

Figure 64-9 Arthroconidia surrounding a hair shaft. Ectothrix hair infection caused by *Microsporum canis* (Gomori methenamine silver-hematoxylin and eosin, ×160.) (From Connor DH, et al: *Pathology of infectious diseases*, Stamford, Conn, 1997, Appleton & Lange.)

humans. Anthropophilic dermatophytes generally infect humans and may be transmitted directly or indirectly from person to person. This classification is quite useful prognostically and emphasizes the importance of identifying the etiologic agent of dermatophytoses. Species of dermatophytes that are considered anthropophilic tend to cause chronic, relatively noninflammatory infections that are difficult to cure. In contrast, the zoophilic and geophilic dermatophytes tend to elicit a profound host reaction, causing lesions that are highly inflammatory and respond well to therapy. In some instances, these infections may heal spontaneously.

The dermatophytes are worldwide in distribution and infection may be acquired from the transfer of arthroconidia or hyphae, or keratinous material containing these elements, from an infected host to a susceptible, uninfected host. Dermatophytes may remain viable in desquamated skin scales or hair for long periods, and infection may be either by direct contact or indirect via fomites. Individuals of both sexes and all ages are susceptible to dermatophytosis; however, tinea capitis is more common in prepubescent children, and tinea cruris and tinea pedis are primarily diseases of adult males. Although dermatophytoses occur worldwide, especially in tropical and subtropical regions, individual dermatophyte species may vary in their geographic distribution and in their virulence for humans. For example, *Trichophyton con-*

centricum, the cause of tinea imbricata, is confined to the islands of the South Pacific and Asia, whereas *T. tonsurans* has replaced *Microsporum audouinii* as the principal agent of tinea capitis in the United States. Infections caused by dermatophytes are generally endemic but may assume epidemic proportions in selected settings (e.g., tinea capitis in school children). On a worldwide scale, *T. rubrum* and *T. mentagrophytes* account for 80% to 90% of all dermatophytoses.

Clinical Syndromes

Dermatophytoses manifest a wide range of clinical presentations, which may be affected by factors such as the species of dermatophytes, the inoculum size, the site of infection, and the immune status of the host. Any given disease manifestation may result from several different species of dermatophytes, as shown in Table 64-1.

The classic pattern of dermatophytosis is the "ringworm" pattern of a ring of inflammatory scaling with diminution of inflammation toward the center of the lesion. Tineas of hair-bearing areas often present as raised, circular or ring-shaped patches of alopecia with erythema and scaling (Figure 64-10) or as more diffusely scattered papules, pustules, vesicles, and kerions (severe inflammation involving the hair shaft) (Figure 64-11). Hairs infected with certain species, such as *M. canis*, *M. audouinii*, and *Trichophyton schoenleinii*, often fluoresce yellow-green when exposed to a Wood light. Infections of smooth skin commonly present as erythematous and scaling patches that expand in a centripetal pattern with central clearing. Dermatophytoses of the foot and hand may often become complicated by onychomycosis (Figure 64-12), in which the nailplate is invaded and destroyed by the fungus. Onychomycosis (tinea unguium) is caused by a variety of dermatophytes (see Table 64-1) and is estimated to affect approximately 3% of the population in most temperate countries. It is a disease seen mostly in adults, with toenails affected more commonly than fingernails. The infection is usually chronic, and the nails become thickened, discolored, raised, friable, and deformed (see Figure 64-12). *T. rubrum* is the most

common etiologic agent in most countries. A rapidly progressive form of onychomycosis that originates from the proximal nailfold and involves the upper

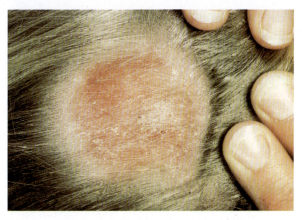

Figure 64-10   Tinea capitis caused by *Microsporum canis*. (From Hay RJ: Cutaneous and subcutaneous mycoses. In Anaissie EJ, McGinnis MR, Pfaller MA, editors: *Clinical mycology*, New York, 2003, Churchill Livingstone.)

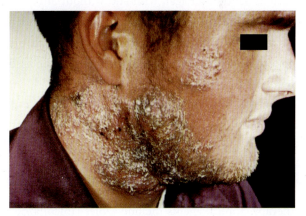

Figure 64-11   Tinea barbae caused by *Trichophyton verrucosum*.(From Chandler FW, Watts JC: *Pathologic diagnosis of fungal infections*, Chicago, 1987, American Society for Clinical Pathology Press.)

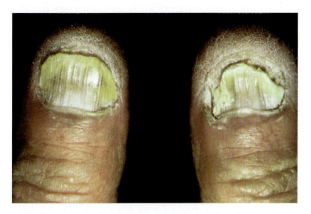

Figure 64-12   Onychomycosis caused by *Trichophyton rubrum*. (From Hay RJ: Cutaneous and subcutaneous mycoses. In Anaissie EJ, McGinnis MR, Pfaller MA, editors: *Clinical mycology*, New York, 2003, Churchill Livingstone.)

and underside of the nail is seen in acquired immunodeficiency syndrome (AIDS) patients.

Laboratory Diagnosis

The laboratory diagnosis of dermatophytoses relies on the demonstration of fungal hyphae by direct microscopy of skin, hair, or nail samples and the isolation of organisms in culture. Specimens are mounted in a drop of 10% to 20% KOH on a glass slide and examined microscopically. Filamentous, hyaline hyphal elements characteristic of dermatophytes may be seen in skin scrapings, nail scrapings, and hairs. In examining specimens for fungal elements, calcofluor white has been used with excellent results.

Cultures are always useful and can be obtained by scraping the affected areas and placing the skin, hair, or nail clippings onto standard mycologic media such as Sabouraud agar, with and without antibiotics, or dermatophyte test medium. Colonies develop within 7 to 28 days. Their gross and microscopic appearance and nutritional requirements can be used in identification.

Treatment

Dermatophytic infections that are localized and that do not affect hair or nails can usually be treated effectively with topical agents; all others require oral therapy. Topical agents include azoles (miconazole, clotrimazole, econazole, tioconazole, and itraconazole), terbinafine, and haloprogin. Whitfield ointment (benzoic and salicylic acids) is an optional agent for dermatophytosis, but responses are usually slower than those seen with agents with specific antifungal activity.

Oral antifungal agents with systemic activity against dermatophytes include griseofulvin, itraconazole, fluconazole, and terbinafine. The azoles and terbinafine are more rapidly and broadly efficacious than griseofulvin, especially for the treatment of onychomycosis.

Onychomycosis Caused by Nondermatophytic Fungi

A number of nondermatophytic molds, as well as Candida species, have been associated with nail infections (see Table 64-1). These organisms include *Scopulariopsis brevicaulis*, *Scytalidium dimidiatum*, *Scytalidium hyalinum*, and a variety of others, including *Aspergillus*, *Fusarium*, and *Candida* species. Among these organisms, *S. brevicaulis* and *Scytalidium* spp. are proven nail pathogens. The other fungi certainly may be the cause of nail pathology; however, the interpretation of nail cultures with these organisms should be done with caution because they may simply represent saprophytic colonization of abnormal nail material. Criteria used to determine an etiologic role for these fungi include isolation on multiple occasions and the presence of abnormal hyphal or conidial structures on microscopic examination of nail material.

Infections caused by *S. brevicaulis*, *S. dimidiatum*, and *S. hyalinum* are notoriously difficult to treat because they are not usually susceptible to any antifungals. Partial surgical removal of infected nails, coupled with oral itraconazole or terbinafine or intensive treatment with 5% amorolfine nail lacquer or Whitfield ointment, may be useful in achieving a clinical response.

SUMMARY

The superficial and cutaneous mycoses are caused by filamentous fungi in the genera *Trichophyton*, *Epidermophyton*, and *Microsporum*. They are able to invade and break down skin, hair, and nails. In infections of skin, hair, and nails, only outermost keratinized layers are invaded. Various forms of dermatophytosis (tineas or "ringworm") are classified according to anatomic site or structure involved. Classification into three categories is based on natural habitat: geophilic, zoophilic, and anthropophilic

KEYWORDS

English	Chinese
Superficial Mycoses	浅部真菌病
Pityriasis Versicolor	花斑癣
Malassezia furfur	糠秕马拉色菌
Cutaneous Mycoses	皮肤真菌病

Dermatophytoses	皮肤癣菌病
Trichophyton	毛癣菌属
Epidermophyton	表皮癣菌属
Microsporum	小孢子菌属

BIBLIOGRAPHY

1. Chandler FW, Watts JC: Pathologic diagnosis of fungal infections, Chicago, 1987, American Society for Clinical Pathology Press.

2. Hay RJ: Cutaneous and subcutaneous mycoses. In Anaissie EJ, McGinnis MR, Pfaller MA, editors: Clinical mycology, New York, 2003, Churchill Livingstone.

3. Hiruma M, Yamaguchi H: Dermatophytes. In Anaissie EJ, McGinnis MR, Pfaller MA, editors: Clinical mycology, New York, 2003, Churchill Livingstone.

4. Summerbell RC: *Trichophyton*, *Microsporum*, *Epidermophyton*, and agents of superficial mycoses. In Versalovic J, et al, editors: Manual of clinical microbiology, ed 10, Washington, DC, 2011, American Society for Microbiology Press.

Subcutaneous Mycoses

Chapter 65

Many fungal pathogens can produce subcutaneous lesions as part of their disease process; however, certain fungi are commonly introduced traumatically through the skin and have a propensity to involve the deeper layers of the dermis, subcutaneous tissue, and bone. Although they may ultimately present clinically as lesions on the skin surface, they rarely spread to distant organs. In general, the clinical course is chronic and insidious; once established, the infections are refractory to most antifungal therapy. The main subcutaneous fungal infections include lymphocutaneous sporotrichosis, chromoblastomycosis, eumycotic mycetoma, subcutaneous zygomycosis, and subcutaneous phaeohyphomycosis.

Although lymphocutaneous sporotrichosis is caused by a single fungal pathogen, *Sporothrix schenckii*, the other subcutaneous mycoses are clinical syndromes caused by multiple fungal etiologies (Table 65-1). The causative agents of subcutaneous mycoses are generally considered to have low pathogenic potential and are commonly isolated from soil, wood, or decaying vegetation. Exposure is largely occupational or related to hobbies (e.g., gardening, wood gathering). Infected patients generally have no underlying immune defect.

LYMPHOCUTANEOUS SPOROTRICHOSIS

Lymphocutaneous sporotrichosis is caused by *S. schenckii*, a dimorphic fungus that is ubiquitous in soil and decaying vegetation. Infection with this organism is chronic and is characterized by nodular and ulcerative lesions that develop along lymphatics that drain the primary site of inoculation (Figure 65-1). Dissem-

ination to the other sites, such as bones, eyes, lungs, and central nervous system, is extremely rare (<1% of all cases) and will not be discussed further. At room temperature, *S. schenckii* grows as a mold (Figure 65-2), and at 37℃ and in tissue, it is a pleomorphic yeast (Figure 65-3, see Table 65-1).

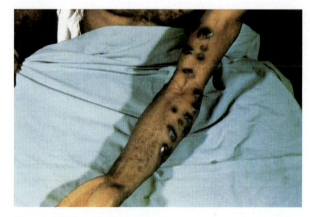

Figure 65-1   Classic lymphocutaneous form of sporotrichosis, demonstrating a chain of subcutaneous nodules along the lymphatic drainage of the arm. (From Chandler FW, Watts JC: *Pathologic diagnosis of fungal infections*, Chicago, 1987, American Society for Clinical Pathology Press.)

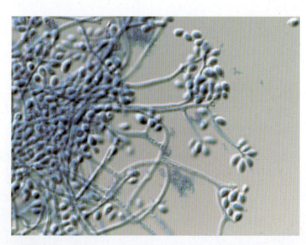

Figure 65-2   Mold phase of *Sporothrix schenckii*.

Table 65-1   Common Agents of Subcutaneous Mycoses.

Disease	Etiologic Agent(s)	Typical Morphology in Tissue	Usual Host Reaction
Sporotrichosis	*Sporothrix schenckii*	Pleomorphic, spheric to oval or cigar-shaped yeasts, 2-10 μm diameter with single or multiple (rare) buds See Figure 65-3	Mixed suppurative and granulomatous Splendore-Hoeppli material surrounds fungus (asteroid body) See Figure 65-4
Chromoblastomycosis	*Cladophialophora* (*Cladosporium*) *carrionii* *Fonsecaea compacta* *Fonsecaea pedrosoi* *Phialophora verrucosa* *Rhinocladiella* spp. *Exophiala* spp.	Large, 6-12 μm diameter, spheric, thick-walled, brown muriform cells (sclerotic bodies) with septations along one or two planes; pigmented hyphae may be present See Figure 65-6	Mixed suppurative and granulomatous Pseudoepitheliomatous hyperplasia
Eumycotic mycetoma	*Phaeoacremonium* spp. *Fusarium* spp. *Aspergillus nidulans* *Scedosporium apiospermum* *Madurella* spp. *Exophiala jeanselmei* among others	Granules, 0.2 to several mm diameter, composed of broad (2-6 μm), hyaline (pale granules) or dematiaceous (black granules), septate hyphae that branch and form chlamydoconidia	Suppurative with multiple abscesses, fibrosis, and sinus tracts; Splendore-Hoeppli material
Subcutaneous entomophthoromycosis	*Basidiobolus ranarum* (*haptosporus*) *Conidiobolus coronatus*	Short, poorly stained hyphal fragments, 6-25 μm diameter, nonparallel sides, pauciseptate, random branches See Figure 65-10	Eosinophilic abscesses and granulation tissue, Splendore-Hoeppli material around hyphae
Subcutaneous phaeohyphomycosis	*Exophiala jeanselmei* *Wangiella dermatitidis* *Bipolaris* spp. *Alternaria* spp. *Chaetomium* spp. *Curvularia* spp. *Phialophora* spp. among others	Pigmented (brown) hyphae, 2-6 μm diameter, branched or unbranched, often constricted at prominent septations, yeast forms and chlamydoconidia may be present See Figure 65-11	Subcutaneous cystic or solid granulomas; overlying epidermis rarely affected

Modified from Chandler FW, Watts JC: *Pathologic diagnosis of fungal infections*, Chicago, 1987, American Society for Clinical Pathology Press.

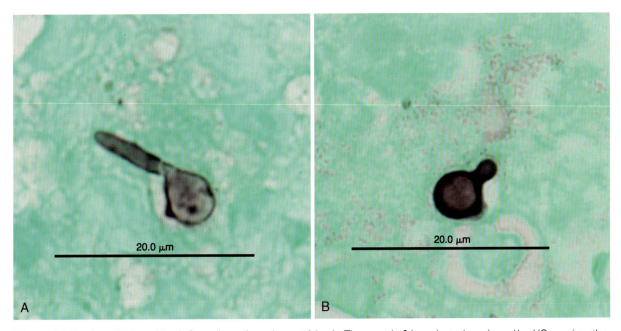

Figure 65-3   **A** and **B,** Lung biopsy from disseminated sporotrichosis. The yeast in **A** has a long cigar-shaped bud (Gomori methenamine silver). (From Anaissie EJ, McGinnis MR, Pfaller MA, editors: *Clinical mycology*, London, 2009, Churchill Livingstone.)

Morphology

S. schenckii is thermally dimorphic. Mycelial form cultures grow rapidly and have a wrinkled membranous surface that gradually becomes tan, brown, or black. Microscopically, the mold form consists of narrow, hyaline, septate hyphae that produce abundant oval conidia (2×3 μm to 3×6 μm) borne on delicate sterigmata or in a rosette or "daisy petal" formation on conidiophores (see Figure 65-2). The yeast form consists of spheric, oval, or elongated ("cigar-shaped") yeastlike cells, 2 to 10 μm in diameter, with single or (rarely) multiple buds (see Table 65-1 and Figure 65-3). Although this is the "tissue phase" of *S. schenckii*, yeast forms are rarely seen on histopathologic examination of tissue.

Epidemiology

Sporotrichosis is usually sporadic and is most common in warmer climates. The major known areas of current endemicity are in Japan and in North and South America, especially Mexico, Brazil, Uruguay, Peru, and Colombia.

Clinical Syndromes

Lymphangitic sporotrichosis classically appears after local trauma to an extremity. The initial site of infection appears as a small nodule, which may ulcerate. Secondary lymphatic nodules appear about 2 weeks after the appearance of the primary lesion and consist of a linear chain of painless, subcutaneous nodules that extend proximally along the course of lymphatic drainage of the primary lesion (see Figure 65-1). With time, the nodules may ulcerate and discharge pus. Primary cutaneous lesions may remain "fixed" without lymphangitic spread. Clinically, these lesions appear nodular, verrucous, or ulcerative and grossly may resemble a malignant process such as squamous cell carcinoma. Other infectious causes of lymphangitic and ulcerative lesions that must be ruled out include mycobacterial and nocardial infections.

Laboratory Diagnosis

Definitive diagnosis usually requires culture of infected pus or tissue. *S. schenckii* grows within 2 to 5 days on a variety of mycologic media and appears as a budding yeast at 35°C and as a mold at 25°C (see Figures 65-2 and 65-3). Laboratory confirmation may be established by converting the mycelial growth to the yeast form by subculture at 37°C or immunologically through the use of the exoantigen test. In tissue, the organism appears as a 2 to 10 μm pleomorphic budding yeast (see Figure 65-3) but is rarely observed in human lesions. The appearance of Splendore-Hoeppli material surrounding yeast cells (asteroid body) may be helpful (Figure 65-4) but is also seen in other types of infection (see Table 65-1).

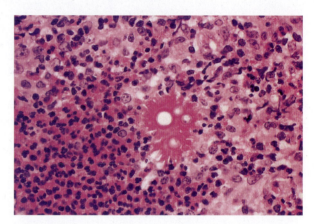

Figure 65-4 Asteroid body in sporotrichosis. The spheric yeastlike cells are surrounded by Splendore-Hoeppli material (hematoxylin and eosin, ×160). (From Connor DH, et al: *Pathology of infectious diseases*, Stamford, Conn, 1997, Appleton & Lange.)

Treatment

The classic treatment for lymphocutaneous sporotrichosis is oral potassium iodide in saturated solution. The efficacy and low cost of this medication makes it a favored option, especially in developing countries; however, it must be given daily over 3 to 4 weeks and has frequent adverse effects (nausea, salivary gland enlargement). Itraconazole has been shown to be safe and highly effective at low doses and is the current treatment of choice. Patients who do not respond may be given a higher dose of itraconazole, terbinafine, or potassium iodide. Fluconazole should be used only if the patient cannot tolerate these other agents. Spontaneous remission is rare but was seen in 13 of the 178 cases in Brazil. The local application of heat has also been shown to be effective.

CHROMOBLASTOMYCOSIS

Chromoblastomycosis (chromomycosis) is a chronic fungal infection affecting skin and subcutaneous tissues. It is characterized by the development of slow-growing verrucous nodules or plaques (Figure 65-5). Chromoblastomycosis is most commonly seen in the tropics, where the warm, moist environment, coupled with the lack of protective footwear and clothing, predisposes individuals to direct inoculation with infected soil or organic matter. The organisms most often associated with chromoblastomycosis are pigmented (dematiaceous) fungi of the genera *Fonsecaea*, *Cladosporium*, *Exophiala*, *Cladophialophora*, *Rhinocladiella*, and *Phialophora* (see Table 65-1).

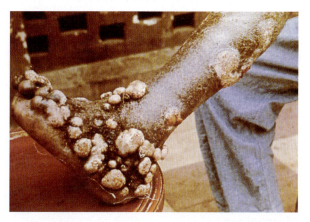

Figure 65-5 Chromoblastomycosis of the foot and leg. (From Connor DH, et al: *Pathology of infectious diseases*, Stamford, Conn, 1997, Appleton & Lange.)

Morphology

The fungi that cause chromoblastomycosis are all dematiaceous (naturally pigmented) molds but are morphologically diverse, and most are capable of producing several different forms when grown in culture. For example, *Exophiala* spp. may grow as a mold and produce conidia-bearing cells called **annelids** and also as a yeastlike form that may appear in freshly isolated colonies. Although the basic form of these organisms is a pigmented septate mold, the different mechanisms of sporulation produced in culture makes specific identification difficult.

In contrast to the diverse morphology seen in culture, in tissue the fungi that cause chromoblastomy-cosis all characteristically form muriform cells (sclerotic bodies, Medlar bodies) that are chestnut brown because of the melanin in their cell walls (Figure 65-6; see Table 65-1). Muriform cells divide by internal septation and appear as cells with vertical and horizontal lines within the same or different planes (see Figure 65-6). In addition to muriform cells, pigmented hyphae may also be present. The fungal cells may be free within the tissue but most often are contained within macrophages or giant cells.

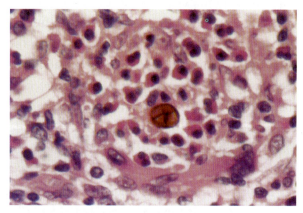

Figure 65-6 Brown-pigmented muriform cell, or Medlar body, of chromoblastomycosis (hematoxylin and eosin, ×250). (From Connor DH, et al: *Pathology of infectious diseases*, Stamford, Conn, 1997, Appleton & Lange.)

Epidemiology

Chromoblastomycosis generally affects individuals working in rural areas of the tropics. The etiologic agents grow on woody plants and in the soil. Most infections have been in men and involve legs and arms, likely the result of occupational exposure.

Clinical Syndromes

Chromoblastomycosis tends to be chronic, pruritic, progressive, indolent, and resistant to treatment. In most instances, patients do not present until the infection is well established. Early lesions are small, warty papules and usually enlarge only slowly. There are different morphologic forms of the disease, ranging from verrucous lesions to flat plaques. Established infections appear as multiple, large, warty, "cauliflower-like" growths that are usually clustered within the same region (see Figure 65-5). Satellite lesions may occur secondary to autoinoculation. Plaquelike lesions often show central scarring as they enlarge. Ulceration and cyst formation may occur. Large lesions are hyperkeratotic, and the limb is grossly distorted because of fibrosis and secondary lymphedema (see Figure 65-5). Secondary bacterial infection may also occur and contribute to regional lymphadenitis, lymph stasis, and eventual elephantiasis.

Laboratory Diagnosis

The clinical presentation (see Figure 65-5), histopathologic findings of chestnut-brown, muriform cells (see Figure 65-6), and isolation in culture of one of the causal fungi (see Table 65-1) confirm the diagnosis. Scrapings obtained from the surface of the warty lesions where small dark dots are observed may result in the demonstration of the characteristic cells when mounted in 20% potassium hydroxide (KOH). Biopsy specimens stained with hematoxylin and eosin (H&E) (see Chapter 68) will also show the organism present in the epidermis or in microabscesses containing macrophages and giant cells. The inflammatory reaction is both suppurative and granulomatous, with dermal fibrosis and **pseudoepitheliomatous hyperplasia.** The organisms are easily cultured from the lesions, although identification may be difficult. There are no serologic tests available for chromoblastomycosis.

Treatment

Treatment with specific antifungal therapy is often ineffective because of the advanced stage of infection upon presentation. The drugs that appear to be most effective are itraconazole and terbinafine. More recently, posaconazole has been used with modest success. These agents are often combined with flucytosine in refractory cases. In an effort to improve the response to treatment, attempts are often made to shrink larger lesions with local heat or cryotherapy before administering antifungal agents. Because of the risk of recurrences developing within the scar, surgery is not indicated. Squamous cell carcinomas may develop in long-standing lesions, and those with atypical areas or fleshy outgrowths should be biopsied to rule out this complication.

EUMYCOTIC MYCETOMA

Eumycotic mycetomas are those caused by true fungi, as opposed to actinomycotic mycetomas, which are caused by aerobic actinomycetes (bacteria). This section will deal only with the eumycotic mycetomas.

As with chromoblastomycosis, most eumycotic mycetomas are seen in the tropics. A mycetoma is defined clinically as a localized, chronic, granulomatous, infectious process involving cutaneous and subcutaneous tissues. It is characterized by the formation of multiple granulomas and abscesses that contain large aggregates of fungal hyphae known as **granules** or **grains.** These grains contain cells that have marked modifications of internal and external structure, ranging from reduplications of the cell wall to the formation of a hard, cement-like extracellular matrix. The abscesses drain externally through the skin, often with extrusion of granules. The process may be quite extensive and deforming, with destruction of muscle, fascia, and bone. The etiologic agents of eumycotic mycetoma encompass a wide range of fungi, including *Phaeoacremonium, Curvularia, Fusarium, Madurella, Exophiala, Pyrenochaeta, Leptosphaeria,* and *Scedosporium* species (see Table 65-1).

Morphology

The granules of eumycotic mycetomas are composed of septate fungal hyphae that are 2 to 6 μm or greater in width and are either dematiaceous (black grain) or hyaline (pale or white grain), depending on the etiologic agent (Figure 65-7). The hyphae are frequently distorted and bizarre in form and size. Large, spheric, thick-walled chlamydoconidia are often present. The hyphae may be embedded in an amorphous cement-like substance. Splendore-Hoeppli material often interdigitates among the mycelial elements at the periphery of the granule. Eumycotic granules may be differentiated from actinomycotic granules based on morphologic (branched filaments versus septate hyphae and chlamydoconidia) and staining (gram-positive beaded rods versus periodic acid-Schiff [PAS]- and Gomori methenamine silver [GMS]-positive hyphae) characteristics (see Chapter 68).

Culture is usually necessary for definitive identification of the fungus (or actinomycete) involved.

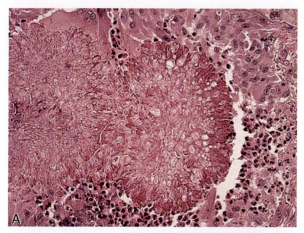

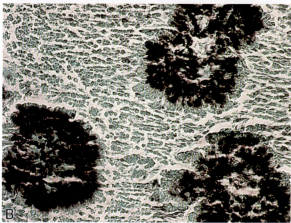

Figure 65-7 A, Mycetoma granule of *Curvularia geniculata.* **B,** Compact dematiaceous hyphae and chlamydoconidia embedded in cement-like substance.

Epidemiology

Mycetomas are primarily seen in tropical areas with low rainfall. Eumycotic mycetomas are more frequent in Africa and the Indian subcontinent but also may be seen in Brazil, Venezuela, and the Middle East. All patients are infected from sources in nature via traumatic percutaneous implantation of the etiologic agent into exposed parts of the body. The foot and hand are most common, but back, shoulders, and chest-wall infections are also seen. Men are more often affected than women. The fungi that cause eumycotic mycetomas differ from country to country, and the agents that are common in one region are rarely reported from others. Mycetomas are not contagious.

Clinical Syndromes

Similar to chromoblastomycosis, patients with eumycotic mycetoma most commonly present with longstanding infection. The earliest lesion is a small, painless, subcutaneous nodule or plaque that increases slowly but progressively in size. As the mycetoma develops, the affected area gradually enlarges and becomes disfigured as a result of chronic inflammation and fibrosis. With time, sinus tracts appear on the skin surface and drain serosanguineous fluid that often contains grossly visible granules. The infection commonly breaches tissue planes and destroys muscle and bone locally. Hematogenous or lymphatic spread from a primary focus to distant sites or viscera is extremely rare.

Laboratory Diagnosis

The key to the diagnosis of eumycotic mycetoma is the demonstration of grains or granules. Grains may be grossly visible in draining sinus tracts or may be expressed onto a glass slide. Material may also be obtained by deep surgical biopsy.

Grains can be visualized microscopically by mounting in 20% KOH. The hyphae are usually clearly visible, as is the presence or absence of pigmentation. Grains can be washed and then cultured or fixed and sectioned for histopathology.

Grains are easily visualized in tissue stained with H&E (see Figure 65-7). Special stains such as PAS and GMS may also be helpful. Although the color, shape, size, and microscopic morphology may be characteristic of a specific causal agent, culture is usually necessary for definitive identification of the organism. Most organisms will grow on standard mycologic medium; however, inclusion of an antibiotic such as penicillin may be useful to inhibit contaminating bacteria, which may overgrow the fungus.

Treatment

Treatment of eumycotic mycetoma is usually unsuccessful. Response of the various etiologic agents to amphotericin B, ketoconazole, or itraconazole is variable and often poor, although such therapy may slow the course of infection. Promising treatment responses have recently been reported for terbinafine, voriconazole, and posaconazole. Local excision is usually ineffective or not possible, and amputation is the only definitive treatment. Because these infections are usually slowly progressive and may be slowed further by specific antifungal therapy, the decision to amputate should take into account the rate of progression, the symptomatology, the availability of adequate prosthetics, and the individual circumstances of the patient. For all of these reasons, it is imperative to differentiate eumycotic mycetoma from actinomycotic mycetoma. Medical therapy is usually effective in cases of actinomycotic mycetoma.

SUMMARY

Sporothrix schenckii is a dimorphic, soil-living fungus grows as a mold at room temperature (e.g., 25℃) and as a pleomorphic yeast at 37℃ and in tissue. It is responsible for infection of the skin, lymphatic vessels and other sites. In tissue, organism appears as a pleomorphic budding yeast. Treatment is with oral itraconazole.

Eumycotic mycetoma is a localized chronic granulomatous infectious process involving cutaneous and subcutaneous tissues. It's caused by a wide array of true fungi (as opposed to actinomycotic mycetomas, which are caused by bacteria) found in soil. Specific antifungal therapy may slow progression by terbinafine, voriconazole, and posaconazole.

KEYWORDS

English	Chinese
Sporothrix schenckii	申克孢子丝菌
Lymphangitic sporotrichosis	淋巴管性孢子丝菌病
Chromoblastomycosis	着色真菌病
Cladosporium	枝孢霉
Phialophora	瓶霉
Exophialajeanselmei	外瓶霉
Rhinocladiella	鼻毛癣菌

BIBLIOGRAPHY

1. Ahmed AOA, De Hoog GS: Fungi causing eumycotic mycetoma. In Versalovic J, et al, editors: Manual of clinical microbiology, ed 10, Washington, DC, 2011, American Society for Microbiology Press.

2. Basto de Lima Barros M, et al: Cat-transmitted sporotrichosis epidemic in Rio de Janeiro, Brazil: description of a series of cases, Clin Infect Dis 38: 529-535, 2004.

3. Chandler FW, Watts JC: Pathologic diagnosis of fungal infections, Chicago, 1987, American Society for Clinical Pathology Press.

4. Connor DH, et al: Pathology of infectious diseases, Stamford, Conn, 1997, Appleton & Lange.

5. Garcia-Hermoso D, et al: Agents of systemic and subcutaneous mucormycosis and entomophthoromycosis. In Versalovic J, et al, editors: Manual of clinical microbiology, ed 10, Washington, DC, 2011, American Society for Microbiology Press.

6. Guarro J, De Hoog GS: *Bipolaris*, *Exophiala*, *Scedosporium*, *Sporothrix*, and other melanized fungi. In Versalovic J, et al, editors: Manual of clinical microbiology, ed 10, Washington, DC, 2011, American Society for Microbiology Press.

7. Kauffman CA, et al: Clinical practice guidelines for the management of sporotrichosis: 2007 update by the Infectious Diseases Society of America, Clin Infect Dis 45: 1255, 2007.

Systemic Mycoses Caused by Dimorphic Fungi

The **dimorphic** fungal pathogens are organisms that exist in a mold form in nature or in the laboratory at 25℃ to 30℃ and in a yeast or spherule form in tissues or when grown on enriched medium in the laboratory at 37℃ (Figure 66-1). The organisms in this group are considered primary **systemic** pathogens because of their ability to cause infection in both "normal" and immunocompromised hosts and for their propensity to involve the deep viscera after dissemination of the fungus from the lungs after its inhalation from nature. The dimorphic pathogens include *Blastomycesdermatitidis, Coccidioidesimmitis* and *Coccidioidesposadasii, Histoplasma capsulatum* var. *capsulatum* and *H. capsulatumvarduboisii, Paracoccidioidesbrasiliensis,* and *Penicilliummarneffei* (Table 66-1). *H. capsulatum, C. immitis (C. posadasii),* and *P. marneffei* have emerged as major opportunistic pathogens in individuals with acquired immunodeficiency syndrome (AIDS) and other forms of immunosuppression. Recognition of these endemic mycoses may be complicated by the fact that they may become manifest only after the patient has left the area of endemicity.

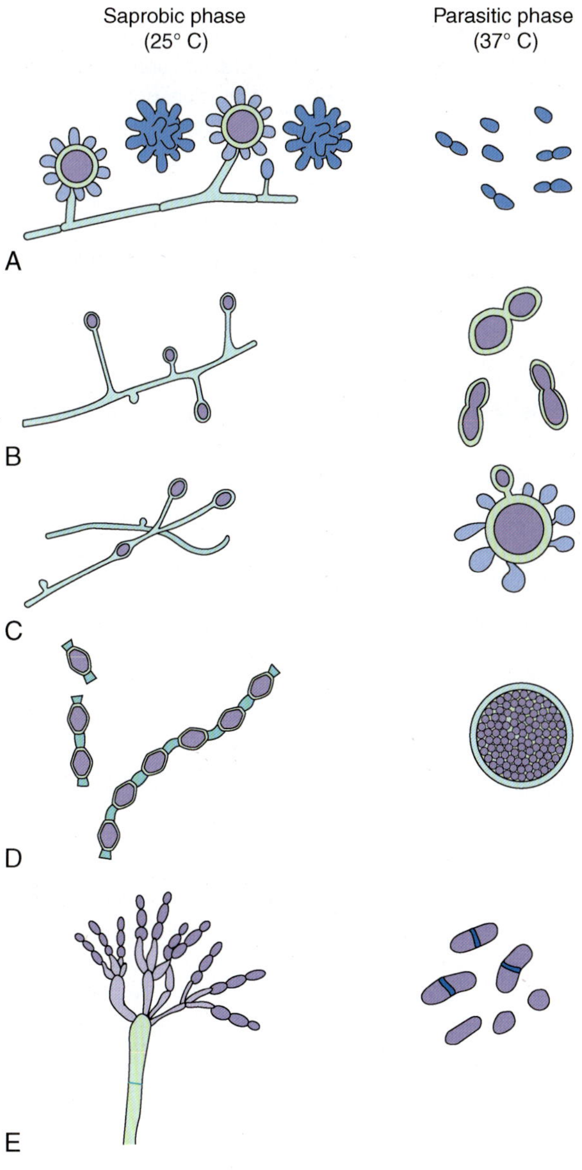

BLASTOMYCOSIS

Blastomycosis is a systemic fungal infection caused by the dimorphic pathogen *Blastomycesdermatitidis.* Like other endemic mycoses, this infection is confined to specific geographic regions, with most infections originating in the Mississippi River basin, around the Great Lakes, and in the southeastern region of the United States (Figure 66-2). Cases have also been

Saprobic phase
(25° C)

Parasitic phase
(37° C)

A

B

C

D

E

Figure 66-1 Saprobic and parasitic phases of endemic dimorphic fungi. **A,** *Histoplasma capsulatum.* **B,** *Blastomycesdermatitidis.* **C,** *Paracoccidioidesbrasiliensis.* **D,** *Coccidioidesimmitis.* **E,** *Penicilliummarneffei.*

553

diagnosed in other parts of the world, including Africa, Europe, and the Middle East.

Morphology

As a thermally dimorphic fungus, *B. dermatitidis* produces nonencapsulatedyeastlike cells in tissue and in culture on enriched media at 37℃ and white to tan, filamentous, mold colonies on standard mycologic media at 25℃. The mold form produces round to oval or pear-shaped conidia (2 to 10 μm) located

Table 66-1 Characteristics of Endemic Dimorphic Mycoses.

Mycosis	Etiology	Ecology	Geographic Distribution	Morphology in Tissue	Clinical Manifestation
Blastomycosis	*Blastomycesdermatitidis*	Decaying organic material	North America (Ohio and Mississippi River valleys) Africa	Broad-based, budding yeasts (8-15 μm in diameter)	Pulmonary disease (<50%) Extrapulmonary: skin, bone, genitourinary, central nervous system Disseminated disease in immunocompromised patients
Coccidioidomycosis	*Coccidioidesimmitis* *Coccidioidesposadasii*	Soil, dust	Southwestern United States, Mexico, Central and South America	Spherules (20-60 μm) containing endospores (2-4 μm)	Asymptomatic pulmonary infection (60%) in normal host Progressive pulmonary infection and dissemination (skin, bone, joints, meninges) in immunocompromised patients
Histoplasmosis capsulati	*Histoplasma capsulatum*var. *capsulatum*	Soil with high nitrogen content (bird/bat droppings)	North America (Ohio and Mississippi River valleys), Mexico, Central and South America	Small (2-4 μm), oval, narrow-based, budding yeasts (intracellular)	Asymptomatic pulmonary infection (90%) in normal host and low-intensity exposure Disseminated disease in immunocompromised host and in children
Histoplasmosis duboisii	*Histoplasma capsulatum* var. *duboisii*	Soil with high nitrogen content	Tropical areas of Africa	Larger (8-15 μm), thick-walled, budding yeast. Prominent isthmus and bud scar	Low rate of pulmonary disease. Higher frequency of skin and bone involvement
Paracoccidioidomycosis	*Paracoccidioidesbrasiliensis*	Likely soil associated	South and Central America	Thin to moderately thick-walled, multiply budding yeast (15-30 μm; pilot wheel)	Self-limited pulmonary disease. Progressive pulmonary infection and dissemination (skin, mucosa, bones, lymph nodes, viscera, and meninges). More common in children and immunocompromised patients
Penicilliosis-marneffei	*Penicillium-marneffei*	Soil Bamboo rat	Southeast Asia	Globose to elongated sausage-shaped yeasts (3-5 μm) that are intracellular and divide by fission	Disseminated infection (skin, soft tissues, viscera) more common in AIDS Resembles histoplasmosis, cryptococcosis, or tuberculosis

AIDS, Acquired immunodeficiency syndrome.
Modified from Anstead GM, Patterson TF: Endemic mycoses. In Anaissie EJ, McGinnis MR, Pfaller MA, editors: *Clinical mycology*, ed 2, New York, 2009, Churchill Livingstone.

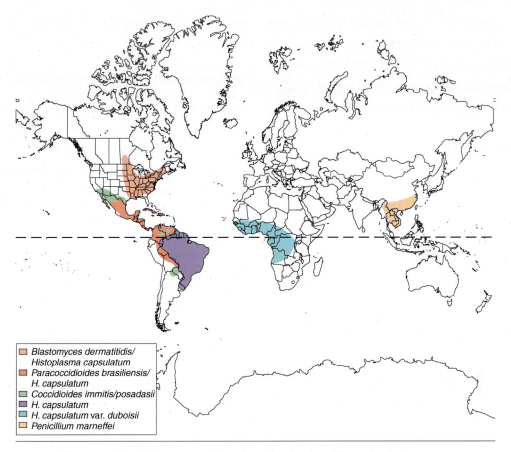

▨	*Blastomyces dermatitidis/ Histoplasma capsulatum*
▨	*Paracoccidioides brasiliensis/ H. capsulatum*
▨	*Coccidioides immitis/posadasii*
▨	*H. capsulatum*
▨	*H. capsulatum* var. *duboisii*
▨	*Penicillium marneffei*

Figure 66-2   Major geographic regional distribution of the endemic mycoses.

on long or short terminal hyphal branches (Figure 66-3). Older cultures may also produce 7- to 18-μm diameter, thick-walled chlamydospores. The yeast form of *B. dermatitidis* is seen in tissue and in culture at 37℃. This form is quite distinctive (Figure 66-4). The yeast cells are spheric, hyaline, 8 to 15 μm in diameter, multinucleated, and have thick "double-contoured" walls. The cytoplasm is often retracted from the rigid cell wall as a result of shrinkage during the fixation process. The yeast cells reproduce by the formation of buds or **blastoconidia.** The buds are usually single and attached to the parent cell by broad bases (see Figure 66-4).

The yeast forms may be visualized in tissue stained with hematoxylin and eosin (H&E); however, the fungal stains, Gomorimethenamine silver (GMS) and periodic acid-Schiff (PAS), help locate the organisms and delineate their morphology.

Epidemiology

Outbreaks of infection have been associated with

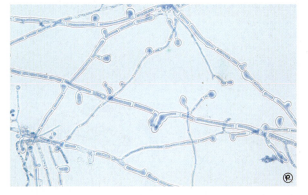

Figure 66-3   *Blastomycesdermatitidis* mold phase.

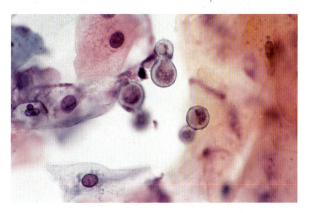

Figure 66-4   Giemsa stain of *Blastomycesdermatitidis* showing broad-based budding yeast.

occupational or recreational contact with soil, and infected individuals include all ages and both genders. Blastomycosis is not transmitted from patient to patient; however, laboratory-acquired primary cutaneous and pulmonary blastomycosis has been reported.

Clinical Syndromes

Pulmonary Disease

The usual route of infection in blastomycosis is inhalation of conidia (Figure 66-5). As with most of the endemic mycoses, the severity of symptoms and course of the disease is dependent on the extent of exposure and the immune status of the exposed individual. Pulmonary blastomycosis may be asymptomatic or present as a mild flulike illness. More severe infection resembles bacterial pneumonia with acute onset, high fever, lobar infiltrates, and cough. Progression to fulminant adult respiratory distress syndrome with high fever, diffuse infiltrates, and respiratory failure may occur. A more subacute or chronic respiratory form of blastomycosis may resemble tuberculosis or lung cancer, with radiographic presentation of pulmonary mass lesions or fibronodular infiltrates.

Extrapulmonary Disseminated Disease

A classic form of blastomycosis is that of chronic cutaneous involvement. The cutaneous form of blastomycosis is almost always the result of hematogenous dissemination from the lung, in most instances without evident pulmonary lesions or systemic symptoms. The lesions may be papular, pustular, or indolent, ulcerative-nodular, and verrucous with crusted surfaces and raised serpiginous borders. They are usually painless and are localized to exposed areas, such as the face, scalp, neck, and hands. They may be mistaken for squamous cell carcinoma. Left untreated, cutaneous blastomycosis takes on a chronic course, with remissions and exacerbations and gradual increase in the size of lesions.

Laboratory Diagnosis

The diagnosis of blastomycosis rests with microscopic detection of the fungus in tissue or other clinical material, with confirmation by culture (Table 66-2). The most useful specimens for the diagnosis of pulmonary blastomycosis include sputum, bronchoalveolar lavage, or lung biopsy. Direct examination of material stained with GMS, PAS, Papanicolaou, or Giemsa stains should be performed. Likewise, fresh wet preparations of sputum, cerebrospinal fluid, urine, pus, skin scrapings, and tissue impression smears may be examined directly using calcofluor white and fluorescence microscopy to detect the characteristic yeast forms. When typical broad-based budding yeast forms are present, a definitive diagnosis may be made.

The mycelial form of the fungus is easily cultured at 25°C to 30°C; however, growth is slow, often requiring 4 weeks or more. The mycelial form (see Figure 66-3) is not diagnostic, and the identity must be confirmed by conversion to the yeast form at 37°C, by exoantigen testing (immunologic detection of cell-free antigen A), or by nucleic acid probe hybridization.

Treatment

The decision to treat patients with blastomycosis must

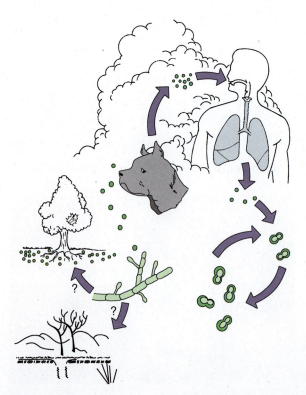

Figure 66-5 Natural history of the mold (saprobic) and yeast (parasitic) cycle of *Blastomyces dermatitidis*.

Table 66-2 Diagnosis of Endemic Dimorphic Mycoses.

Mycosis	Culture	Morphology in Culture 25℃	Morphology in Culture 37℃	Histopathology	Serology
Blastomycosis	Sputum, BAL, lung tissue, skin biopsy, CSF	Mold, round to oval or pear-shaped conidia (2-10 μm diameter)	Thick-walled, broad-based budding yeast (8-15 μm)	Broad-based, budding yeast	Antibody: CF, ID, EIA (poor sensitivity and specificity) Antigen: serum and urine (performance undefined)
Coccidioidomy-cosis	Sputum, BAL, tissue, CSF	Mold with barrel-shaped arthroconidia (3-6 μm)	NA	Spherules (20-60 μm) containing endo-spores	Antibody: TP, CF, ID, LPA (diagnostic and prognostic) Antigen: urine (performance undefined)
Histoplasmosis capsulati	Sputum, BAL, blood, bone marrow, tis-sue, CSF	Mold with tuberculate macroconidia (8-15 μm) and small, oval micro-conidia (2-4 μm)	Small (2-4 μm), budding yeast	Intracellular bud-ding yeast	Antibody: CF, ID Antigen: serum and urine (92% sensi-tive in dissemi-nated disease)
Paracoccidioido-mycoses	Sputum, BAL, tissue	Mold, round microco-nidia (2-3 μm) and inter-calary chlamydospores	Large (15-30 μm), multiple, bud-ding yeast	Large, multiply budding yeasts	Antibody: ID, CF (variable speci-ficity; CF useful for monitoring response)
Penicilliosis-marneffei	Blood, bone marrow, tis-sue, CSF	Mold with diffusible red pigment Conidiophores terminat-ing in conspicuous, penicillus-bearing, ellip-soidal, smooth conidia	Pleomorphic, elongated yeast (1-8 μm) with transverse septa	Intracellular elongated yeast with transverse septa	Under develop-ment

BAL, Bronchoalveolar lavage; *CF*, complement fixation; *CSF*, cerebrospinal fluid; *EIA*, enzyme immunoassay; *ID*, immunodiffusion; *LPA*, latex particle agglutination; *NA*, not applicable; *TP*, tube precipitin.

take into consideration the clinical form and severity of disease, as well as the immune status of the patient and the toxicity of antifungal agents. Clearly, pulmonary blastomycosis in immunocompromised patients and those with progressive pulmonary disease should be treated. Likewise, all patients with evidence of hematogenous dissemination (e.g., skin, bone, all nonpulmonary sites) require antifungal therapy. Amphotericin B, preferably a lipid formulation, is the agent of choice for the treatment of life-threatening or meningeal disease. Mild or moderate disease may be treated with itraconazole. Fluconazole, posaconazole, or voriconazole may be alternatives for those patients unable to tolerate itraconazole. Depending upon the severity of the disease and the status of the host, therapeutic success rates with amphotericin B or azole therapy range from 70% to 95%. Survival for AIDS patients and other immunocompromised patients is about half this figure. The latter patients may require long-term suppressive therapy with itraconazole in an effort to avoid relapses of the infection.

COCCIDIOIDOMYCOSIS

Coccidioidomycosis is an endemic mycosis caused by either of two indistinguishable species, Coccidioidesimmitis and *C. posadasii*. The disease is caused by the inhalation of infectious arthroconidia (Figure 66-6) and may range from asymptomatic infection (in most people) to progressive infection and death.

Like syphilis and tuberculosis, coccidioidomycosis causes a wide variety of lesions and has been called "the great imitator."

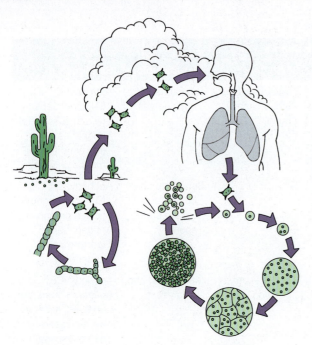

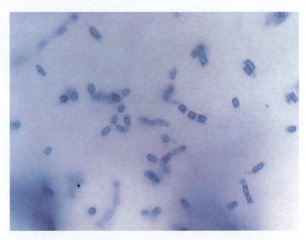

Figure 66-7 *Coccidioidesimmitis* mold phase.

Figure 66-6 Natural history of the mold (saprobic) and spherule (parasitic) cycle of *Coccidioidesimmitis*.

Morphology

C. immitis (*C. posadasii*) is a dimorphic fungus that exists as a mold in nature and when cultured in the laboratory at 25°C and as an endosporulating spherule in tissue and under very specific conditions in vitro (Figures 66-7 and 66-8; see Table 66-2 and Figure 66-1). Microscopically, the vegetative hyphae give rise to fertile hyphae that produce alternating (separated by disjunctor cells) hyaline arthroconidia (see Figure 68-7). Upon inhalation, the arthroconidia (2.5 to 4 μm wide) become rounded as they convert to spherules in the lung (see Figure 66-8). At maturity, the spherules (20 to 60 μm in diameter) produce endospores by a process known as progressive cleavage. Rupture of the spherule walls releases the endospores, which in turn form new spherules (see Figure 66-6). In approximately 10% to 30% of pulmonary cavities associated with coccidioidomycosis, branched, septate hyphae and arthroconidia may be produced.

Epidemiology

Coccidioidomycosis is endemic to the desert southwestern United States, northern Mexico, and scattered areas of Central and South America (see Figure 66-2).

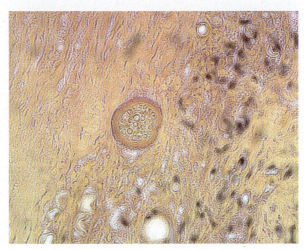

Figure 66-8 *Coccidioidesimmitis* spherule filled with endospores.

C. immitis is found in soil, and the growth of the fungus in the environment is enhanced by bat and rodent droppings. Acquisition of coccidioidomycosis occurs principally by inhalation of arthroconidia, and in endemic areas, infection rates may be 16% to 42% by early adulthood. The incidence of coccidioidomycosis is approximately 15 cases per 100,000 population annually in the endemic area; however, it is known to disproportionately affect persons 65 years of age and older (≈36 per 100,000) and those with human immunodeficiency virus (HIV) infection (≈20 per 100,000).

Clinical Syndromes

C. immitis is probably the most virulent of all human mycotic pathogens. The inhalation of only a few arthroconidia produces primary coccidioidomycosis, which may include asymptomatic pulmonary disease (≈60% of patients) or a self-limited flulike illness marked by fever, cough, chest pain, and weight loss. Patients with primary coccidioidomycosis may have a variety of allergic reactions (≈10%) as a result of immune complex formation, including an erythematous macular rash, erythema multiforme, and erythema nodosum.

Laboratory Diagnosis

The diagnosis of coccidioidomycosis includes the use of histopathologic examination of tissue or other clinical material, isolation of the fungus in the culture, and serologic testing (see Table 66-2). Direct microscopic visualization of endosporulating spherules in sputum, exudates, or tissue is sufficient to establish the diagnosis (see Figure 66-8) and is preferred over culture because of the highly infectious nature of the mold when grown in culture. Clinical exudates should be examined directly in 10% to 20% potassium hydroxide (KOH) with calcofluor white, and tissue from biopsy can be stained with H&E or specific fungal stains such as GMS or PAS (see Figure 66-8).

Treatment

Most individuals with primary coccidioidomycosis do not require specific antifungal therapy. For those with concurrent risk factors (see Table 66-3), such as organ transplant, HIV infection, high doses of corticosteroids, or when there is evidence of unusually severe infection, treatment is necessary. Primary coccidioidomycosis in the third trimester of pregnancy or during the immediate postpartum period requires treatment with amphotericin B.

HISTOPLASMOSIS

Histoplasmosis is caused by two varieties of *Histoplasma capsulatum*: *H. capsulatumvar. capsulatum* and *H. capsulatum* var. *duboisii* (see Table 66-1).

Morphology

Both varieties of H. capsulatum are thermally dimorphic fungi existing as a hyaline mold in nature and

Table 66-3 Risk Factors for Disseminated Coccidioidomycosis.

Risk Factor	Highest Risk
Age	Infants and elderly
Sex	Male
Genetics	Filipino > African American > Native American > Hispanic > Asian
Serum CF antibody titer	>1:32
Pregnancy	Late pregnancy and postpartum
Skin test	Negative
Depressed cell-mediated immunity	Malignancy, chemotherapy, steroid treatment, HIV infection

CF, Complement fixation; *HIV*, human immunodeficiency virus.
From Mitchell TG: Systemic fungi. In Cohen J, Powderly WG, editors: *Infectious diseases*, ed 2, St Louis, 2004, Mosby.

in culture at 25℃ and as an intracellular budding yeast in tissue and in culture at 37℃ (Figures 66-9, 66-10, and 66-11; see Table 66-2). In culture, the mold forms of H. capsulatum var. capsulatum and var. duboisii are indistinguishable macroscopically and microscopically. The mold form produces two types of conidia: (1) large (8 to 15 μm), thick-walled, spheric macroconidia with spikelike projections (tuberculate macroconidia) that arise from short conidiophores (Figure 66-12, see Figure 66-1) and (2) small, oval microconidia (2 to 4 μm) with smooth or slightly rough walls that are sessile or on short stalks (see Figures 66-1 and 66-12). The yeast cells are thin walled, oval, and measure 2 to 4 μm (var. capsulatum)

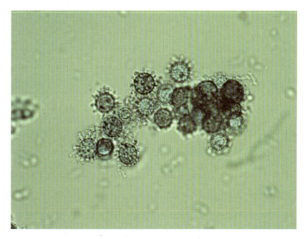

Figure 66-9 *Histoplasma capsulatum* mold phase showing tuberculate macroconidia.

(see Figure 66-10) or thicker walled and 8 to 15 μm (var. duboisii) (see Figure 66-11). The yeast cells of both varieties of H. capsulatum are intracellular in vivo and are uninucleated (see Figures 66-10 and 66-11).

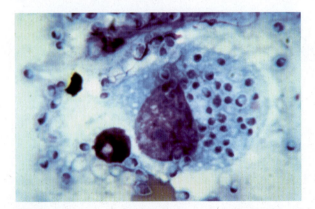

Figure 66-10   Giemsa-stained preparation showing intracellular yeast forms of *Histoplasma capsulatum* var. *capsulatum*.

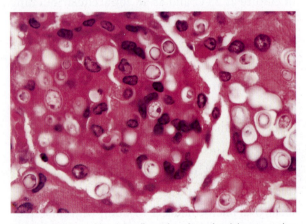

Figure 66-11   Hematoxylin and eosin-stained tissue section showing intracellular yeast forms of *Histoplasma capsulatum* var. *duboisii*.(From Connor DH, et al: *Pathology of infectious diseases*, Stamford, Conn, 1997, Appleton & Lange.).

Epidemiology

Histoplasmosis capsulati is localized to the broad regions of the Ohio and Mississippi River valleys in the United States and occurs throughout Mexico and Central and South America (see Figure 66-2 and Table 66-1). Histoplasmosis duboisii, or African histoplasmosis, is confined to the tropical areas of Africa, including Gabon, Uganda, and Kenya (see Figure 66-2 and Table 66-1).

Aerosolization of microconidia and hyphal fragments in the disturbed soil, with subsequent inhalation by exposed individuals, is considered to be the basis for these outbreaks (see Figure 66-12). Although attack rates may reach 100% in certain of these exposures, most cases remain asymptomatic and are detected only by skin testing. Immunocompromised individuals and children are more prone to develop symptomatic disease with either variety of Histoplasma. Reactivation of the disease and dissemination is common among immunosuppressed individuals, especially those with AIDS.

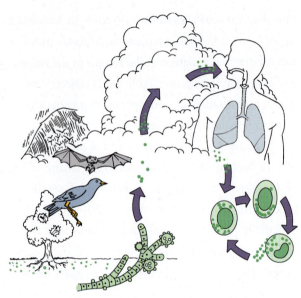

Figure 66-12   Natural history of the mold (saprobic) and yeast (parasitic) cycle of *Histoplasma capsulatum*.

Clinical Syndromes

The usual route of infection for both varieties of histoplasmosis is via inhalation of microconidia, which in turn germinate into yeasts within the lung and may remain localized or disseminate hematogenously or by the lymphatic system (see Figure 66-12). The microconidia are rapidly phagocytosed by pulmonary macrophages and neutrophils, and it is thought that conversion to the parasitic yeast form takes place intracellularly.

Histoplasmosis Capsulati

The clinical presentation of histoplasmosis caused by H. capsulatum var. capsulatum is dependent upon the intensity of exposure and immunologic status of the host. Asymptomatic infection occurs in 90% of individuals after a low-intensity exposure. In the event of an exposure to a heavy inoculum, however, most individuals exhibit some symptoms.

Progressive Pulmonary Histoplasmosis

Chronic pulmonary symptoms are associated with apical cavities and fibrosis and are more likely to occur in patients with prior underlying pulmonary disease. It may follow acute infection in approximately 1 in 100,000 cases per year.

Disseminated Histoplasmosis

Chronic disseminated histoplasmosis is characterized by weight loss and fatigue, with or without fever. Oral ulcers and hepatosplenomegaly are common. It follows acute infection in 1 in 2000 adults and is much higher in children and immunocompromised adults.

Subacute Disseminated Histoplasmosis

Subacute disseminated histoplasmosis is marked by fever, weight loss, and malaise. Oropharyngeal ulcers and hepatosplenomegaly are prominent. Bone marrow involvement may produce anemia, leukopenia, and thrombocytopenia. Other sites of involvement include the adrenals, cardiac valves, and the CNS. Untreated subacute disseminated histoplasmosis will result in death in 2 to 24 months.

Acute Disseminated Histoplasmosis

Acute disseminated histoplasmosis is a fulminant process that is most commonly seen in severely immunosuppressed individuals, including those with AIDS, organ transplant recipients, and those receiving steroids or other immunosuppressive chemotherapy. In contrast to the other forms of histoplasmosis, acute disseminated disease may present with a septic shock-like picture, with fever, hypotension, pulmonary infiltrates, and acute respiratory distress. Oral

and gastrointestinal ulcerations and bleeding, adrenal insufficiency, meningitis, and endocarditis may also be seen. If untreated, acute disseminated histoplasmosis is fatal within days to weeks.

Histoplasmosis Duboisii

In contrast to classic histoplasmosis, pulmonary lesions are uncommon in African histoplasmosis. The localized form of histoplasmosis duboisii is a chronic disease characterized by regional lymphadenopathy, with lesions of skin and bone. Skin lesions are papular or nodular and eventually progress to abscesses, which then ulcerate. About one third of patients will exhibit osseous lesions characterized by osteolysis and involvement of contiguous joints. The cranium, sternum, ribs, vertebrae, and long bones are most frequently involved, often with overlying abscesses and draining sinuses.

Laboratory Diagnosis

The diagnosis of histoplasmosis may be made by direct microscopy, culture of blood, bone marrow, or other clinical material, and by serology, including antigen detection in blood and urine (Table 66-4; see Table 66-2). In tissue sections, cells of H. capsulatum var. capsulatum are yeastlike, hyaline, spheric to oval, 2 to 4 μm in diameter, and uninucleate and have single buds attached by a narrow base. The cells are usually intracellular and clustered together. The cells of H. capsulatum var. duboisii are also intracellular, yeastlike, and uninucleate but are much larger (8 to 15 μm) and have thick "double-contoured" walls. They are usually in macrophages and giant cells (see Figure 66-11). Because of the high organism burden in patients with disseminated disease, cultures of

Table 66-4 Laboratory Tests for Histoplasmosis.

Test	Sensitivity (% True Positives) in Disease States		
	Disseminated	**Chronic Pulmonary**	**Self-Limited***
Antigen	92	21	39
Culture	85	85	15
Histopathology	43	17	9
Serology	71	100	98

*Includes acute pulmonary histoplasmosis, rheumatologic syndrome, and pericarditis.
From Wheat LJ: Endemic mycoses. In Cohen J, Powderly WG, editors: *Infectious diseases*, ed 2, St Louis, 2004, Mosby.

respiratory specimens, blood, bone marrow, and tissue are of value. They are less useful in self-limited or localized disease (see Table 66-4).

Serologic diagnosis of histoplasmosis employs tests for both antigen and antibody detection (see Table 66-2). Antibody detection assays include a CF assay and an ID test. These tests are usually used together to maximize sensitivity and specificity, but neither is useful in the acute setting; CF and ID are often negative in immunocompromised patients with disseminated infection.

Detection of *Histoplasma* antigen in serum and urine by enzyme immunoassay has become very useful, particularly in diagnosing disseminated disease (see Tables 66-2 and 66-4). The sensitivity of antigen detection is greater in urine specimens than in blood and ranges from 21% in chronic pulmonary disease to 92% in disseminated disease. Serial measurements of antigen may be used to assess response to therapy and for establishing relapse of the disease.

Treatment

In cases of severe acute pulmonary histoplasmosis with hypoxemia and acute respiratory distress syndrome, amphotericin B should be administered acutely, followed by oral itraconazole to complete a 12-week course.

Chronic pulmonary histoplasmosis also warrants treatment because it is known to progress if left untreated. Treatment with amphotericin B, followed by itraconazole for 12 to 24 months, is recommended.

Disseminated histoplasmosis usually responds well to amphotericin B therapy. Once stabilized, the patient may be switched to oral itraconazole to be administered over 6 to 18 months. Patients with AIDS may require lifelong therapy with itraconazole. Alternative azole agents include posaconazole, voriconazole, or fluconazole; however, secondary resistance to fluconazole has been described in patients on long-term maintenance therapy.

Histoplasmosis of the CNS is universally fatal if not treated. The therapy of choice is amphotericin B followed by fluconazole for 9 to 12 months.

Patients with severe obstructive mediastinal histoplasmosis require amphotericin B therapy. Itraconazole may be used for outpatient therapy.

PARACOCCIDIOIDOMYCOSIS

Paracoccidioidomycosis is a systemic fungal infection caused by the dimorphic pathogen Paracoccidioidesbrasiliensis. This infection is also known as South American blastomycosis and is the major dimorphic endemic fungal infection in Latin American countries.

Morphology

The mold phase of *P. brasiliensis* grows slowly in vitro at 25℃. The characteristic yeast form is seen in tissue and in culture at 37℃. Variable-sized (3 to 30 μm or more in diameter), oval to round, yeastlike cells with double refractile walls and single or multiple buds (blastoconidia) are characteristic of this fungus (Figure 66-13). The blastoconidia are connected to the parent cell by a narrow isthmus, and six or more of various sizes may be produced from a single cell: the so-called "mariner's" or "pilot-wheel" morphology. The variability in size and number of blastoconidia and their connection to the parent cell are identifying features (see Figure 66-13). These features are best disclosed by the GMS stain but may also be seen in H&E-stained tissues or in KOH mounts of clinical material.

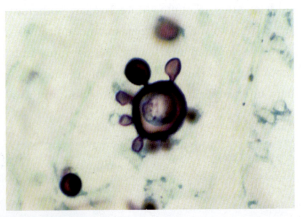

Figure 66-13 Gomorimethenamine silver-stained yeast form of *Paracoccidioidesbrasiliensis* showing multiple budding "pilot wheel" morphology. (From Connor DH, et al: *Pathology of infectious diseases*, Stamford, Conn, 1997, Appleton & Lange.)

Epidemiology

Paracoccidioidomycosis is endemic throughout Latin America but is more prevalent in South America than in Central America (see Figure 66-2). The highest incidence is seen in Brazil, followed by Colombia, Venezuela, Ecuador, and Argentina. The portal of entry is thought to be either by inhalation or traumatic inoculation (Figure 66-14), although even this is poorly understood. Natural infection has only been documented in armadillos. Although infection occurs in children (peak incidence 10 to 19 years), overt disease is uncommon in both children and adolescents. In adults, disease is more common in men aged 30 to 50 years. Most patients with clinically apparent disease live in rural areas and have close contact with the soil. There are no reports of epidemics or human-to-human transmission. Depression of cell-mediated immunity correlates with the acute progressive form of the disease.

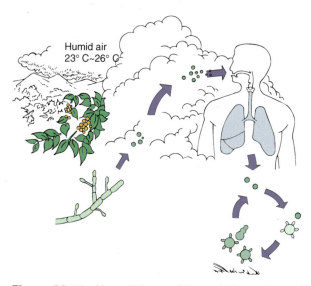

Figure 66-14 Natural history of the mold (saprobic) and yeast (parasitic) cycle of *Paracoccidioidesbrasiliensis.*

Clinical Syndromes

Paracoccidioidomycosis may be subclinical or progressive with acute or chronic pulmonary forms or acute, subacute, or chronic disseminated forms of the disease.A subacute disseminated form is seen in younger patients and immunocompromised individuals with marked lymphadenopathy, organomegaly, bone marrow involvement, and osteoarticular

manifestations mimicking osteomyelitis. Recurrent fungemia results in dissemination and frequent skin lesions. Pulmonary and mucosal lesions are not seen in this form of the disease.

Although 25% of patients exhibit only pulmonary manifestations of the disease, the infection can disseminate to extrapulmonary sites in the absence of diagnosis and treatment. Prominent extrapulmonary locations include skin and mucosa, lymph nodes, adrenal glands, liver, spleen, CNS, and bones. The mucosal lesions are painful and ulcerated and usually are confined to the mouth, lips, gums, and palate. More than 90% of these individuals are male.

Laboratory Diagnosis

The diagnosis is established by the demonstration of the characteristic yeast forms on microscopic examination of sputum, bronchoalveolar lavage fluid, scrapings or biopsy of ulcers, pus draining from lymph nodes, cerebrospinal fluid, or tissue (see Table 66-2). The organism may be visualized by a variety of staining methods, including calcofluor white fluorescence, H&E, GMS, PAS, or Papanicolaou stains (see Figure 66-13). The presence of multiple buds distinguishes *P. brasiliensis* from *Cryptococcus neoformans* and *B. dermatitidis.*

Isolation of the organism in culture requires confirmation by demonstration of thermal dimorphism or exoantigen testing (detection of exoantigen 1, 2, and 3). Cultures should be manipulated in a biosafety cabinet.

Serologic testing using either ID or CF to demonstrate antibody may be helpful in suggesting the diagnosis and in evaluating response to therapy (see Table 66-2).

Treatment

Itraconazole is the treatment of choice for most forms of the disease and generally must be given for at least 6 months. More severe or refractory infections may require amphotericin B therapy, followed by either itraconazole or sulfonamide therapy. Relapses are common with sulfonamide therapy, and both dose and duration require adjustment based on clinical and mycologic parameters. Fluconazole has some activity against this organism, although frequent relapses have limited its use for the treatment of this disease.

PENICILLIOSIS MARNEFFEI

Penicilliosis marneffei is a disseminated mycosis caused by the dimorphic fungus *Penicillium marneffei*. This infection involves the mononuclear phagocytic system and occurs primarily in HIV-infected individuals in Thailand and southern China (see Figure 66-2).

Morphology

In its mold phase in culture at 25°C, it exhibits sporulating structures that are typical of the genus (see Figure 66-1). Identification is aided by the formation of a soluble red pigment that diffuses into the agar (see Table 66-3).

At 37°C in culture and in tissue, *P. marneffei* grows as a yeastlike organism that divides by fission and exhibits a transverse septum (Figure 66-15). The yeast form is intracellular in vivo and, in this way, resembles *H. capsulatum*, although it is somewhat more pleomorphic and elongated and does not bud (see Table 66-2 and Figures 66-10 and 66-15).

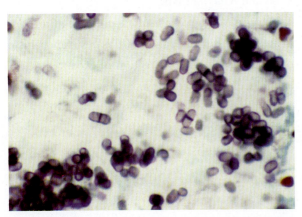

Figure 66-15   Gomorimethenamine silver-stained yeast forms of *Penicilliummarneffei*, including forms with single, wide, transverse septa (center). (From Connor DH, et al: *Pathology of infectious diseases*, Stamford, Conn, 1997, Appleton & Lange.)

Epidemiology

P. marneffei has emerged as a prominent mycotic pathogen among HIV-infected individuals in Southeast Asia

(see Figure 66-2). *Penicilliosis marneffei* has become an early indicator of HIV infection in that part of the world. *P. marneffei* has been isolated from bamboo rats and occasionally from soil. Laboratory-acquired infection has been reported in an immunocompromised individual exposed to the mycelial form in culture.

Clinical Syndromes

The infection may mimic tuberculosis, leishmaniasis, and other AIDS-related opportunistic infections, such as histoplasmosis and cryptococcosis. Patients present with fever, cough, pulmonary infiltrates, lymphadenopathy, organomegaly, anemia, leukopenia, and thrombocytopenia. Skin lesions reflect hematogenous disseminatidis and appear as molluscumcontagiosum-like lesions on the face and trunk.

Laboratory Diagnosis

P. marneffei is readily recovered from clinical specimens, including blood, bone marrow, bronchoalveolar lavage specimens, and tissue. In culture at 25°C to 30°C, isolation of a mold that exhibits typical Penicillium morphology and a diffusible red pigment is highly suggestive. Conversion to the yeast phase at 37°C is confirmatory. Microscopic detection of the elliptic fission yeasts inside phagocytes in buffy coat preparations or smears of bone marrow, ulcerative skin lesions, or lymph nodes is diagnostic (see Figure 66-15). Serologic tests are under development.

Treatment

Amphotericin B with or without flucytosine is the treatment of choice. Administration of amphotericin B for 2 weeks should be followed by itraconazole for another 10 weeks. AIDS patients may require lifelong treatment with itraconazole to prevent relapses of the infection. Fluconazole therapy has been associated with a high rate of failure and is not recommended.

SUMMARY

Blastomyces dermatitidis

Blastomyces dermatitidis is thermally dimorphic fungus, large nonencapsulated budding yeast cells in tissue and in culture at 37℃; mold colonies form in culture at 25℃. Usual route of infection is inhalation of conidia. Severity of symptoms and course of disease depends on extent of exposure and immune status of exposed individual; most are asymptomatic. Classic form of blastomycosis is chronic cutaneous involvement.

Coccidioides immitis and C. posadasii

Coccidioidomycosis is caused by two indistinguishable species: *C. immitis* and *C. posadasii*. Disease is caused by inhalation of infectious arthroconidia, which is symptomatic or subclinical, self-limited flulike illness, acute and chronic pulmonary disease, single or multisystem dissemination. It is dimorphic fungus; endosporulating spherule in tissue, mold in culture at 25℃ and in nature.

Histoplasma capsulatum

Histoplasmosis is caused by two varieties of *Histoplasma capsulatum*. *H. capsulatum var. capsulatum* causes pulmonary and disseminated infections. *H. capsulatum var. dubosisii*: causes predominantly skin and bone lesions. Disease is caused by inhalation of infectious microconidia. Severity of symptoms and course of disease depend on extent of exposure and immune status of infected individual; most are asymptomatic, self-limited; flulike illness also occurs. **Histoplasma capsulatum** is thermically dimorphic fungus, hyaline mold in nature and in culture at 25℃, budding yeast in tissue (intracellular) and in culture at 37℃.

Paracoccidioides brasiliensis

Paracoccidioides brasiliensis is thermally dimorphic fungus, slowly growing mold phase in nature and at 25℃, yeast phase (variable sized with single or multiple buds) in tissue and in culture at 37℃. Usual route of infection is inhalation or possible traumatic inoculation of conidia or hyphal fragments. Paracoc-

cidioidomycosis may be subclinical or progressive with acute or chronic pulmonary forms or acute, subacute, or chronic disseminated forms.

KEYWORDS

English	Chinese
Blastomyces dermatitidis	皮炎芽生菌
Blastomycosis	芽生菌病
Coccidioides immitis	粗球孢子菌
Coccidioidomycosis	环孢子菌病
Histoplasma capsulatum	荚膜组织胞浆菌
Paracoccidioides brasiliensis	巴西副球孢子菌
Penicillium marneffei	马尔尼菲青霉菌

BIBLIOGRAPHY

1. Anstead GM, Patterson TF: Endemic mycoses. In Anaissie EJ, McGinnis MR, Pfaller MA, editors: Clinical mycology, ed 2, New York, 2009, Churchill Livingstone.

2. Brandt ME, et al: Histoplasma, Blastomyces, Coccidioides, and other dimorphic fungi causing systemic mycoses. In Versalovic J, et al, editors: Manual of clinical microbiology, ed 10, Washington, DC, 2011, American Society for Microbiology Press.

3. Chu JH, et al: Hospitalization for endemic mycoses: a population-based national study, Clin Infect Dis 42: 822, 2006.

4. Connor DH, et al: Pathology of infectious diseases, Stamford, Conn, 1997, Appleton & Lange.

5. Kauffman CA: Histoplasmosis: a clinical and laboratory update, ClinMicrobiol Rev 20: 115, 1997.

6. Mitchell TG: Systemic fungi. In Cohen J, Powderly WG, editors: Infectious diseases, ed 2, St Louis, 2004, Mosby.

7. Vanittanakom N, et al: Penicilliummarneffei infection and recent advances in the epidemiology and molecular biology aspects, ClinMicrobiol Rev 19: 95, 2006.

8. Wheat LJ: Endemic mycoses. In Cohen J, Powderly WG, editors: Infectious diseases, ed 2, St Louis, 2004, Mosby.

Opportunistic Mycoses

Chapter

67

The frequency of invasive mycoses caused by opportunistic fungal pathogens has increased significantly over the past two decades. The most well-known causes of opportunistic mycoses include *Candida albicans*, *Cryptococcus neoformans*, and *Aspergillus fumigatus*. High-risk infections include individuals undergoing blood and marrow transplantation (BMT), solid organ transplantation, major surgery (especially gastrointestinal [GI] surgery), those with acquired immunodeficiency syndrome (AIDS), neoplastic disease, immunosuppressive therapy, advanced age, and premature birth (Table 67-1). Given the complexity of the patients at risk for infection and the diverse array of fungal pathogens, opportunistic mycoses pose a considerable diagnostic and therapeutic challenge.

CANDIDIA SPP

Morphology

All *Candida* species exist as oval yeastlike forms (3 to 5 μm) that produce buds or blastoconidia. Species of *Candida* other than *C. glabrata* also produce pseudohyphae and true hyphae (Figure 67-1). In addition, *C. albicans* forms germ tubes and terminal, thick-walled chlamydoconidia (Figure 67-2). *C. glabrata*, the second most common species of *Candida* in many settings, is incapable of forming pseudohyphae, germ tubes, or true hyphae under most conditions. In culture, most *Candida spp.* form smooth, white, creamy, domed colonies. *C. albicans* and other species may also undergo phenotypic switching, in which a single strain of *Candida* may change reversibly among several different morphotypes, ranging from the typical smooth, white colony composed of predominantly

budding yeastlike cells to very "fuzzy" or "hairy" colonies composed primarily of pseudohyphal and hyphal forms.

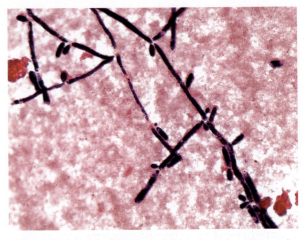

Figure 67-1 *Candida tropicalis* blastoconidia and pseudohyphae (Gram stain, ×1000).

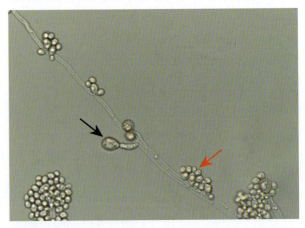

Figure 67-2 *Candida albicans*, microscopic morphology in cornmeal agar showing large chlamydospores (*black arrow*), blastoconidia (*red arrow*), hyphae, and pseudohyphae.

Epidemiology

Candida spp. are known colonizers of humans and other warm-blooded animals. The primary site of

Table 67-1 Predisposing Factors for Opportunistic Mycoses.

Factor	Possible Role in Infection	Major Opportunistic Pathogens
Antimicrobial agents (number and duration)	Promote fungal colonization Provide intravascular access	*Candida* spp., other yeastlike fungi
Adrenal corticosteroid	Immunosuppression	*Cryptococcus neoformans, Aspergillus* spp., Mucormycetes, other molds, *Pneumocystis*
Chemotherapy	Immunosuppression	*Candida* spp., *Aspergillus* spp., *Pneumocystis*
Hematologic/solid organ malignancy	Immunosuppression	*Candida* spp., *Aspergillus* spp., Mucormycetes, other molds and yeastlike fungi, *Pneumocystis*
Previous colonization	Translocation across mucosa	*Candida* spp.
Indwelling catheter (central venous, pressure transducer, Swan-Ganz)	Direct vascular access Contaminated product	*Candida* spp., other yeastlike fungi
Total parenteral nutrition	Direct vascular access Contamination of infusate	*Candida* spp., *Malassezia* spp., other yeastlike fungi
Neutropenia (WBC < 500/mm³)	Immunosuppression	*Aspergillus* spp., *Candida* spp., other molds and yeastlike fungi
Extensive surgery or burns	Route of infection Direct vascular access	*Candida* spp., *Fusarium* spp., Mucormycetes
Assisted ventilation	Route of infection	*Candida* spp., *Aspergillus* spp.
Hospitalization or intensive care unit stay	Exposure to pathogens Exposure to additional risk factors	*Candida* spp., other yeastlike fungi, *Aspergillus* spp.
Hemodialysis, peritoneal dialysis	Route of infection Immunosuppression	*Candida* spp., *Rhodotorula* spp., other yeastlike fungi
Malnutrition	Immunosuppression	*Pneumocystis, Candida* spp., *Cryptococcus neoformans*
HIV infection/AIDS	Immunosuppression	*Cryptococcus neoformans, Pneumocystis, Candida* spp.
Extremes of age	Immunosuppression Numerous comorbidities	*Candida* spp.

AIDS, Acquired immunodeficiency syndrome; *HIV,* human immunodeficiency virus; *WBC,* white blood cells.

colonization is the GI tract from mouth to rectum. They may also be found as commensals in the vagina and urethra, on the skin and under the fingernails and toenails.

It is estimated that 25% to 50% of healthy persons carry Candida as part of the normal flora of the mouth, with *C. albicans* accounting for 70% to 80% of isolates. Oral carriage rates are increased substantially in hospitalized patients; those with human immunodeficiency virus (HIV) infection, dentures, and diabetes; patients receiving antineoplastic chemotherapy; those receiving antibiotics; and children. Virtually all humans may carry one or more Candida species throughout their GI tract, and the levels of carriage may increase to that detectable in illness or other circumstances in which the host's microbial

suppression mechanisms become compromised.

The predominant source of infection caused by *Candida spp.,* from superficial mucosal and cutaneous disease to hematogenous dissemination, is the patient. That is, most types of candidiasis represent endogenous infection in which the normally commensal host flora take advantage of the "opportunity" to cause infection. To do so, there must be a lowering of the host's anti-*Candida* barrier. In the cases of *Candida* BSI, transfer of the organism from the GI mucosa to the bloodstream requires prior overgrowth of the numbers of yeasts in their commensal habitat, coupled with a breach in the integrity of the GI mucosa.

Exogenous transmission of *Candida* may also account for a proportion of certain types of candidiasis. Examples include the use of contaminated irrigation solutions, parenteral nutrition fluids, vascular pressure transducers, cardiac valves, and corneas. Transmission of *Candida spp.* from health care workers to patients and from patient to patient has been well documented, especially in the intensive care unit environment. The hands of health care workers serve as potential reservoirs for nosocomial transmission of *Candida spp.*

Among the various species of *Candida* capable of causing human infection (Table 67-2), *C. albicans* predominates in most types of infection. Infections of genital, cutaneous, and oral sites always involve *C. albicans*. A wider array of *Candida spp.* is seen causing BSI and other forms of invasive candidiasis, and although *C. albicans* usually predominates (see Table 67-2), the frequency with which this and other species of *Candida* are isolated from blood varies considerably according to the clinical service (see Table 67-2), the age of the patient (Figure 67-3), and the local, regional, or global setting (Table 67-3). Whereas *C. albicans* and *C. parapsilosis* predominate as causes of BSI among infants and children, a decrease in *C. albicans* and *C. parapsilosis* infections and a prominent increase in *C. glabrata* infections is seen among older individuals (see Figure 67-3). Likewise, although *C. glabrata* is the second most common species causing BSI in North America, it is seen at a lower frequency in Latin America, where *C.*

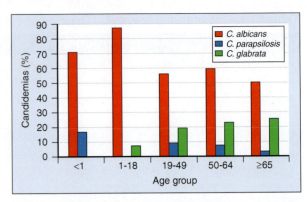

Figure 67-3 Percentage of all candidemias caused by selected *Candida* species in each age group. Data are from the Emerging Infections and the Epidemiology of Iowa Organisms Survey, 1998 to 2001. (Data from Pfaller MA, Diekema DJ: Epidemiology of invasive candidiasis: a persistent public health problem, *Clin Microbiol Rev* 20: 133, 2007.)

parapsilosis and *C. tropicalis* are more common (see Table 67-3). The differences in the number and types of *Candida spp.* causing infections may be influenced by numerous factors, including patient age, increased immunosuppression, antifungal drug exposure, or differences in infection-control practices. Each one of these factors, alone or in combination, may affect the prevalence of different *Candida spp.* in each institution. For example, the use of azoles (e.g., fluconazole) for antifungal prophylaxis in hematologic malignancy patients and recipients of stem cell transplantation, may increase the likelihood of infections caused by *C. glabrata* and *C. krusei*, two species with decreased susceptibility to this class of antifungals

Table 67-2 Species Distribution of *Candida* Bloodstream Infection Isolates by Clinical Service in the United States[*]

Species	% of Isolates by Species and Clinical Service (No. Tested)								
	GMED (1339)	**HEME** (197)	**SCT** (58)	**NICU** (26)	**SOT** (166)	**ST** (351)	**SURG** (662)	**HIV/AIDS** (41)	**Total** (2019)
C. albicans	46.3	27.4	22.4	69.2	39.2	47.6	47.9	43.9	45.6
C. glabrata	26.6	25.9	32.8	0.0	38.6	26.8	24.0	29.3	26.0
C. parapsilosis	15.7	11.7	15.5	26.9	12.0	12.8	17.7	9.8	15.7
C. tropicalis	7.5	17.3	8.6	0.0	6.0	7.4	7.3	7.3	8.1
C. krusei	1.9	13.7	15.5	0.0	1.8	2.6	1.4	4.9	2.5
Other[†]	2.0	4.0	5.2	3.9	2.4	2.8	1.7	4.8	2.1

GMED, General medicine; *HEME*, hematologic malignancy; *HIV/AIDS*, human immunodeficiency virus/acquired immunodeficiency syndrome; *NICU*, neonatal intensive care unit; *SCT*, stem cell transplant; *SOT*, solid organ transplant; *ST*, solid tumor; *SURG*, surgical (nontransplant).

[*]Data compiled from Horn DL, et al: Clinical characteristics of 2,019 patients with candidemia: data from the PATH Alliance Registry, *Clin Infect Dis* 48: 1695-1703, 2009.

[†]Other: 17 cases of *C. lusitaniae*, 5 of *C. guilliermondii*, 7 of *C. dubliniensis*, 11 other, and 3 unknown *Candida* spp.

Table 67-3   Species Distribution of *Candida* Bloodstream Infection Isolates by Geographic Region.

Region	No. of Isolates	% of Isolates by Species				
		CA	CG	CP	CT	CK
Asia-Pacific	1064	49.1	12.1	13.8	17.3	2.5
Europe	2151	58.5	14.8	9.8	8.5	4.7
Latin America	1348	46.0	6.8	18.5	18.5	4.5
North America	2116	51.8	20.3	14.4	8.5	1.9
Total	7191	52.7	14.2	13.9	11.8	3.3

CA, *C. albicans*; CG, *C. glabrata*; CK, *C. krusei*; CP, *C. parapsilosis*; CT, *C. tropicalis*.
Modified from Diekema DJ, et al: A global evaluation of voriconazole activity tested against recent clinical isolates of *Candida* spp, *Diagn Microbiol Infect Dis* 63: 233-236, 2009.

(see Table 67-2). Likewise, breaks in infection-control precautions and in the proper care of vascular catheters may lead to more infections with *C. parapsilosis*, the predominant species isolated from the hands of health care workers and a frequent cause of catheter-related fungemia.

The consequences of *Candida* BSI in the hospitalized patient are severe. Hospitalized patients with candidemia have been shown to be at a twofold greater risk of death in hospital than those with non-candidal BSI. Among all patients with nosocomial (hospital-acquired) BSI, candidemia was found to be an independent predictor of death in hospital. Although estimates of mortality may be confounded by the serious nature of the underlying diseases in many of these patients, matched cohort studies have confirmed that the mortality directly attributable to the fungal infection is quite high (Table 67-4). Notably, the excess or attributable mortality resulting from candidemia has not decreased from that observed in the mid-1980s to that observed in the present day, despite the introduction of new antifungal agents with good activity against most species of *Candida*.

Clearly, more is known about the epidemiology of nosocomial candidemia than any other fungal infection. The accumulated evidence allows one to propose a general view of nosocomial candidemia (Figure 67-4). Certain hospitalized individuals are clearly at increased risk of acquiring candidemia during hospitalization because of their underlying medical condition: patients with hematologic malignancies and/or neutropenia, those undergoing GI surgery, premature infants, and patients older than 70 years (see Table 67-1 and Figure 67-4). Compared to control subjects without the specific risk factors or exposures, the likelihood of these already high-risk patients contracting candidemia in hospital is approximately 2 times greater for each class of antibiotics they receive, 7 times greater if they have a central venous catheter, 10 times greater if Candida has been found to be colonizing other anatomic sites, and 18 times greater if the patient has undergone acute hemodialysis. Hospitalization in the intensive care unit setting provides the opportunity for transmission of Candida among patients and has been shown to be an additional independent risk factor.

The outcome for almost half of those patients with candidemia could be improved by more effective means of prevention, diagnosis, and therapy.

Table 67-4   Excess Mortality Attributable to Nosocomial Infections with *Candida* and *Aspergillus*.

Type of Mortality Rate	Percent Mortality		
	Candida[*]		Aspergillus[†]
	1988	2001	1991
Crude mortality			
Cases	57	61	95
Controls	19	12	10
Attributable mortality	38	49	85

[*]Patients with candidemia. Data from Wey SB, et al: Hospital-acquired candidemia: attributable mortality and excess length of stay, *Arch Intern Med* 148: 2642-2645, 1988; and Gudlagson O, et al: Attributable mortality of nosocomial candidemia, revisited, *Clin Infect Dis* 37: 1172-1177, 2003.
[†]Bone marrow transplant patients with invasive pulmonary aspergillosis. Data from Pannuti CS, et al: Nosocomial pneumonia in adult patients undergoing bone marrow transplantation: a 9-year study, *J Clin Oncol* 9: 1, 1991.

Clearly the most desirable of these is prevention, which is best approached by rigorous control of the exposures—especially limiting the use of broad-spectrum antibiotics, improving catheter care, and adhering to infection-control practices.

Clinical Syndromes

Given the right setting, *Candida spp.* can cause clinically apparent infection of virtually any organ system (Table 67-5). Infections range from superficial mucosal and cutaneous candidiasis to widespread hematogenous dissemination involving target organs, such as the liver, spleen, kidney, heart, and brain. In the latter situation, the mortality directly attributable to the infectious process approaches 50% (see Table 67-4 and Figure 67-4).

Non-Invasive Infections

Mucosal Infections

Candida spp. (known as "thrush") are limited to the oropharynx or extend to the esophagus and the entire GI tract, the vaginal mucosa. These infections are generally seen in individuals with local or generalized immunosuppression or in those settings in which candidal overgrowth is favored (see Table 67-5). These infections usually present as white "cottage cheese"-like patches on the mucosal surface. Other presentations include the pseudomembranous type, which reveals a raw bleeding surface when scraped; the erythematous type—flat, red, occasionally sore areas; candidal leukoplakia—nonremovable white thickening of epithelium caused by *Candida* spp.; and angular cheilitis—sore fissures at the corners of the mouth.

Onychomycosis and Paronychia

The infection may occur in the setting of a mixed microbial flora, including *Candida*. The species most commonly involved are *C. albicans, C. parapsilosis,* and *C. guilliermondii.*

Chronic Mucocutaneous Candidiasis

It is a rare condition marked by a deficiency in T-lymphocyte responsiveness to *Candida* spp. These patients suffer from severe, unremitting mucocutaneous *Can-*

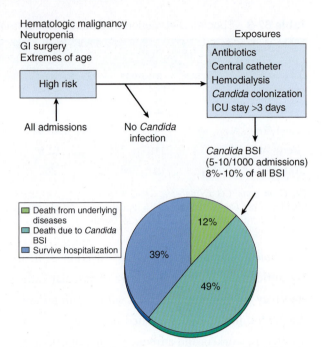

Figure 67-4   Global view of hospital-acquired candidemia. *BSI,* Bloodstream infections; *GI,* gastrointestinal; *ICU,* intensive care unit.(Modified from Lockhart SR, et al: The epidemiology of fungal infections. In Anaissie EJ, McGinnis MR, Pfaller MA, editors: *Clinical mycology,* ed 2, New York, 2009, Churchill Livingstone.)

dida lesions, including extensive nail involvement and vaginitis. The lesions may become quite large, with a disfiguring granulomatous appearance.

Invasive Infections

Urinary Tract Infection

Bladder colonization with *Candida spp.* is essentially not seen unless a patient requires an indwelling bladder catheter, has diabetes, suffers from urinary obstruction, or has had prior urinary procedures. Benign colonization of the bladder is most common in these settings, but urethritis and/or cystitis may occur. Hematogenous seeding of the kidney may result in renal abscess, papillary necrosis, or "fungus ball" of the ureter or renal pelvis.

Candida peritonitis may be seen in the setting of chronic ambulatory peritoneal dialysis or after GI surgery, anastomotic leak, or intestinal perforation. These infections may remain localized to the abdomen, involve adjacent organs, or lead to hematogenous candidiasis.

Candida peritonitis may be seen in the setting of chronic ambulatory peritoneal dialysis or after GI

Table 67-5 Types of *Candida* Infection and Associated Predisposing Factors.

Type of Disease	Predisposing Factors	Type of Disease	Predisposing Factors
Oropharyngeal infection	Age extremes Denture wearers Diabetes mellitus Antibiotic use Radiotherapy for head and neck cancer Inhaled and systemic steroids Cytotoxic chemotherapy HIV infection Hematologic malignancies Stem cell or solid organ transplantation	Endocarditis	Major surgery Previous valvular disease Prosthetic valve Intravenous drug use Long-term central venous catheter
		Pericarditis	Thoracic surgery Immunosuppression
		CNS infection	CNS surgery Ventriculoperitoneal shunt Ocular surgery
Esophagitis	Systemic corticosteroids AIDS Cancer Stem cell or solid organ transplantation	Ocular infection	Trauma Surgery
		Bone and joint infection	Trauma Intraarticular injections Diabetic foot
Vulvovaginal infection	Oral contraceptives Pregnancy Diabetes mellitus Systemic corticosteroids HIV infection Antibiotic use	Abdominal infection	Perforation Abdominal surgery Anastomotic leaks Pancreatitis Continuous ambulatory peritoneal dialysis
Infections of the skin and nails	Local moisture and occlusion Immersion of hands in water Peripheral vascular disease	Hematogenous infection	Solid organ transplantation Colonization Prolonged antibiotic use Abdominal surgery Intensive care support Total parenteral nutrition Hemodialysis Immunosuppression Extremes of age Stem cell transplantation
Chronic mucocutaneous candidiasis	T-lymphocyte defects		
Urinary tract infection	Indwelling urinary catheter Urinary obstruction Urinary procedures Diabetes mellitus		
Pneumonia	Aspiration		

AIDS, Acquired immunodeficiency syndrome; *CNS*, central nervous system: *HIV*, human immunodeficiency virus.
Modified from Dignani MC, Solomkin JS, Anaissie EJ: *Candida.* In Anaissie EJ, McGinnis MR, Pfaller MA, editors: *Clinical mycology,* New York, 2003, Churchill Livingstone.

surgery, anastomotic leak, or intestinal perforation. These infections may remain localized to the abdomen, involve adjacent organs, or lead to hematogenous candidiasis.

Hematogenous candidiasis may be acute or chronic and usually results in seeding of deep tissues, including the abdominal viscera, heart, eyes, bones and joints, and brain. Chronic hepatosplenic candidiasis may occur after overt or occult fungemia and presents as an indolent process marked by fever, elevated alkaline phosphatase, and multiple lesions in the liver and spleen.

Central nervous system (CNS) candidiasis may occur secondary to hematogenous disease or be associated with neurosurgical procedures and ventriculoperitoneal shunts. This process may mimic bacterial meningitis, or the course may be indolent or chronic.

Laboratory Diagnosis

The laboratory diagnosis of candidiasis involves the procurement of appropriate clinical material followed by direct microscopic examination and culture (see Chapter 67). Scrapings of mucosal or cutaneous lesions may be examined directly after treatment with 10% to 20% potassium hydroxide (KOH) containing calcofluor white. The budding yeastlike forms and pseudohyphae are easily detected upon examination with a fluorescence microscope. Culture on standard mycologic medium will allow the isolation of the organism for subsequent identification to species. Increasingly, such specimens are plated directly on a selective chromogenic medium such as CHROMagar *Candida*, which allows the detection of mixed species of *Candida* within the specimen and the rapid identification of *C. albicans* (green colonies) and *C. tropicalis* (blue colonies) based on their morphologic appearance (Figure 67-5).

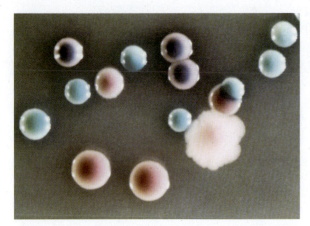

Figure 67-5 Differentiation of *Candida* species by isolates on CHROMagar Candida. The green colonies are *C. albicans*, the blue-gray colonies are *C. tropicalis*, and the large, rough, pale pink colony is *C. krusei*. The smooth, pink or mauve colonies are another yeast species (only *C. albicans*, *C. tropicalis*, and *C. krusei* can be reliably recognized on this media; other species have colonies ranging from white, to pink, to mauve). (From Anaissie EJ, McGinnis MR, Pfaller MA, editors: *Clinical mycology*, ed 2, New York, 2009, Churchill Livingstone.)

Whenever possible, skin lesions should be biopsied and histologic sections stained with GMS or another fungal-specific stain. Visualization of characteristic budding yeasts and pseudohyphae is sufficient for the diagnosis of candidiasis (Figure 67-6). Cultures of blood, tissue, and normally sterile body fluids should also be performed. Identification of Candida isolates to species level is important, given the differences in response to the various antifungal agents. This can be accomplished as described in Chapter 67, using the germ-tube test (*C. albicans*), various chromogenic media/tests (see Figure 67-5), peptide nucleic acid-fluorescence in situ hybridization (PNA-FISH), and commercially available sugar assimilation panels.

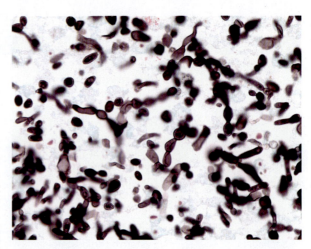

Figure 67-6 *Candida* stained with Gomori methenamine silver demonstrating budding yeasts and pseudohyphae (×1000).

Treatment, Prevention, and Control

There are a wide variety of treatment options for candidiasis. Mucosal and cutaneous infections may be treated with a number of different topical creams, lotions, ointments, and suppositories containing various azole antifungal agents. Oral systemic therapy of these infections may also be accomplished with either fluconazole or itraconazole.

Bladder colonization or cystitis may be treated with either instillation of amphotericin B directly into the bladder (bladder wash) or by oral administration of fluconazole. Both of these measures will likely be unsuccessful if the bladder catheter cannot be removed.

More deep-seated infections require systemic therapy, the choice of which depends upon the type of infection, the infecting species, and the overall status of the host. In many instances, oral fluconazole may be quite effective in treating candidiasis. It may be used in the treatment of peritonitis, as well as in more long-term maintenance therapy of invasive disease after an initial intravenous course of therapy. Fluconazole is efficacious when administered intravenously for the treatment of candidemia in non-neutropenic patients. Those patients who become candidemic while on fluconazole prophylaxis or those with documented infection caused by C. krusei or fluconazole-resistant C. *glabrata* require treatment with either amphotericin B (conventional or lipid formulation) or an echinocandin (anidulafungin, caspofungin, or micafungin). In those clinical settings where *C. glabrata* or *C. krusei* are plausible etiologic agents (e.g., prior fluconazole therapy/prophylaxis or an endemic situation), initial therapy with either an echinocandin or an amphotericin B formulation is advised, with a switch to fluconazole (less toxic than amphotericin B, less expensive, and orally available versus echinocandins) based upon final species identification and susceptibility test results. In every instance, care should be taken to remove the nidus of infection if possible. Thus vascular catheters should be removed or changed, abscesses should be drained, and other potentially infected implanted materials should be removed to the extent possible. Likewise, efforts should be directed toward immune reconstitution.

As in most infectious diseases, prevention is clearly preferable to the treatment of an established candidal infection. Avoidance of broad-spectrum antimicrobial agents, meticulous catheter care, and rigorous adherence to infection-control precautions are a must. Decreased colonization achieved by fluconazole prophylaxis has been shown to be efficacious when employed in specific high-risk groups, such as BMT patients and liver transplant patients. Such prophylaxis carries with it the potential for selecting for, or creating, strains or species that are resistant to the agent administered. This in fact has been seen with the emergence of fluconazole-resistant *C. glabrata* and *C. krusei* in certain institutions, but the overall benefit in the high-risk patient groups outweighs the risk. Transfer of this approach to other patient groups, however, is fraught with problems and should not be undertaken without careful study and risk stratification to identify those individuals most likely to benefit from antifungal prophylaxis.

OPPORTUNISTIC MYCOSES CAUSED BY CRYPTOCOCCUS NEOFORMANS AND OTHER NONCANDIDAL YEASTLIKE FUNGI

In the same manner that *Candida* species have taken advantage of immunocompromising conditions,

indwelling devices, and broad-spectrum antibiotic use, so too have a number of non-*Candida* yeastlike fungi found an "opportunity" to colonize and infect immunocompromised patients. These organisms may occupy environmental niches or be found in food and water and can be normal human microbial flora. The list of these opportunistic yeasts is long, but we will limit this discussion to two major pathogens, *C. neoformans* and *Cryptococcus gattii*, and four genera that pose particular problems as opportunistic pathogens: *Malassezia spp.*, *Trichosporon spp.*, *Rhodotorula spp.*, and *B. capitatus* (teleomorph, *Dipodascus capitatus*).

Cryptococcosis

Cryptococcosis is a systemic mycosis caused by the encapsulated, basidiomycetous, yeastlike fungi *C. neoformans* and *C. gattii. C. neoformans* is worldwide in distribution and is found as a ubiquitous saprophyte of soil, especially that which is enriched with pigeon droppings. *C. neoformans* includes capsular serotypes A, D, and AD, and *C. gattii* includes serotypes B and C. *C. neoformans* is further divided into two varieties, *var. grubii* (serotype A) and *var. neoformans* (serotype D).

Morphology

Microscopically, *C. neoformans* and *C. gattii* are spheric to oval, encapsulated, yeastlike organisms, 2 to 20 μm in diameter. Replication is by budding from a relatively narrow base. Single buds are usually formed, but multiple buds and chains of budding cells are sometimes present (Figure 67-7). In tissue and upon staining with India ink, the cells are variable in size, spheric, oval, or elliptic, and are surrounded by optically clear, smoothly contoured, spheric zones or "halos" that represent the extracellular polysaccharide capsule (Figure 67-8). The capsule is a distinctive marker, which may have a diameter of up to five times that of the fungal cell and is readily detected with a mucin stain, such as Mayer mucicarmine (Figure 67-9). The organism stains poorly with H&E but is easily detected with PAS and GMS stains. The cell wall of *C. neoformans* contains mela-

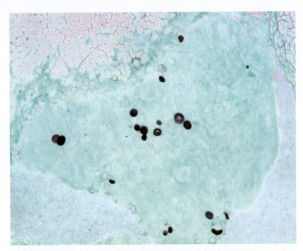

Figure 67-7 *Cryptococcus neoformans.* Microscopic morphology, Gomori methenamine silver stain.

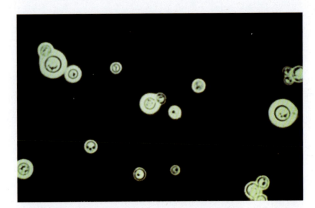

Figure 67-8 *Cryptococcus neoformans.* India ink preparation demonstrating the large capsule surrounding budding yeast cells (×1000).

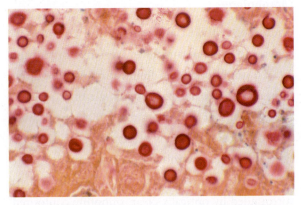

Figure 67-9 *Cryptococcus neoformans* stained with mucicarmine (×1000).

nin, which may be demonstrated by staining with the Fontana-Masson stain.

Epidemiology

Cryptococcosis is usually acquired by inhaling aerosolized cells of *C. neoformans* and *C. gattii* from the environment (Figure 67-10). Subsequent dissemination from the lungs, usually to the CNS, produces clinical disease in susceptible individuals. Primary cutaneous cryptococcosis may occur after transcutaneous inoculation but is rare. *C. neoformans* is most often encountered as an opportunistic pathogen. It is the most common cause of fungal meningitis and tends to occur in those patients with defective cellular immunity. *C. gattii* is generally found in tropical and subtropical climates in association with Eucalyptus trees. Recently, however, an endemic focus of *C. gattii* has been identified in Vancouver Island, British Columbia, and in Oregon and Washington State. *C. neoformans* is a major opportunistic pathogen of patients with AIDS. Those individuals with CD4+ lymphocyte counts of less than 100/mm (usually <200/mm2) are at high risk for CNS and disseminated cryptococcosis.

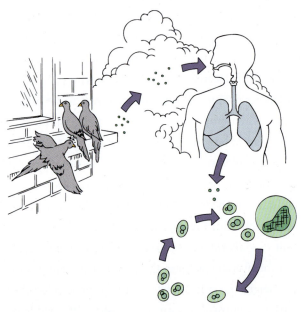

Figure 67-10 Natural history of saprobic and parasitic cycle of *Cryptococcus neoformans.*

Clinical Syndromes

Cryptococcosis may present as a pneumonic process or, more commonly, as a CNS infection secondary to hematogenous and lymphatic spread from a primary pulmonary focus. Less often, a more widely disseminated infection may be seen with cutaneous, mucocutaneous, osseous, and visceral forms of the disease.

Laboratory Diagnosis

The diagnosis of infection caused by *C. neoformans* and *C. gattii* may be made by culture of blood, cerebrospinal fluid (CSF), or other clinical material. Microscopic examination of CSF may reveal the characteristic encapsulated budding yeast cells. The cells of C. neoformans, when present in CSF or other clinical material, may be visualized with Gram stain, as well as with India ink (see Figure 67-8) or other stains (see Figure 67-7). Most commonly, however, the diagnosis of cryptococcal meningitis is made by direct detection of the capsular polysaccharide antigen in serum or CSF (Table 67-6). Detection of cryptococcal antigen is accomplished by using one of several commercially available latex agglutination or enzyme immunoassay kits. These assays have been shown to be rapid, sensitive, and specific for the diagnosis of cryptococcal disease (see Table 67-6).

Table 67-6 Sensitivity of Antigen Detection, India Ink Microscopy, and Culture of Cerebrospinal Fluid in the Diagnosis of Cryptococcal Meningitis.

	% Sensitivity	
Test	**AIDS Patients**	**Non-AIDS Patients**
Antigen	100	86-95
India ink	82	50
Culture	100	90

AIDS, Acquired immunodeficiency syndrome.
Modified from Viviani MA, Tortorano AM: *Cryptococcus*. In Anaissie EJ, McGinnis MR, Pfaller MA, editors: *Clinical mycology*, ed 2, New York, Churchill Livingstone, 2009.

Treatment

Cryptococcal meningitis (and other disseminated forms of cryptococcosis) is universally fatal if left untreated. In addition to the prompt administration of appropriate antifungal therapy, effective management of CNS pressure is crucial to the successful treatment of cryptococcal meningitis. All patients should receive amphotericin B plus flucytosine acutely for 2 weeks (induction therapy), followed by 8-week consolidation with either oral fluconazole (preferred) or itraconazole. AIDS patients generally require lifelong maintenance therapy with either fluconazole or itraconazole. In non-AIDS patients,

treatment may be discontinued after the consolidation therapy; however, relapse may be seen in up to 26% of these patients within 3 to 6 months after discontinuation of therapy. Thus a prolonged consolidation treatment with an azole for up to 1 year may be advisable, even with patients without AIDS.

Treatment of these patients should be followed both clinically and mycologically. Mycologic follow-up requires repeat lumbar puncture to be performed (1) at the end of the 2-week induction therapy to ensure sterilization of the CSF, (2) at the end of the consolidation therapy, (3) whenever indicated by a change in clinical status during follow-up. CSF samples collected during follow-up must be cultured. Determination of CSF protein, glucose, cell count, and cryptococcal antigen titer are helpful in assessing the response to therapy but are not highly predictive of outcome. Failure to sterilize the CSF by day 14 of therapy is indicative of a much higher probability that the consolidation therapy will fail.

Other Mycoses Caused by Yeast-like Fungi

Among the non-*Candida*, non-*Cryptococcus* yeastlike pathogens, nosocomial infections caused by *Malassezia spp.*, *Trichosporon spp.*, *Rhodotorula spp.*, and *B. capitatus* are most prominent, either because they are difficult to detect or because they may pose particular problems with respect to antifungal resistance.

Infections caused by *Malassezia spp.* (*M. furfur* and *M. pachydermatis*) are usually catheter-related and tend to occur in premature infants or in other patients receiving lipid infusions. Both of these organisms are budding yeasts (Figure 67-11). *M. furfur* is a common skin colonizer and is the etiologic agent of tinea (pityriasis) versicolor, whereas *M. pachydermatis* is a frequent cause of otitis in dogs, as well as a human skin commensal. *Malassezia spp.* should be considered when yeasts are seen microscopically in blood culture bottles or clinical material but no organisms are recovered on routine agar medium. To isolate *Malassezia spp.*, especially *M. furfur*, on agar medium, the plates must be inoculated and then overlaid with sterile olive oil. Olive oil provides the lipid requirement, and growth should be detected in

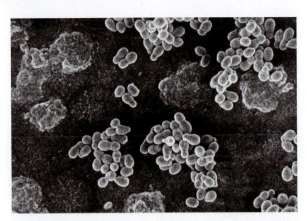

Figure 67-11   Scanning electron micrograph of *Malassezia furfur* adhering to the lumen of a central venous catheter. (Courtesy of S.A. Messer.)

3 to 5 days. Treatment of fungemia caused by *Malassezia spp.* does not usually require the administration of antifungal agents. The infection subsides once the lipid infusion is stopped and the intravascular lines are removed.

The genus *Trichosporon* currently consists of six species that are of clinical significance: *T. asahii* and *T. mucoides* are known to cause deep invasive infections, *T. asteroides* and *T. cutaneum* cause superficial skin infections, *T. ovoides* causes white piedra of the scalp, and *T. inkin* causes that of the pubic hair. Confusingly, most of the literature regarding deep-seated trichosporonosis refers to the older nomenclature of *T. beigelii*. Morphologically, these organisms are similar and appear in clinical material as hyphae, arthroconidia, and budding yeast cells. Susceptibility to amphotericin B is variable, and this agent lacks fungicidal activity against *Trichosporon*. Clinical failures with amphotericin B, fluconazole, and combinations of the two have been reported, and the outcome is generally dismal in the absence of neutrophil recovery. *Trichosporon* species are resistant to the echinocandins but appear to respond clinically to treatment with voriconazole.

Rhodotorula include *R. glutinis*, *R. mucilaginosa* (syn. *R. rubra*), and *R. minuta*. These yeastlike fungi are found as commensals on skin, nails, and mucous membranes, as well as in cheese and milk products and environmental sources, including air, soil, shower curtains, bathtub grout, and toothbrushes. *Rhodotorula* species are emerging as important human pathogens in immunocompromised patients and those with indwelling devices. *Rhodotorula* has been implicated as a cause of central venous catheter infection and fungemia, ocular infections, peritonitis, and meningitis. Amphotericin B has excellent activity against *Rhodotorula* and, coupled with catheter removal, is an optimal approach to infections with this organism. Flucytosine has excellent activity as well but should not be considered for monotherapy. Neither fluconazole nor the echinocandins should be used to treat infections caused by *Rhodotorula* species, and the role of the new extended-spectrum triazoles (e.g., voriconazole and posaconazole) is uncertain pending clinical data.

B. capitatus (teleomorph *D. capitatus*) is a rarely described fungus that produces severe systemic infection in immunocompromised patients, especially those with hematologic malignancies. This organism produces hyphae and arthroconidia, is widely distributed in nature, and may be found as part of the normal skin flora. Infection with *B. capitatus* presents similar to that with *Trichosporon* in neutropenic patients, with frequent fungemia and multiorgan (including brain) dissemination and a mortality rate of 60% to 80%. Rapid removal of central venous catheters, adjuvant immunotherapy, and novel antifungal therapies (e.g., voriconazole or high-dose fluconazole plus amphotericin B) are recommended for treatment of this rare but devastating infection.

ASPERGILLOSIS

Aspergillosis comprises a broad spectrum of diseases caused by members of the genus Aspergillus. The majority of infections are caused by *A. fumigatus*, *A. flavus*, *A. niger*, and *A. terreus*. Molecular taxonomic studies have shown that all of the aforementioned species are actually species complexes that contain morphologically indistinguishable cryptic species, some of which may exhibit important antifungal resistance profiles and pathogenic features.

Morphology

Aspergillus spp. grow in culture as hyaline molds. On a gross level, the colonies of Aspergillus may be black, brown, green, yellow, white, or other colors, depending upon the species and the growth conditions. Colonial appearance may provide an initial suggestion as to the species of Aspergillus, but definitive identification requires microscopic examination of the hyphae and the structure of the conidial head. A conidial head consists of a conidiophore with a terminal vesicle, on which are borne one or two layers of phialides, or sterigmata. Identification of individual species of Aspergillus depends in part on the difference in their conidial heads, including the arrangement and morphology of the conidia (Figures 67-12 and 67-13). In tissue, the hyphae of *Aspergillus spp.* stain poorly with H&E but are well visualized by the PAS, GMS, and Gridley fungal stains (Figure 67-14). The hyphae are homogeneous,

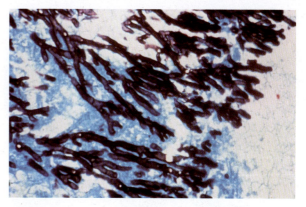

Figure 67-14 *Aspergillus* in tissue showing acute-angle branching, septate hyphae (Gomori methenamine silver, ×1000).

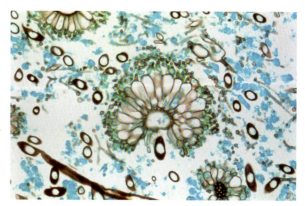

Figure 67-15 *Aspergillus niger* in a cavitary lung lesion showing both hyphae and conidial head (Gomori methenamine silver, ×1000).

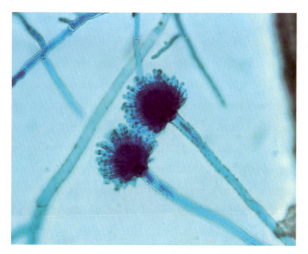

Figure 67-12 *Aspergillus fumigatus.* Lactophenol cotton blue preparation showing conidial heads.

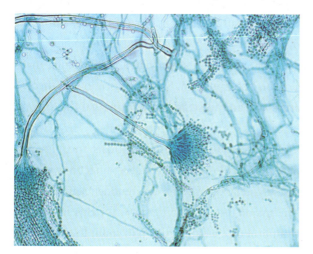

Figure 67-13 *Aspergillus terreus.* Lactophenol cotton blue preparation showing conidial head.

uniform in width (3 to 6 μm), with parallel contours, regular septations, and a progressive, treelike pattern of branching (see Figure 67-14). The branches are dichotomous and usually arise at acute (≈45°) angles. The hyphae may be seen within blood vessels (angioinvasion), causing thrombosis. The conidial heads are rarely seen in tissue but may arise within a cavity (Figure 67-15). The important species *A. terreus* can be identified in tissue by its spheric or oval aleurioconidia that develop from the lateral walls of the mycelium (Figure 67-16). Otherwise, the hyphae of pathogenic *Aspergillus* spp. are morphologically indistinguishable from one another in tissue.

Epidemiology

Aspergillus spp. are common throughout the world. Their conidia are ubiquitous in air, soil, and decaying matter. Within the hospital environment, *Aspergil-*

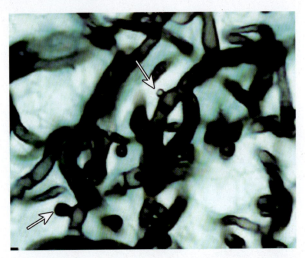

Figure 67-16 *Aspergillus terreus* in tissue. Arrows point to aleurioconidia (Gomori methenamine silver, ×1000). (From Walsh TJ, et al: Experimental pulmonary aspergillosis due to *Aspergillus terreus*: pathogenesis and treatment of an emerging fungal pathogen resistant to amphotericin B, *J Infect Dis* 188: 305-319, 2003.)

lus spp. may be found in air, showerheads, hospital water storage tanks, and potted plants. As a result, they are constantly being inhaled. The type of host reaction, the associated pathologic findings, and the ultimate outcome of infection depend more on host factors than on the virulence or pathogenesis of the individual *Aspergillus* spp. The respiratory tract is the most frequent, and most important, portal of entry.

Clinical Syndromes

The allergic manifestations of aspergillosis constitute a spectrum of presentations based on the degree of hypersensitivity to *Aspergillus* antigens. In the bronchopulmonary form, asthma, pulmonary infiltrates, peripheral eosinophilia, elevated serum IgE, and evidence of hypersensitivity to *Aspergillus* antigens (skin test) may be seen. Allergic sinusitis shows laboratory evidence of hypersensitivity to go along with upper respiratory symptoms of nasal obstruction and discharge, headache, and facial pain.

Both the paranasal sinuses and the lower airways may become colonized with *Aspergillus* spp., resulting in obstructive bronchial aspergillosis and true aspergilloma ("fungus ball"). Obstructive bronchial aspergillosis usually occurs in the setting of underlying pulmonary disease, such as cystic fibrosis, chronic bronchitis, or bronchiectasis. The condition is marked by the formation of bronchial casts or plugs composed of hyphal elements and mucinous material. The symptoms remain those of the underlying disease; no tissue injury results, and no treatment is necessary. An aspergilloma can form either in the paranasal sinuses or in a preformed pulmonary cavity secondary to old tuberculosis or other chronic cavitary lung disease. Aspergillomas may be seen on radiographic examination but usually are asymptomatic. Treatment is generally not warranted unless pulmonary hemorrhage occurs. In the event of pulmonary hemorrhage, which may be severe and life threatening, surgical excision of the cavity and fungus ball is indicated. Likewise, radical debridement of the paranasal sinuses may be necessary to alleviate any symptomatology or hemorrhage caused by a fungus ball of the sinuses.

Forms of invasive aspergillosis run the gamut from superficially invasive disease that may occur in the setting of mild immunosuppression (e.g., low-dose steroid therapy, collagen vascular disease, or diabetes) to destructive, locally invasive pulmonary or disseminated aspergillosis. The more limited forms of invasion generally include necrotizing pseudomembranous bronchial aspergillosis and chronic necrotizing pulmonary aspergillosis. Bronchial aspergillosis may cause wheezing, dyspnea, and hemoptysis. Most patients with chronic necrotizing pulmonary aspergillosis have underlying structural pulmonary disease, which may be treated with low-dose corticosteroids. This is a chronic infection that may be locally destructive, with the development of infiltrates and fungus balls seen on radiographic examination. It is not associated with vascular invasion or dissemination. Surgical resection of affected areas and administration of antifungal therapy are efficacious in treating this condition.

Invasive pulmonary aspergillosis and disseminated aspergillosis are devastating infections seen in severely neutropenic and immunodeficient patients. The major predisposing factors for this infectious complication include neutrophil count less than 500/mm3, cytotoxic chemotherapy, and corticosteroid therapy. Patients present with fever and pulmonary infiltrates, often accompanied by pleuritic chest pain and hemoptysis. Definitive diagnosis is often delayed because sputum and blood cultures are usually negative. The mortality of this infection despite specific antifungal therapy is quite high, usually exceeding 70% (see Table 67-4). Hematogenous dissemination of infection to extrapulmonary sites is common because of the angioinvasive nature of the fungus. Sites most often involved include brain, heart, kidneys, GI tract, liver, and spleen.

Laboratory Diagnosis

As with other ubiquitous fungi, the diagnosis of aspergillosis necessitates caution when evaluating the isolation of an *Aspergillus* species from clinical specimens. Recovery from surgically removed tissue or sterile sites, accompanied by positive histopathology (moniliaceous, septate, dichotomously branching hyphae) should always be considered significant; isolation from normally contaminated (e.g., respiratory) sites requires closer scrutiny. Most etiologic agents of aspergillosis grow readily on routine mycologic media lacking cycloheximide. Species-level identification of the major human pathogens can be made by observing cultural and microscopic characteristics from growth on potato dextrose agar. Microscopic morphology (conidiophores, vesicles, metulae, phialides, and conidia) is best observed with a slide culture and is necessary for species identification. The β-D-glucan test has been applied to the diagnosis of invasive aspergillosis, but it suffers from a lack of specificity. In contrast, PCR-based assays have proven to be both sensitive and specific for the diagnosis of invasive aspergillosis, and efforts to standardize this method are ongoing.

Treatment and prevention

Prevention of aspergillosis in high-risk patients is paramount. Neutropenic and other high-risk patients are generally housed in facilities where the air is filtered to minimize exposure to Aspergillus conidia.

Specific antifungal therapy of aspergillosis usually involves the administration of voriconazole or one of the lipid formulations of amphotericin B. It is impor-

tant to realize that A. terreus is considered resistant to amphotericin B and should be treated with an alternative agent such as voriconazole. The introduction of voriconazole provides a treatment option that is more efficacious and less toxic than amphotericin B. Concomitant efforts to decrease immunosuppression and/or reconstitute host immune defenses are important components of the treatment of aspergillosis. Likewise, surgical resection of involved areas is recommended if possible.

MUCORMYCOSIS

Mucormycosis refers to diseases caused by fungi of the subphyla *Mucoromycotina* and *Entomophthoromycotina*. The principal human pathogens among the Mucormycetes are encompassed by two orders: the *Mucorales* and the *Entomophthorales*. The order *Entomophthorales* contains two pathogenic genera, *Conidiobolus* and *Basidiobolus.*.

In the order *Mucorales*, pathogenic genera include *Rhizopus, Mucor, Lichtheimia* (formerly *Absidia*), *Rhizomucor, Saksenaea, Cunninghamella, Syncephalastrum*, and *Apophysomyces*. Infections caused by Mucormycetes are rare, occurring at an annual rate of 1.7 infections per million population in the United States. Unfortunately, when they do occur, infections caused by these agents are generally acute and rapidly progressive, with mortality rates of 70% to 100%.

Morphology

Macroscopically, the pathogenic *Mucorales* grow rapidly, producing gray to brown woolly colonies within 12 to 18 hours. Microscopically, the Mucormycetes are molds with broad, hyaline, sparsely septate, coenocytic hyphae. The asexual spores of the order *Mucorales* are contained within a sporangium and are referred to as sporangiospores. The sporangia are borne at the tips of stalklike sporangiophores that terminate in a bulbous swelling called the columella (Figure 67-17). The presence of rootlike structures, called rhizoids, is helpful in identifying specific genera within the *Mucorales*. In tissue, Mucormycetes (order *Mucorales*) are seen as ribbon-like, aseptate or sparsely septate, moniliaceous (nonpigmented) hyphae (Figure 67-18). In contrast to *Aspergillus spp.* and other hyaline molds, the diameter of the hyphae often exceeds 10 μm, and the hyphae are irregularly contoured and pleomorphic, often folding and twisting back upon themselves. The pattern of hyphal branching is haphazard and nonprogressive, and branches typically arise from the parent hyphae at right angles. The walls of the hyphae are thin, stain weakly with GMS and other fungal stains, and are often more easily detected with H&E (see Figure 67-18). The Mucormycetes are typically angioinvasive.

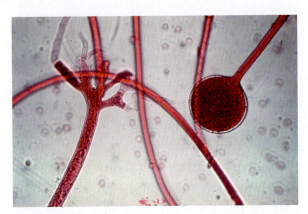

Figure 67-17   *Rhizopus* sp. showing sporangium and rhizoids.

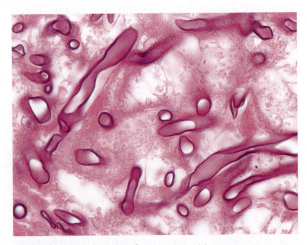

Figure 67-18   *Rhizopus* sp. in tissue showing broad, ribbon-like, aseptate hyphae (hematoxylin and eosin, ×1000).

Epidemiology

Mucormycosis is a sporadic disease that occurs worldwide. *Rhizopus arrhizus* is the most common cause of human mucormycosis; however, additional species of *Rhizopus, Rhizomucor, Lichtheimia,* and *Cunninghamella* are known to cause invasive disease in hospitalized individuals. The organisms are ubiquitous in soil and decaying vegetation, and infection may be acquired by inhalation, ingestion, or contamination of wounds with sporangiospores from the environment. As with *Aspergillus spp.*, nosocomial spread of Mucormycetes may occur by way of air-conditioning systems, particularly during construction. Focal outbreaks of mucormycosis have also been associated with the use of contaminated adhesive bandages or tape in surgical wound dressings, resulting in primary cutaneous mucormycosis.

Invasive mucormycosis occurs in immunocompromised patients and is similar clinically to aspergillosis. It is estimated that Mucormycetes may cause infection in 1% to 9% of solid organ transplants, especially those with underlying diabetes mellitus. Risk factors include corticosteroid and deferoxamine therapy, diabetic ketoacidosis, renal failure, hematologic malignancy, myelosuppression, and exposure to hospital construction activity. Recently, mucormycosis has been seen after BMT in patients receiving antifungal prophylaxis with voriconazole, an agent that is not active against the Mucormycetes.

Clinical Syndromes

There are several clinical forms of mucormycosis caused by members of the order Mucorales.

Rhinocerebral mucormycosis is an acute invasive infection of the nasal cavity, paranasal sinuses, and orbit that involves the facial structures and extends into the CNS, involving the meninges and the brain.

Pulmonary mucormycosis: The pulmonary lesions are infarctive as a result of hyphal invasion and subsequent thrombosis of large pulmonary vessels. Chest radiographs show a rapidly progressive bronchopneumonia, segmented or lobar consolidation, and signs of cavitation. Fungus-ball formation mimicking aspergilloma may be seen. Pulmonary hemorrhage with fatal hemoptysis may be seen as a result of vascular invasion by the fungus.

Disseminated infection: Symptoms at presentation point to neurologic, pulmonary, or GI involvement. Involvement of the GI tract often results in massive hemorrhage or perforation.

Cutaneous mucormycosis: Primary cutaneous mucormycosis may occur after traumatic injury, in surgical dressings, or as colonization of burn wounds. The infection may be superficial or extend rapidly into the subcutaneous tissues. The aftermath of the devastating tornados of 2011 in the United States saw several cases of deeply invasive mucormycosis in non-immunocompromised individuals secondary to cutaneous inoculation by flying debris.

Laboratory Diagnosis

The Mucormycetes are an extremely ubiquitous group of fungi, so demonstration of characteristic fungal elements in tissue merits considerably more importance than simple isolation in culture. Appropriate specimens include scrapings of nasal mucosa, aspirates of sinus contents, bronchial alveolar lavage fluid, and biopsy of any and all necrotic infected tissue. Direct examination of material mounted in KOH with calcofluor white may reveal the broad, aseptate hyphae. Histopathologic sections stained with H&E or PAS are most useful (see Figure 67-18). Broad, irregularly branched, pauciseptate, twisted hyphae can be observed.

Treatment

Amphotericin B remains the first-line therapy for mucormycosis, often supplemented by surgical debridement and immune reconstitution. Among the extended-spectrum triazoles, however, posaconazole stands out, in that it appears to be active against most of the Mucormycetes. Posaconazole has documented efficacy in murine models of mucormycosis and in limited experience in the treatment of infections in humans.

Mycoses Caused by Other Hyaline Molds

The list of hyaline molds, also known as hyalohyphomycetes, is quite long, and it is well beyond the scope of this chapter to discuss them all. In this chapter,

the discussion of specific genera is limited to selected clinically important hyaline molds: *Fusarium spp.*, *Scedosporium spp.*, *Acremonium spp.*, *Paecilomyces spp.*, *Trichoderma spp.*, and *Scopulariopsis spp.* These organisms tend to cause infections in neutropenic patients, are often disseminated in nature, and are almost uniformly fatal in the absence of immune reconstitution. Several of these organisms are capable of adventitious conidiation (generation of spores in tissue) with concomitant hematogenous dissemination, positive blood cultures, and multiple cutaneous lesions.

Fusarium spp.

Morphology

Fusarium is also an important cause of fungal keratitis, especially among contact lens wearers. The most common species isolated from clinical specimens include *Fusarium moniliforme, F. solani*, and *F. oxysporum*. The hallmark of disseminated fusariosis is the appearance of multiple purpuric cutaneous nodules with central necrosis. Biopsy of these nodules generally reveals branching, hyaline, septate hyphae invading dermal blood vessels (Figure 67-19). Microscopically, *Fusarium spp.* are characterized by the production of both macroconidia and microconidia. Microconidia are single or double celled, ovoid to cylindric, and generally borne as mucous balls or short chains. Macroconidia are fusiform or sickle

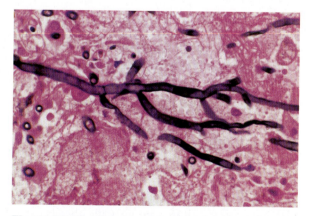

Figure 67-19 *Fusarium* sp. in tissue showing acute-angle branching, septate hyphae that are indistinguishable from that of *Aspergillus* spp. (From Chandler FW, Watts JC: *Pathologic diagnosis of fungal infections*, Chicago, 1987, American Society for Clinical Pathology Press.)

shaped and many celled (Figure 67-20). In culture, colonies of *Fusarium spp.* are rapidly growing, cottony to woolly, flat, and spreading.

Colors may include blue-green, beige, salmon, lavender, red, violet, and purple.

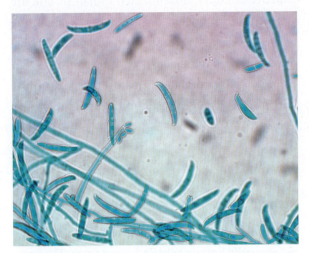

Figure 67-20 *Fusarium oxysporum,* lactophenol cotton blue preparation.

Epidemiology

Fusarium species have been recognized with increased frequency as causes of disseminated infection in immunocompromised patients. *Fusarium* is also an important cause of fungal keratitis, especially among contact lens wearers. The most common species isolated from clinical specimens include *Fusarium moniliforme, F. solani,* and *F. oxysporum.*

Clinical Syndromes

The hallmark of disseminated fusariosis is the appearance of multiple purpuric cutaneous nodules with central necrosis. Biopsy of these nodules generally reveals branching, hyaline, septate hyphae invading dermal blood vessels (see Figure 67-19).

Laboratory Diagnosis

Cultures of biopsy material and of blood are useful in establishing the diagnosis of Fusarium infection. Although blood cultures are virtually always negative in invasive infections caused by *Aspergillus* spp., approximately 75% of patients with fusariosis will have positive blood cultures. In culture, colonies of

Fusarium spp. are rapidly growing, cottony to woolly, flat, and spreading. Colors may include blue-green, beige, salmon, lavender, red, violet, and purple.

Treatment

Primary therapy with a lipid formulation of amphotericin B, voriconazole, or posaconazole, plus vigorous efforts at immune reconstitution, are recommended for treatment of fusariosis.

Scedosporium spp.

S. apiospermum (teleomorph *Pseudallescheria boydii*) and *S. prolificans* represent two important antifungal-resistant opportunistic pathogens.

Morphology

In culture, colonies are woolly to cottony and are initially white, becoming smoky brown to green. Microscopically, conidia are one celled, elongate, and pale brown and are borne singly or in balls on either short or long conidiophores (Figure 67-21).

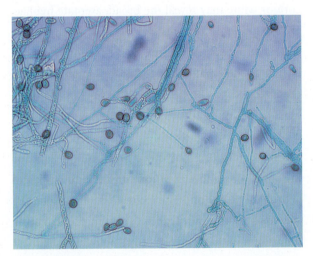

Figure 67-21 *Scedosporium apiospermum (Pseudallescheria boydii).* Lactophenol cotton blue preparation showing conidia and septate hyphae.

Epidemiology, Clinical Syndromes and Treatment

S. apiospermum may be readily isolated from soil and is an occasional cause of mycetoma worldwide; however, it is also the cause of serious disseminated and localized infection in immunocompromised patients. In addition to widespread disseminated disease, *S. apiospermum* has been reported to cause corneal ulcers, endophthalmitis, sinusitis, pneumonia, endocarditis, meningitis, arthritis, and osteomyelitis. *S. apiospermum* is indistinguishable from *Aspergillus spp.* and other agents of hyalohyphomycosis on histopathologic examination. Such distinction is important clinically because *S. apiospermum* is resistant to amphotericin B and susceptible to voriconazole and posaconazole.

S. prolificans

It is a potentially virulent and highly aggressive emerging agent of hyalohyphomycosis.

Morphology

S. prolificans resembles *S. apiospermum* in macroscopic and microscopic morphology.

Epidemiology, Clinical Syndromes and Treatment

Although far less important than Fusarium or *S. apiospermum*, infections caused by *S. prolificans* are associated with soft-tissue trauma and are characterized by widespread local invasion, tissue necrosis, and osteomyelitis. The formation by *S. prolificans* of annelloconidia in wet clumps at the apices of annellides with swollen bases is the most useful characteristic in differentiating this organism from *S. apiospermum*. *S. prolificans* is considered to be resistant to virtually all of the systemically active antifungal agents, including the extended-spectrum triazoles and the echinocandins. Surgical resection remains the only definitive therapy for infection by *S. prolificans*.

Acremonium spp.

Morphology

Colonies of *Acremonium spp.* are whitish gray or rose, with a velvety to cottony surface. The conidia may be single celled in chains or a conidial mass arising from short, unbranched, tapered phialides.

Epidemiology, Clinical Syndromes and Treatment

Invasive infections caused by *Acremonium spp.* are almost exclusively seen in patients with neutropenia, transplantation, or other immunodeficiency conditions and occur in a manner similar to that of Fusarium, with hematogenously disseminated skin lesions and positive blood cultures. Species of Acremonium are commonly found in soil, decaying vegetation, and decaying food. The optimal treatment for infections caused by *Acremonium spp.* has not been established. Resistance is seen to amphotericin B, itraconazole, and the echinocandins. A recent report of successful treatment of a pulmonary infection caused by Acremonium strictum with posaconazole suggests that the new triazoles may be useful in treatment of Acremonium infections.

Paecilomyces spp.

Morphology

Microscopically, the *Paecilomyces spp.* conidia are unicellular, ovoid to fusiform, and form chains. Phialides have a swollen base and a long, tapered neck.

Epidemiology, Clinical Syndromes and Treatment

Paecilomyces spp. may cause invasive disease in organ and hematopoietic stem cell recipients, individuals with AIDS, and other immunocompromised patients. The portal of infection is often through breaks in the skin or intravascular catheters. Dissemination of the infection may be aided by adventitious conidiation that takes place within the tissues. The two most common species are *P. lilacinus* and *P. variotti*. Susceptibility to amphotericin B is variable, with resistance seen with *P. lilacinus*. Voriconazole has been used successfully to treat both severe cutaneous infection and disseminated disease.

Trichoderma spp.

Trichoderma spp. are excellent examples of fungi previously labeled as nonpathogenic that have emerged as important opportunistic pathogens in immunocompromised patients and in patients undergoing peritoneal dialysis. Fatal disseminated disease caused by *T. longibrachiatum* occurs in patients with hematologic malignancies, after BMT or solid organ transplantation. Most Trichoderma spp. show decreased susceptibility to amphotericin B, itraconazole, fluconazole, and flucytosine. Voriconazole appears to be active against the few isolates tested.

Scopulariopsis spp.

Scopulariopsis spp. are ubiquitous soil saprobes that have been rarely implicated in invasive human disease. *S. brevicaulis* is the most frequently isolated species.

Morphology

Scopulariopsis spp. grow moderately to rapidly on standard mycologic media. Colonies are initially smooth, becoming granular to powdery with age. Conidiophores are simple or branched; the conidiogenous cells are annellides that form singly or in clusters or may form a broomlike structure, or scopula, similar to that seen with *Penicillium spp.* The annelloconidia are smooth initially, become rough at maturity, are shaped like light bulbs, and form basipetal chains.

Epidemiology, Clinical Syndromes and Treatment

Infection is usually confined to the nails; however, serious deep infection has been noted in neutropenic leukemia patients and after BMT. Both local and disseminated infections have been described, with involvement of the nasal septum, skin and soft tissues, blood, lungs, and brain. Diagnosis is made by culture and histopathology. Scopulariopsis spp. are usually resistant to itraconazole and moderately susceptible to amphotericin B. Invasive infections may require surgical and medical treatment and are often fatal.

PHAEOHYPHOMYCOSIS

Phaeohyphomycosis is defined as tissue infection caused by dematiaceous (pigmented) hyphae and/or yeasts. The dematiaceous fungi that have been documented to cause human infection encompass a large number of different genera; however, the more common causes of human infection include *Alternaria*, *Bipolaris*, *Cladosporium*, *Curvularia*, and *Exserohilum* species. In addition, several of the dematiaceous fungi appear to be neurotropic: *Cladophialophora bantiana*, *Bipolaris spicifera*, *Exophiala spp.*, *Wangiella dermatitidis*, *Ramichloridium obovoideum*, and *Chaetomium atrobrunneum*. Brain abscess is the most common CNS presentation. *Bipolaris spp.* and *Exserohilum spp.* infections may present initially as sinusitis, which then extends into the CNS.

Alternaria spp. are important causes of paranasal sinusitis in both healthy and immunocompromised individuals. Other sites of infection include skin and soft tissue, cornea, lower respiratory tract, and peritoneum. *Alternaria alternata* is the best-documented human pathogen in this genus. In tissue, hyphae with or without yeast forms are present. Most often, the pale brown to dark melanin-like pigment within the cell wall is apparent in H&E- or Papanicolaou-stained tissue (Figure 67-22). Staining with the Fontana-Masson technique (a melanin-specific stain) may help visualize the dematiaceous elements. In culture, *Alternaria* colonies are rapidly growing, cottony, and gray to black. The conidiophores are usually solitary and simple or branched. The conidia develop in branching chains and are dematiaceous, muriform, and smooth or rough and taper toward the distal end with a short beak at their apices (Figure 67-23).

Cladosporium spp. usually cause superficial cutaneous infections but may cause deep infections as well. These fungi are rapidly growing with a velvety, olive gray to black colony. The conidiophores arise from the hyphae and are dematiaceous, tall, and branching. The conidia may be smooth or rough and single to several celled and form branching chains at the apex of the conidiophore.

Curvularia spp. are ubiquitous inhabitants of the soil and have been implicated in both disseminated and local infections. Sites of infection include endocarditis, local catheter-site infections, nasal septum and paranasal sinuses, lower respiratory tract, skin and subcutaneous tissues, bones, and cornea. In tissue, the hyphae may appear nonpigmented. Common species found to be etiologic agents of human infection include *C. geniculata*, *C. lunata*, *C. pallescens*, and *C. senegalensis*. In culture, colonies are rapidly growing, woolly, and gray to grayish black. Microscopically, the conidia are dematiaceous, solitary or in groups, septate, simple or branched, sympodial, and geniculate.

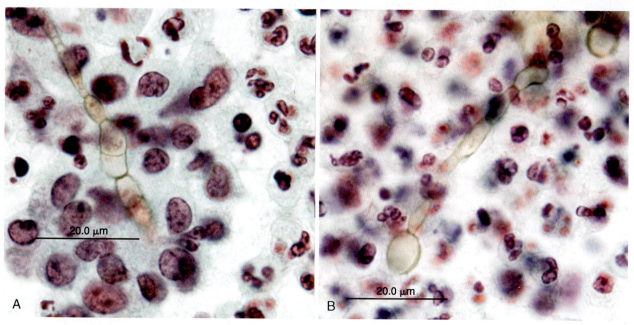

Figure 67-22 **A** and **B,** Fine-needle aspirate of a fluctuant mass showing the pigmented hyphae of *Phialophora verrucosa* (Papanicolaou). (From Anaissie EJ, McGinnis MR, Pfaller MA, editors: *Clinical mycology*, ed 2, New York, 2009, Churchill Livingstone.)

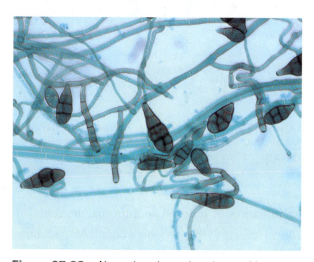

Figure 67-23 *Alternaria* sp. Lactophenol cotton blue preparation showing darkly pigmented chains of muriform conidia.

Infections caused by the genera Bipolaris and Exserohilum present similarly to those of *Aspergillus* spp., except that the disease progresses more slowly. Clinical presentations include dissemination with vascular invasion and tissue necrosis, involvement of the CNS and paranasal sinuses, and association with allergic bronchopulmonary disease. These organisms cause sinusitis in "normal" (atopic or asthmatic) hosts and more invasive disease in immunocompromised hosts. In culture, both Bipolaris and Exserohilum form rapidly growing, woolly, gray to black colonies.

Microscopically, the conidiophores are sympodial and geniculate. The conidia are dematiaceous, oblong to cylindric, and multicelled (Figure 67-24).

The optimal treatment of deep-seated phaeohyphomycosis has not yet been established, although it most often includes early administration of amphotericin B and aggressive surgical excision. Despite these efforts, phaeohyphomycosis does not respond well to treatment and relapses are common. Posaconazole has been used successfully to treat disseminated infec-

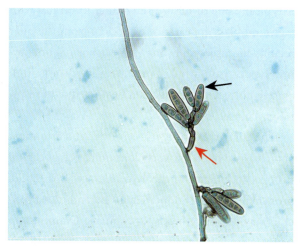

Figure 67-24 *Bipolaris* sp. Lactophenol cotton blue preparation showing pigmented conidia *(black arrow)* borne on geniculate conidiophores *(red arrow).*

tion caused by *Exophiala spinifera*. In those patients with brain abscesses, complete excision of the lesion has been associated with improved survival. Long-term triazole (posaconazole or voriconazole) therapy coupled with repeated surgical excision may prevent recurrences.

PNEUMOCYSTOSIS

Pneumocystis jirovecii (formerly *Pneumocystis carinii*) is an organism that causes infection almost exclusively in debilitated and immunosuppressed patients, especially those with HIV infection. It is the most common opportunistic infection among individuals with AIDS; however, the incidence has decreased considerably in recent years with the use of highly active antiretroviral therapy.

During the course of human infection, *P. jirovecii* may exist as free trophic forms (1.5 to 5 μm in diameter), as a uninucleate sporocyst (4 to 5 μm), or as a cyst (5 μm) containing up to eight ovoid to fusiform intracystic bodies (Figure 67-25). After rupture of the cyst, the cyst wall may be seen as an empty, collapsed structure (Figure 67-26).

The hallmark of *P. jirovecii* infection is an interstitial pneumonitis with a mononuclear infiltrate composed predominantly of plasma cells. The onset of disease is insidious, with signs and symptoms including dyspnea, cyanosis, tachypnea, nonproductive cough, and fever. The radiographic appearance is typically one of diffuse interstitial infiltrates with a ground-glass appearance extending from the hilar region, but radiographs may appear normal or show nodules or cavitation. The mortality rate is high among untreated patients, and death is due to respiratory failure.

The diagnosis of *P. jirovecii* infection is almost entirely based upon microscopic examination of clinical material, including bronchoalveolar lavage (BAL) fluid, bronchial brushing, induced sputum, and transbronchial or open-lung biopsy specimens. Examination of BAL fluid has been shown to have a sensitivity of 90% to 100% and usually precludes the need for transbronchial or open-lung biopsy. Microscopic

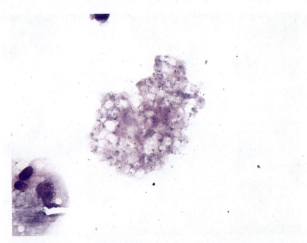

Figure 67-25 *Pneumocystis jirovecii* in bronchoalveolar lavage fluid. Giemsa stain shows intracystic forms (×1000).

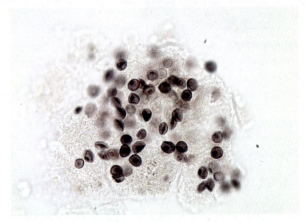

Figure 67-26 *Pneumocystis jirovecii* in bronchoalveolar lavage fluid. Gomori methenamine silver stain shows typical intact and collapsed cysts (×1000).

examination of induced sputum may be useful in AIDS patients with a very high organism load; however, it has a 20% to 25% false-negative rate. A variety of histologic and cytologic stains have been used to detect *P. jirovecii*: GMS, Giemsa, PAS, toluidine blue, calcofluor white, and immunofluorescence. The Giemsa stain demonstrates the trophic forms but does not stain the cyst wall (see Figure 67-25), whereas the GMS stain is specific for the cyst wall (see Figure 67-26). Immunofluorescent techniques stain both trophic forms and the cyst wall.

The cornerstone for both prophylaxis and treatment is trimethoprim-sulfamethoxazole. Alternative therapies have been used in AIDS patients; they include pentamidine, trimethoprim-dapsone, clindamycin-primaquine, atovaquone, and trimetrexate.

SUMMARY

Candidiasis

Opportunistic yeasts are causing infections ranging from superficial mucosal and cutaneous disease to hematogenously disseminated, often fatal infections. Vast majority of infections are due to five major species: *C. albicans*, *C. glabrata*, *C. parapsilosis*, *C. tropicalis*, and *C. krusei*. Morphology ranges from budding yeasts to peudohyphae and true hyphae. Reproduction is by formation of blastoconidia (buds). Candida is the most important group of opportunistic fungal pathogens, and may be community acquired (mucosal infections) or hospital associated (invasive disease).

Cryptococcosis

Systemic mycosis caused by the fungi *Cryptococcus neoformans* and *C. gatti*. *C. neoformans* includes capsular serotypes A, D, and AD; *var. grubii* (serotype A) and *var. Neoformans* (serotype D). *C. gatti* includes serotypes B and C. Spherical to oval, encapsulated, yeastlike organisms that replicate by budding. Both species may cause pulmonary, hematogenously disseminated, and central nervous system (CNS) disease.

Aspergillosis

Broad spectrum of diseases caused by filamentous fungi (molds) of genus Aspergillus. Exposure to spores in environment may cause allergic reactions in hypersensitized hosts or destructive, invasive, pulmonary, and disseminated disease in highly immunocompromised hosts. Vast majority of infections caused by *A. fumigatus* (most common), *A. flavus*, *A. niger*, and *A. terreus*. Hyaline molds that produce vast amounts of spores (conidia) that serve as infectious propagules upon inhalation by host. Invasive aspergillosis marked by angioinvasion and tissue destruction due to infarction.

KEYWORDS

English	Chinese
Candida spp.	念珠菌
Candida albicans	白色念珠菌
Cryptococcosis	隐球菌病
Crytococcus neoformans	新型隐球菌
Aspergillosis	曲霉病
Mucormycosis	毛霉(菌)病
Fusarium	镰刀菌属
Scedosporium	足放线菌属

BIBLIOGRAPHY

1. Anaissie EJ, McGinnis MR, Pfaller MA: Clinical mycology, ed 2, New York, 2009, Churchill Livingstone.

2. Chandler FW, Watts JC: Pathologic diagnosis of fungal infections, Chicago, 1987, American Society for Clinical Pathology Press.

3. Diekema DJ, et al: A global evaluation of voriconazole activity tested against recent clinical isolates of Candida spp, Diagn Microbiol Infect Dis 63: 233-236, 2009.

4. Dignani MC, Solomkin JS, Anaissie EJ: Candida. In Anaissie EJ, McGinnis MR, Pfaller MA, editors: Clinical mycology, ed 2, New York, 2009, Churchill Livingstone.

5. Gudlagson O, et al: Attributable mortality of nosocomial candidemia, revisited, Clin Infect Dis 37: 1172-1177, 2003.

6. Hidron AI, et al: Antimicrobial-resistant pathogens associated with healthcare-associated infections: annual summary of data reported to the National Healthcare Safety Network at the Centers for Disease Control and Prevention, 2006-2007, Infect Control Hosp Epidemiol 29: 996-1011, 2008.

7. Horn DL, et al: Clinical characteristics of 2,019 patients with candidemia: data from the PATH Alliance Registry, Clin Infect Dis 48: 1695-1703, 2009.

8. Lockhart SR, et al: The epidemiology of fungal infections. In Anaissie EJ, McGinnis MR, Pfaller MA, editors: Clinical mycology, ed 2, New York, 2009, Churchill Livingstone.

9. Pannuti CS, et al: Nosocomial pneumonia in adult patients undergoing bone marrow transplantation: a 9-year study, J Clin Oncol 9: 1, 1991.

10. Pfaller MA, Diekema DJ: Epidemiology of invasive candidiasis: a persistent public health problem, Clin Microbiol Rev 20: 133-163, 2007.

11. Pfaller MA, Diekema DJ: Epidemiology of invasive mycoses in North America, Crit Rev Microbiol 36: 1-53, 2010.

12. Viviani MA, Tortorano AM: Cryptococcus. In Anaissie EJ, McGinnis MR, Pfaller MA, editors: Clinical mycology, ed 2, New York, 2009, Churchill Livingstone.

13. Wey SB, et al: Hospital-acquired candidemia: attributable mortality and excess length of stay, Arch Intern Med 148: 2642-2645, 1988.

Fungal and Fungal-Like Infections of Unusual or Uncertain Etiology

Chapter

68

Thus far we have discussed mycotic processes caused by reasonably well characterized fungi that may serve as colonizers, opportunistic pathogens, or true pathogens. Although many of these organisms have undergone minor taxonomic reclassification over time, they all share the characteristics of the kingdom Fungi. In this chapter, we will discuss several infections that historically have been considered to represent fungal or "fungal-like" processes based on clinical and histopathologic presentation, but have been difficult to classify because they cannot be grown on artificial media. In addition to being unusual, as well as uncommon, these infections are all diagnosed based on detection of characteristic structures on histopathologic examination of tissue. A listing of the infections, the etiologic agents, and the typical morphology in tissue is provided in Table 68-1.

ADIASPIROMYCOSIS

In humans, adiaspiromycosis is a rare, self-limited, pulmonary infection caused by inhalation of the asexual conidia of the soil saprophytes *Emmonsia crescens* and *Emmonsia parva*. Synonyms include haplomycosis or adiasporosis.

Morphology

The fungi, *E. crescens* and *E. parva*, grow as molds in culture at room temperature and in nature. The hyphae are septate and branched. The small (2 to 4 μm) aleurioconidia are borne on conidiophores that arise at right angles to the vegetative hyphae. Upon incubation at 40℃ *in vitro*, or when introduced into the lungs, the conidia transform into adiaconidia, which

then undergo massive enlargement but show no evidence of replication (e.g., budding, endospore formation).

When mature, the adiaconidia are thick-walled spherules measuring 200 to 400 μm or more in diameter (Figure 68-1; see Table 68-1). The walls of the spherule are refractile, 20 to 70 μm thick, and when stained with hematoxylin and eosin (H&E) stain, comprise two layers: a narrow, outer, eosinophilic layer containing periodic fenestrations and a broad, hyaline, inner layer composed predominantly of chitin (see Figure 68-1). The conidial walls stain with Gomori methenamine silver (GMS), periodic acid-Schiff (PAS), and the Gridley fungus stains but not with mucicarmine (Table 68-2). In human lung tissue, the adiaconidia are usually empty but may contain small eosinophilic globules along the inner surface of the walls (see Figure 68-1).

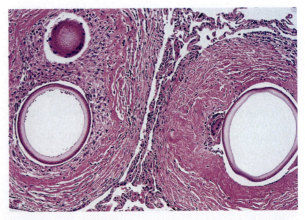

Figure 68-1 Pulmonary adiaspiromycosis. The hematoxylin and eosin (H&E) stain defines two layers in the wall of the adiaconidium. Each adiaconidium has evoked a fibro-granulomatous response (H&E, ×40). (From Connor DH, et al: *Pathology of infectious diseases*, vol 2, Stamford, Conn, 1997, Appleton & Lange.)

Table 68-1 Morphologic Features of Fungal and Fungal-Like Infections of Unusual or Uncertain Etiology.

Disease	Etiologic Agent(s)	Typical Morphology in Tissue	Usual Host Reaction
Adiaspiromycosis	*Emmonsia* spp.	Large adiaconidia, 200-400 µm diameter with thick (20-70 µm) walls; see Figure 74-1	Granulomatous fibrotic and noncaseating
Chlorellosis	*Chlorella* sp. (chlorophyllous green alga)	Unicellular, endosporulating, round organisms, 4-15 µm diameter, containing multiple cytoplasmic granules (chloroplasts); lesions are green pigmented; see Figure 74-2	Pyogranulomatous
Lacaziosis (Lobomycosis)	*Lacazia loboi (Loboa loboi)*	Spheric, budding yeasts, 5-12 µm diameter, that form chains of cells connected by tubelike structures; secondary budding may be present; see Figure 74-3	Granulomatous
Protothecosis	*Prototheca wickerhamii, Prototheca zopfii* (achlorophyllous green algae)	Spheric, oval, or polyhedral spherules, 2-25 µm diameter, containing 2-20 endospores when mature; see Figure 74-5	Variable; no reaction to granulomatous
Pythiosis insidiosi	*Pythium insidiosum* (not a true fungus; belongs to the protistal kingdom Straminopila)	Hyphae and short hyphal fragments that are hyaline, thin-walled, pauciseptate, irregularly branched, 5-7 µm wide with nonparallel contours; angioinvasive; see Figure 74-6	Granulomatous, necrotizing, suppurative, arteritis
Rhinosporidiosis	*Rhinosporidium seeberi* (aquatic protistan parasite of the Mesomycetozoa clade)	Large sporangia (100-350 µm diameter) with thin walls (3-5 µm) that enclose numerous endospores (6-8 µm diameter) with a zonal distribution; see Figures 74-7 and 74-8	Nonspecific chronic inflammatory or granulomatous

Data from Chandler FW, Watts JC: *Pathologic diagnosis of fungal infections*, Chicago, 1987, American Society for Clinical Pathology Press; and Connor DH, et al: *Pathology of infectious diseases*, vol 2, Stamford, Conn, 1997, Appleton & Lange.

Table 68-2 Comparative Morphologic Features of Fungi and Fungal-Like Organisms That Appear as Large Spherules in Tissue.

Feature	Organisms		
	Coccidioides immitis	*Rhinosporidium seeberi*[*]	*Emmonsia* spp.[†]
External diameter of spherule (µm)	20-200	10-350	200-400
Thickness of spherule wall (µm)	1-2	3-5	20-70
Diameter of endospores (µm)	2-5	6-10[‡]	None
Pigmentation	None	None	None
Hyphae or arthroconidia	Rare	None	None
Host reaction	Necrotic granulomas	Mucosal polyps with acute and chronic inflammation	Fibrotic granulomas
Growth in culture	+	−	±[§]
Special stain reactions			
Gomori methenamine silver	+	+	+
Periodic acid-Schiff	+	+	+
Mucicarmine	−	+	−

[*]Not a fungus. Newly classified as an aquatic protistan parasite of the Mesomycetozoa clade.
[†]Adiaconidia.
[‡]Endospores arranged in characteristic zonal distribution. Mature endospores contain distinctive eosinophilic globules.
[§]Grows as a mold on agar medium. Organism not recoverable from tissue.
Modified from Chandler FW, Watts JC: *Pathologic diagnosis of fungal infections*, Chicago, 1987, American Society for Clinical Pathology Press.

Epidemiology

Although human adiaspiromycosis is uncommon, the infection is prevalent in rodents worldwide. Likewise, the fungus may be found in nature, predominantly in temperate zones. Human disease has been reported from France, Czechoslovakia, Russia, Honduras, Guatemala, Venezuela, and Brazil. Rodents may serve as a zoonotic reservoir for the disease. The likely mode of infection is by inhalation of fungal conidia aerosolized by contaminated soil.

Clinical Syndromes

As with many fungal infections, most cases of documented adiaspiromycosis have been asymptomatic. Three forms of human adiaspiromycosis have been recognized: solitary granuloma, localized granulomatous disease, and diffuse, disseminated granulomatous disease. Patients with the disseminated granulomatous form of pulmonary adiaspiromycosis may experience fever, cough, and progressive dyspnea caused by compression and displacement of distal airways and alveolar parenchyma by the expanding granulomas. Fungal replication in the lungs does not occur, and dissemination to extrapulmonary sites has not been reported. The severity of the disease appears to be entirely commensurate with the number of conidia inhaled.

Laboratory Diagnosis

The diagnosis of adiaspiromycosis is established by histopathologic examination of affected lung and identification of the characteristic adiaconidia. Each adiaconidium is surrounded by an epithelioid and giant-cell granulomatous response, which is further encompassed by a dense capsule of fibrous tissue (see Figure 68-1). All of the granulomas are at a similar stage of development, reflecting a one-time exposure without subsequent replication within the lung.

The spherules represented by the adiaconidia should not be confused with those of *C. immitis* or *R. seeberi*, two other organisms that produce large spherules in tissue (see Table 68-2). In contrast to *C. immitis*, the adiaconidia of *Emmonsia spp.* are much larger, have a thicker wall, and do not contain endospores. The sporangia of *R. seeberi* are distinguished by the zonation of the sporangiospores and the distinctive eosinophilic globules seen within the mature sporangiospores (see Table 68-2). No other fungus of medical importance has walls as thick as those of the adiaconidia of *Emmonsia spp.* Culture of infected tissue is not useful because the adiaconidia do not represent a replicative form of the fungus.

Treatment

Human pulmonary adiaspiromycosis is a self-limited infection. Specific antifungal therapy is not necessary.

CHLORELLOSIS

Chlorellosis is an infection of humans and animals caused by a unicellular green alga of the genus *Chlorella*. In contrast to *Prototheca*, another alga that causes human infection, *Chlorella* contains chloroplasts, which give the lesions of chlorellosis a distinct green color. Most infections with this organism occur in sheep and cattle. A single human infection has been reported thus far.

Morphology

Chlorella spp. are unicellular, ovoid, spheric, or polygonal, and 4 to 5 μm in diameter. They reproduce by endosporulation. The organisms contain numerous green chloroplasts that appear as cytoplasmic granules. The chloroplasts contain starch granules, which stain intensely with GMS, PAS, and Gridley fungal stains. The cell walls may appear doubly contoured (Figure 68-2; see Table 68-1). *Chlorella* spp. reproduce asexually by internal septation and cytoplasmic cleavage, producing up to 20 daughter cells (sporangiospores) within the sporangium (parent cell). Upon maturation, the outer wall of the sporangium ruptures, releasing the sporangiospores, each of which goes on to produce sporangiospores of its own.

Epidemiology

The single human case took place in Nebraska and resulted from exposure of a surgical wound to river

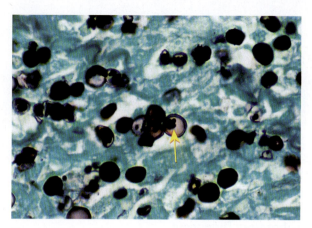

Figure 68-2   *Chlorella* sp. showing intracellular chloroplasts and doubly contoured cell wall (Gomori methenamine silver, ×400). (From Connor DH, et al: *Pathology of infectious diseases*, vol 2, Stamford, Conn, 1997, Appleton & Lange.)

water. Infections in domestic (sheep and cattle) and wild animals (beaver) range from lymph node and deep organ involvement to cutaneous and subcutaneous lesions, presumably related to exposure to water containing the organism.

Clinical Syndromes

As noted above, the human case of chlorellosis involved a healing surgical wound contaminated with river water. The wound subsequently drained a greenish yellow exudate. The infection was cured by repeated surgical debridement over a 10-month period. In animals, fresh lesions in liver, lymph nodes, and subcutaneous tissue are green on gross examination, and smears reveal organisms that contain green refractile granules (chloroplasts).

Laboratory Diagnosis

Infections caused by *Chlorella spp.* may be diagnosed by culture and by histopathologic examination of infected tissue. The organism grows well on most solid media, producing bright green colonies. Wet mounts of wound exudate or touch preparations of infected tissue reveal ovoid, endosporulating cells with characteristic green cytoplasmic granules representing chloroplasts. In tissue, the cells stain well with GMS and PAS but not H&E stains. They may be distinguished histopathologically from Prototheca by the intracellular chloroplasts.

Treatment

Treatment in the only human case of chlorellosis consisted of repeat debridement, irrigation with Dakin solution, and gauze packing and removal for drainage and granulation. Alternatively, amphotericin B therapy combined with administration of tetracycline has proven efficacious in the treatment of protothecosis and may be useful for chlorellosis as well.

LACAZIOSIS (LOBOMYCOSIS)

Lacaziosis is a chronic fungal infection of the skin caused by *Lacazia loboi* (formerly *Loboa loboi*). *L. loboi* is currently classified as an ascomycete fungus in the order Onygenales and the family Ajellomycetaceae. The disease is seen primarily in the South and Central American tropics. Natural infection occurs only in humans and dolphins, although it has been reproduced experimentally by injecting infected tissue into hamsters and armadillos. The organism has never been cultured in vitro.

Morphology

L. loboi is spheric to oval and yeastlike in appearance. The fungi are 6 to 12 μm in diameter and have a thick, double-refractile cell wall. *L. loboi* reproduces by sequential budding and usually forms chains of cells connected by narrow, tubelike bridges (Figure 68-3).

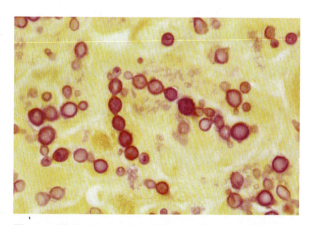

Figure 68-3   *Lacazia loboi.* The fungi form a single chain with individual cells joined by tubelike bridges (Gridley, ×400). (From Chandler FW, Watts JC: *Pathologic diagnosis of fungal infections*, Chicago, 1987, American Society for Clinical Pathology Press.)

Epidemiology

The human disease is endemic in the tropical regions of Central and South America. L. loboi is believed to be a saprophyte of soil or vegetation, and lacaziosis predominates in tropical regions with thick vegetation, such as the Amazon rain forests. Cutaneous trauma is believed to be the mode of infection. A plant reservoir has not been identified. Infection among dolphins has been reported for Florida, the Texas coast, the Spanish-French coast, the South Brazilian coast, and the Surinam River estuary. One instance of dolphin-to-human transmission has been reported; however, there is no evidence of human-to-human transmission. Farmers, miners, hunters, and rubber plant workers have an increased incidence of disease. There is no racial predilection, and lobomycosis affects all age groups, with the peak age of onset being 20 to 40 years.

Clinical Syndromes

Lacaziosis is characterized by slowly developing cutaneous nodules of varying size and shape (Figure 68-4). The dermal lesions are polymorphic, ranging from macules, papules, keloidal nodules, and plaques to verrucous and ulcerated lesions, all of which may be present in a single patient (see Figure 68-4). The nodular keloid-like lesion is the most common. The disease is characterized by a long dormancy period of months to years. The increase in the number and

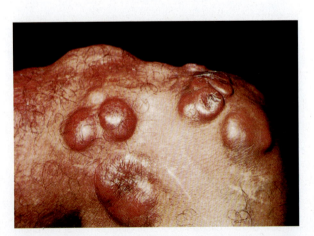

Figure 68-4   Multiple keloid-like lesions of lacaziosis. (From Chandler FW, Watts JC: *Pathologic diagnosis of fungal infections*, Chicago, 1987, American Society for Clinical Pathology Press.)

size of lesions is also a slow process, progressing over a period of 40 to 50 years. Lesions tend to arise on traumatized areas of skin, such as the face, ears, arms, legs, and feet. The disease does not involve mucous membranes or internal organs. Local cutaneous spread may occur through autoinoculation. Aside from occasional pruritus and hypesthesia or anesthesia of the affected area, patients are asymptomatic. There are no systemic manifestations of the disease.

Laboratory Diagnosis

Diagnosis is based on demonstrating the presence of the characteristic yeast cells in lesion exudate or tissue sections. Biopsy reveals a dispersed granulomatous infiltrate, along with numerous fungal forms in the dermis and subcutaneous tissue. The granuloma consists primarily of giant cells, macrophages, and epithelioid cells. Both the giant cells and macrophages contain fungi that have been phagocytosed. *L. loboi* stains intensely with both GMS and PAS stains. H&E stain reveals the thick, doubly contoured, hyaline cell wall and one or more hematoxylinophilic nuclei.

Treatment

Surgical excision of localized lesions is the optimal therapy. More widespread disease usually recurs when treated surgically and does not respond to antifungal therapy. Clofazimine has been used in these situations, but at this time medical treatment of lacaziosis is not satisfactory.

PROTOTHECOSIS

Protothecosis is an infection of humans and animals caused by achlorophyllous algae of the genus *Prototheca*. These organisms belong to the same family as the green algae of the genus *Chlorella*. Two species, *P. wickerhamii* and *P. zopfii*, are known to cause infection. Three forms of human protothecosis have been described: (1) cutaneous, (2) olecranon bursitis, and (3) disseminated.

Morphology

The protothecae are unicellular, oval or spheric organisms that reproduce asexually by internal septation and irregular cleavage within hyaline sporangia. Each sporangium contains between 2 and 20 sporangiospores arranged in a "morula" configuration (Figure 68-5). The sporangiospores are released after rupture of the sporangium and in turn develop into mature endosporulating forms. The cells measure 3 to 30 μm in diameter and differ from those of *Chlorella* by the lack of chloroplasts. *Prototheca* differ from fungi by the lack of glucosamine in their cell walls. The two species of Prototheca that cause human disease differ from one another in size: *P. wickerhamii* measures 3 to 15 μm in diameter, whereas *P. zopfii* measures 7 to 30 μm in diameter. Both species are readily stained with PAS, GMS, and the Gridley fungus stain (see Figure 68-5) and are gram-positive organisms.

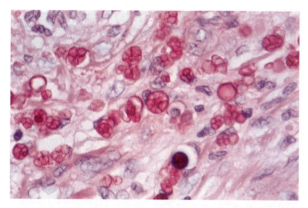

Figure 68-5 *Prototheca wickerhamii.* Single and endosporulating algal cells that are readily demonstrated with the periodic acid-Schiff stain. A classic "morula" form is present (×1000).

Epidemiology

Prototheca spp. are ubiquitous environmental saprobes that have been isolated from grass, soil, water, and both wild and domestic animals. Human protothecosis has been reported on all continents with the exception of Antarctica.

Clinical Syndromes

At least half of all cases of protothecosis are simple cutaneous infections. For the most part, these infections occur in patients who are immunocompromised because of immunosuppressive therapy, acquired immunodeficiency syndrome (AIDS), malnutri-

tion, renal or hepatic disease, cancer, or autoimmune disorders. Disseminated protothecosis is rare but has been reported in individuals with no known immunologic deficiency. One patient with visceral protothecosis presented with abdominal pain and abnormal liver function studies that were initially considered to be the result of cholangitis. The patient had multiple peritoneal nodules that resembled metastatic cancer but were in fact manifestations of protothecosis. Another patient presented with protothecal lesions on the forehead and nose.

Laboratory Diagnosis

Prototheca spp. grow easily on a wide variety of solid media at 30°C to 37°C. Colonies are yeastlike, white, and creamy in appearance and consistency. The organisms are quite metabolically active and may be identified to species using one of several commercially available yeast identification panels to determine the carbohydrate assimilation profile. On histopathologic examination of infected tissue, *Prototheca spp.* appear as sporangiospores that are wedge shaped and arranged in a radial or "morula" pattern within the sporangium (see Figure 68-5). The organisms are best visualized by stains used to demonstrate fungi in tissue: the GMS, PAS, and Gridley fungus procedures. In addition to the size differences noted above, the two species of *Prototheca* differ in that *P. wickerhamii* tends to form very symmetric morula forms, whereas these forms are rare with *P. zopfii*, which exhibits more random internal divisions. The inflammatory response in protothecosis is predominantly granulomatous.

Treatment

Treatment of olecranon bursitis usually involves bursectomy. Repeated drainage has failed; however, drainage coupled with local instillation of amphotericin B was curative in one patient. Local excision coupled with topical amphotericin B, systemic tetracycline, and systemic ketoconazole has proven useful, despite ketoconazole-related hepatotoxicity. Disseminated protothecosis has been treated with systemic antifungal agents; both amphotericin B and ketoconazole have been used.

PYTHIOSIS INSIDIOSI

Pythiosis insidiosi is a "fungal-like" infection of humans and animals caused by the plant pathogen *P. insidiosum*. It belongs to the protistal kingdom *Stramenopila* near the green algae and some lower plants in the evolutionary tree.

Morphology

P. insidiosum grows as white colonies with submerged vegetative hyphae and short aerial hyphae on solid culture medium. In nature, it produces biflagellate zoospores that attach and penetrate the leaves of various grasses and water lilies. In tissue, *P. insidiosum* exists as hyaline, pauciseptate, thin-walled hyphae or hyphal fragments that branch infrequently. The hyphal elements are 5 to 7 μm wide with nonparallel contours and superficially resemble those of Mucormycetes (Figure 68-6). Like the Mucormycetes, *P. insidiosum* is angioinvasive. In tissue the hyphal elements of *P. insidiosum* stain with GMS but not with H&E or other fungal stains.

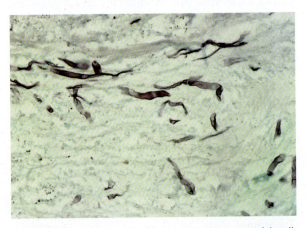

Figure 68-6 *Pythium insidiosum* invading an arterial wall. Infrequently septate, weakly stained hyphae, and hyphal fragments resemble those of Mucormycetes (Gomori methenamine silver, ×160). (From Connor DH, et al: *Pathology of infectious diseases*, vol 2, Stamford, Conn, 1997, Appleton & Lange.)

Epidemiology

P. insidiosum grows in aquatic to wet environments in tropical to subtropical regions. Reports of pythiosis have come from Australia, Costa Rica, India, Japan, New Guinea, Thailand, and the United States.

Clinical Syndromes

Human disease caused by *P. insidiosum* has occurred in patients with thalassemia who developed pythiosis insidiosi of the lower limbs. The disease process was marked by progressive ischemia of the lower limbs, necrosis, thrombosis of major arteries caused by fungal invasion, gangrene, aneurism formation, and ultimately fatal hemorrhage. Orbital pythiosis has been misdiagnosed as a mucormycotic fungal infection. Less serious forms of the infection include keratitis and localized cutaneous infections after injury.

Laboratory Diagnosis

The organism may be isolated from fresh clinical material seeded onto mycologic medium such as Sabouraud glucose agar. Demonstration of biflagellate zoospores may be accomplished using water cultures with grass or lily bait incubated at 37℃ for 1 hour. Serologic assays using either the enzyme-linked immunosorbent assay or Western blot technologies have been useful in the early detection of the disease in humans and animals.

Histopathologic examination of infected tissue shows a necrotizing arteritis and thrombosis. Vascular invasion by sparsely septate, irregularly branched hyphae is seen (see Figure 68-6). The acute perivascular inflammatory reaction is eventually replaced by granulomas that contain sparse hyphae and hyphal fragments. The hyphal elements of *P. insidiosum* may be surrounded by the eosinophilic Splendore-Hoeppli phenomenon. Pythiosis insidiosi in humans must be differentiated from cutaneous and subcutaneous mucormycosis, sporotrichosis, mycetoma, and neoplasms.

Treatment

Although potassium iodide has been used to treat cutaneous infections, medical treatment of pythiosis insidiosi is generally not effective. Surgical debridement and excision of infected tissue has been used with some success. There is some evidence that azole antifungal agents, such as fluconazole, ketoconazole, itraconazole, and miconazole, exhibit in vitro activity against this organism. A case of orbital pythiosis responded well to a combination of itraconazole and terbinafine, although this combination has not been useful in other cases of pythiosis. Immunotherapy has been useful in the treatment of equine pythiosis and has a 55% cure rate in human disease.

RHINOSPORIDIOSIS

Rhinosporidiosis is a granulomatous disease of humans and animals that is characterized by the development of polyps that primarily affect the nasopharynx and the ocular conjunctiva of infected individuals, which is caused by *R. seeberi*.

Morphology

Given that *R. seeberi* will not grow on artificial media, the morphologic descriptions are entirely based on the organism as it appears in infected tissue. Two developmental forms of R. seeberi are seen in tissue: the large spheric form, or sporangia, and the smaller trophocyte. The sporangium is considered the mature form of the organism and measures 100 to 350 µm in diameter. The sporangial wall is 3 to 5 µm thick and is composed of an inner hyaline layer and thin outer eosinophilic layer. The sporangium contains numerous endoconidia arranged in a characteristic zonal formation, whereby the small, flattened, uninucleate immature endoconidia (1 to 2 µm) form a crescentic

mass at the periphery of one wall of the sporangium, with the larger maturing and mature endoconidia arranged sequentially toward the center (Figure 68-7).

The trophocytes are considered to develop directly from endoconidia that have been released from the sporangium. The trophocytes range in size from 10 to 100 µm in diameter and have refractile eosinophilic walls (2 to 3 µm thick), granular cytoplasm, and a round, pale nucleus with a prominent nucleolus. Ultimately, the trophocytes enlarge and transform into mature sporangia through a process of endosporulation.

The walls of both the sporangia and endoconidia stain with both GMS and PAS fungal stains. In addition, the walls of the endoconidia and the inner wall of the sporangium stain positively with the mucin stain, mucicarmine (Figure 68-8; see Table 68-2).

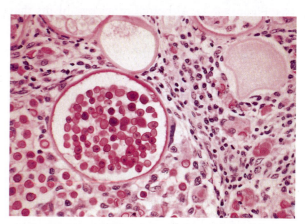

Figure 68-8   Mature sporangium of *R. seeberi*. The walls of the mature endoconidia are carminophilic (Mayer mucicarmine, ×100). (From Connor DH, et al: *Pathology of infectious diseases*, vol 2, Stamford, Conn, 1997, Appleton & Lange.)

Epidemiology

Approximately 90% of all known cases of rhinosporidiosis occur in India and Sri Lanka. The disease also occurs in the Americas, Europe, and Africa. The natural habitat and the extent of distribution of *R. seeberi* in nature are unknown. The disease occurs primarily in young men 20 to 40 years old and appears to be associated with both rural and aquatic environments. There is no evidence that rhinosporidiosis is contagious.

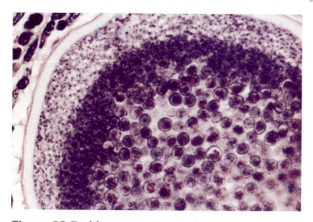

Figure 68-7   Mature sporangium of *Rhinosporidium seeberi* showing the zonal arrangement of immature, maturing, and fully mature endoconidia (hematoxylin and eosin, ×480). (From Chandler FW, Watts JC: *Pathologic diagnosis of fungal infections*, Chicago, 1987, American Society for Clinical Pathology Press.)

Clinical Syndrome

Rhinosporidiosis manifests as slow-growing polypoid or tumor-like masses, usually of the nasal mucosa or conjunctiva. Lesions may also be seen in the paranasal sinuses, larynx, and external genitalia. Secondary spread to surrounding skin is thought to result from autoinoculation by scratching. In most patients, the disease remains localized, and symptoms are primarily nasal obstruction and bleeding resulting from polyp formation. Limited systemic dissemination has been reported, but is rare.

Laboratory Diagnosis

The diagnosis of rhinosporidiosis is made by histopathologic examination of the affected tissue. The distinctive appearance of the trophocytes and sporangia in routine H&E-stained sections is diagnostic (see Figure 68-7). Although other organisms that occur in tissue in the form of large spherules may be mistaken for *R. seeberi*, they are usually easily differentiated from this organism by consideration of the tissue involved and the morphologic and staining characteristics of the spherule and the endoconidia (see Table 68-2).

Treatment

The only effective form of treatment is surgical excision of the lesions. Recurrences are common, especially in mucosal sites such as the oropharynx and paranasal sinuses, where complete excision is often difficult to achieve.

SUMMARY

Chlorellosis

Infection of humans and animals is caused by a unicellular green alga of genus Chlorella. Chlorella: unicellular, ovoid, spherical or polygonal, reproduce by endosporulation. Fresh lesions in liver, lymph nodes, cutaneous tissue are green on gross examination. Smears reveal organisms that contain green refractile granules (chloroplasts). A single human infection has been reported thus far; most infections occur in sheep and cattle.

Lacaziosis

Lacaziosis is a chronic fungal skin infection caused by *Lacazia loboi*. *L. loboi*: ascomycete fungus reproduces by sequential budding, forms chains of spherical to oval cells connected by narrow tube-like bridges. Nodular keloid-like lesions are most common that occur on the face, ears, arms, legs, feet. Leisions increase in size and number over a period of 40 to 50 years. Most patients are asymptomatic; no systemic manifestations of disease.

Rhinosporidiosis

Granulomatous disease of humans and animals are caused by *Rhinosporidium seeberi*. It can be characterized by development of nasopharyngeal and ocular conjunctival polyps. Two developmental forms are seen in tissue: a large spherical form (sporangia) and a smaller trophic form.

KEYWORDS

English	Chinese
Adiaspiromycosis	大孢子菌病
Chlorella	小球藻属
Lobomycosis	瘢痕芽生菌病
Protothecosis	原壁菌病
Pythium	腐霉属
Rhinosporidiosis	鼻孢子菌病

BIBLIOGRAPHY

1. Burns RA, et al: Report of the first human case of lobomycosis in the United States, J Clin Microbiol 38: 1283-1285, 2000.
2. Chandler FW, Watts JC: Pathologic diagnosis of fungal infections, Chicago, 1987, American Society for Clinical Pathology Press.
3. Connor DH, et al: Pathology of infectious diseases, vol 2, Stamford, Conn, 1997, Appleton & Lange.
4. Fredericks DN, et al: Rhinosporidium seeberi: a human pathogen from a novel group of aquatic protistan parasites, Emerg Infect Dis 6: 273-282, 2000.
5. Herr RA, et al: Phylogenetic analysis of Rhinosporidium seeberi's 18S small-subunit ribosomal DNA groups this pathogen among members of the protoctistan Mesomycetozoa clade, J Clin Microbiol 37: 2750-2754, 1999.

6. Krajaejun T, et al: Clinical and epidemiological analysis of human pythiosis in Thailand, Clin Infect Dis 43: 568, 2006.

7. Lass-Florl C, Mayr A: Human protothecosis, Clin Microbiol Rev 20: 230-242, 2007.

8. Mendoza L, et al: Orbital pythiosis: a nonfungal disease mimicking orbital mycotic infections, with a retrospective review of the literature, Mycoses 47: 14, 2004.

9. Mendoza L, Vilela R: Lacazia, Pythium, and Rhinosporidium. In Versalovic J, et al, editors: Manual of clinical microbiology, ed 10, Washington, DC, 2011, American Society for Microbiology Press.

10. Taborda PR, et al: Lacazia loboi gen. nov., comb. nov., the etiologic agent of lobomycosis, J Clin Microbiol 37: 2031-2033, 1999.

Mycotoxins and Mycotoxicoses

Chapter 69

In addition to their role as opportunistic pathogens, filamentous fungi can produce toxins that have been implicated in a variety of illnesses and clinical syndromes in humans and in animals. These mycotoxins are secondary fungal metabolites that cause diseases, known collectively as mycotoxicoses, after ingestion, inhalation, or direct contact with the toxin (Figure 69-1). In the remainder of this chapter, we will discuss those mycotoxins that have been implicated in human disease, as well as metabolites that are produced by molds that may be associated with human foods or living/working environments. Although mushroom poisoning is a form of mycotoxicosis, it will not be discussed herein. A listing of

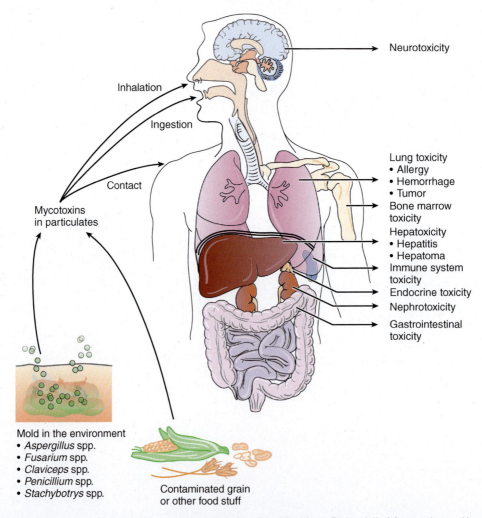

Figure 69-1 Various exposures and influences of mycotoxins. (Modified from Richard JL: Mycotoxins and human disease. In Anaissie EJ, McGinnis MR, Pfaller MA, editors: *Clinical mycology*, ed 2, New York, 2003, Churchill Livingstone.)

mycotoxicoses where there is considerable evidence for the involvement of a specific mycotoxin is provided in Table 69-1.

AFLATOXINS

The aflatoxins are produced primarily by *Aspergillus flavus* and *Aspergillus parasiticus*, but many other species of *Aspergillus* produce aflatoxins as well. *A. flavus* is the most common aflatoxin-producing

species found in agriculture and may produce as much as 106 mg/kg. Aflatoxin B1 is the most potent natural carcinogen known and is the major aflatoxin produced by toxigenic strains; however, there are more than a dozen other aflatoxins that have been described. Aflatoxin is associated with both toxicity and carcinogenicity in human and animal populations. Acute aflatoxicosis results in death, whereas chronic aflatoxicosis results in more prolonged pathologic changes, including cancer and immunosup-

Table 69-1 Mycotoxin-Related Illnesses Postulated to Affect Humans, Based on Analytic or Epidemiologic Data.

Disease	Toxin	Substrate	Fungus	Clinical Presentation
Akakabi-byo (red mold disease)	*Fusarium* metabolites	Wheat, barley, oats, rice	*Fusarium* spp.	Headaches, vomiting, diarrhea
Alimentary toxic aleukia (ATA)	Trichothecenes (T-2 toxin, diacetoxyscirpenol [DAS])	Cereal grains (toxic bread)	*Fusarium* spp.	Vomiting, diarrhea, angina, skin inflammation
Balkan endemic nephropathy (BEN)	Ochratoxin	Cereal grains	*Aspergillus* spp. *Penicillium* spp.	Chronic nephritis
Cardiac beriberi	Citreoviridin	Rice	*Penicillium* spp.	Palpitations, vomiting, mania, respiratory failure
Ergotism (gangrenous and convulsive)	Ergot alkaloids	Rye, cereal grains	*Claviceps purpurea* *Claviceps fusiformis*	Gangrenous: vasoconstriction, edema, pruritus, necrosis of extremities Convulsive: numbness, tingling, pruritus, cramps, seizures, hallucinations
Esophageal cancer	Fumonisins	Corn	*Fusarium moniliforme*	Dysphagia, pain, hemorrhage
Hepatitis and hepatic cancer	Aflatoxins	Cereal grains, peanuts	*Aspergillus flavus* *Aspergillus parasiticus*	Acute and chronic hepatitis, liver failure
Kodua poisoning	Cyclopiazonic acid	Millet	*Penicillium* spp. *Aspergillus* spp.	Somnolence, tremors, giddiness
Moldy sugarcane poisoning	3-Nitropropionic acid	Sugarcane	*Arthrinium* spp.	Dystonia, seizures, carpopedal spasms, coma
Onyalai disease	*Fusarium* metabolites	Millet	*Fusarium* spp.	Thrombocytopenia, purpura
Stachybotryotoxicosis	Trichothecenes (T-2 toxin, DAS)	Hay, cereal grains, fodder (skin contact, inhaled hay dust)	*Stachybotrys, Fusarium, Myrothecium, Trichoderma, Cephalosporium* spp.	Tremors, loss of vision, dermonecrosis, gastrointestinal bleeding (horses and cattle), nasal inflammation, dermatitis, headache, fatigue, respiratory symptoms (humans), idiopathic pulmonary hemorrhage of infants (?)
Yellow rice disease	Citrinin	Wheat, oats, barley, rice	*Penicillium* spp. *Aspergillus* spp.	Nephropathy

Data from Kuhn DM, Ghannoum MA: Indoor mold, toxigenic fungi, and *Stachybotrys chartarum*: infectious disease perspective, *Clin Microbiol Rev* 16: 144-172, 2003; Smith M, McGinnis MR: Mycotoxins and their effect on humans. In Anaissie EJ, McGinnis MR, Pfaller MA, editors: *Clinical mycology*, ed 2, New York, 2009, Churchill Livingstone; and Bennett JW, Klich M: Mycotoxins, *Clin Microbiol Rev* 16: 497-516, 2003.

pression. The liver is the primary target organ, and liver damage has been documented in rodents, poultry, and nonhuman primates following ingestion of aflatoxin B1.

The primary mode of human exposure to aflatoxins is the consumption of contaminated foods, such as peanuts and cereal grains. Aflatoxins can be aerosolized and have been detected in air near farm sources, as well as in dust. Aflatoxin is a pulmonary carcinogen in experimental animals; however, the evidence that airborne aflatoxin exposure leads to cancer in humans is generally weak.

The mechanism of aflatoxin-induced carcinogenesis is thought to involve tumor promotion or progression. There is evidence that aflatoxin is involved in the activation of protooncogenes (c-MYC, c-Ha-RAS, Ki-RAS, and N-RAS) and also may cause mutations in the tumor suppressor gene TP53. Aflatoxin exposure and TP53 mutations have been tightly linked in epidemiologic studies in Africa and China. Specifically, aflatoxin has been linked to a TP53 mutation, whereby a G-to-T transversion at codon 249 occurs. This particular mutation has been called the first example of a "carcinogen-specific" biomarker that remains fixed in the human tissue. This biomarker has been used in epidemiologic studies to establish the link between aflatoxins and hepatic cancer and also to show that cofactors, such as infection with hepatitis B virus, increase the risk of hepatocellular cancer substantially.

CITRININ

Citrinin is produced by several species of *Penicillium* and *Aspergillus*, including strains used to produce cheese (*P. camemberti*) and sake (*A. oryzae*). Citrinin acts as a potent nephrotoxin in all animal species tested and has been associated with yellow rice disease in Japan (see Table 69-1). Citrinin may act synergistically with another nephrotoxin, ochratoxin A. *Citrinin* is regularly associated with human foods, including wheat, oats, rye, corn, barley, and rice; however, its significance as a cause of human disease is unknown.

ERGOT ALKALOIDS

The ergot alkaloids constitute a family of compounds that are derived from a tetracyclic ergoline ring system. Mixtures of these alkaloids are produced within the sclerotia, or ergots, of common grass pathogens of the genus Claviceps. The ergots are ingested when the contaminated grain is used to make bread or in cereals. The two forms of ergotism, convulsive and gangrenous (see Table 69-1), are thought to result from different modes of action of the various alkaloids produced by different species of Claviceps.

The gangrenous form, marked by peripheral vasoconstriction and necrosis of the distal extremities, is associated primarily with the ingestion of wheat and rye contaminated with *Claviceps purpurea* and containing alkaloids of the ergotamine group. In addition to tissue infarction and necrosis, the gangrenous form of ergotism is associated with edema, pruritus, and sensations varying from pricking to severe muscle pain.

Apparently, different species of *Claviceps* produce different alkaloids, although it is likely that the substrate also plays a role in the composition of the secondary metabolites. Although modern methods of grain cleaning have virtually eliminated ergotism as a human disease, it is still an important veterinary problem. Cattle, pigs, sheep, and poultry are the animals at highest risk. Clinical symptoms of ergotism among these animals include gangrene, abortion, seizures, and ataxia.

FUMONISINS

Fumonisins are produced by a number of *Fusarium* species. The major species of economic importance is *F. moniliforme* (*F. verticilloides*), a corn pathogen. Fumonisins, especially fumonisin B1, interfere with sphingolipid metabolism and cause leukoencephalomalacia (severe necrotizing brain disease) in horses, pulmonary edema and hydrothorax in pigs, and hepatotoxic and carcinogenic effects in the liver of rats. Fumonisin B1 has been associated with a higher incidence of esophageal cancer in people living in South

Africa, China, and Italy. It may be isolated in high concentrations in cornmeal and corn grits. Although this evidence is intriguing, multiple factors, including other mycotoxins, have been implicated in the etiology of human esophageal cancer.

Acute intoxication with fumonisin B1 has been observed in India, where consumption of unleavened bread made from moldy corn caused transient abdominal pain and diarrhea. Fumonisins have also been shown to cause neural tube defects in experimental animals and may have a role in human cases. Fumonisins have been classified as group 2B carcinogens (probably carcinogenic) by the International Agency for Research on Cancer.

OCHRATOXIN

Ochratoxin belongs to a group of secondary metabolites produced by *Aspergillus* and *Penicillium* species found on cereals, coffee, bread, and foods of animal origin (e.g., pork). OchratoxinA (OA) is the most common and most toxic chemical in its class. OA is nephrotoxic, teratogenic, and carcinogenic in all animals tested. It has been implicated in porcine nephropathy, as well as urinary tract tumors, and may cause cholinergic responses, such as bronchospasm, vasodilation, and smooth muscle contraction.

Ochratoxin has been linked to a disease known as Balkan endemic nephropathy (BEN), which is a chronic, progressive nephritis seen in populations living in areas bordering the Danube River in parts of Romania, Bulgaria, and the former Yugoslavia. In addition, individuals with BEN also suffer from a high frequency of renal tumors. Ochratoxin contamination of food and the presence of OA in human serum have been shown to be more common in families with BEN and those with urinary tract tumors than in unaffected families. Despite this evidence, a number of other factors, such as genetics, heavy metals, and possible occult infectious agents, may also contribute to this disease. Although much of the evidence for the cause of BEN leans toward ochratoxin, the evidence is not conclusive. Regardless, its acute nephrotoxicity, immunosuppressive action, and

teratogenic effects in animals, coupled with its propensity to be carried through the food chain, merit concern and further investigation.

TRICHOTHECENES

The trichothecenes are all tricyclic sesquiterpinoid metabolites that are produced by a number of fungi, including *Fusarium*, *Myrothecium*, *Stachybotrys*, *Trichoderma*, and *Cephalosporium spp.* (see Table 69-1). There are more than 148 natural trichothecenes, of which at least 40 are mycotoxins. Trichothecenes act by inhibiting various aspects of protein synthesis in eukaryotic cells. The most potent of these mycotoxins are T-2 toxin, diacetoxyscirpenol (DAS), deoxynivalenol (vomitoxin), and fusarenon-X. These mycotoxins are commonly found as food and feed contaminants, the consumption of which can result in gastrointestinal hemorrhage and vomiting; direct contact causes dermatitis.

T-2 toxin and DAS appear to be the most potent and exhibit both cytotoxic and immunosuppressive activity. They cause a wide range of gastrointestinal, dermatologic, and neurologic symptoms and also decrease host resistance to infection with various microbes. Both T-2 toxin and DAS have been implicated in a human disease known as alimentary toxic aleukia (ATA).

OTHER MYCOTOXINS AND PURPORTED MYCOTOXICOSES

Cyclopiazonic acid is an indole tetramic acid that is a specific inhibitor of calcium-dependent ATPase and induces alterations in ion transport across cell membranes. It is produced by many species of *Penicillium* and *Aspergillus*, including A. flavus. Consumption of millet that was heavily contaminated with molds and contained high levels of cyclopiazonic acid produced a condition known as Kodua poisoning, characterized by giddiness and nausea (see Table 69-1).

Cardiac beriberi, a condition seen in Japan and other Asian countries in the early 20th century, has been associated with the yellow rice toxins, citreoviridin, citrinin, and related compounds. This disease is characterized by palpitations, nausea, vomiting, respiratory distress, hypotension, and violent mania, leading to respiratory failure and death. The neurologic symptoms and respiratory failure have been reproduced in animals given citreoviridin.

Several rare and obscure diseases have been purported to be mycotoxicosis, often with minimal objective evidence. These include Kashin-Beck disease in Russia, Onyalai disease in Africa, and moldy sugar cane disease in China (see Table 69-1).

It is difficult to prove that a disease is a mycotoxicosis. Even known toxigenic molds may be present in foods or the environment and not produce toxin. The mere isolation of mold from cultures of a given substrate is not the same as detection of a specific mycotoxin. Likewise, even when mycotoxins are detected, it is difficult to prove conclusively that they are the cause of specific acute or chronic disease states. Regardless, valid concerns do exist with respect to the relationship between mycotoxins and human disease. Examples of certain fungus-disease associations are reasonably well documented in the literature, including ATA from *Fusarium*, liver disease from *Aspergillus*, and ergotism from *Claviceps* spp. Other than these examples, the evidence is tenuous. It is likely that mycotoxins do pose an important danger to the health of humans and animals, the extent of which can only be determined by rigorous, well-designed clinical and laboratory studies.

SUMMARY

Mycotoxin and Mycotoxicoses

Mycotoxins are secondary fungal metabolites that cause diseases, known collectively as mycotoxicoses, after ingestion, inhalation or direct contact with the toxin. Among the most important mycotoxins and their primary toxic effects are: aflatoxins (carcinogens), citrinin (nephrotoxin), ergot alkaloids (convulsive and gangrenous), fumonsins (carcinogens), ochratoxin (nephrotoxin), trichothecenes (bone marrow toxicity), stachybotryotoxins (neurotoxin). Mycotoxins are produced by filamentous fungi (molds), many of which may also serve as opportunistic pathogens that cause invasive disease in immunocompromised individuals. Mycotoxicoses may manifest as acute or chronic disease, ranging from rapid death to tumor formation. There are more than 100 toxigenic fungi and more than 300 compounds recognized as mycotoxins.

KEYWORDS

English	Chinese
Aflatoxins	黄曲毒素类
Citrinin	橘霉素
Ergot Alkaloids	麦角生物碱类
Fumonisins	烟曲霉毒素
Mycotoxins	真菌毒素
Ochratoxin	赭曲霉素
Trichothecenes	单端孢霉烯族毒素类

BIBLIOGRAPHY

1. Bennett JW, Klich M: Mycotoxins, Clin Microbial Rev 16: 497-516, 2003.

2. Isham NC, et al: Mycotoxins. In Versalovic J, et al, editors: Manual of clinical microbiology, ed 10, Washington, DC, 2011, American Society for Microbiology Press.

3. Kuhn DM, Ghannoum MA: Indoor mold, toxigenic fungi, and Stachybotryschartarum: infectious disease perspective, ClinMicrobiol Rev 16: 144-172, 2003.

4. Smith M, McGinnis MR: Mycotoxins and their effect on humans. In Anaissie EJ, McGinnis MR, Pfaller MA, editors: Clinical mycology, ed 2, New York, 2009, Churchill Livingstone.

Local and system infections

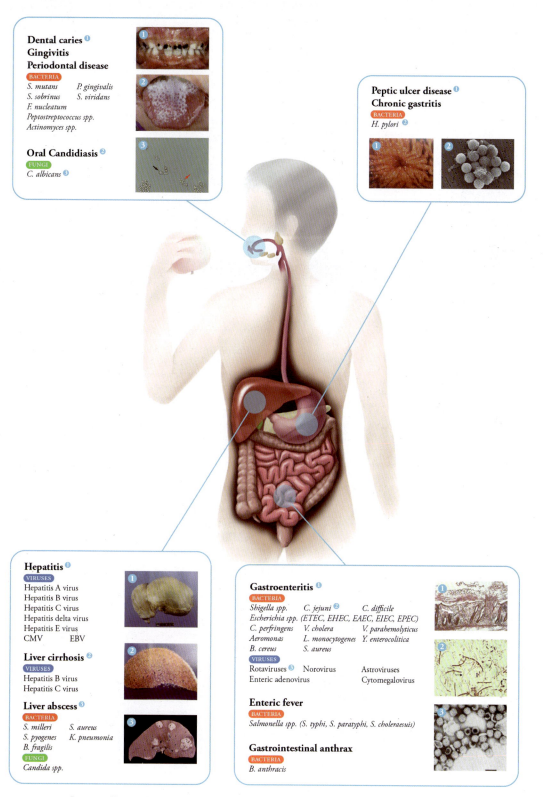

Dental caries ❶
Gingivitis
Periodontal disease
`BACTERIA`
S. mutans   *P. gingivalis*
S. sobrinus   *S. viridans*
F. nucleatum
Peptostreptococcus spp.
Actinomyces spp.

Oral Candidiasis ❷
`FUNGI`
C. albicans ❸

Peptic ulcer disease ❶
Chronic gastritis
`BACTERIA`
H. pylori ❷

Hepatitis ❶
`VIRUSES`
Hepatitis A virus
Hepatitis B virus
Hepatitis C virus
Hepatitis delta virus
Hepatitis E virus
CMV   EBV

Liver cirrhosis ❷
`VIRUSES`
Hepatitis B virus
Hepatitis C virus

Liver abscess ❸
`BACTERIA`
S. milleri   *S. aureus*
S. pyogenes   *K. pneumonia*
B. fragilis
`FUNGI`
Candida spp.

Gastroenteritis ❶
`BACTERIA`
Shigella spp.   *C. jejuni* ❷   *C. difficile*
Escherichia spp. (ETEC, EHEC, EAEC, EIEC, EPEC)
C. perfringens   *V. cholera*   *V. parahemolyticus*
Aeromonas   *L. monocytogenes* *Y. enterocolitica*
B. cereus   *S. aureus*
`VIRUSES`
Rotaviruses ❸   Norovirus   Astroviruses
Enteric adenovirus   Cytomegalovirus

Enteric fever
`BACTERIA`
Salmonella spp. (S. typhi, S. paratyphi, S. choleraesuis)

Gastrointestinal anthrax
`BACTERIA`
B. anthracis

Appendix-1   Microbial Infections of the Digestive System (Le Sun, Xiao-kui Guo)

Common cold
VIRUSES
Rhinoviruses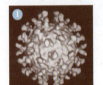
Coronaviruses
Influenza viruses
Respiratory syncytial virus
Parainfluenza viruses
Adenoviruses
Enteroviruses

Sinusitis
BACTERIA
S. pneumoniae
H. influenza
M. catarrhalis
S. aureus
Anaerobes
Streptococcus spp.
VIRUSES
Rhinovirus
Influenza viruses
Parainfluenza viruses

Bronchitis
BACTERIA
K. pneumoniae
H. influenzae
C. pneumoniae
M. pneumoniae
Streptococcus spp.
VIRUSES
Influenza viruses
RSV

Bronchitis
VIRUSES
RSV
Adenovirus
Rhinovirus
Influenza viruses
Parainfluenza viruses
Measles virus
Mumps virus
VZV
CMV
BACTERIA
B. pertussis
M. pneumoniae
Nocardia

Pertussis
BACTERIA
B. pertussis

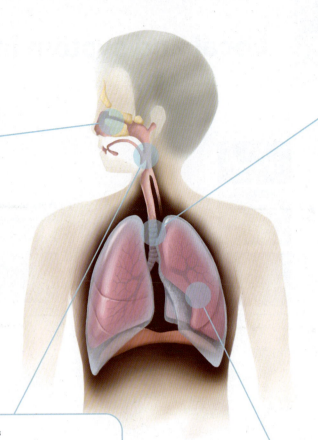

Pharyngitis and tonsillitis
BACTERIA

Group A,C,G streptococcus	*N.gonorrheae*	
A. haemolyticum	*C. diphtheriae*	

VIRUSES

Rhinovirus	Adenovirus	Influenza A and B viruses
Parainfluenza virus	Coxsackievirus	Coronavirus
Echovirus	HSV RSV	EBV CMV
Metapneumovirus		

Epiglottitis
BACTERIA

H. influenzae	*H. parainfluenzae*	*S. pneumoniae* *S. aureus*
Group A,B,C,F,G streptococcus	*P. multocida*	*M. catarrhalis*
K. pneumoniae *Neisseria spp.*	*E·coli*	*P. aeruginosa*

VIRUSES

HSV-1	VZV	Parainfluenza virus type 3
Influenza B viruses		EBV

FUNGI
Candida spp.

Herpangina
Hand-foot-and-mouth disease
VIRUSES
Coxsackievirus A6   Enterovirus A71

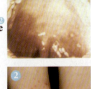

Pharyngo-conjunctival fever
VIRUSES
Adenovirus

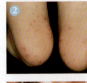

Diphtheria
BACTERIA
C. diphtheriae

Flu
VIRUSES
Influenza virus

Scarlet fever
BACTERIA
S. pyogenes

Mumps
VIRUSES
Mumps virus

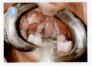

Pneumonia
BACTERIA

S. pneumonia	*M. pneumonia*	*K. pneumonia*	*H. influenzae*
L. pneumophila	*S. aureus*	*P. aeruginosa*	*A. baumanii*
E. cloacae	*E. aerogenes*	*C. pneumoniae*	*Acinetobacter spp.*

VIRUSES

Influenza virus	Parainfluenza virus
Adenovirus	Hantavirus Cytomegalovirus
Respiratory syncytial virus	Human Metapneumovirus (hMPV)

FUNGI

C. neoformans	*C. immitis*	*B. dermatitidis*
H. capsulatum	*P. pneumonia*	*P. jirovecii*

Coronavirus respiratory syndromes
VIRUSES
Coronaviruses

Tuberculosis
BACTERIA
M. tuberculosis

Inhalation anthrax
BACTERIA
B. anthracis

Other lung infections
BACTERIA
L. interrogans   *C. burnetii*

Pulmonary abscess
BACTERIA

S. aureus	*E·coli*
K. pneumonia	*P. aeruginosa*
S. pneumonia	*Prevotella spp.*
Peptostreptococcus	*F. nucleatum*
F. necrophorum	*B. fragilis*
N. asteroids	

Non-tuberculous mycobacterial infections
BACTERIA
non-tuberculous mycobacterium
(*M. avium, M. kansasii, M. sinense*)

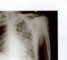
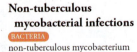

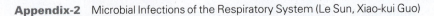

Appendix-2   Microbial Infections of the Respiratory System (Le Sun, Xiao-kui Guo)

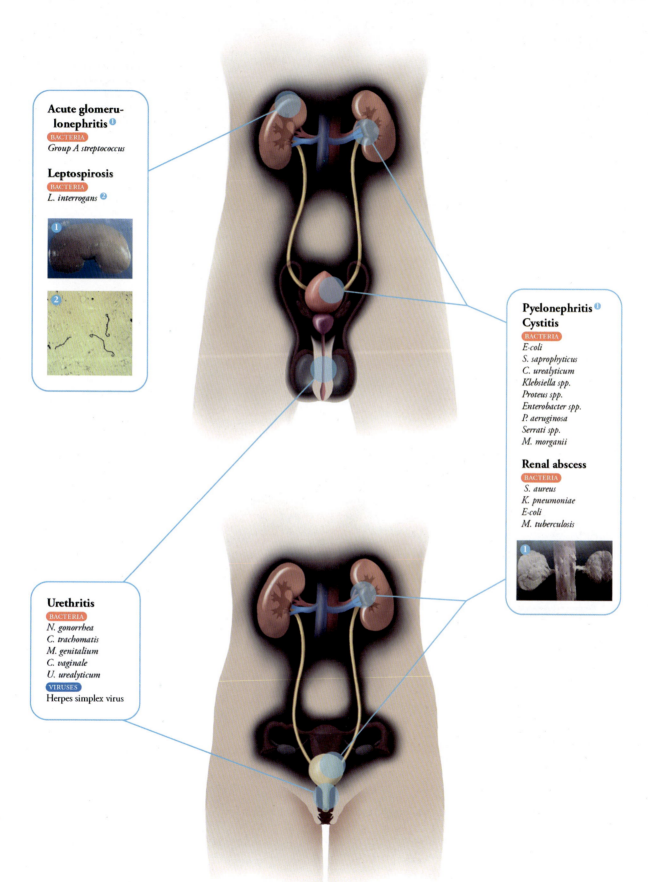

Acute glomeru-lonephritis ❶
BACTERIA
Group A streptococcus

Leptospirosis
BACTERIA
L. interrogans ❷

Pyelonephritis ❶
Cystitis
BACTERIA
E·coli
S. saprophyticus
C. urealyticum
Klebsiella spp.
Proteus spp.
Enterobacter spp.
P. aeruginosa
Serrati spp.
M. morganii

Renal abscess
BACTERIA
S. aureus
K. pneumoniae
E·coli
M. tuberculosis

Urethritis
BACTERIA
N. gonorrhea
C. trachomatis
M. genitalium
C. vaginale
U. urealyticum
VIRUSES
Herpes simplex virus

Appendix-3   Microbial Infections of the Urinary System (Le Sun, Xiao-kui Guo)

Prostatitis
BACTERIA
E.coli
Proteus spp.
C. trachomatis
Enterobacteriaceae
  (Klebsiella,
  Enterobacter,
  Serratia species)
P. aeruginosa
Enterococci
S. aureus
N. gonorrhea

Epididymitis
BACTERIA
M. hominis
C. trachomatis
E.coli

Pelvic inflammatory disease (endometritis, salpingitis)
BACTERIA
N. gonorrhea
C. trachomatis
M. genitalium
M. hominis
Groups A and B streptococci
E.coli
Klebsiella spp.
P. mirabilis
Prevotella spp.
Peptococcus
Bacteroides spp.
Peptosptreptococcus spp.

Cervicitis
BACTERIA
N. gonorrhea
C. trachomatis
M. genitalium
Group B streptococcus
M. tuberculosis
Actinomyces spp.
VIRUSES
HSV-2

Cervical neoplasm
VIRUSES
HSV 16, 18, 33, 45

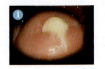

STDs
BACTERIA
N. gonorrhea   *T. pallidum*
C. trachomatis   *M. hominis*
M. genitalium   *U. urealyticum*
H. ducreyi
VIRUSES
HSV-2   HPV 6,11,42
HIV   HTLV-1
HBV(?)   HCV(?)
HDV(?)

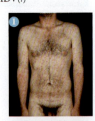

Bacterial vaginitis
BACTERIA
G. vaginalis
Prevotella spp.
Bacteroides spp.
Peptostreptococcus spp.
M. hominis
U. urealyticum
Mobiluncus spp.
Fusobacterium spp.
A. vaginae

Vaginal candidiasis
BACTERIA
C. albicans

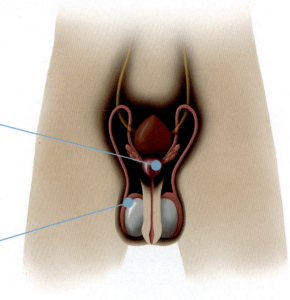

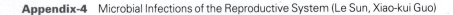

Appendix-4 Microbial Infections of the Reproductive System (Le Sun, Xiao-kui Guo)

Conjunctivitis ❶

BACTERIA ❷

C. trachomatis ❷	S. aureus	S. pneumoniae
H. influenzae	M. catarrhalis	N. gonorrhea ❸
H. aegyptius	P. aeruginosa	F. tularensis

VIRUSES
Adenovirus

Keratitis

BACTERIA

S. aureus	P. aeruginosa	
Coagulase-negative staphylococcus		Diphtheroids
S. pneumoniae	Group A streptococcus	
N. gonorrhea	P. mirabilis	Bacillus spp.

VIRUSES
HSV   Adenovirus

Endophthalmitis

BACTERIA

Coagulase-negative Staphylococci	
S. aureus	Streptococcus spp.
B. cereus	P. aeruginosa
Corynebacterium spp.	
Propionibacterium spp.	

FUNGI
Candida spp.   Aspergillus spp.

Chorioretinitis

BACTERIA

T. pallidum   B. henselae

VIRUSES
Herpes virus
Cytomegalovirus West Nile virus

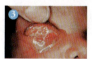
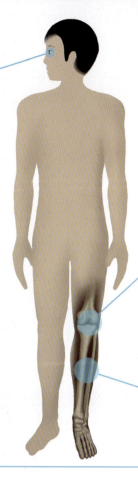

Osteomyelitis

BACTERIA

S. aureus
Coagulase-negative staphylococci
Aerobic gram-negative bacilli
Streptococcus spp.

P. aeruginosa	Salmonella spp.
H. influenza	Enterococcus spp.
Anaerobes	Mycobacteria
E.coli	

Arthritis

BACTERIA

S. aureus	Streptococcus spp.
N. gonorrhea	Salmonella spp.
Aerobic gram-negative bacteria	
Anaerobic gram-negative bacteria	
B. melitensis	Mycobacterium spp.
B. burgdorferi	M. hominis
P. multocida	

FUNGI

| Sporotrichosis | Cryptococcus |
| Blastomycosis | Coccidioidomycosis |

Infectious diseases of the skin

BACTERIA

Folliculitis

S. aureus	P. aeruginosa
Klebsiella	Enterobacter
Proteus spp.	A. hydrophila

Skin abscesses
Furuncle
Carbuncle

| S. aureus | S. pyogenes |
| Pseudomonas | |

Cellulitis
Erysipelas ❶

Groups A, B, C, G, F Streptococci	
S. aureus ❷	H. influenzae
Clostridium spp.	Pneumococcus
Meningococcus	Propionibacterium
Bartonella	Pseudomonas

Impetigo ❸

S. aureus   Group A streptococcus

Necrotizing fasciitis
Myositis

Bacteroides	Clostridium
Peptostreptococcus	S. aureus
E.coli	Enterobacter
Klebsiella	Proteus
Fusobacteria	Anaerobic streptococci
Spirochetes	

Acne vulgaris
P. acnes

Rosacea

| B. oleronius | Malassezia |
| S. epidermidis | C. pneumoniae |

Syphilis
T. pallidum

Endemic typhus
R. prowazekii   R. typhi

Spotted fever rickettsiosis
R. rickettsii

Cat scratch disease
B. henselae

Catinomycosis
Actinomyces spp.

Mycetoma
N. brasiliensis

Gas gangrene
C. perfringens

Leprosy
M. leprae

Cutaneous anthrax
B. anthracis

Wound infection

| P. multocida | Aeromonas | C. tetani |
| C. botulinum | P. aeruginosa | |

FUNGI

Dermatohyte(tinea) infections
- **Tinea captis**
Trichophyton spp.
Microsporum spp.
- **Tinea corporis**
Trichophyton spp.
- **Tinea pedis**
Trichophyton spp.

Onychomycosis
T. rubrum
C. albicans
Nondermatophyte molds

Pityriasis versicolor
Malassezia spp.

Candidiasis
Candida spp.

Chromoblastomycosis
F. pedrosoi
F. compacta
P. verrucosa
C. carrionii;

Sporotrichosis
S. schenckii

Malassezia folliculitis ❹
Malassezia spp.

VIRUSES

Herpes simplex ❺
HSV-1
HSV-2

Viral rashes
- **Chickenpox and shingles** ❻
VZV
- **Rubella**
Rubella virus
- **Measles**
Measles virus
- **Erythema infectiosum**
Human Parvovirus B19
- **Roseola**
HHV-6

Warts and condyloma acuminatum
HPV

Molluscum contagiosum
MCV-1
MCV-2

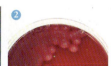

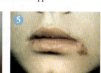
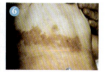

Appendix-5   Microbial Infections of the Eyes, Skin, Bones and Joints (Le Sun, Xiao-kui Guo)

Septicemia
Bacteremia
Toxemia ❶

BACTERIA

E.coli
S. aureus
Coagulase-negative Staphylococcus
P. aeruginosa
N. meningitides
S. pneumonia
S. pyogenes
Salmonella spp.
Bacteroides spp.
Enterococcus spp.
Klebsiella spp.
B. fragilis
Peptostreptococcus spp.
Citrobacter
Aeromonas
S. agalactiae
B. anthracis

Fungemia/(Candidemia?)

FUNGI

Candida spp.

Infectious mononucleosis

VIRUSES

Epstein-Barr virus ❷

Lymphocytic leukemia

VIRUSES

HTLV

AIDS

VIRUSES

HIV

Anaplasmosis

BACTERIA

A. phagocytophilum

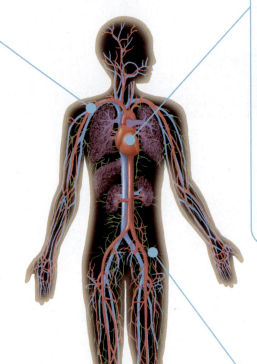

Endocarditis ❶

BACTERIA

S. aureus
Viridans streptococci
Enterococcus spp.
Coagulase-negative
  staphylococci
S. bovis
S. epidermidis
S. pneumonia   *Escherichia*
Neisseria   *Pseudomonas spp.*
Bartonella   *Mycobacterium*
Mycoplasma   *C. burnetii*
Bartonella spp.   *Chlamydia spp.*
Legionella spp.   *Brucella*
HACEK organsims
(*H. aphrophilus, A. actinomycetemcomitans,*
C. hominis, E. corrodens, K. kingae)

Myocarditis

VIRUSES

Coxsackie B virus   Adenovirus
Hepatitis C   Cytomegalovirus
Echovirus   Influenza virus
Parvovirus B19

Prosthetic valve endocarditis

BACTERIA

Viridans streptococci
S. epidermidis   *S. aureus*
Coagulase-negative staphylococci
Enterococci   *C. burnetiid*
M. chimaera

Lymphangitis
Lymphadenitis

BACTERIA

S. pyogenes   *S. aureus*
P. multocida
Non-tuberculous mycobacterium

Other systemic diseases

BACTERIA

Brucellosis
B. melitensis

Tularemia
F. tularensis ❶

Bubonic plague
Pneumonic plague
Y. pestis

Lyme disease ❷
B. burgdorferi

Ehrlichiosis
Anaplasmosis
E. chaffeensis
A. phagocytophilum

Scrub typhus
O. tsutsugamushi

VIRUSES

Cytomegalovirus disease
Cytomegalovirus (CMV) ❸

Yellow fever
Yellow fever virus

Dengue fever
Dengue viruses

African viral hemorrhagic fevers
Ebolavirus ❹   Marburgvirus

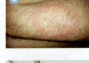
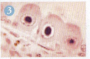

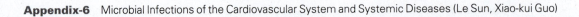

Appendix-6 Microbial Infections of the Cardiovascular System and Systemic Diseases (Le Sun, Xiao-kui Guo)

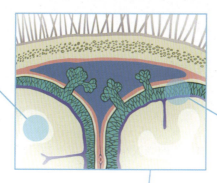

Encephalitis ❶

Epidemic type B encephalitis virus ❷
Eastern equine encephalitis (EEE)
Western equine encephalitis (WEE)
Venezuelan equine encephalitis (VEE)
St. Louis encephalitis
West Nile encephalitis
California encephalitis
(HSV-1   Rabies virus
Picornaviruses   Togavirus
Flavivirus
Bunya encephalitis viruses)

Brain abscess ❸

BACTERIA

S. aureus   Fusobacterium spp.
Peptostreptococcus spp.
P. aeruginosa   Viridens Streptococcus
N. asteroids
Gram-negative anaerobes

Creutzfeldt-Jakob disease ❹

Prion

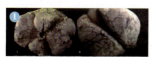
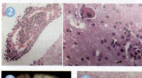
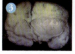

Leprosy

BACTERIA
M. leprae

Meningitis

BACTERIA
N. meningitidis ❶   S. pneumoniae
S. aureus   H. influenzae
L. monocytogenes ❷   S. agalactiae
Enterococcus   E·coli
Group B Streptococcus

VIRUSES
Enteroviruses (Coxsackie A virus
Coxsackie B virus   Echovirus)
Herpesviruses   Mumps virus

FUNGI
C. neoformans

Tetanus ❶

BACTERIA
C. tetani

Poliomyelitis

VIRUSES
Poliovirus

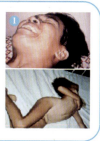

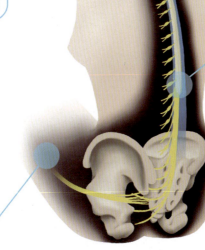

Botulism

BACTERIA
C. botulinum

Rabies

VIRUSES
Rabies virus ❶

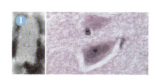
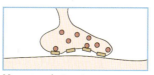

Neuromuscular junction

Appendix-7   Microbial Infections of the Nervous System (Le Sun, Xiao-kui Guo)

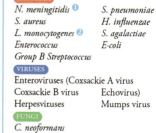

图书在版编目（CIP）数据

医学微生物学/郭晓奎主编. —北京：人民卫生
出版社，2019
临床医学专业英文版教材
ISBN 978-7-117-25651-3

Ⅰ. ①医…　Ⅱ. ①郭…　Ⅲ. ①医学微生物学－医学院
校－教材－英文　Ⅳ. ①R37

中国版本图书馆 CIP 数据核字（2017）第 299985 号

人卫智网　www.ipmph.com	医学教育、学术、考试、健康，购书智慧智能综合服务平台	
人卫官网　www.pmph.com	人卫官方资讯发布平台	

医学微生物学

主　　编：郭晓奎
出版发行：人民卫生出版社（中继线 010-59780011）
地　　址：北京市朝阳区潘家园南里 19 号
邮　　编：100021
E - mail：pmph @ pmph.com
购书热线：010-59787592　010-59787584　010-65264830
印　　刷：三河市宏达印刷有限公司（胜利）
经　　销：新华书店
开　　本：889×1194　1/16　　印张：39.5
字　　数：1168 千字
版　　次：2019 年 8 月第 1 版　2019 年 8 月第 1 版第 1 次印刷
标准书号：ISBN 978-7-117-25651-3
定　　价：158.00 元

打击盗版举报电话：**010-59787491　E-mail：WQ @ pmph.com**
（凡属印装质量问题请与本社市场营销中心联系退换）